Wound, Ostomy and Continence Nurses Society™

Core Curriculum

OSTOMY MANAGEMENT

Wound, Ostomy and Continence Nurses Society™

Core Curriculum

OSTOMY MANAGEMENT

EDITED BY

Jane E. Carmel, MSN, RN, CWOCN
Program Co-Director
Harrisburg Area Wound Ostomy Continence Nurse
Education Program
Mechanicsburg, Pennsylvania

Janice C. Colwell, MS, RN, CWOCN, FAAN
Advanced Practice Nurse Ostomy Care Services
The University of Chicago Medicine
Chicago, Illinois

Margaret T. Goldberg, MSN, RN, CWOCN
Delray Wound Treatment Center
Delray Beach, Florida

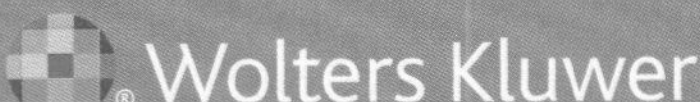

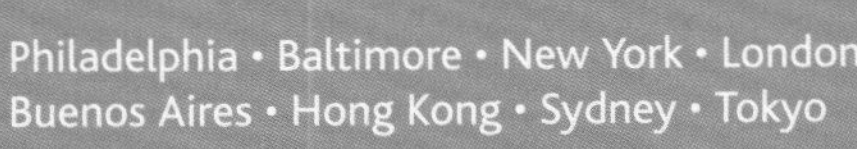

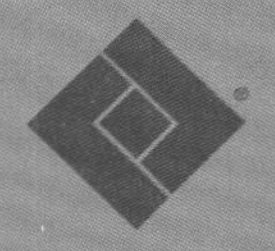
Wound
Ostomy and
Continence
Nurses
Society®

Executive Editor: Shannon W. Magee
Senior Product Development Editor: Emilie Moyer
Senior Marketing Manager: Mark Wiragh
Senior Production Project Manager: Cynthia Rudy
Design Coordinator: Teresa Mallon
Manufacturing Coordinator: Kathleen Brown
Prepress Vendor: SPi Global

9 8 7 6 5 4 3

Printed in China

Cataloging-in-Publication Data available on request from the Publisher.
ISBN: 978-1-4511-9439-5

LWW.com

CONTRIBUTORS

Jean Asburn, MD
Medical Director, WOC Nursing Education
Staff Surgeon, Colorectal Surgery/
Digestive Disease Institute
Cleveland Clinic
Cleveland, Ohio

Janice Beitz, PhD, RN, CS, CNOR, CWOCN, CRNP, APN-C, MAPWCA, FAAN
Director, WOC Nursing Education Program
Professor, Rutgers University School of Nursing-Camden
Camden, New Jersey

Greta V. Bernier, MD
General Surgery Resident
Department of Surgery
University of Washington Medical Center
Seattle, Washington

Ruth A. Bryant, MS, RN, CWOCN
Scholar in Residence
Washington State University
Providence Health Care
Spokane, Washington

Jane E. Carmel, MSN, RN, CWOCN
Program Co-Director
Harrisburg Area Wound Ostomy Continence Nurse
Education Program
Mechanicsburg, Pennsylvania

Russell D. Cohen, MD
Professor of Medicine, Pritzker Medical School
Director, Inflammatory Bowel Disease Center
Section of Gastroenterology, Department of Medicine
The University of Chicago Medicine
Chicago, Illinois

Janice C. Colwell, MS, RN, CWOCN, FAAN
Advanced Practice Nurse Ostomy Care Services
The University of Chicago Medicine
Chicago, Illinois

JoAnn Ermer-Seltun, MS, RN, ARNP, FNP-BC, CWOCN
Co-Director and Faculty, webWOC Nursing Education
Program
Minneapolis, Minnesota
Mercy Medical Center Advanced Wound Center and
Continence Clinic
Bladder Control Solutions, LLC
Mason City, Iowa

Jane Fellows, MSN, RN, CWOCN
Ostomy/Wound Clinical Nurse Specialist
Duke University Health System
Durham, North Carolina

Alessandro Fichera, MD
Professor and Chief, Section of Gastrointestinal Surgery
Department of Surgery
University of Washington Medical Center
Seattle, Washington

Margaret T. Goldberg, MSN, RN, CWOCN
Delray Wound Treatment Center
Delray Beach, Florida

Barbara Hocevar, MSN, RN, CWOCN
Assistant Director, R.B. Turnbull, Jr. MD WOC
Nursing Education Program
Digestive Disease Institute
Cleveland Clinic
Cleveland, Ohio

Mary F. Mahoney, MSN, RN, CWON
Wound and Ostomy Nurse
WOC Nursing Department
UnityPoint at Home
Des Moines, Iowa

Kimberly McIltrot, DNP, CPNP, CWOCN
Pediatric Nurse Practitioner
Department of Pediatric Surgery
Johns Hopkins Hospital
Baltimore, Maryland

Debra S. Netsch, DNP, APRN-CNP, FNP-BC, CWOCN
Nurse Practitioner and WOC Nurse, Mankato Clinic, Ltd
Mankato, Minnesota
Co-Director and Faculty, webWOC Nursing Education Program
Minneapolis, Minnesota

Denise Nix, MS, RN, CWOCN
Consultant
Minnesota Hospital Association
Minneapolis, Minnesota

Joseph J. Pariser, MD
Urology Resident
Section of Urology, Department of Surgery
The University of Chicago Medicine
Chicago, Illinois

Sanjay G. Patel, MD
Urologic Oncology Fellow
Section of Urology, Department of Surgery
The University of Chicago Medicine
Chicago, Illinois

Joyce Pittman, PhD, ANP-BC, FNP-BC, CWOCN
Nurse Practitioner, Team Lead WOC Team
Indiana University Health-Methodist
Adjunct Assistant Professor
Indiana University School of Nursing
Indianapolis, Indiana

Michelle C. Rice, MSN, RN, CWOCN
Ostomy/Wound Clinical Nurse Specialist
Duke University Hospital
Durham, North Carolina

Michele Rubin, APN, CNS, CGRN
IBD Clinical Nurse Specialist
Department of Colorectal Surgery
The University of Chicago Medicine
Chicago, Illinois

Ginger Salvadalena, PhD, RN, CWOCN
Principal Scientist, Global Clinical Affairs
Hollister Incorporated
Libertyville, Illinois

Jody Scardillo, DNP, RN, ANP-BC, CWOCN
Clinical Nurse Specialist/Nurse Practitioner
Albany Medical Center
Albany, New York

Adam C. Stein, MD
Assistant Professor in Medicine—Gastroenterology and Hepatology
Northwestern University Feinberg School of Medicine
Chicago, Illinois

Gary D. Steinberg, MD
Bruce and Beth White Family Professor of Surgery
Director of Urologic Oncology
Vice Chairman, The University of Chicago Section of Urology
Chicago, Illinois

Linda Stricker, MSN, RN, CWOCN
Director, R.B. Turnbull, Jr. MD WOC Nursing Education Program
Digestive Disease Institute
Cleveland Clinic
Cleveland, Ohio

FOREWORD

It is an honor to be invited to write the foreword to the *Wound, Ostomy and Continence Nurses Society™ Core Curricula*. Having served 22 years as a Wound, Ostomy and Continence (WOC) Nursing Program Director, I can attest as to how valuable a resource these books will be to students, faculty, preceptors, and all clinicians caring for people with wounds, ostomies, and incontinence.

Terms currently popular in health care refer to patient-centered and patient-focused care. For those of you entering the wonderful WOC nursing specialty, know this: the patient has always been the focus of WOC nursing! In fact, our specialty grew from a need identified by patients themselves. As colorectal and urologic surgeries advanced, so did the number of people living with ostomies. In 1958, Akron, Ohio native Norma N. Gill joined her surgeon, Rupert B. Turnbull, Jr., MD, in founding what was then coined by Dr. Turnbull as enterostomal therapy (ET).

Beginning in 1948, when she was a 28-year-old mother of two young children, Norma began a long odyssey battling mucosal ulcerative colitis. She manifested all the gastrointestinal symptoms, including massive bouts of bloody diarrhea associated with this disease, along with many of the extraintestinal manifestations, such as uveitis, iritis, and extensive pyoderma gangrenosum on her face, chest, abdomen, and legs. During a brief remission in 1951, much to the amazement of Norma and her husband Ted, she became pregnant. The pregnancy was fraught with complications, the need for numerous blood transfusions, and fear for the lives of both mother and child throughout. Despite all of these life-threatening occurrences, in June 1952, Norma gave birth to a healthy baby girl. The complications continued after her baby's birth, and Norma's response to treatment was spotty at best. In October 1954, she was admitted to the Cleveland Clinic, and there her life was saved and history forever changed. Dr. Turnbull operated to remove Norma's colon and create an ileostomy. Her postoperative course after ileostomy was rocky, and she had to undergo some additional operations to remove her rectum and have plastic surgery performed on her face.

Despite all of this, Norma began to feel better—incredibly better. As she was resuming her role as a wife and mother, she felt the need, as we now say, to "pay it forward." Norma wanted to help others who were facing the same challenges she had endured and emerged stronger than she had been before her illness. Her journey began with the Akron physicians and hospital she had come to know well during her illness. Norma started from scratch and cobbled together an inventory of the limited equipment available at the time. Soon she had many referrals from the surgeons and knew she had found her calling. In 1958, during an appointment with Dr. Turnbull, she told him what she was doing in Akron to help people with new ostomies and fistulae. He was impressed and called her a couple of months later to offer her a job at the Cleveland Clinic.

August 1958 is when the seeds for the modern specialty of WOC nursing were planted. It was not long before the word was out, and surgeons began requesting that their staff come to train with Norma and Dr. Turnbull. The R.B. Turnbull, Jr. School of Enterostomal Therapy (now WOC Nursing) was established. After her long work day in Cleveland, Norma would return to Akron and see patients in hospitals there before heading home to her family and doing it all again the next day.

There was a child in an Akron hospital who always remembered her first encounter with Norma. Here was a woman who commanded respect. The surgeon, head nurse, and staff nurses, as well as the girl's mom, crowded around the bed as Norma taught the proper way to care for a new ileal conduit. That child grew up well adjusted to her new stoma, and thanks to a great family and the one and only Norma Gill, that child grew up to be me! The baby who was predicted never to be born to Norma and Ted is Sally Gill-Thompson—one of my best friends and a famous ET practitioner in her own right.

After establishment of the formal program in Cleveland, other ET schools soon opened, and graduates from the United States and abroad spread the word across the globe. Professional organizations were established, and admission criteria became more stringent as health care became more complex. ET nurses became well respected for their skills and experience caring for people with complex ostomies and fistulae. It was a natural extension of our practice to embrace wound and continence care, and with a painful good-bye to our ET designation in the 1990s, we became known as WOC nurses to better reflect our practice. As you embark on your studies of WOC nursing, take time to reflect and appreciate the wonderful legacy you are continuing with your specialty practice.

Norma will be watching.

Paula Erwin-Toth, MSN, RN, CWOCN, CNS, FAAN

PREFACE

This text was developed for the student who will receive instruction in a Wound, Ostomy and Continence Nursing Education Program (WOCNEP). The WOCNEP Directors have developed a curriculum blueprint that was approved by the Wound, Ostomy and Continence Nurses Society™ (WOCN®) Accreditation Committee and Board of Directors. The curriculum objectives have been used to develop the content for this book. Each chapter begins with an outline and ends with review questions that highlight the important issues in each chapter. The text has been written by experts in the field who provide care to patients undergoing ostomy surgery. As the editors, we have supported their work and edited this content to ensure it reflects the curriculum outline and current clinical practice.

The information in this book will help the future clinicians of ostomy services to provide a high level of care to their patients. We believe that the person with an ostomy should have the services of an educated nurse specialist and continued access to those services as they live their lives with a stoma. Once educated in ostomy care, the specialty nurse has a unique role to contribute to the care of a person with an ostomy. It is our hope that this book will provide the foundation that helps deliver optimal care to all individuals with fecal and urinary diversions.

ACKNOWLEDGMENTS

The Wound, Ostomy and Continence Nurses Society™ (WOCN®) wishes to thank all of the clinical experts who munificently shared their time and expertise to create this textbook. The Society would like to especially acknowledge the consulting editors, Jane Carmel, Jan Colwell, and Margaret Goldberg, for their inspiration, knowledge, and unwavering commitment to the development of this resource and to the field of wound, ostomy, and continence nursing.

The WOCN Society would like to acknowledge Hollister Incorporated for providing a commercially supported educational grant for the development of this textbook.

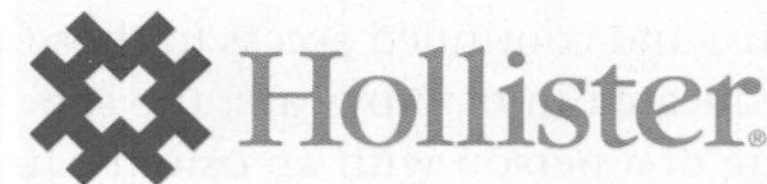

AUTHOR ACKNOWLEDGMENTS

A special thank you to the contributing authors, colleagues, and the WOCN Society for supporting this project. Without their help this book would not have been possible.

Thank you to our patients, families, and caregivers, who inspire us to provide our best care.

To future WOC students, may this book be a valuable resource as you embark on your journey to become a WOC nurse.

Jane, Jan, and Margaret

CONTENTS

CHAPTER 1

Anatomy and Physiology of the Gastrointestinal Tract

Debra S. Netsch

OBJECTIVE

Apply knowledge of normal anatomy and physiology of the GI system in nursing management and education of the patient with a fecal diversion.

Topic Outline

The gastrointestinal (GI) system coordinates complex processes to prepare ingested food for cellular absorption and utilization, provide the body with water, and eliminate waste products. The physical state and chemical composition of the ingested food or liquid are changed through digestive, secretory, absorptive, and excretory functions to provide essential nutrition. This system is comprised of the GI (alimentary) tract and accessory organs (salivary glands, liver, gallbladder, and exocrine pancreas; **Fig. 1-1**) (Patton & Thibodeau, 2014). It is through understanding normal anatomy and physiology of the GI system that pathological and surgical changes are more thoroughly appreciated. This chapter discusses the normal anatomy and physiology of the GI system.

Overview

The digestive process begins in the mouth with chewing and continues in the stomach. In the stomach, food is mixed with enzymes, mucus, acid, and other secretions. The partially digested food and fluid pass from the stomach into the small intestine. The liver and exocrine pancreas secrete biochemicals and enzymes into the small intestine causing further breakdown into absorbable monosaccharides, amino acids, and fatty acids.

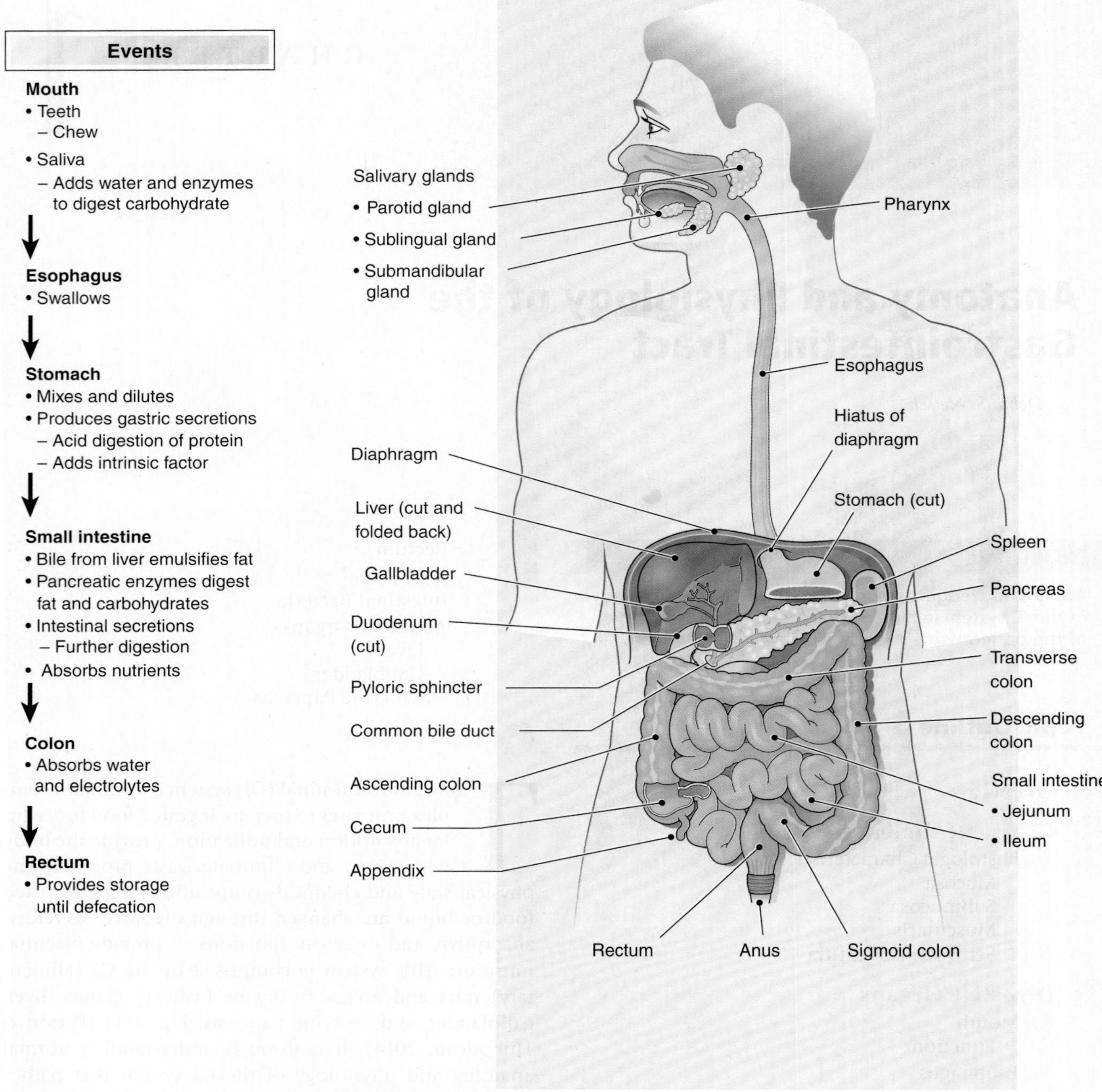

FIGURE 1-1. Normal anatomy of the digestive system.

These nutrients are transported through the small intestinal wall into blood vessels and lymphatics, which carry them to the liver for storage or further processing. The ingested food components not absorbed in the small intestine pass into the large intestine, which continues to absorb water. The fluid waste products are transported to the kidneys for elimination in the urine. Solid waste products pass into the rectum for elimination as stool through the anus.

The GI system functions with little conscious effort. The GI motility, other than chewing, swallowing, and defecation, is controlled by hormones and the autonomic nervous system (sympathetic and parasympathetic). The autonomic nervous system is controlled in the brain and by local stimuli mediated by intramural bundles of nerve fibers (plexuses) within the GI walls. The GI motility regulatory hormones particularly affect the small intestine. These are peptide and nonpeptide hormones. The peptide hormones including gastrin, cholecystokinin (CCK), secretin, insulin, and gastric inhibitory peptide (GIP) are produced and released throughout the GI tract to either stimulate or inhibit peristalsis and to facilitate digestion.

TABLE 1-1 Digestive Secretions

Source	Daily Volume	pH	Sodium (mmol)	Potassium (mmol)	Chloride (mmol)	Bicarbonate (mmol)	Water
Saliva	1.5 L	6.7–7.0	20–80	16–23	24–44	20–60	1 L
Gastric juice	2.0 L	1.0–3.5	20–100	4–12	52–124	0	2 L
Pancreatic	1.5 L	8.0–8.3	120–150	2–7	54–95	70–110	1.2 L
Bile	0.5 L	7.8	120–200	3–12	80–120	30–50	0.8L
Intestinal juice	1.5 L	7.8–8.9	80–130	12–21	48–116	23–30	3.0 L

Modified from Bryant, R. (2004). Anatomy and physiology of the gastrointestinal tract. In J. Colwell, M. Goldberg & J. Carmel (Eds.), *Fecal & urinary diversions: Management principles*. St. Louis, MO: Mosby-Elsevier; Ireland, A. P. (2004). Surgical fluids and electrolytes. http://surgstudent.org/lectures/flud/flud_centre_html.html

Nonpeptide hormones include vitamin D, aldosterone, hydrocortisone, nitric oxide, and serotonin (Bryant, 2004; Doig & Huether, 2012; Reed & Wickham, 2009).

GI Tract (Alimentary Canal)

The GI tract is essentially a hollow muscular tube from the mouth to the anus. It is composed of the mouth, esophagus, stomach, small intestine, large intestine, rectum, and anus. The digestive processes performed by the GI tract include (1) ingestion of food and fluids; (2) propulsion of food and waste products throughout the GI tract; (3) secretion of mucus, water, and digestive enzymes; (4) mechanical digestion of food particles; (5) chemical digestion of food particles; (6) absorption of nutrients; and (7) elimination of solid waste products by defecation (**Table 1-1**).

Histologic Characteristics

The alimentary canal has essentially the same four tissue layers from innermost to outermost: the mucosa, submucosa, muscularis, and serosa or adventitia (esophagus only; **Fig. 1-2**). These tissue layers vary in thickness and have sublayers.

Mucosa

The innermost tissue layer of the gut wall is the mucosal layer with sublayers of epithelium, lamina propria, and muscularis mucosa. The epithelium sublayer tissue is differentiated along the GI tract correlating with the regional specific function. The mucosal epithelium is composed of protective stratified squamous epithelial cells at the beginning and end of the GI tract (mouth, esophagus, and anal canal). Simple columnar or glandular epithelial cells constitute the mucosal epithelium of the stomach, small intestine, and colon and secrete protective or digestive mucus, enzymes, and other biochemicals. This layer essentially provides lubrication and moisture, which facilitates the forward movement of food bolus while protecting the mucosa from abrasions. The mucosal lamina propria is the next sublayer outside the mucosal epithelium.

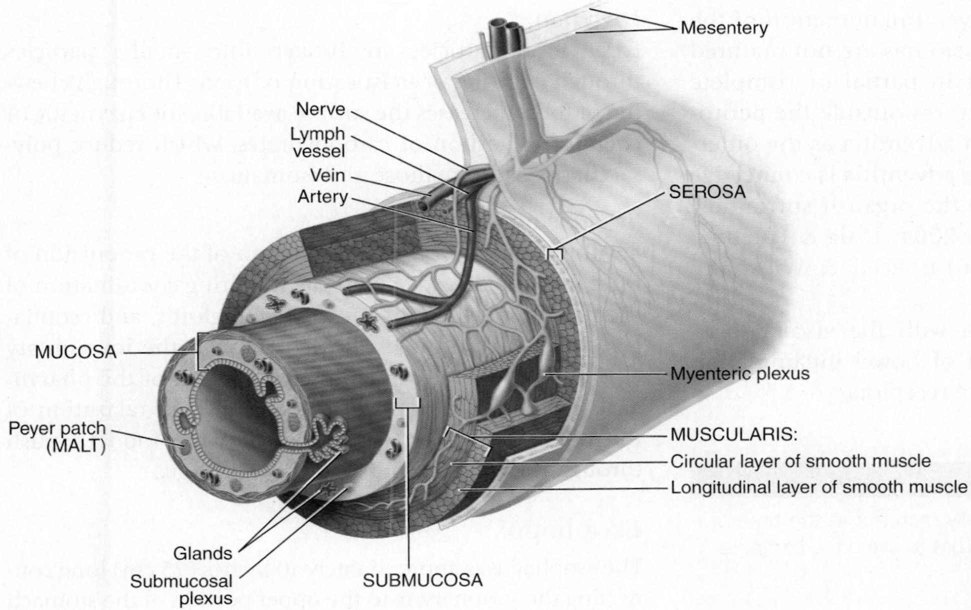

FIGURE 1-2. Layers of the GI tract.

It is primarily connective tissue containing blood vessels and lymphatics providing nutrients to the mucosal epithelium, transportation of hormones secreted by endocrine epithelium, and absorption of digestive end products from the lumen of the GI tract. The outermost mucosal sublayer is the muscularis mucosa. It is a thin layer of smooth muscle separating the mucosa and submucosa layers. Networks of widely distributed interstitial cells of Cajal (ICC) are considered the GI tract pacemaker cells. The ICC networks are present within the submucosal (ICC-SM), intramuscular (ICC-IM, ICC-DMP), and intermuscular layers (ICC-MY) of the GI tract from the esophagus to the internal anal sphincter.

Submucosa

The submucosa is the second tissue layer of the gut wall. It is a connective tissue layer containing blood vessels, lymphatics, submucosal glands, Meissner plexus (a submucosal nerve network affecting the muscularis smooth muscle), and a number of reticuloendothelial cells.

Muscularis

The muscularis is the third layer of the gut wall. It consists of two smooth muscle layers, a circular inner layer and longitudinal outer layer. The Auerbach (myenteric) plexus lies between these two muscle layers and coordinates rhythmic peristaltic contractions of the muscles resulting in the mixing and forward propulsion of the food bolus through the stomach and intestine.

Serosa or Adventitia

The outermost layer of the GI tract is a serous membrane. Structures within the peritoneal cavity are covered with serosa, which is connective tissue covered by the visceral peritoneum. This is continuous with the visceral peritoneum and is a factor in severe abdominal pain associated with transmural inflammatory bowel disease. If the serosa is exposed to air, it can lead to necrosis and sloughing of the serosal layer. Inflammation of the serosa (serositis) such as when stomas are not matured (everted) in surgery can result in partial or complete obstruction of the stoma. Structures outside the peritoneal cavity are surrounded with adventitia as the outermost layer instead of serosa. The adventitia is connective tissue that provides support to the organ it surrounds, such as the esophagus (Bryant, 2004; Doig & Huether, 2012; Patton & Thibodeau, 2014; Reed & Wickham, 2009; Takaki, 2003).

The continuity of the serosa with the visceral peritoneum is associated with pain of bowel inflammation despite the bowel not having pain receptors.

CLINICAL PEARL

One reason why stomas are typically matured at the time of surgery (primary matured or everted) is to avoid the complication of serositis.

Digestive Organs

Mouth

The mouth is the beginning or proximal end of the GI tract. The digestive process begins in the mouth through chewing and mixing of the food with saliva. This process is facilitated by the 32 teeth contained in the mouth. The tongue is muscular covered by moist squamous epithelium with the anterior surface covered by papillae containing thousands of taste buds. The taste buds or chemoreceptors differentiate between salty, sour, bitter, and sweet tastes. As the taste buds and olfactory nerves are stimulated, salivation is initiated and gastric juice is secreted in the stomach. Three pairs of salivary glands (submandibular, sublingual, and parotid glands) are located in the mouth. The salivary glands produce approximately 1 to 1.5 L of saliva per day. Saliva consists primarily of water and of a combination of mucus and sodium, bicarbonate, chloride, potassium, and salivary α-amylase (ptyalin), which is an enzyme that initiates carbohydrate digestion. It also contains immunoglobulin A and other antimicrobial substances, which prevent infection. Saliva sustains an alkaline pH around 7.4, which aids in neutralizing bacterial acids and preventing tooth decay.

Function

The functions performed by the structures of the mouth include speech, food ingestion, initiation of digestion, and swallowing.

Speech

The tongue and teeth are integral in the formation of words necessary for clear speech.

Ingestion

Nutrition is normally taken into the body through the mouth, which stimulates the taste buds and creates a pleasant sensation for future ingestion.

Digestion

Large food particles are broken into smaller particles through chewing or mastication of food. Thorough chewing of food increases the surface available for enzymatic or chemical digestion of carbohydrates, which reduce polysaccharides into maltose and isomaltose.

Swallowing

Swallowing is an important function of the propulsion of food into the digestive pathway requiring coordination of the mouth, palate, tongue, larynx, epiglottis, and esophagus. Ingested food is swallowed through the involuntary closing of the larynx opening, contraction of the pharyngeal muscles, inhibition of respiration, and relaxation of the upper esophageal sphincter allowing food to push through the pharynx and into the esophagus.

Esophagus

The esophagus is approximately 10 inches (25 cm) long connecting the oropharynx to the upper portion of the stomach traversing through the diaphragm. The esophagus is divided into three sections: the upper, middle, and lower. The upper third of the esophagus is composed of voluntary striated muscle. The lower two thirds contain involuntary smooth muscle innervated by preganglionic cholinergic fibers, with innervation of the entire esophagus originating from the vagus nerve. The vascular supply to the esophagus is from the esophageal branch of the thoracic aorta and the left gastric artery branching from the celiac trunk of the abdominal aorta. Each section of the esophagus has different venous return with the upper esophagus venous drainage through the superior vena cava; midesophagus venous return by the azygos vein; and the lower esophagus venous drainage by the gastric veins, which empty into the portal system. Sphincters are present in the proximal and distal sections of the esophagus. The upper esophageal sphincter (cricopharyngeal muscle) prevents entry of air into the esophagus during respiration and prevents reflux from the esophagus into the oropharynx. The lower esophageal sphincter (cardiac sphincter) prevents reflux from the stomach with caustic injury to the esophagus. The esophagus is further protected from caustic injury by thick mucus produced in the submucosal layer delivered via ducts to coat the mucosal surface.

Function

The esophagus facilitates transport of food from the mouth and oropharynx into the stomach, completing swallowing. Swallowing starts in the oropharynx area, which was aforementioned. The esophageal phase of swallowing occurs when the bolus of food enters the esophagus and the esophagus relaxes preparing for the bolus to move. Peristalsis occurs through rhythmic waves of muscular contractions moving the food bolus forward causing relaxation of the lower esophageal sphincter and allowing the food bolus to enter into the stomach (Bryant, 2004; Doig & Huether, 2012; Hall & Guyton, 2011; Patton & Thibodeau, 2014; Reed & Wickham, 2009).

Abdominal Cavity Organs and Peritoneum

The abdominal cavity is located below the diaphragm and is continuous with the pelvic cavity. The majority of the GI tract organs are contained in the abdominal cavity, with portions of the colon being contained in the pelvic cavity. The peritoneum is a serous membrane lining much of the abdominal cavity (the parietal peritoneum) and covering most of the abdominal organs (visceral peritoneum). The parietal peritoneum nerve supply is adjacent to the body wall with sensitivity for pain. The visceral peritoneum is insensate. Retroperitoneal organs lie outside the peritoneum. A double layer of peritoneum with a central layer of loose connective tissue constitutes the mesentery. It surrounds most of the small intestine, connecting it to the posterior abdominal wall. The mesentery is vital to the intestine providing blood supply to the bowel and nerve fibers for bowel innervation. The

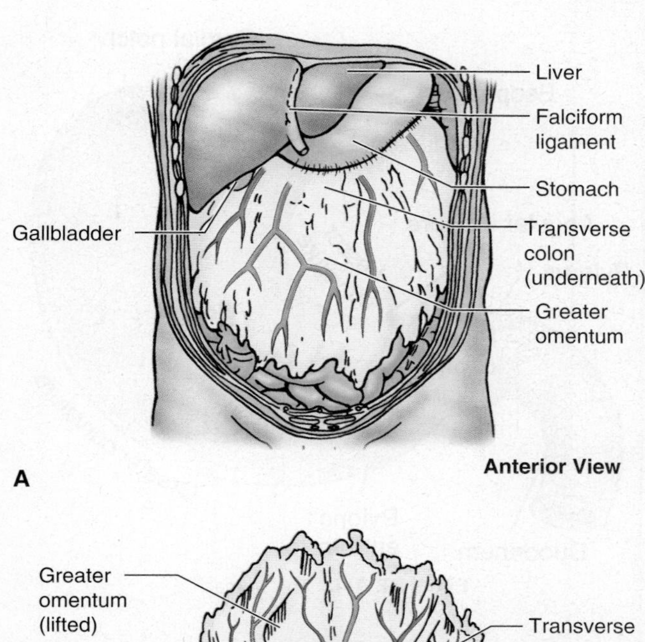

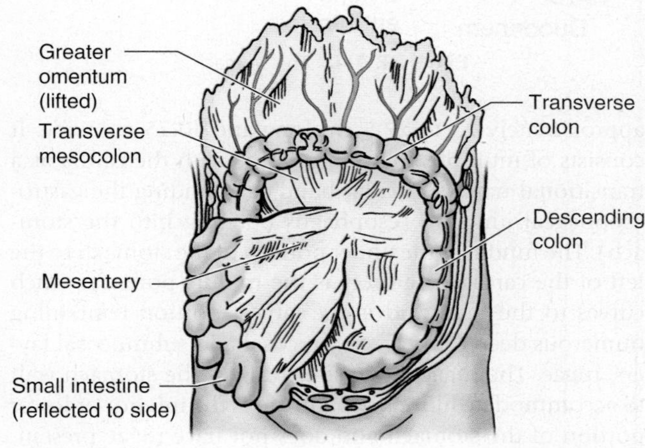

FIGURE 1-3. **A.** Omentum. **B.** Mesentery.

greater omentum is mesentery with a double fold that attaches the anterior stomach to the transverse colon and connects the stomach to the posterior abdominal wall (**Fig. 1-3**). This is also known as the "fatty apron" since large amounts of fat are present between and among the double folds. Much of the lesser omentum lies posteriorly to the stomach extending among the liver, the stomach, and the duodenum (Bryant, 2004; O'Rahilly et al., 2008; Patton & Thibodeau, 2014).

> **CLINICAL PEARL**
>
> Stoma viability and function relies upon enough mesentery being kept with the bowel utilized to create a stoma since the mesentery is vital to providing blood supply to the bowel and nerve fibers for bowel innervation.

Stomach

The stomach is a hollow, J-shaped muscular organ located just below the diaphragm (**Fig. 1-4**). The size and shape vary somewhat with a capacity of 1 to 1.5 L, measuring

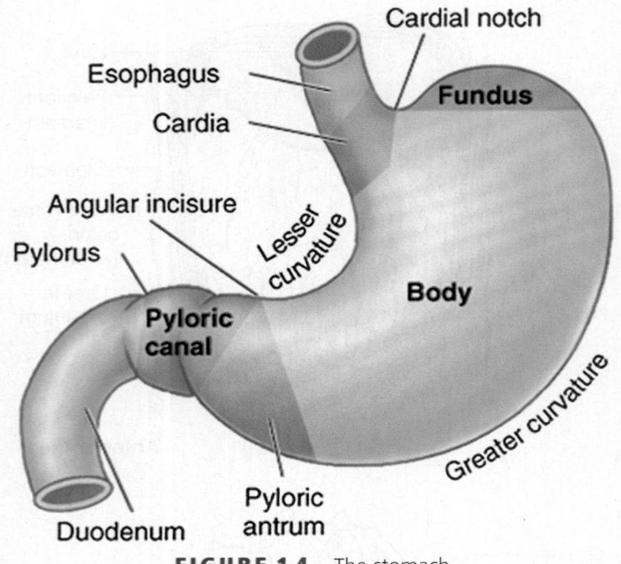

FIGURE 1-4. The stomach.

approximately 25 to 27.5 cm long and 10.25 cm wide. It consists of multiple anatomical areas with the cardia as a transitional narrow circular band surrounding the gastroesophageal junction (esophagus opening into the stomach). The fundus is the upper portion of the stomach to the left of the cardia. The body is the middle portion, which curves to the right and is the largest portion containing numerous deep folds of the mucosal and submucosal layers, rugae. The rugae allow stretching of the stomach wall to accommodate filling. The antrum is the inferior or lower portion of the stomach and does not have rugae present, which are present in the rest of the stomach. The pylorus is the most distal stomach structure. The muscularis layer of the stomach has a circular muscle layer, oblique muscle layer, and a longitudinal muscle layer. The oblique muscle lies between the submucosa and the circular muscle layer. This is one more muscle layer than the rest of the GI tract, as a way to increase the ability to churn or mix the gastric contents.

The muscular layer becomes progressively thicker in the body and antrum of the stomach. The blood supply is abundant to the stomach supplied by the branches of the celiac trunk. Venous drainage is from the splenic vein for the right side of the stomach and the gastric vein for the left side of the stomach both emptying into the portal vein. Innervation of the stomach is through the autonomic nervous system, with parasympathetic innervation provided by the vagus nerve and sympathetic innervation provided by the celiac plexus.

Columnar epithelial cells line the stomach and the gastric glands penetrating as gastric pits into the mucosal layer. The mucous cells secrete a protective viscous alkaline mucus. The mucus is approximately 1 to 1.5 mm thick blanketing the mucosa to neutralize acid with the mucosal bicarbonate, thus protecting the undisturbed innermost layer of mucus. The pH in the stomach itself is 2.0, while the innermost layer of mucus pH is 7.0. The gastric gland parietal cells produce hydrochloric acid (HCl), intrinsic factor, and TGF-α. The HCl creates the low pH, which inactivates salivary amylase and inhibits carbohydrate digestion. This also activates pepsin, a proteolytic enzyme, which initiates protein digestion and forms polypeptides in the stomach. The pepsin is inactivated when it enters the alkaline environment of the duodenum. The intrinsic factor binds with vitamin B_{12} and is key to the absorption of vitamin B_{12} in the terminal ileum (Bryant, 2004; Doig & Huether, 2012).

Function

Digestion

Swallowing relaxes the fundus (receptive relaxation) in preparation of a food bolus to be received from the esophagus. The food enters the stomach, which serves as a reservoir with controlled emptying into the duodenum. Peristaltic contractions mix the food with gastric secretions until it is chyme, a semifluid consistency. The mechanical mixing with chemical secretions in the stomach contributes to the digestive process. The more solid the food, the more mixing is required. The consistency of gastric contents, acidity, chyme fat content, vagal stimuli, osmolality, temperature, and emotional state all affect the rate of gastric emptying of the chyme into the duodenum through the pyloric sphincter.

Secretion

The stomach secretes 2 to 3 L/day of gastric juices and secretions (Table 1-1). These include mucus, acid enzymes, hormones, intrinsic factor, and gastroferrin. The gastric gland parietal cells produce HCl, intrinsic factor, and TGF-α. The HCl creates the low pH (high acidity), which inactivates salivary amylase and inhibits carbohydrate digestion. This also activates pepsin, which initiates protein digestion. The intrinsic factor binds with vitamin B_{12} (cyanocobalamin) and is key to the absorption of vitamin B_{12} in the terminal ileum. Lifelong injections of B_{12} will be necessary to prevent pernicious anemia if the stomach is removed. Gastroferrin facilitates iron absorption in the small intestine. Hormones secreted by the stomach also affect gastric secretion with secretin and gastric inhibitory polypeptides inhibiting stomach emptying through decreased gastric motor activity and gastric acid secretion. G cells make gastrin, which stimulates secretion of HCl promoting pepsinogen secretion and gastric motility. D cells secrete somatostatin, which inhibits secretion of gastric acid, gastrin, and intrinsic factor. Enterochromaffin (EC) cells produce serotonin. The zymogenic chief cells secrete lipase and pepsinogen, a precursor of pepsin. The amount of gastric secretions vary according to the time of day with the lowest volume and rate being in the morning, whereas the highest is in the afternoon and evening. The three phases of gastric secretion (cephalic, gastric, and intestinal phases) are influenced by multiple factors. The cephalic phase is stimulated by the thought, smell, and taste of food. The gastric phase is stimulated by food distention in the stomach. The intestinal phase is stimulated by chyme in the intestine. Gastric secretion is additionally stimulated by moderate amounts of alcohol and caffeine and interestingly by anger and hostility. Inversely, gastric secretion is inhibited by unpleasant odors, tastes, and the emotions of fear and depression.

Absorption

The role in nutrient absorption is limited in the stomach to include some partially chemically digested carbohydrates, alcohol, and some medications such as aspirin.

Elimination of Ingested Bacteria

The antibacterial effect of the stomach is provided by the extremely low pH, thus eliminating most of the ingested bacteria (Bryant, 2004; Doig & Huether, 2012; Hall & Guyton, 2011; Patton & Thibodeau, 2014; Reed & Wickham, 2009).

A patient with a large portion of the stomach resected may require lifelong vitamin B_{12} supplementation to avoid pernicious anemia since not enough intrinsic factor may be available to bind with vitamin B_{12} and facilitate absorption of vitamin B_{12}.

Small Intestine

The small intestine is divided into three functioning sections, the duodenum, jejunum, and the ileum. Essentially, it stretches from the gastric pylorus to the ileocecal valve and is in total approximately 6.7 m (22 feet) varying from 5 to 8 m long. The duodenum starts at the pylorus and joins the jejunum at the ligament of Treitz, a suspension ligament. There is no line of separation to distinguish the jejunum from the ileum. The ileum ends at the ileocecal valve, which controls the flow of digested material from the small intestine into the large intestine and prevents reflux into the ileum. The duodenum lies retroperitoneal and attaches to the posterior abdominal wall. The jejunum and ileum are suspended from the posterior abdominal wall by the mesentery (**Fig. 1-5**). A branch of the celiac trunk provides the blood supply to the proximal (first portion) duodenum with the branches of the superior mesenteric artery supplying the majority of the small intestine, including the distal duodenum, jejunum, and ileum. The venous return is by the superior mesenteric vein, which joins the splenic vein and empties into the portal circulation. Both the parasympathetic and sympathetic components of the autonomic nervous system innervate the small intestine. The parasympathetic nerves mediate secretion, motility, pain sensation, and intestinal reflexes, that is, relaxation of sphincters. The sympathetic nerves inhibit motility and cause vasoconstriction. Intrinsic motor innervation is mediated by both the Auerbach plexus (myenteric plexus) and the Meissner plexus (submucosal plexus).

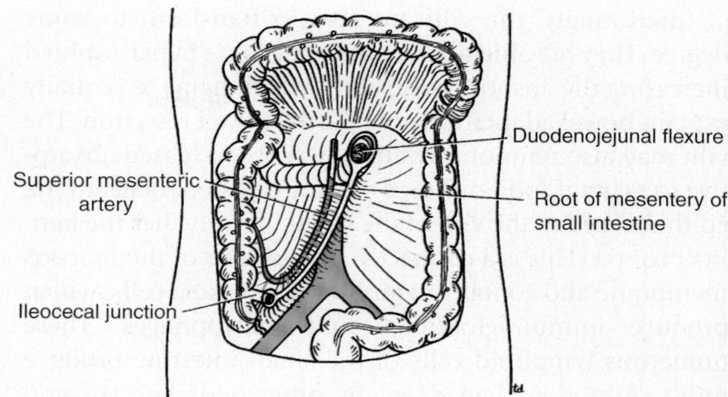

FIGURE 1-5. Attachment of the root of the mesentery of the small intestine to the posterior abdominal wall. The ileocecal junction is identified.

The submucosal and mucosal layers are unique in the small intestine being arranged in folds (plicae circulares), which increase the absorptive surface along with the villi (**Fig. 1-2**). The mucosal layer of the small intestine is lined with simple columnar epithelium. The epithelium contains enterocytes (absorptive cells) primarily with scattered goblet cells and occasional enteroendocrine cells. The lamina propria lies beneath the epithelial cell of the villi. This is a connective tissue layer of the mucous membrane and contains lymphocytes; plasma cells, which produce immunoglobulins; and macrophages. These numerous lymphoid cells of the small intestine produce more antibodies than does any other body site. This protects the mucosa from pathogens and ingested noxious substances. Peptides are also produced from the mucosal layer.

The villi are small intestinal structures of the mucosal layer, which are finger-like projections that cover the mucosal surface and increase the absorptive area of the small intestine, creating a velvety appearance of the lumen being 0.5 to 1 mm in length. Each villus contains a capillary network, lymph vessel, numerous white blood cells, and smooth muscle fibers. This protects the mucosa from pathogens and ingested noxious substances. Each villus has absorptive columnar cells and mucus-secreting goblet cells of the mucosal epithelium. Each villus is covered with absorptive cytoplasmic extensions (microvilli). Together, the villi and microvilli create the brush border, which, combined with the plicae circulares, increases the absorptive surface of the mucosa by 600 times what would be expected from a tube with the same diameter. The brush border has enzymes present including peptidases, disaccharidases, and nucleases. Between the villi are simple tubular glands (crypts of Lieberkühn). These crypts contain undifferentiated (stem) cells, mucus-secreting goblet cells, Paneth cells, and endocrine paracrine cells. Undifferentiated (stem) cells rise from the base of the crypts to the top of the villus, maturing as they rise reproducing mucosal cells on a continual basis with mucosal cell turnover between 48 and 72 hours and in entirety replaced every 4 to 7 days.

Interestingly, the villi are able to transform to some degree. They are able to elongate or become hypertrophied increasing the absorptive capacity, which helps to partially explain bowel adaptation after partial bowel resection. The villi may also temporarily atrophy with decreased absorptive capacity if food or fluids are not ingested. Beneath the epithelial cell of the villi of the small intestine lies the lamina propria. This is a connective tissue layer of the mucous membrane and contains lymphocytes; plasma cells, which produce immunoglobulins; and macrophages. These numerous lymphoid cells of the small intestine produce more antibodies than does any other body site (Bryant, 2004; Doig & Huether, 2012; Hall & Guyton, 2011; Patton & Thibodeau, 2014; Reed & Wickham, 2009).

CLINICAL PEARL

Because the villi are able to transform to some degree and elongate or become hypertrophied, they are able to increase the absorptive capacity taking on some of the function of the colon when the colon is surgically removed.

As the villi atrophy and flatten, decreased absorption occurs. Additionally, as gut atrophy progresses, there is increased risk of bacterial translocation and the immune functions of the GI tract are impaired.

Function

The small intestine is the organ responsible for much of the digestive process, absorption of nutrients, electrolytes, vitamins, minerals, and miscellaneous substances. It is a major contributor to maintaining fluid and electrolyte balance. The specific functions contributing to the digestive process include intestinal motility, secretion, and absorption.

Motility

The motility of the small intestine facilitates both digestion and absorption. Chyme arriving in the duodenum from the stomach stimulates intestinal mixing of secretions from the liver, pancreas, and intestinal glands containing enzymes as well as bile salts. The luminal contents are brought into contact with the absorbing villi through a churning motion (short segmental contractions). The plicae or mucosal folds slow the motility of the chyme allowing for more time for digestion and absorption. The chyme is pushed further through the small intestine toward the large intestine by propulsive movements (peristaltic waves). Distention of the intestinal wall by the luminal contents stimulates the peristalsis. The myenteric plexus (Auerbach plexus) lies between the longitudinal and circular muscle layers and is primarily responsible for control of peristalsis and segmentation. Food entering into the stomach causes the ileum to empty into the large intestine (gastroileal reflex). The average normal transit time from the mouth to the colon is 4 to 9 hours with 3 to 5 hours of that time spent continually mixing the chyme in the small intestine (Bryant, 2004; Doig & Huether, 2012; Hall & Guyton, 2011; Reed & Wickham, 2009).

Secretion

Extensive amounts of mucus are secreted within only the first few centimeters of the duodenum by the Brunner glands (compound mucous glands). These glands secrete mucus to protect the duodenal wall from being digested by the highly acidic chyme emptying into the duodenum from the stomach. The mucus neutralizes the HCl contained in the chyme as the mucus contains a large amount of bicarbonate ions, which combine with the bicarbonate ions from pancreatic secretion and liver bile. The epithelium covering villi and Lieberkühn crypts contains secretory cells of two types, goblet cells and enterocytes. Large amounts of mucus are secreted by goblet cells, which serve to lubricate and protect the intestinal surfaces. The enterocytes secrete approximately 3 L of extracellular fluid into the small bowel lumen each day. The pH of this fluid is slightly alkaline 7.5 to 8 (Table 1-1). This watery intestinal fluid is almost all extracellular fluid and contains no enzymes. It promotes the absorptive process by providing a flow of fluid from the crypts into the villi for osmotic absorption of substances from the chyme as it contacts the villi.

The enterocytes of the villi contain digestive enzymes that digest food substances while they are being absorbed through the epithelium. These digestive enzymes include (1) peptidases, which split small peptides into amino acids; (2) four enzymes, sucrase, maltase, isomaltase, and lactase, which split disaccharides into monosaccharides; and (3) intestinal lipase in small amounts, which split neutral fats into glycerol and fatty acids (Bryant, 2004; Doig & Huether, 2012; Hall & Guyton, 2011; O'Rahilly et al., 2008; Patton & Thibodeau, 2014; Reed & Wickham, 2009).

Absorption

The digestive processes break down complex molecules into substances that are more easily absorbed into the bloodstream. The vast amount of absorption occurs in the proximal small intestine (duodenum and jejunum) where the villi and brush border are ample. The ileum can absorb a substantial amount if necessary. The amount of bowel necessary to absorb enough nutrition to sustain life is difficult to determine due to variations in measurement techniques. However, digestion and absorption of nutrients is more than 90% completed within the first 100 cm of the small intestine. The absorption of intraluminal fluid is significant with as much as 5 to 6 L/day received by the proximal small bowel, an additional 3 L/day produced (Table 1-1). Of this total 8 to 9 L, 7 to 8 L is reabsorbed back into the small intestine. Only 1 to 2 L of fluid per day is passed through the ileocecal valve (Bryant, 2004; Hall & Guyton, 2011; Patton & Thibodeau, 2014).

Duodenum

The duodenum is the first section of the small intestine; being C shaped, the concavity encloses the head of the pancreas. It is 20 to 25 cm long extending from the pylorus to the duodenojejunal flexure. It lies retroperitoneally in close proximity to the stomach, the accessory organs (liver, gallbladder, and pancreas), and the transverse colon. The common bile duct and pancreatic duct empty into the duodenum at Vater ampulla. The flow of secretions through Vater ampulla into the duodenum is controlled by the sphincter of Oddi. The ligament of Treitz separates the duodenum and the jejunum. This ligament suspends the duodenum at an angle facilitating passage of the contents.

The major function of the duodenum is to neutralize acidic gastric contents as they enter the duodenum. The acidic chyme is partially neutralized by alkaline mucus secreted by Brunner glands located in the submucosal layer of the duodenum, as previously discussed. Additionally, secretin is released as the acid chyme enters the duodenum. The secretin stimulates the pancreas to secrete high concentrations of bicarbonate ions draining through the pancreatic duct and emptying into the duodenum at Vater ampulla helping to neutralize the chyme. The presence of fats in the duodenum stimulates delivery of alkaline bile, which further neutralizes gastric acids.

The second function of the duodenum is to continue the digestive processes. The presence of fatty acids and amino acids in the duodenum stimulates CCK release, which in turn contracts the gallbladder and secretion of pancreatic enzymatic juices. Bile is delivered to the duodenum to emulsify the fats, making them more susceptible to enzymatic breakdown. The pancreatic juice contains many digestive enzymes: amylase, to continue carbohydrate digestion; lipases, to continue lipid digestion; and the trypsin precursor of proteolytic enzymes, which is activated in the duodenum by enterokinase. Once trypsin is activated, it then activates the other proteolytic enzymes: chymotrypsin and carboxypeptidase.

Absorption is also another function of the duodenum. Substances absorbed include carbohydrates and minerals including iron, calcium, and magnesium. The villi are flatter with less frequent plicae in the duodenum compared to the jejunum (Bryant, 2004; O'Rahilly et al., 2008; Patton & Thibodeau, 2014).

Jejunum

The jejunum is the middle section of the small intestine. The ligament of Treitz is considered the division of the ileum and jejunum though it is difficult to distinguish between the distal part of the jejunum and the ileum. It is approximately 40 cm long with a diameter of 2.5 to 3.8 cm. The jejunum is the primary organ of nutritional absorption of most fats, proteins, vitamins, and the remaining carbohydrates. Digestion is finalized by the enzymes of the ample villi brush border. Absorption is through the carrier systems and the large volume of intestinal secretions. Additionally, absorption is facilitated through prominent villi and frequent plicae circulares (Bryant, 2004; O'Rahilly et al., 2008; Patton & Thibodeau, 2014).

Ileum

The third and most distal section of the small intestine is the ileum. It is 60 cm in length extending from the ligament of Treitz to the ileocecal valve. The width of the ileum is approximately 2.5 cm. The ileum has proportionately the most goblet cells of the small bowel. Increased amounts of mucosal lymphoid tissue are also present in the ileum with conspicuous cluster called Peyer patches. The Peyer patches together with the tonsils, appendix, and other diffuse lymphoid tissue constitute gut-associated lymphoid tissues (GALTs). The ileum is narrower than the jejunum with less prominent villi and no plicae circulares. The ileum absorbs nutrients not absorbed previously by the duodenum or jejunum. The terminal ileum contains the only receptors to absorb the intrinsic factor–vitamin B_{12} complex and bile salts. Patients who have had significant lengths of the terminal ileum resected may require lifelong vitamin B_{12} replacement to prevent pernicious anemia, improve fat intolerance, and reduce weight loss. Fat intolerance occurs when the bile salts in the terminal are not reabsorbed, which reduces bile production in the liver. Bile is produced in the liver and stored concentrated in the gallbladder until CCK stimulates the gallbladder to contract and deliver bile into the duodenum. Fats are emulsified by the bile, and the residual bile salts continue to pass further through the bowel until they are reabsorbed in the terminal ileum. Recycling of bile salts is known as the enterohepatic circulation, which promotes bile production and thus fat absorption (Bryant, 2004; Doig & Huether, 2012; Hall & Guyton, 2011; O'Rahilly et al., 2008; Patton & Thibodeau, 2014).

CLINICAL PEARL

The terminal ileum is the only site that absorbs vitamin B_{12} and bile salts. Patients who have had significant lengths of the terminal ileum resected may require lifelong vitamin B_{12} replacement to prevent pernicious anemia, improve fat intolerance, and reduce weight loss.

Ileocecal Valve

The ileocecal valve is a one-way valve separating the ileum and the cecum (separates the small intestine from the large intestine; **Fig. 1-5**). The ileocecal valve (sphincter) is 2 to 3 cm of smooth muscle intrinsically regulated. It typically remains closed until peristaltic waves occur in the last few centimeters relaxing or opening the ileocecal valve and allows controlled amounts of chyme to pass through to the large intestine. Distention of the cecum causes increased contractions and constriction of the ileocecal valve, which protects the small bowel from distention and reflux (Bryant, 2004; Doig & Huether, 2012; O'Rahilly et al., 2008; Patton & Thibodeau, 2014).

CLINICAL PEARL

As a native one-way valve, the ileocecal valve is used at times as continence mechanism for continent diversions.

Large Intestine (Colon)

The large intestine consists of the cecum with appendix appendage, ascending colon, transverse colon, descending colon, sigmoid colon, rectum, and anal canal. It is approximately 122 to 152 cm (4 to 5 feet) long and is somewhat horseshoe shaped. The diameter is 2.5 to 5.5 cm, being largest at the cecum with the caliber decreasing distally (further down the colon).

Unique to the colon are several features of the tissue layers from the rest of the GI tract. The outer layer (serosa) forms peritoneal sacs, which enclose fat and hang from the bowel (epiploic appendices). The longitudinal muscle of the colon unlike that of the small intestine is gathered into three muscular bands, or taeniae. The taeniae coli extend from the appendix to the rectosigmoid junction where the taeniae fuse into one continuous, circumferential longitudinal muscle. The taeniae are shorter than the colon, which causes a sacculated or gathered appearance (haustra). Colonic contractions and relaxation of the circular muscle make the haustra more or less prominent. The mucosa of the colon has many features different from the mucosa of the small intestine. The mucosa has folds (rugae) between the haustra. Villi are not present in the large intestine (colon). Lieberkühn crypts are deeper extending into the muscularis mucosae. Paneth cells are scattered throughout the cecum and ascending colon but absent in the rest of the colon.

The Lieberkühn crypts along with goblet cells produce colonic secretions of water, mucus, potassium, and bicarbonate. The bicarbonate secretion creates alkaline fecal matter with a pH of 7.8. Mucus produced by the goblet cells provides (1) lubrication to facilitate transportation of the fecal bolus and (2) protection from mucosal injury and (3) serves as a binding agent for the fecal material. Mucus production is stimulated by colonic irritants (bacterial, mechanical, or chemical) and the parasympathetic nervous system. Mucus secretion is decreased with anxiety and tension. The superior mesenteric artery provides the blood supply to the cecum, the right colon, and the transverse colon to the splenic flexure (**Fig. 1-6**). The inferior mesenteric artery provides the blood supply to the descending colon, the sigmoid colon, and the proximal portion of the rectum. The middle and inferior hemorrhoidal arteries, arising from the internal iliac arteries, supply the remainder of the rectum. The venous return is from the veins corresponding to the arteries supplying the colon. The superior mesenteric vein provides venous drainage for the cecum, the right colon, and the transverse colon to the splenic flexure. The inferior mesenteric vein provides venous drainage to the descending colon, the

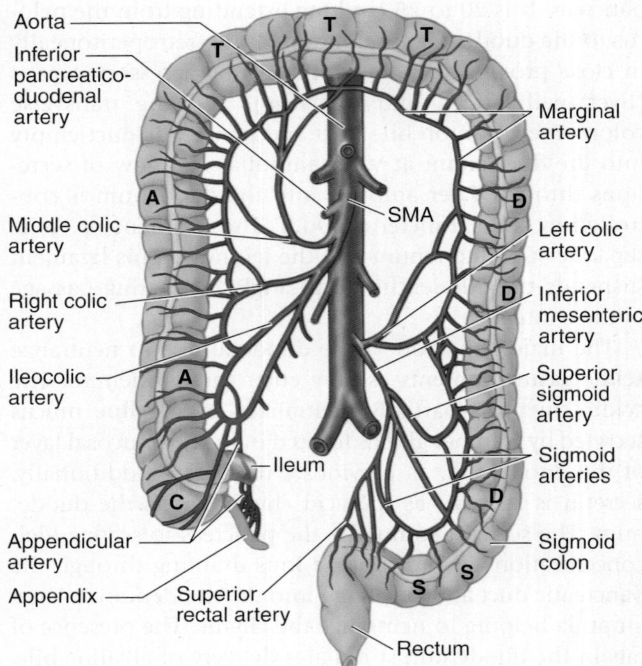

FIGURE 1-6. Blood supply to the large intestine, cecum, and appendix. A, ascending colon; C, cecum; D, descending colon; S, sigmoid colon; SMA, superior mesenteric artery; T, transverse colon.

sigmoid colon, and the proximal portion of the rectum. The blood from these veins is delivered to the liver as part of the portal vein system. The middle and inferior hemorrhoidal veins drain the remainder of the rectum and drains into the iliac veins as part of the systemic circulation (Bryant, 2004; Doig & Huether, 2012).

Function

The functions of the colon are collection, concentration, transportation, and elimination of fecal waste materials. The proximal half of the colon concerns essentially absorption, and the distal half of the colon concerns primarily storage. The intestinal materials pass into the cecum through the ileocecal valve totaling 1 to 1.5 L/day. Water, electrolytes (sodium and chloride), glucose, and urea are absorbed from this material. As the intestinal matter progresses through the colon, more fluid is absorbed from the fecal material and the consistency thickens from being fluid (in the ascending colon) to semifluid or soft (in the transverse colon) to solid (in the descending colon). Once the intestinal content reaches the sigmoid colon, it becomes feces, a collection of solid fecal waste products.

Transportation of the fecal material is through synchronous longitudinal and circular muscle movements that propel the fecal material forward primarily through segmentation (kneading) but also through several types of peristalsis. Historically, this was referred to gastrocolic reflex and is stimulated when chyme enters from the ileum (most commonly during or immediately after eating).

This reflex stimulates propulsion of the fecal material rapidly into the sigmoid colon and rectum, stimulating elimination. Relaxation of the colon is important to moving fecal material through the colon. The cecum fills with receptive relaxation, the fecal material accumulates and is stored with adaptive relaxation, pendulum movements (continuous back and forth movement) aid in absorption, and mass movement (en masse contraction of the left colon) propels the fecal bolus into the rectum to be evacuated. In summary, the cecum, ascending colon, transverse colon, and descending colon provide absorption and epithelial transport. When the fecal material mass reaches the sigmoid colon, it is entirely composed of waste products (undigested food residue, unabsorbed GI secretions, epithelial cells, and bacteria) and is considered feces or stool. The rectosigmoid section serves essentially as storage until it is time to defecate (Bryant, 2004; Doig & Huether, 2012).

CLINICAL PEARL

The colon's main functions of fluid absorption, fecal material transportation and storage, and elimination of feces lend the colon to be considered by some as an "organ of convenience" and not necessary to sustain life.

Colon Segments

The *cecum* is the first section of the colon essentially forming a pouch below the ileocecal valve. It measures 6 to 7.6 cm in length containing the ileocecal valve. The *ileocecal valve* lies between the cecum and the ascending colon preventing reflux of colonic material and bacteria into the small intestine. The *appendix* is a finger-like appendage of the cecum lying 1 to 2 cm below the ileum. The mucosa of the appendix is laden with lymphoid tissue. The *ascending colon* extends from the cecum to the right hepatic flexure, being the segment that is in a vertical position on the right side of the colon. It is 15 cm long and slightly smaller in diameter than is the cecum. The ascending colon is covered with peritoneum on the front and sides. The *hepatic flexure* is a sharp 90-degree left turn in the colon as it continues as the transverse colon. The *transverse colon* lies horizontally across the upper portion of the abdomen and is approximately 45 to 50 cm in length.

At the distal or furthest end, the transverse colon makes an extremely sharp (almost 180 degree) downward turn, which is the *splenic flexure*. The transverse colon is only fixed at two points (hepatic and splenic flexures) so it is quite mobile and may sag downward. In front of the transverse colon lies the greater omentum. The splenic flexure lies higher than the hepatic flexure. The *descending colon* is the next segment, extending from the splenic flexure to the true pelvic brim. The descending colon lies vertically on the left side of the abdomen. The front and both sides of the descending colon are covered with peritoneum. As the descending colon passes over the psoas muscle, the *sigmoid colon* starts and continues in an S-shaped curve to the left and continues to the upper end of the rectum. The length of the sigmoid colon is varied on average 40 cm. The sigmoid colon is covered with peritoneum on the front, posterior, and sides. The remaining portions include the *rectum* and *anal canal*, which follow (Bryant, 2004; Doig & Huether, 2012; Hall & Guyton, 2011; O'Rahilly et al., 2008).

CLINICAL PEARL

The S-shaped curve to the left of the sigmoid colon is the reason why patients are positioned on their left side for endoscopic exams or enemas.

Rectum

The rectum is distensible as an angulated hollow structure 12 to 15 cm (6 inches) in length (**Fig. 1-7**). It is slightly wider or the same in diameter than the preceding sigmoid colon segment and is similar anatomically. The rectum begins where the sigmoid colon terminates and is marked by the third sacral vertebra following the curve of the sacrum and coccyx. It angles sharply downward and backward in a straight manner. The rectum does not have haustra or epiploic appendices. It is normally collapsed being surrounded by strong muscular longitudinal fibers of the merging of the taeniae coli.

The rectal mucosa creates three transverse folds, which are the valves of Houston (two on the left and one on the right). The valves of Houston are composed of mucosa,

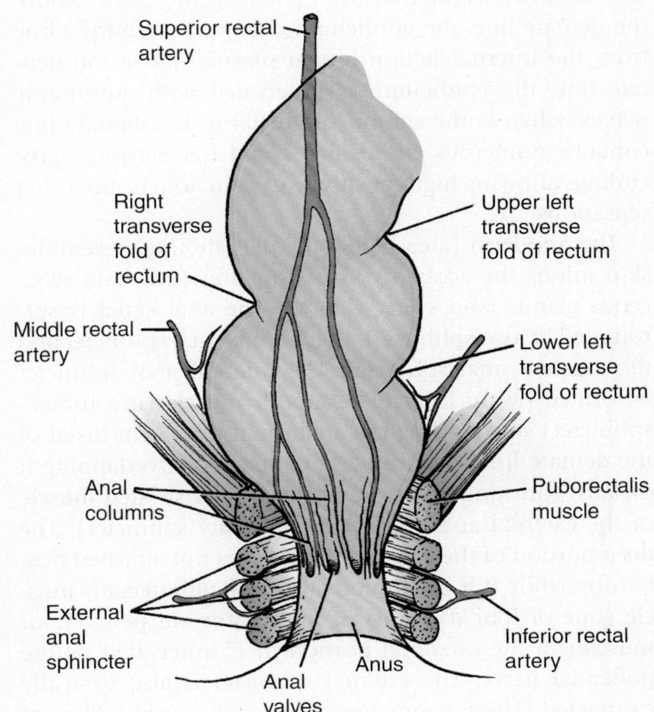

FIGURE 1-7. The rectum.

muscularis mucosa, submucosa, and circular muscle, which help support the weight of the fecal matter and reduce the frequency of the urge to defecate. Rectal compliance (resistance of the rectal wall to stretch or the amount of stiffness of the rectal wall) is related to rectal capacity (volume). Together, they are integral components of continence. In clinical practice, stool frequency and rectal compliance are correlated in patients with an ileal pouch. Poor outcomes are found when compliance of the ileal pouch fails to increase postoperatively.

The rectum becomes the anal canal as it passes through the levator ani muscle (Bryant, 2004; Doig & Huether, 2012; Fox et al., 2006; Hall & Guyton, 2011; O'Rahilly et al., 2008).

Anal Canal

The anal canal is a short canal approximately 3 to 4 cm in length and is the last portion of the colon positioned from the anorectal junction to the anal verge (typically the portion visible at skin level). A distinction in tissue types occurs at the midpoint of the anal canal known as the dentate line (also known as the pectinate line). Proximal (above) the dentate line, the mucosa has a pleated appearance referred to as the columns of Morgagni. These longitudinal folds occur as the rectum narrows into the anal canal. The anal canal is lined with columnar epithelium above the dentate line. Below the dentate line, to the anal verge, the anal canal is lined with modified squamous epithelium. The transition of tissue types from columnar epithelium to the squamous epithelium occurs gradually, approximately 6 to 12 mm proximal to the dentate line, and is known as the transition (cloacogenic) zone. Above the dentate line, the epithelium changes to a purple hue from the internal hemorrhoidal plexus. Above the dentate line, the epithelium is innervated with autonomic nerves, whereas the submucosa distal to the dentate line contains numerous encapsulated and free sensory nerve endings allowing high sensitivity to pain, touch, and other sensations.

The anoderm (area below the dentate line) resembles skin minus the accessory skin structures (i.e., hair, sebaceous glands, and sweat glands). The anal canal is surrounded by two sphincters, the internal anal sphincter and the external anal sphincter. The internal anal sphincter is formed by thick circular smooth muscle (involuntary sphincter) surrounding the anal canal to 1.5 cm distal of the dentate line. It is tonically contracted. Overlapping it distally, surrounding the anal canal is the striated muscle of the external anal sphincter (voluntary sphincter). The deep portion of the external sphincter is not attached posteriorly while it is continuous with the puborectalis muscle (one of four divisions of the levator ani pelvic floor muscle) in the proximal portion. It is innervated by the pudendal nerve. The external sphincter is also tonically contracted. These sphincters along with coordination of the pelvic floor muscles and voluntary efforts maintain continence and allow voluntary defecation. The anal verge is the level where the anal canal walls make contact in their normal resting state and have a puckered appearance. The perianal skin is considered the 5-cm radius of skin around the anal verge.

A mass movement of feces is delivered to the rectum, causing distention. Rectosigmoid distention causes stimulation of the mechanoreceptors, which elicit a reflex causing internal sphincter relaxation (rectoanal inhibitory reflex) while simultaneously the external anal sphincter contracts. The sensitive anal canal epithelium "samples" the contents to determine if the composition is air, liquid, or solid (sampling reflex). If defecation is desired and straining occurs to push the fecal mass into the rectum, intrarectal pressures increase. The increased pressure is sufficient to overcome the external sphincter contraction except at times of micturition or voluntary contraction of the external sphincter. Simultaneously, the external sphincter and pelvic floor muscles relax, causing straightening of the rectum and eliminating resistance by Houston valves or rectal angles. The squatting position also reduces rectal angles. Fecal mass stimulation of the anal canal mucosa allows continued relaxation of the external sphincter (Bryant, 2004; Doig & Huether, 2012; Hall & Guyton, 2011; Heitkemper, 2006; Reed & Wickham, 2009).

CLINICAL PEARL

The cell type differences lining above and below the dentate line in the anal canal are associated with common types of cancer above and below the dentate line (adenocarcinoma above the dentate line associated with colorectal cancer and squamous cell carcinoma below the dentate line associated with anal cancer).

Intestinal Bacteria

The presence of bacteria in the GI tract increases from the stomach to the distal colon. The stomach is rather sterile due to the high acidity that obliterates ingested pathogens or inhibits bacterial growth. The duodenum and jejunum have a relatively low aerobic bacterial concentration (10^{-1} to 10^{-4}) since in the duodenum, bile acid secretion, intestinal motility, and antibody production reduce bacterial growth. The aerobic bacteria that are present include streptococci, lactobacilli, staphylococci, and enterobacteria. Anaerobic bacteria are not found proximal to the ileocecal valve but are found distal of the ileocecal valve in the colon. Bacteria are quite prevalent in the colon and are vital to many functions. The anaerobes found from the ileocecal valve to the cecum include *Bacteroides*, clostridia, anaerobic lactobacilli, and coliforms.

Anaerobic bacteria decompose remaining proteins and indigestible residue; synthesize folic acid, vitamin K, nicotinic acid, riboflavin, and some B vitamins; and convert urea salts into ammonium salts and ammonia absorption into the portal circulation. *Escherichia coli, Enterobacter aerogenes*, *Clostridium perfringens*, and *Lactobacillus bifidus* are common colonic bacteria. The bacteria become more concentrated the further or more distal in the colon. Anaerobic bacteria compose approximately 95% of colonic fecal flora and contribute one third of the solid bulk of feces. Together, these bacteria are responsible to some degree for fecal odor and intestinal gas production.

The normal intestinal bacteria flora is not virulent or pathogenic. Endogenous infections of the GI tract occur through three major methods: bacterial overgrowth, intestinal perforation, and contamination of nearby structures. Prebiotics are plant fibers that promote healthy bowel flora growth. Probiotics are probiotic bacteria that arrive to the bowel in an active state. They interact with epithelial and immune cells boosting systemic immune activity and epithelial function. Synbiotics are synergistic combinations of both probiotics and prebiotics. The use of probiotics decreases bacterial overgrowth and reestablishes a healthy bowel flora. They are clinically used mainstream as therapeutic treatment of many GI disorders and disease processes, that is, irritable bowel syndrome, inflammatory bowel disease, antibiotic associated diarrhea, and *Clostridium difficile* colitis and diarrhea (Beisner et al., 2010; Bryant, 2004; Doig & Huether, 2012; Fedorak & Madsen, 2004).

Bacterial concentration increases distally in the bowel. This is the reason why there is more gas and odor for a sigmoid colostomy compared to an ileostomy.

CLINICAL PEARL

The ability of probiotics and symbiotics to promote healthy bowel flora, facilitate epithelial transport, and boost the immune system is the rationale behind the accepted therapeutic use to treat pouchitis of continent diversions.

Accessory Organs

The accessory organs of digestion include the liver, gallbladder, and exocrine pancreas, all of which secrete substances that are necessary for the digestion of chyme. The secretions are delivered in the duodenum. The liver provides bile for the digestion and absorption of fats. The bile produced by the liver is stored in the gallbladder when food is not being digested. The exocrine pancreas provides enzymes necessary for digestion of three main types of food: carbohydrates, proteins, and fats. The exocrine pancreas produces an alkaline fluid that contains large amounts of bicarbonate ions helping to neutralize acidic chyme leaving the stomach as it empties into the duodenum.

The liver metabolizes or synthesizes nutrients absorbed by the small intestine into forms that can be more readily absorbed by the body's cells. These nutrients are then either released into the bloodstream or stored for later use (Bryant, 2004; Doig & Huether, 2012; Hall & Guyton, 2011; Patton & Thibodeau, 2014; Reed & Wickham, 2009).

Liver

The liver is the largest internal organ of the body and weighs between 1,200 and 1,600 g. It lies under the right diaphragm. The liver is divided into right and left lobes, with the larger right lobe subdivided into the caudate and quadrate lobes. The liver is suspended from the anterior abdominal wall, the inferior diaphragmatic surface by the falciform ligament, the coronary ligament, and the round ligament. The liver is unique in having a blood supply of both arterial and venous sources (the hepatic artery and the portal vein). The hepatic artery is a branch of the abdominal aorta and provides the liver with oxygenated blood at the rate of 400 to 500 mL/minute or 25% to 33% of the cardiac output.

The portal vein receives nutrient-rich, deoxygenated blood from the splenic, inferior, and superior mesenteric veins (blood from the intestines, pancreas, spleen, stomach, and mesentery) at the rate of 1,000 to 1,200 mL/minute or 70% to 75% of the liver's blood supply. The portal vein branches into the sinusoids supplying each of the lobules. The sinusoids empty the venous blood into the intralobular vein, which eventually empties into the hepatic vein and the inferior vena cava. The volume of the liver's blood supply and proximity to the cells individually is thought to allow for the liver's ability to regenerate. On average, regeneration is believed to occur within 3 weeks functioning normally within 4 weeks.

Blood vessels, lymphatics, and nerves are supplied to the liver by the Glisson capsule, which covers the liver. If the liver is diseased or swollen, the distention of this capsule causes pain and the lymphatics may ooze fluid into the peritoneal space.

The lobules are the functional units of the liver that are formed from hepatocytes. The plates of hepatocytes contain capillaries or sinusoids and small channels (bile canaliculi) that are adjacent to the hepatocytes. Hepatocytes secrete electrolytes, lipids, lecithin, bile acids, and cholesterol into the small channels (bile canaliculi). Bile is also secreted via the hepatocytes and contains these substances as well as bilirubin (a by-product of destroyed red blood cells), which provides the bile pigment. The alkaline bile (7.5 pH) flows through the canaliculi channels to bile ducts that drain into the common bile duct and empties into the duodenum through the sphincter of Oddi (the major duodenal papilla). Bile salts are conjugated bile acids required for intestinal fat emulsification and absorption. Most bile salts are absorbed in the terminal ileum and returned to the liver via the portal circulation with this recycling of bile salts termed the enterohepatic circulation. Vitamin B_{12} is likewise absorbed in the terminal ileum and returned to the liver for storage.

The liver lobules sinusoids are lined with highly permeable endothelium. This allows the transport of nutrients into the hepatocytes for metabolism. The liver lobules sinusoids are also lined with phagocytic Kupffer cells (tissue macrophages), which destroy foreign substances, kill bacteria from the blood, and play a role in bilirubin production. Interstitial fluid is drained into the hepatic lymphatic system by Disse space (the endothelial lining of the sinusoid and hepatocyte) (Bryant, 2004; Doig & Huether, 2012; Hall & Guyton, 2011; Patton & Thibodeau, 2014; Reed & Wickham, 2009). The liver's ability to regenerate is significant allowing for up to 70% liver destruction before becoming symptomatic.

Gallbladder

The gallbladder is sac-like and pear shaped and is located on the inferior aspect of the liver. Bile flows through the cystic duct into the gallbladder from the liver. The bile is stored in the gallbladder and concentrated until it is needed for digestion. The bile concentrates as it is stored through absorption of water and electrolytes through the gallbladder wall, which creates a highly concentrated mixture of bile salts, bile pigments, and cholesterol, changing the pH of the bile to 7. Bile flows from the liver and gallbladder into the duodenum through the major duodenal papilla (sphincter of Oddi) into the duodenum as chyme enters the duodenum. After the duodenum empties, the major duodenal papilla closes, causing the gallbladder to fill with bile until the cycle begins again (Bryant, 2004; Doig & Huether, 2012; Hall & Guyton, 2011; Patton & Thibodeau, 2014; Reed & Wickham, 2009).

Exocrine Pancreas

The pancreas is fish shaped weighing approximately 85 g and approximately 20 cm long by 5 cm wide with four sections (head, neck, body, and tail). Its head is tucked into the C-shaped curve of the duodenum near the pyloric valve, the body is behind the stomach, and the tail touches the spleen at the level of the first and second lumbar vertebrae. The blood supply to the pancreas is supplied from branches of the celiac, splenic, and superior mesenteric arteries. The venous return is through the splenic and superior mesenteric veins, which drain blood into the portal circulation. The pancreas is innervated by sympathetic and parasympathetic fibers.

The pancreas uniquely has both exocrine and endocrine functions. Endocrine pancreatic cells are located within the islets of Langerhans and directly secrete hormones into the bloodstream. The hormones are insulin (secreted by beta cells), glucagon (alpha cells elucidate), somatostatin (produced by delta cells), and pancreatic polypeptide (produced by PP cells).

The exocrine (digestive) pancreas is composed of acinar cells and networks of ducts lined with columnar epithelial cells that secrete enzymes and aqueous bicarbonate fluids important to digestive functions secreting 700 to 1,000 mL daily. The clusters of the acinar cells for an acinus will form lobules. Connective tissue joins each lobule together forming the pancreas. Each acinus contains small ducts that empty into lobules where the secretions from the acinar cells are received and empty into the Wirsung duct. The Wirsung duct runs the entire length of the pancreas and connects to the duodenum through the Vater ampulla being surrounded by the sphincter of Oddi. The alkaline pancreatic juice (pH of 8.3) neutralizes the acidic chyme as it enters the duodenum and creates an optimal environment to active digestive enzymes (Bryant, 2004; Doig & Huether, 2012; Hall & Guyton, 2011; Patton & Thibodeau, 2014; Reed & Wickham, 2009).

Conclusions

This chapter has covered the normal anatomy and physiology of the GI tract including the structures, functions, blood supply, and innervation of the different organs involved throughout the entire process. The GI tract is complex with many interrelated functions and structures. It is through a better understanding of normal anatomy and physiology that more thorough comprehension of physiologic or surgical changes can occur.

REFERENCES

Beisner, J., Stange, E., & Wehkamp, J. (2010). Innate antimicrobial immunity in inflammatory bowel diseases. *Expert Review of Clinical Immunology, 6*(5), 809–818.

Bryant, R. (2004). Anatomy and physiology of the gastrointestinal tract. In J. Colwell, M. Goldberg, & J. Carmel (Eds.), *Fecal & urinary diversions: Management principles*. St. Louis, MO: Mosby-Elsevier.

Doig, A., & Huether, S. (2012). Structure and function of the digestive system. In S. Huether & K. McCance (Eds.), *Understanding pathophysiology* (5th ed.). St Louis, MO: Mosby-Elsevier.

Fedorak, R., & Madsen, M. (2004). Probiotics and prebiotics in gastrointestinal disorders. *Current Opinion in Gastroenterology, 20*, 146–155.

Fox, M., Thumshirn, M., & Fried, M. (2006). Barostat measurement of rectal compliance and capacity. *Diseases of the Colon & Rectum, 49*, 360–370.

Hall, J., & Guyton, A. (2011). *Guyton and hall textbook of medical physiology* (12th ed.). St Louis, MO: Elsevier.

Heitkemper, M. (2006). Physiology of bowel function. In D. Doughty (Ed.), *Urinary & fecal incontinence: Current management concepts* (3rd ed.). St Louis, MO: Mosby-Elsevier.

Ireland, A. P. (2004). Surgical fluids and electrolytes. http://surgstudent.org/lectures/flud/flud_centre_html.html

O'Rahilly, R., Muller, F., Carpenter, S., et al. (2008). Basic human anatomy: A regional study of human structure. Online version developed at: Dartmouth Medical School. http://www.dartmouth.edu/~humananatomy/index.html, accessed initially on September 1, 2014.

Patton, K., & Thibodeau, G. (2014). *Mosby's handbook of anatomy & physiology* (2nd ed.). St. Louis, MO: Mosby.

Reed, K., & Wickham, R. (2009). Review of the gastrointestinal tract: From macro to micro. *Seminars in Oncology Nursing, 25*(1), 3–14.

Takaki, M. (2003). Gut pacemaker cells: the interstitial cells of Cajal (ICC). *Journal of Smooth Muscle & Research, 39*(5), 137–161.

QUESTIONS

1. A WOC nurse is explaining to a student how digestion occurs. Which step in this process immediately follows the propulsion of food and waste products throughout the GI tract?
A. Elimination of waste product by defecation
B. Secretion of mucus, water, and digestive enzymes
C. Chemical digestion of food particles
D. Absorption of nutrients

2. Which tissue layer of the alimentary canal coordinates rhythmic peristaltic contractions of the muscles, which results in the mixing and forward propulsion of the food bolus through the stomach and intestine?
A. Mucosa
B. Submucosa
C. Muscularis
D. Serosa

3. Which tissue layer of the alimentary canal is involved when a patient is experiencing the pain of bowel inflammation?
A. Mucosa
B. Submucosa
C. Muscularis
D. Serosa

4. What complication may be avoided when stomas are matured (everted) at the time of surgery?
A. Serositis
B. Bowel perforation
C. Polyps
D. Stoma prolapse

5. Which postsurgical patient would the WOC nurse monitor for pernicious anemia due to impaired absorption of vitamin B_{12}?
A. A patient with an ileostomy
B. A patient with a large part of the stomach resected
C. A patient with a bowel resection
D. A patient with a colostomy

6. Which structure of the small intestine may take on some of the functions of the colon when the colon is surgically removed?
A. Crypts of Lieberkühn
B. Villi
C. Paneth cell
D. Epithelium

7. A patient is undergoing surgery for a continent diversion. Which structure of the small intestine may be used as a continence mechanism for this patient?
A. Terminal ileum
B. Ligament of Treitz
C. Ileocecal valve
D. Duodenojejunal flexure

8. Of all the organs of the digestive tract, which one is considered by some to be an "organ of convenience" and is not necessary to sustain life?
A. Ileum
B. Jejunum
C. Duodenum
D. Colon

9. Patient should be positioned on their left side for a colonoscopy because of an S shaped curve to the
A. Sigmoid colon
B. Rectum
C. Anal canal
D. Duodenum

10. Which organ has the ability to regenerate for up to 70% destruction before becoming symptomatic?
A. Liver
B. Pancreas
C. Gallbladder
D. Appendix

ANSWERS: 1.**B**, 2.**C**, 3.**D**, 4.**A**, 5.**A**, 6.**B**, 7.**C**, 8.**D**, 9.**A**, 10.**A**

CHAPTER 2

Anatomy and Physiology of the Urinary System

JoAnn Ermer-Seltun

OBJECTIVE

Apply knowledge of anatomy and physiology of the renal and urologic system in nursing management and education of the patient with a urinary diversion.

Topic Outline

A fundamental understanding of the urinary system and the changes in urine filling, storage and elimination associated with urinary reconstruction is essential in providing care for a person with a urinary diversion. This complex system provides homeostasis to maintain a stabilized internal environment for optimal cell and tissue metabolism. This arduous task is accomplished through excretion of water and waste; fluid and electrolyte balance; regulation of acid–base balance, and endocrine function by secreting hormones: erythropoietin (EPO) to promote red blood cell production and renin–angiotensin–aldosterone to regulate blood volume and pressure; and activation of vitamin D to promote ossification of bones and teeth. The urinary system consists of the upper urinary tract, which is responsible for urine formation and transportation (pair of kidneys, renal pelves, and ureters), and lower urinary tract (urinary bladder, urethra, and support structures), which provides urine storage and elimination (Fig. 2-1). This chapter concentrates on the normal structure and function of the urinary system.

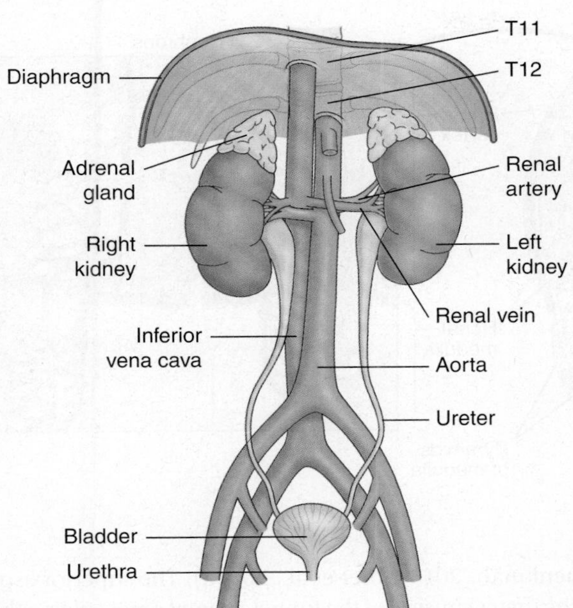

FIGURE 2-1. Kidneys, ureters, and bladder.

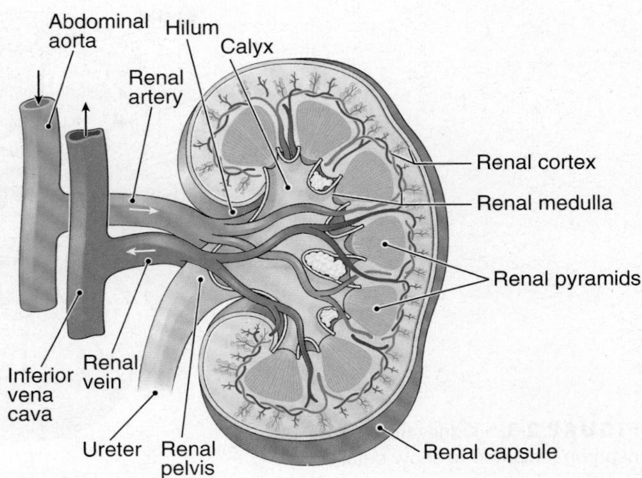

FIGURE 2-2. Structure of the kidney.

Kidney Location and Structure

The kidneys are a pair of reddish brown, bean-shaped organs situated near the twelfth thoracic (T-12) and third lumbar (L-3) vertebrae, lying on either side of the vertebral column. They are located against the deep muscles of the back in the retroperitoneal space. The right kidney is lower than the left to accommodate the liver. The lateral aspect of the kidney is convex, while the medial surface is quite concave. The hilum is located at the resulting medial depression that leads into a hollow chamber called the renal sinus, which contains blood vessels, nerves, lymphatic vessels, and the proximal ureter. The renal pelvis is a funnel-shaped sac, which is the superior end of the expanded ureter that is created by the convergence of two or three tubes called major calyces.

A bisected kidney discloses two distinct regions: an inner medulla and outer cortex, which is often referred as the parenchyma or "meat of the kidney" (Fig. 2-2). The inner medulla is made up of conical masses of tissue called renal pyramids. The base of the pyramids orientate toward the convex surface, whereas their apices form the renal papillae, which arise from the calyces approaching the hilum. The renal papilla is a valvular-like system that promotes outward (antegrade) flow from the nephron (functional unit of the kidney) into the renal pelvis to prevent reflux (retrograde flow) into the renal cortex. The renal cortex is granular in nature and forms a shell around the medulla. It dips into the medulla to fill the space between the pyramids forming renal columns and lobules. The cortex is protected by a dense adherent covering (renal capsule) and embedded in a mass of fat tissue. In addition, a double layer of renal fascia over the perinephric fat and other fibrous tissue helps protect and anchor the kidneys to the posterior abdominal wall. Therefore, the renal capsule, fat cushion, and perirenal and Gerota fascia, as well as the abdominal muscles, diaphragm, quadratus lumborum muscles, and ribs, offer protection and absorb shock if a blow occurs from the abdomen or flank region (Huether, 2011; Shier et al., 2013a).

The functional unit of the kidney is the nephron (Fig. 2-3). Its primary function is to remove waste and toxic products from the plasma and control the composition of body fluids. There are about 1 million nephrons in each renal parenchyma, so one can envision how tiny and condensed each unit must be. The nephron is a tubelike structure subdivided into the renal corpuscle (glomerulus and Bowman capsule) and a renal tubule. The glomerulus begins as a complex filtering unit composed of a tangled collection of blood capillaries that is surrounded by a thin-walled, cuplike structure called a Bowman capsule. It continues with a proximal convoluted (highly coiled) tubule, loop of Henle, and ends with the distal convoluted tubule, which empties into a collecting duct where multiple distal convoluted tubules merge. The fluid (glomerular filtrate) then drains into the top of the renal pyramid, and then to the renal papillae (prevents retrograde flow) where it joins the minor calyx and major calyx and lastly empties into the renal pelvis.

Blood supply to the nephron enters by an afferent arteriole, which gives rise to the glomerus's tangled capillaries and exits the glomerus via the efferent arteriole. It continues through the peritubular and vasa recta capillary system near the nephron loop where it joins blood from other peritubular capillary systems and ultimately unites with the kidney's venous system. The intricate adjacent capillary system of the nephron is crucial for renal filtration and urine formation.

There are two types of nephrons, cortical and juxtamedullary (Huether, 2011; Shier et al., 2013a). The kidney is a highly vascular organ. Although the kidneys account for

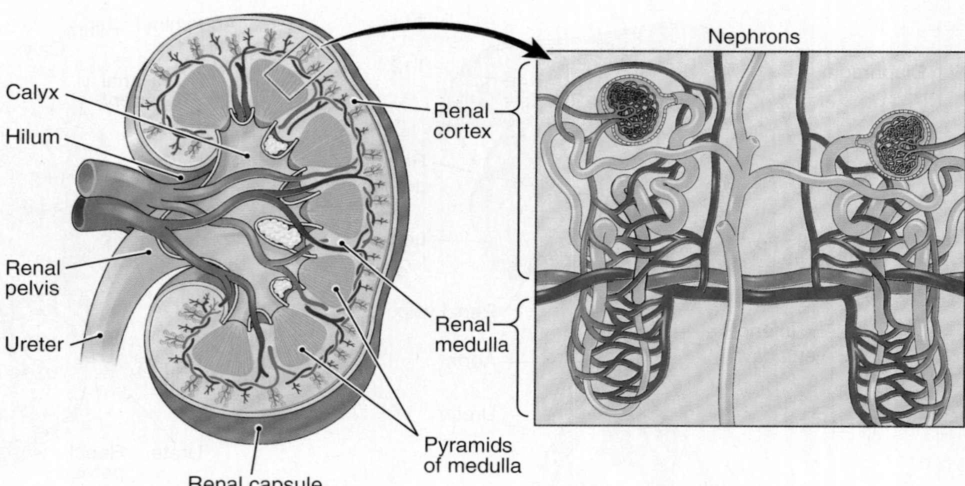

FIGURE 2-3. Kidney (**left**) with nephron (enlarged to show detail, **right**).

only 1% of a person's body weight, it receives over 15% to 30% (1,000 to 1,200 mL/min) of the total cardiac output when a person is at rest (Shier et al., 2013a). Blood is supplied to the kidney from usually a single (pairing can occur) renal artery, which directly branches off from the abdominal aorta. The position of the artery may vary in individuals; therefore, best surgical approach may need to be determined by the urologist prior to reconstruction. As the renal artery enters the hilum, it splits into the interlobar arteries, which pass through the renal pyramids and then branch to form a series of incomplete arches at the junction between the medulla and cortex called arcuate arteries. These arteries in turn branch into cortical radiate arteries, which finally give rise to the afferent arterioles that lead to the functional kidney units called nephrons. Venous return follows the same flow series as does the arterial return.

Elimination of Urine

Urine forms as the result of glomerular filtration of the blood plasma, tubular reabsorption, and minus tubular secretion. Once the glomerular filtrate passes through the collecting ducts, the urine remains unchanged. It exits the collecting ducts, drains into the minor and major renal calyces, and enters the renal pelvis, which is formed from the convergence of two to three major calyces. The renal pelvis is the funnel-shaped portion of the proximal ureter. The urine is transported from the kidney and ureters to a saclike muscle (bladder) in an antegrade fashion (efflux) while avoiding retrograde (reflux) movement of the urine through peristalsis. The bladder serves as a reservoir for urine and exits the body through a tubular structure called the urethra.

Ureters

The ureter is a long, tubular organ with an approximate length of 24 to 30 cm, with the left ureter slightly longer due to the inferior location of the right kidney (Huether, 2011; Schenkman, 2013; Shier et al., 2013a). The superior aspect of the ureter consists of the funnel-shaped renal pelvis, which holds approximately 15 to 20 mL of urine and tapers to 2 mm where it becomes officially the ureter, known as the ureteropelvic junction (UPJ). The UPJ is a common site for congenital or acquired obstruction, i.e., stones. The ureter continues in an inverted "S" shape in a downward and medial fashion until it terminates into the posterior base of the bladder (trigone) called the ureterovesical junction (UVJ).

A variety of sources supply arterial blood to the ureters, and these vary among people. Branches of the renal, gonadal, or adrenal arteries supply the upper ureters, while branches of the obturator artery, deferential artery in men, or uterine artery in women supply the lower (pelvic) ureter region. Venous return parallels the arterial supply as well as lymphatic drainage channels.

CLINICAL PEARL

The ureteropelvic junction (UPJ) obstruction is a common congenital condition.

Ureter Function

The main function of the ureter is to transport urine to the bladder in a fashion that promotes emptying without reflux. Several mechanisms promote antegrade urine flow: peristalsis through mechanical distention; neurologic, endocrine, and pharmacologic stimulation; as well as the UVJ structure. The renal pelvis holds about 15 to 20 mL of urine, and this distension initiates muscular peristaltic waves at a rate consistent with amount of urine present in the renal pelvis. For instance, if urine is formed quickly (i.e., diuretic therapy), then the peristaltic wave may occur every few seconds; in contrast, if glomerular filtration rate is slow (i.e., dehydration), the peristalsis may occur every few minutes (Shier et al., 2013a). In recent research, it appears that interstitial cells of Cajal (ICC) are more likely the modulators of smooth muscle activity involved in ureteral peristalsis (Hurtado et al., 2014; Lang et al., 2007).

Resting intraluminal pressure is elevated with each peristaltic contraction (r), which pushes the bolus of urine before it is at relatively low pressure. Because urine transport is at low pressure, any disorder that increases bladder pressure (i.e., low bladder wall compliance or bladder outlet obstruction) can elevate the risk of upper tract damage such as hydroureteronephrosis, recurrent urinary tract infections (UTIs), vesicoureteral reflux, and potentially irreversible renal damage. Gap junctions (electrochemical communication between ureteral muscle cells) allow the ureter to function as a single unit to propel urine forward through the entire ureter to the bladder in one single peristaltic contraction, even if innervation to the ureter is compromised or the ureter is transplanted (Gray, 2006; Gray & Moore, 2009). In addition to mechanical distention, neurologic, endocrine, and pharmacologic factors aid in ureteral peristaltic action. Sympathetic stimulation within the ureteral wall of the alpha adrenergic receptors cause increase strength and number of contractions, while beta adrenergic stimulation causes relaxation of the ureter. Parasympathetic stimulation of cholinergic receptors with medications such as epinephrine (catecholamine) creates strong peristaltic action.

CLINICAL PEARL

Since urine transport is at low pressure, any disorder that increases bladder pressure (i.e., low bladder wall compliance or bladder outlet obstruction) can elevate the risk of upper tract damage such as hydroureteronephrosis, recurrent UTIs, vesicoureteral reflux, and potentially irreversible renal damage.

The UVJ plays a pivotal role in promoting antegrade urine flow from the kidney into the bladder and preventing reflux (retrograde movement) from the bladder to the upper tracts. It consists of the distal ureter, the adjoining bladder wall, and the trigone of the bladder, which acts together as a unit to prevent retrograde urine movement by three methods (Gray, 2004; Gray & Moore, 2009). First, the terminal ureter tunnels the adjacent bladder wall and trigone at a gentle angle for about 1.5 cm. This layout promotes sealing of the ureter when the bladder or trigone contract. The outer layer (adventitia) of the intramural (tunneled) ureter contains three sheaths known as Waldeyer sheath, to provide limited mobility and solid attachment to the bladder. Second, the smooth muscle bundles arranged in a circular and longitudinal manner within the bladder offer additional support as well as promotion of UVJ closure during urination. Lastly, the trigone is a triangular-shaped smooth muscle at the base of the bladder with the apex extending into the bladder neck in women and the verumontanum (an elevation in the floor of the prostrate where seminal ducts enter) in men.

The trigone is divided into two distinct segments, superficial and deep (Gray & Moore, 2009). Urine is expelled into the bladder following a peristaltic contraction through a flaplike fold of the mucous membrane. This fold acts like a valve at the UVJ in that it allows urine to enter the bladder but prevents backing up of urine from the bladder to the ureter even during coughing, sneezing, and physical exertion (Shier et al., 2013a). As the bladder fills with urine, both the detrusor and trigone regions are relaxed due to sympathetic nerve stimulation to allow urine to pass through the UVJ. Beta adrenergic receptors in the bladder cause smooth muscle relaxation, while alpha adrenergic receptors in the bladder neck cause the smooth muscle to contract to prevent urine leakage while filling and storage.

In contrast, during micturition, the bladder contracts due to parasympathetic stimulation of the cholinergic receptors and indirectly inhibits sympathetic stimulation of the bladder neck (causes relaxation of bladder neck) to promote urine elimination. The contraction of the bladder and trigone raises the closing pressure of the intramural ureter (UVJ) to prevent reflux. Moreover, the trigone contracts an additional approximately 20 seconds after micturition to further lessen the risk of reflux (Gray & Moore, 2009).

CLINICAL PEARL

The UVJ prevents retrograde urine flow from the lower to upper urinary tract.

Structure and Function of the Lower Urinary Tract

The lower urinary tract consists of the bladder, urethra, and pelvic floor muscles. These structures work together as a unit to maintain continence through storage and elimination of urine at a desirable time.

Urinary Bladder

The urinary bladder is a hollow, muscular organ that has a fixed base and quite a dispensable body designed to fill with urine at low pressures, store approximately 300 to 600 mL in the healthy adult, and eliminate urine. The bladder lies within the pelvic cavity and is located posterior to the symphysis pubis and inferior to the parietal peritoneum. In females, the anterior uterine wall and vagina come in contact with the bladder, while in males, the posterior bladder neighbors the rectum (Shier et al., 2013a). The pressure of surrounding organs modifies the spherical shape of the bladder, but the size and shape of the bladder are dependent upon the amount of urine being stored. Often, anatomic drawings inaccurately depict an air bubble in the bladder; however, as the bladder empties, the walls collapse down upon the fixed base creating a tetrahedron (triangular pyramid)-like shape.

As the bladder fills, the superior surface expands upward into a dome; it pushes above the pubic crest if distended and near the umbilicus if greatly distended (Shier et al., 2013a). The trigone is the anterior floor of the bladder with an inlet at each of the angles, the UVJ orifices as described above and a funnel-shaped extension into the apex of the trigone is called the bladder neck or UVJ. There are four histological layers in the wall of the bladder: mucosa, lamina propria or submucosa, muscularis, and serous coat or adventitia (Gray & Moore, 2009; Shier et al., 2013). The mucosa coat is composed of several thicknesses of the transitional epithelial cells or uroepithelium that are similar to the lining of the renal pelvis and ureters as well as the upper portion of the urethra. The thickness of this layer becomes reduced (only one to two cells deep) as the bladder fills and distends and returns to five to seven cells deep with urine elimination.

The uroepithelium is impermeable to the contents of the urine and manufactures a very thick, mucoid-like substance called glycosaminoglycans (GAG layer) to protect the mucosa from irritants in the urine. The second layer, lamina propria, is loosely connected to the uroepithelium but firmly attached to the third layer, muscularis. It contains connective tissue, nerves, blood vessels, as well as interstitial cells that communicate considerably by gap junctions. The third layer consists of a complex meshwork of smooth muscle bundles (unlike the organized circular and longitudinal layers of the intestine) known as the detrusor muscle. The muscle layer contains collagen and elastin to provide structural integrity to the bladder.

Unfortunately, some lower urinary tract disorders such as seen in specific types of denervation and obstruction result in excessive collagen deposition. This consequence creates trabeculation (thickening or hypertrophy of bladder muscle) and ineffective contractility of the bladder leading to elevated urine residuals, elevated risk for UTIs, and compromised upper tract urine production and drainage (Casey, 2011; Gray & Moore, 2009). The muscularis also contains interstitial cells connected by gap junctions to provide communication and coordination of detrusor activity.

The fourth layer is the serosal coat or adventitia. It covers most of the bladder with fibroelastic connective tissue except the upper portion of the bladder where simple squamous epithelium covers the area along with a small amount of connective tissue. Perivesical fat covers beyond the serosa/adventitia. The bladder receives its arterial blood supply via the superior, inferior, and medial vesical arteries, in addition to branches of the obturator, inferior gluteal, or internal iliac arteries. Females also receive arterial blood to the bladder from uterine and vaginal arteries.

CLINICAL PEARLS

The urinary bladder is also known as the detrusor muscle. The detrusor smooth muscle contains collagen and elastin.

Urethra

Urine is expelled from the bladder through a collapsible tube called the urethra. Like the upper urinary tract and bladder, the urethra is composed of the same four histological layers (urothelium, lamina propria, muscularis, and serosa or adventitia) but differs in that it is composed of both smooth and specialized striated muscle that aids in maintaining continence. The urethra has specialized striated muscle that contains both fast-twitch and short-twitch muscle fibers that aid in tone of the urethra during periods of sudden increase in abdominal pressure (i.e., cough) and prolong periods needed for continence between voids. In females, the urethra is about 4 cm in length (3.5 to 5.5 cm), which begins at the bladder neck and terminates at the urethral meatus between the vagina and clitoris.

To promote female continence further, the anterior vaginal wall is fused with the distal two thirds of the urethra and shares vascular components, muscular and endopelvic fascial support (Gray & Moore, 2009; Pradidarcheep et al., 2011; Sampselle & DeLancey, 1998). The female urethra is obviously short compared to the male urethra but acts as a continence mechanism almost the entire length. In contrast, the male urethra is approximately 23 cm in length and acts as a passageway to transport not only urine but cells and secretions from the reproductive organs. It can be divided into three sections: prostatic urethra approximately 3 cm, membranous urethra approximately 2.5 cm, and penile urethra approximately 15 cm (Shier et al., 2013a).

The male urethra is composed of uroepithelium, lamina propria, muscularis, and adventitia but devoid of the muscularis layer in the distal portion. The proximal urethra wall contains both smooth and striated muscle that contributes to the continence sphincter mechanism. Females receive their urethral arterial blood supply from the vaginal artery while males receive theirs from the pudendal artery. Venous return occurs from the venous pelvic plexus in females; in males, venous return occurs through the deep dorsal vein. Lymphatic drainage takes place through the superficial and deep inguinal nodes, hypogastric, obturator, as well as internal and external iliac nodes.

Pelvic Floor

The pelvic floor consists of several muscle groups and ligaments that help support the pelvic viscera and deliver sphincter-like action in the anal canal and vagina (Ashton-Miller & DeLancey, 2007; Perucchini & DeLancey, 2008; Sampselle & DeLancey, 1998).

CLINICAL PEARL

The lower urinary tract is also supported by the perineal membrane and anal sphincter.

Female Pelvic Floor

Female functional continence mechanism is complex and depends on the integrity of the pelvic floor. The pelvic floor is made of three primary layers: (1) endopelvic fascia, (2) levator ani muscle, and (3) perineal membrane and external anal sphincter. The pelvic floor layers must anchor to the bony structures of the pelvis in order to provide optimal support. The female pelvis is a ring of bones composed of the sacrum and fusion of paired bones of the iliac, ischial, and pubic bones. The female pelvis accommodates both locomotion and childbirth by being larger and broader than that of a male (tall, narrow, and compact) as well as having an ovoid-shaped inlet in contrast to the male heart-shaped inlet. The second layer and the principal source of support of the pelvic floor is the levator ani (Gray & Moore, 2009; Pradidarcheep et al., 2011; Sampselle & DeLancey, 1998).

Male Pelvic Floor

The pelvic floor of the male is also made up of three primary layers: endopelvic fascia, levator ani, and perineal membrane/anal sphincter. The endopelvic fascia is analogous to that of the female, but condensations of the fascia provide specific support to the prostate gland, bladder base, and urethra. The levator ani is separated into two muscles as seen in females (iliococcygeus and pubovisceral) but is a thicker and larger U-shaped muscle as well as the primary support structure for the bladder and urethra. The perineal membrane and anal sphincter also provide secondary support (Gray & Moore, 2009; Pradidarcheep et al., 2011).

Adrenal Glands and Adjacent Organs

The adrenal glands are pyramid shaped, superior to each kidney, and entrenched in adipose tissue as well as Gerota fascia that encompasses the kidney. Although the adrenal glands are closest in proximity to the kidneys, they are functionally and anatomically distinct. They consist of two parts that secrete different hormones: adrenal medulla (central portion) and adrenal cortex (the outer portion).

The other organs adjacent to the kidneys include the duodenum, pancreas tail, hepatic flexure of the large intestine, ascending colon, and descending and sigmoid colon. Therefore, identification and protection of these adjacent organs by the surgeon during urinary reconstruction surgery are crucial to prevent life-threatening inter- and postoperative complications.

Function of the Kidneys

The function of the renal system is to maintain homeostasis of the body's internal environment through the regulation of body fluid volume, pH, and composition. This vital task is accomplished through (1) excretion of water and waste through urine production, (2) fluid and electrolyte balance, (3) regulation of acid–base balance, and (4) endocrine function by secreting hormones such as EPO to promote red blood cell production and renin and aldosterone to regulate blood volume and pressure and activation of vitamin D to promote bone growth and preservation (Huether, 2011; Shier et al., 2013b).

Urine Formation

Urine is an end product of glomerular filtration plus tubular secretion minus tubular reabsorption. Urine is composed of wastes, excess water, and electrolytes and is excreted from the body by the lower urinary tract. The nephrons are responsible for filtering 180 L of fluid every 24 hours with a formation of 1 to 2 L of urine per day, depending upon health, hydration, activity, and environmental factors. Excessive or poor urine production requires further medical evaluation.

Glomerular filtration rate (GFR) is the amount of filtrate through the nephron system per minute and often used as a marker reflecting kidney health. Filtration begins as the glomerular capillaries that filter the water dissolve molecules and ions out of the capillary plasma and into the glomerular capsules. The resulting glomerular filtrate composition is mostly water, glucose, amino acids, urea, uric acid, creatine, creatinine, sodium, chloride, potassium, calcium, bicarbonate, phosphate, and sulfate ions. Three forces affect the GFR favorably or negatively: hydrostatic pressure, filtration pressure, and plasma oncotic pressure. The sum of these three forces is net filtration pressure and normally is positive, causing filtration. The GFR is directly proportional to the net filtration pressure. Therefore, anything affecting hydrostatic pressure of the glomerulus capillaries or Bowman capsule and capillary oncotic pressure will also affect the GFR.

CLINICAL PEARL

The greatest factor that drives net filtration and GFR is the glomerular hydrostatic pressure.

Urine Concentration and Volume

The average GFR for a healthy adult is 125 mL/min, which translates into 45 gallons of protein-free filtrate in a 24-hour period (Shier et al., 2013). Obviously, to maintain homeostasis, this filtrate is not excreted as urine but reabsorbed by the renal tubular system. Once the filtrate reaches the loop of Henle, over 60% to 70% of filtered water and sodium have been reabsorbed. In addition, over half of the urea and more than 90% of the potassium, glucose, bicarbonate, calcium, and phosphate have been reabsorbed as well (Gray & Moore, 2009). Glomerular filtrate is isotonic (equal in concentration) when it reaches the loop of Henle.

CLINICAL PEARLS

The primary purpose of the loop of Henle is to determine urine concentration and hydration needs by the body.

Urine pH

Urine pH is approximately 4.6 to 8.0. Under normal conditions, the urine is more acidic but can vary depending upon dietary intake and acid–base balance mechanism. A higher pH may be due to large intake of citrus fruits, legumes, and vegetables, and an acidic pH may be due to a robust diet of meat or cranberry. Upon rising in the morning, urine is more acidic due to a slower respiratory rate (more CO_2 [acid] retained) during sleep. Urea is a by-product of protein metabolism, and the amount eliminated in the urine reflects the amount of ingested dietary protein. Eighty percent of the filtered urea is reabsorbed by the renal tubules. Uric acid is a by-product of purine and guanine metabolism from the intake of meat and seafood. Only 10% is excreted in the urine. If in excess, uric acid may precipitate in the blood and cause painful deposits in joints called gout.

Some species of bacteria (especially *Proteus* strains, *Klebsiella*, *Staphylococcus*, and *Pseudomonas*) produce an enzyme called urease. Urease converts urea into ammonia and carbon dioxide, which leads to a significant rise in urine pH. Unfortunately, phosphate will precipitate in an alkaline urine environment and create struvite crystals made of magnesium–phosphate–ammonium. Struvite stones account for about 15% to 20% of the renal calculi (Gray & Moore, 2009). Stone formation can occur in both high alkaline (calcium phosphate, calcium carbonate, magnesium phosphate stones) and acidic urine environments (uric acid, cystine, and calcium oxalate stones). However, under general circumstances, it is thought that an acidic urine pH is beneficial. Any conditions that alter the H^+ balance (vomiting, diarrhea, uncontrolled diabetes, COPD, dehydration, diet, some medications, etc.) will alter urine pH values to compensate and bring about homeostasis in acid–base balance as described below (Berkowitz, 2007).

CLINICAL PEARL

High urine pH in a urinary diversion can cause peristomal lesions.

Fluid and Electrolyte Balance

The second function of the renal system is to balance the body's fluid volume and electrolytes to maintain homeostasis since they are interdependent. Four key points to remember when discussing fluid and electrolyte balance are as follows: (1) Aldosterone causes reabsorption of sodium (Na^+) and secretion of potassium (K^+); (2) antidiuretic hormone (ADH) causes water reabsorption; (3) Na^+ is the main ion outside the cell (interstitial and vascular), while K^+ is the main ion within the actual cell; and (4) Water easily diffuses through a membrane readily from low to high solute concentration, while other ions need active or passive transport to cross membranes.

Water Regulation

The distribution of body fluids is not uniform and occupies different compartments in varying compositions. The body has approximately 40 L of water with 63% (25 L) of this total body water volume occupying the intracellular fluid compartment, while 37% (15 L) is in the extracellular fluid compartment. A seemingly simplistic yet complex equilibrium must exist; water intake must equal water output. The average oral intake is approximately 2,500 mL with approximately 60% (1,500 mL) lost in urine and 6% (150 mL) in feces and sweat (150 mL), while 28% (700 mL) will be lost in evaporation from the skin and lungs.

Life-sustaining measures of water balance are primarily regulated through the renal system and urine production since the other avenues (feces, sweat, skin, lungs) of water output are less in volume and variability. The primary effectors for the regulation of water output in the urine are the renal distal convoluted tubules and collecting ducts, although water reabsorption starts in the proximal renal tubules (Shier et al., 2013). The renal convoluted tubules and collecting ducts are impermeable to water unless ADH is present. ADH stimulates the cells in these structures to become greatly permeable to water, so water rapidly leaves the tubules/ducts through osmosis into the pericapillary system and the hypertonic medulla. This process creates a more concentrated urine, and water is conserved in the internal environment.

Dehydration is the epitome of excess water loss via sweat, water deprivation, and illnesses that cause prolonged vomiting and/or diarrhea. Infants and the elderly are at higher risk for water imbalance. Infants have less efficient water conservation by the kidneys, while the elderly have a reduced thirst mechanism, possible immobility issues, and lack of autonomy to obtain adequate fluid intake. In contrast, water intoxication can occur with excessive oral intake of fluids that leads to low serum sodium levels and intravascular water diffusion into the cells by osmosis leading to cellular swelling that can increase intracranial pressure, central nervous system (CNS) symptoms, and death in rare cases.

Electrolyte Balance and Renin–Angiotensin–Aldosterone System

Electrolyte balance, like water equilibrium, occurs when ionic gains equal losses. The kidneys regulate important electrolytes (sodium, chloride, potassium, calcium, phosphate, magnesium, bicarbonate, and hydrogen) that are essential in cell membrane permeability, impulse conduction along an axon, muscle fiber contraction, and pH balance. The intake and regulation of intake of electrolytes usually is satisfied by ingestion of foods and beverages in response to thirst and hunger as well as existing as by-products of metabolic reactions.

Electrolyte loss or output is reflected in perspiration and feces, but the greatest output arises from the end result of kidney function and urine production. Remember, sodium ions represent 90% of the positively charged ions in the extracellular fluid. In contrast, potassium positively charged ions predominate in the intracellular fluid. In review, most of the Na^+ (60% to 70%) and 90% of K^+ and other electrolytes are reabsorbed by the proximal convoluted tubule and loop of Henle. In addition, aldosterone regulates both Na^+ and K^+. Low serum Na^+ and low renal artery pressure and $beta_1$ adrenergic receptor stimulation (within the JGA) incite the juxtaglomerular cells to secrete the enzyme renin.

The renin–angiotensin–aldosterone system (RAAS) plays a critical role in influencing cardiac output and arterial pressure by regulating blood volume and systemic vascular resistance (Klabunde, 2014). Renin reacts with angiotensinogen (a blood protein), which releases angiotensin I. This reacts with angiotensin-converting enzyme (ACE) that is supplied from lung endothelial blood vessels, which in turn changes angiotensin I into angiotensin II.

Angiotensin II (a potent vasoconstrictor) travels in the bloodstream to stimulate the adrenal gland to release aldosterone (in the presence of adrenocorticotropic hormone [ACTH]) as well as ADH (also called vasopressin for its mild vascular constricting properties) from the posterior pituitary to conserve water. Aldosterone then stimulates the distal convoluted tubules and collecting ducts to reabsorb Na^+ and water and secrete K^+. Angiotensin II also stimulates the thirst centers in the brain to help increase fluid volume and facilitates norepinephrine release from adrenergic receptor sites to promote sympathetic function. Renin secretion is inhibited by normalization of blood pressure and plasma sodium concentration. In summary, Na^+, water, and blood volume regulation is primarily controlled by renal tubule system in response to fluid and Na^+ concentrations, the RAAS, and ANP (Berkowitz, 2007; Huether, 2011; Shier et al., 2013).

Potassium Regulation

In addition to previous content discussing potassium regulation, an elevated K^+ level is a powerful stimulus for the adrenal gland to secrete aldosterone to reduce K^+ concentrations by distal tubular secretion (as well as reabsorption of Na^+ and water). Diuretic therapy (K^+ sparing or loop), presence of aldosterone, dietary intake, and hydrogen ion concentration for acid–base balance are primarily controlled by potassium balance (Berkowitz, 2007; Huether, 2011; Shier et al., 2013).

Calcium, Phosphate, and Magnesium Regulation

Minerals account for about 4% of the total body weight and are primarily located in bone and teeth. Calcium and phosphorus contribute up to 75% of that weight (Huether, 2011; Shier et al., 2013b). As in Na^+ and K^+ reabsorption, calcium, phosphate, and magnesium are resorbed mostly by the proximal convoluted tubules and loop of Henle (approximately 85%), while the distal convoluted tubule actively makes the final adjustments in concentration through the effect of parathyroid hormone (PTH), calcitonin, and glucagon hormones (Gray & Moore, 2009). In addition, dietary intake, H^+ ion concentration (regulated by acid–base balance), and vitamin D may influence homeostasis of these minerals. Noteworthy, Ca-sparing diuretics (thiazides) promote reabsorption of calcium thereby reducing urinary excretion, while loop diuretics promote calcium urinary excretion to reduce serum calcium.

Vitamin D

Vitamin D is obtained through the diet or made in the skin but must be converted to a metabolic active form by the liver and then kidneys (Huether, 2011; Shier et al., 2013b). In addition to enhancing absorption of calcium and phosphate from the gut, vitamin D increases bone reabsorption, which releases calcium and phosphate into the blood and augments phosphate reabsorption in the kidneys.

Calcitonin

The C cells of the thyroid secrete calcitonin in the response to elevated calcium serum levels. It acts as an antagonist compared to vitamin D and PTH by decreasing serum Ca through promotion of bone development and reduction of renal reabsorption of calcium. Calcitonin plays a lesser role in calcium metabolism than do PTH and vitamin D (Berkowitz, 2007).

Magnesium

Often labeled the forgotten cation, magnesium plays a critical role in intracellular and extracellular function, which prevents cardiac arrhythmias, hypertension, possible CAD, neuromuscular and neuropsychiatric disturbances, and osteoporosis (Fulop, 2013; Fulop, 2014). Some emerging studies report that low levels of magnesium may be a central factor in the development of type 2 diabetes, asthma, migraines, and nephrolithiasis (Fulop, 2013). Moreover, calcium and magnesium antagonize each other's gut absorption; high calcium intake reduces magnesium absorption, while low magnesium intake promotes calcium absorption. Mainly poor renal function; alteration in PTH, calcium, and possible vitamin D levels; as well as gut malabsorption and poor intake may alter magnesium homeostasis. In summary, PTH and vitamin D increase serum calcium, while calcitonin reduced serum calcium. PTH promotes excretion of phosphate, while vitamin D promotes reabsorption. Presence of calcium in the gut reduces magnesium absorption in contrast to the presence of PTH and vitamin D, which promote magnesium absorption. Diseases that affect the bone, kidney, and parathyroid gland, as well as altered vitamin D levels may lead to hypo or hyper conditions of calcium, phosphate, and magnesium.

Acid–base Balance

An acid is an electrolyte that releases hydrogen ions (H^+) in water; in contrast, an electrolyte that releases ions that combine with a hydrogen ion is called a base. Buffers are substances that assist in normalizing pH change by donating a hydrogen ion when depleted or combining with a hydrogen ion when in excess. Normal blood pH is 7.35 to 7.45, whereas acidosis is 7.0 to 7.3, and alkalosis is 7.5 to 7.8. Homeostatic mechanisms to maintain this narrow pH range is primarily done by the kidneys and lungs to maintain hydrogen (H^+) balance. Bicarbonate (HCO_3-base) is regulated by the kidneys and normally reabsorbed by the proximal tubules and a small amount in the distal tubules, while carbon dioxide (CO_2-acid) is blown off by the lungs as a by-product of respiratory metabolic processes. Both of these systems help maintain H^+ balance to regulate or buffer the pH when acid–base disturbances occur that cannot be compensated.

If the acidosis or alkalosis is caused by the respiratory system, then the kidneys will compensate. For instance, if the patient has an exacerbation of COPD, which leads to an excess of H^+ ions (respiratory acidosis) from the retained CO_2, the kidneys will buffer the system by retaining more HCO_3 to soak up the excess H^+ ions to balance the blood pH. Likewise, if a patient develops respiratory alkalosis as seen in hyperventilation (excess loss of CO_2), the kidneys will compensate by increasing excretion of HCO_3 to normalize the H^+ ion balance. If the kidneys cause the metabolic acidosis or alkalosis, the lungs will buffer the system through regulation of CO_2.

Metabolic acidosis can occur if there is too much acid (H^+) or too little base (HCO_3). If a patient is suffering from diarrhea, then bicarbonate (HCO_3) is lost, leaving an acid environment behind. The lungs will compensate by decreasing CO_2 (blowing off more CO_2). In metabolic alkalosis as seen in hyperaldosteronism, H^+ ions are secreted, which leaves behind a basic environment (remember that aldosterone causes reabsorption of Na^+ and secretion of K^+ and H^+) (Berkowitz, 2007).

Metabolic alkalosis is also seen in hypokalemia. The lungs will compensate for loss of H^+ and excess HCO_3 by increasing CO_2. Notice that if the kidney HCO_3 is in excess, then the lungs compensate by increasing CO_2, and conversely if kidney HCO_3 is low, then the lungs compensate by reducing CO_2. So the compensating organ always buffers the system with the substance it makes (kidneys, HCO_3; lungs, CO_2) in the same direction as the molecules causing the abnormality.

CLINICAL PEARL

Metabolic acidosis can occur with urinary diversions.

Endocrine Function

The kidneys possess endocrine-like function by secreting hormones: EPO to promote red blood cell production and renin–angiotensin–aldosterone to regulate blood volume and pressure, and activation of vitamin D to promote ossification of bones and teeth.

Erythropoietin

EPO is a glycoprotein hormone that stimulates the bone marrow through cytokine properties to create red blood cells in the response to hypoxia due to reduced renal blood flow (bleeding) or exposure to high altitudes (reduced oxygen levels). EPO is created mainly by fibroblast cells lining the peritubular capillary system near the renal tubules and minimally by the liver except during fetal gestation. Chronic kidney disease can drastically reduce EPO production and may lead to anemia and reduced hematocrit. Recumbent human EPO is often used to treat anemia produced by renal failure, inflammatory bowel disease, and myelodysplasia occurring from cancer treatment involving chemotherapy or radiation.

Renin–Angiotensin–Aldosterone System

As previously discussed, the kidneys monitor blood pressure and take a corrective action by producing renin in response to low afferent arteriole pressure caused by either systemic hypotension or renal artery stenosis. In short, renin acts upon angiotensinogen, which creates angiotensin I. Angiotensin I is cleaved by a peptidase (ACE) generated by blood vessels in the lung to create angiotensin II. Angiotensin II causes multiple reactions to help elevate low blood pressure and volume including constriction of arterioles to reduce capillary bed flow, thereby enhancing vascular resistance; stimulation of the proximal tubules to reabsorb sodium (thus water); stimulation of the adrenal gland to produce aldosterone, which promotes Na^+ reabsorption and K^+ secretion at the distal convoluted tubes; excitation of the posterior pituitary gland to release ADH (vasopressin) to promote water reabsorption at the collecting ducts; and increase in the strength of the heartbeat (Huether, 2011; Klabunde, 2014; Shier et al., 2013b).

Vitamin D_3

The inactive form of vitamin D_3 (calciferol) is synthesized in the skin when ultraviolet rays trigger the conversion of dehydrocholesterol into calciferol or is supplied through diet or supplementation. It is then changed into an active form of vitamin D_3 through a two-step process. Vitamin D_3 plays a vital role in intestinal calcium and phosphate absorption from food and promotes healthy bones and teeth through ossification.

Conclusions

The role of the renal system is to provide homeostasis to maintain a stabilized internal environment for optimal cell and tissue metabolism. It accomplishes this vital task through filtration of toxins from the blood and excretion of water and waste. Moreover, it provides homeostasis through fluid, electrolyte, and acid–base balance as well as hormonal secretion. The created filtrate (urine) leaves the kidneys through the renal pelves and ureters and is then transported to the bladder where it is stored and eliminated depending upon physiologic, psychological, and social influences that create a desire to urinate. The renal and urologic system is multifaceted where essential knowledge of the anatomy and physiology is imperative for optimal care of a patient who is a candidate for a urinary diversion due to a urological disorder. Depending upon the type of urinary diversion, alteration in the functions of the kidney may occur such as fluid and electrolyte and acid–base imbalances, urinary reflux, hydronephrosis, and renal failure. The primary goal when creating a urinary diversion is to preserve the function of the upper urinary tract.

REFERENCES

Ashton-Miller, J. A., & DeLancey, J. O. (2007). Functional anatomy of the female pelvic floor. *The Annals of the New York Academy of Sciences, 1101*, 266–296.

Berkowitz, A. (2007). *Clinical pathophysiology made ridiculously simple* (pp. 47–70). Miami, FL: MedMaster.

Casey, G. (2011). Incontinence and retention: How the bladder misfunctions. *Nursing New Zealand, 7*(7), 26–31.

Fulop, T. (2013). Hypomagnesemia. Retrieved from http://emedicine.medscape.com/article/2038394-overview

Fulop, T. (2014). Hypermagnesium. Retrieved from http://emedicine.medscape.com/article/246489-overview#aw2aab6b5

Gray, M. (2004). Anatomy and physiology of the urinary system. In J. C. Colwell, M. T. Goldberg, & J. E. Carmel (Eds.), *Fecal & urinary diversions: Management principles* (pp. 163–204). St. Louis, MO: Mosby.

Gray, M. (2006). Physiology of voiding. In D. B. Doughty (Ed.), *Urinary & fecal incontinence: Current management concepts* (3rd ed., pp. 21–54). St. Louis, MO: Elsevier.

Gray, M., & Moore, K. N. (2009). Atlas of genitourinary anatomy and physiology. In M. Gray & K. N. Moore (Eds.), *Urologic disorders: Adult and pediatric care* (pp. 12–43). St. Louis, MO: Mosby.

Huether, S. E. (2011). Structure and function of the renal and urologic system. In S. E. Huether & K. L. McCance (Eds.), *Understanding pathophysiology* (5th ed.). St. Louis, MO: Mosby.

Hurtado, R., Bub, G., & Herzlinger, D. (2014). A molecular signature of tissues with pacemaker activity in the heart and upper urinary tract involves coexpressed hyperpolarization-activated cation and T-type Ca2+ channels. *FASEB Journal, 28(2)*, 730–739.

Klabunde, R. (2014). Cardiovascular physiology concepts: Renin-angiotensin-aldosterone system. Retrieved from http://cvphysiology.com/Blood%20Pressure/BP015.htm

Lang, R. J., Hashitani, H., Tonta, M. A., et al. (2007). Spontaneous electrical and Ca^{2+} signals in typical and atypical smooth muscle cells and interstitial cell of Cajal-like cells of mouse renal pelvis. *The Journal of Physiology, 583*(Pt 3), 1049–1068. Published online 2007, July 26. doi: 10.1113/jphysiol.2007.137034

Perucchini, D., & DeLancey, J. (2008). Functional anatomy of the pelvic floor and lower urinary tract. In K. Baessler, et al. (Eds.), *Pelvic floor re-education* (2nd ed.). London, UK: Springer Verlag.

Pradidarcheep, W., Wallner, C., Dabhoiwala, N. F., et al (2011). Anatomy and histology of the lower urinary tract. In K. E. Andersson & M. C. Michel (Eds.), *Urinary tract, handbook of experimental pharmacology* (pp. 117–148). Berlin/Heidelberg, Germany: Springer-Verlag.

Sampselle, C. A., & DeLancey, O. L. (1998). Anatomy of female continence. *Journal of Wound, Ostomy, and Continence Nursing, 25(2)*, 63–74.

Schenkman, N. S. (2013). Ureter anatomy. Retrieved from http://emedicine.medscape.com/article/949127-overview

Shier, D., Butler, J., & Lewis, R. (2013a). Urinary system. In D. Shier, J. Butler, & R. Lewis (Eds.), *Hole's human anatomy & physiology* (13th ed., pp. 767–802). New York, NY: McGraw-Hill.

Shier, D., Butler, J., & Lewis, R. (2013b). Water, electrolyte, and acid–base balance. In D. Shier, J. Butler, & R. Lewis (Eds.), *Hole's human anatomy & physiology* (13th ed., pp. 767–802). New York, NY: McGraw-Hill.

QUESTIONS

1. The functional unit of the kidney is the nephron. What is the primary function of this structure?
   A. Removing waste and toxic products from the plasma
   B. Secreting mucus, water, and enzymes
   C. Forming urine
   D. Absorbing nutrients

2. Which structure of the urinary system assists with urine storage and elimination?
   A. Kidneys
   B. Renal pelves
   C. Ureters
   D. Bladder

3. Which structure of the urinary system is a common site for congenital or acquired obstruction, such as stones?
   A. Kidney
   B. Urinary bladder
   C. Ureteropelvic junction (UPJ)
   D. Urethra

4. The urethra is composed of both smooth and specialized striated muscle. What is an important function of this structure?
   A. Maintaining homeostasis
   B. Maintaining continence
   C. Storing excess urine
   D. Providing perfusion

5. Which of the organs adjacent to the kidneys needs to be protected by the surgeon during urinary reconstruction?
   A. Adrenal glands
   B. Abdominal aorta
   C. Liver
   D. Gallbladder

6. Which of the following statements accurately describes a function of the renal system when maintaining homeostasis of the body's internal environment?
   A. The kidneys secrete renin–angiotensin–aldosterone to regulate blood volume and pressure.
   B. Erythropoietin (EPO) causes multiple reactions to help elevate low blood pressure and volume.
   C. Carbon dioxide (CO_2-acid) is regulated by the kidneys and normally reabsorbed by the proximal tubules and a small amount in the distal tubules
   D. Vitamin K plays a vital role in intestinal calcium and phosphate absorption from food and promotes healthy bones and teeth through ossification.

7. The renal system controls urine concentration and volume. Which statement accurately describes this process?
   A. The average GFR for a healthy adult is 75 mL/min.
   B. Once filtrate reaches the loop of Henle over 75% of filtered water and sodium have been reabsorbed.
   C. Over half the urea is reabsorbed once the filtrate reaches the loop of Henle.
   D. More than 50% of potassium, glucose, bicarbonate, calcium, and phosphate are excreted in the urine.

8. What condition might occur when an excess of uric acid is precipitated in the blood?
   A. Hypertension
   B. Diabetes mellitus
   C. Diabetes insipidus
   D. Gout

9. What important point should be emphasized when explaining how the renal system works to regulate the body's fluid and electrolyte balance?
   A. Aldosterone causes secretion of sodium (Na^+) and reabsorption of potassium (K^+).
   B. Antidiuretic hormone (ADH) causes water reabsorption.
   C. Potassium (K^+) is the main ion outside the cell, while sodium (Na^+) is the main ion within the actual cell.
   D. Water needs active or passive transport to cross membranes.

10. What is the primary goal when creating a urinary diversion?
   A. Preserve the function of the upper urinary tract.
   B. Preserve the function of the lower urinary tract.
   C. Maintain acid–base balance.
   D. Prevent damage to the kidneys.

11. What condition might occur when erythropoietin (EPO) production is suppressed by chronic kidney disease?
   A. Elevated hematocrit
   B. Anemia
   C. Urinary incontinence
   D. Acid–base imbalances

ANSWERS: 1.**A**, 2.**D**, 3.**C**, 4.**B**, 5.**A**, 6.**A**, 7.**C**, 8.**D**, 9.**B**, 10.**A**, 11.**B**

CHAPTER 3

Diseases that Lead to a Fecal Stoma

Colorectal Cancer

Greta V. Bernier and Alessandro Fichera

OBJECTIVE

Describe the disease states that lead to creation of a fecal stoma: colorectal cancer.

Topic Outline

In the United States, colorectal cancer (CRC) is the fourth most common malignancy and second most common cause of cancer-related death (Howlander et al., 2014). Fortunately, due to significant efforts in both screening and treatment, those rates are decreasing on the order of 3.1% and 2.8% yearly for CRC incidence and deaths, respectively (National Cancer Institute, 2014). Despite these promising trends, there will be an estimated 136,830 new cases of colon cancer in 2014, making care of the colorectal patient in need of either temporary or permanent stoma a very common occurrence in clinical practice.

Colorectal Adenocarcinoma

Etiology

Adenocarcinoma accounts for the majority of cancers in the colon and rectum. The development of these tumors is believed to be from a single transformed cell that undergoes abnormal growth and division leading to formation of an adenoma and ultimately adenocarcinoma. In order to progress to carcinoma, the cell must undergo a series of genetic mutations causing inactivation of tumor suppressor genes such as *APC*, *DDC*, and *p53* or activation of protooncogenes like *K-ras*, which is associated with poor prognosis (Conlin et al., 2005).

Risk Factors

There are both modifiable and nonmodifiable risk factors for CRC development. Modifiable risk factors include high-fat and/or low-fiber diet, decreased physical activity, and associated obesity (American Cancer Society, 2014). Nonmodifiable risk factors include age >50 years, patient disease, family history of polyps or CRC, and genetic predisposition. Patients suffering from inflammatory bowel disease (i.e., Crohn's disease or ulcerative colitis) are at increased risk of developing CRC with a lifetime risk of 3.7% to 5.4% (Eaden et al., 2001). Their risk is proportional to the duration of inflammation, extent of colonic involvement, and age of onset. Personal history of neoplastic polyps (i.e., adenomas) carries a two- to fivefold increased risk of carcinoma, which is not surprising given the natural history of CRC development. A family history of adenoma or CRC yields a two- to fourfold increased risk of CRC, with greater risk for CRC over adenoma, family age of diagnosis at <50 years, and multiple affected family members (Johns & Houlston, 2001).

CLINICAL PEARL

People with a history of colorectal cancer in one or more first-degree relatives (parents, siblings, or children) are at increased risk.

While the majority of CRCs are sporadic, approximately 15% are associated with an inherited colon cancer predisposition via a germline genetic mutation. Such syndromes include familial adenomatous polyposis (FAP) and hereditary nonpolyposis colon cancer (HNPCC). FAP is caused by mutations in the oncogene *APC* and is inherited in an autosomal dominant pattern with a 100% risk of developing colon cancer by age 40 years. Individuals with FAP develop hundreds to thousands of adenomatous polyps in the colon and in the duodenum and stomach. Each of these is at risk for malignant transformation. Individuals with FAP should undergo total colectomy or proctocolectomy for treatment and risk reduction rather than segmental resection alone. There is a high risk of recurrence in the rectum if proctectomy is not performed, and therefore these individuals must continue rectal screening postoperatively.

HNPCC (Lynch Syndrome) is inherited by mutations in one of several mismatch repair genes (*MLH1*, *MSH2*, *MSH6*, and *PMS2*) leading to microsatellite instability. It is estimated that HNPCC accounts for 5% of CRCs. The lifetime CRC risk is slightly lower than with FAP at a rate of 70% to 90%. These individuals do not develop diffuse adenomatous disease as with FAP, and the cancers are typically flat and difficult to detect by colonoscopy. These tumors have a predilection for the right colon and can be treated with total colectomy alone without proctectomy as with FAP. Additionally, they are at risk for extracolonic cancers such as endometrial, ovarian, stomach, small bowel, and bladder. Women with HNPCC are counseled to undergo surveillance if premenopausal or consider prophylactic total abdominal hysterectomy and bilateral salpingo-oophorectomy if done with childbearing.

Screening

CRC screening has been a mainstay of health maintenance therapy for decades. The two primary studies are the fecal occult blood test (FOBT) and endoscopy. FOBT is limited in that not all CRCs cause bleeding and only 10% to 15% of individuals with positive FOBT have CRC (Umar et al., 2004). Despite this limitation, even 50% compliance with annual FOBT is estimated to decrease the incidence of CRC by approximately 20% (Hardcastle et al., 1986; Umar et al., 2000). Endoscopic evaluation of the colon is the other primary means of CRC screening, through either sigmoidoscopy or colonoscopy. These have the advantage of increased sensitivity and specificity as compared to FOBT, but are invasive studies and carry a risk of iatrogenic perforation. Additionally both diagnostic biopsies and therapeutic procedures can be performed. CT colonography and virtual colonoscopy are additional screening modalities that have the benefit of improved visualization of the colonic mucosa without the risks of an invasive procedure. Thus far, these are not routinely used. Current National Comprehensive Cancer Network (NCCN) guidelines recommend colonoscopy, annual FOBT, or combination of flexible sigmoidoscopy with FOBT starting age 50 for average-risk individuals (National Comprehensive Cancer Network, 2014a).

CLINICAL PEARL

The National Comprehensive Cancer Network has Colon Cancer Guidelines for Patients (http://www.nccn.org/patients/guidelines/colon/index.html#1).

Presentation/Workup

If not diagnosed through a screening modality, patients with CRC may present with a variety of symptoms including blood per rectum, decreased stool caliber, nonspecific abdominal pain, weight loss, and fatigue. Initial evaluation includes endoscopy if not previously performed, to assess tumor location and obtain biopsies to confirm suspected diagnosis of CRC. Once the diagnosis is confirmed, further studies are used to evaluate extent of tumor invasion and tumor spread including CT chest, abdomen and pelvis, CEA, and MRI or endoscopic ultrasound for rectal cancers. Based on this information, the cancer is staged using tumor invasion, spread to lymph nodes, and distant metastatic spread (TNM classification, Table 3-1) (Edge et al., 2010).

Treatment Algorithms

Based on staging information, specifically local tumor invasion and metastatic disease, patients may be treated with preoperative neoadjuvant therapy or go directly to surgical resection, followed by adjuvant therapy if indicated.

Surgical Management: Colon Cancer

Surgical resection is commonly a first step in the treatment of CRC depending on stage (Figs. 3-1 and 3-2) (National Comprehensive Cancer Network, 2014b, 2014c). It is estimated that over 200,000 colectomies are performed yearly in the United States, making it one of the most commonly performed procedures (Bal, 1992; Etzioni et al., 2009). A preoperative evaluation must be performed to determine the patient's fitness for the planned operation. The steps of resection include ligation of the feeding artery with en bloc

TABLE 3-1 TNM Classification

AJCC Stage	TNM Classification	Definition
0	Tis (carcinoma in situ)	Tis: Tumor involves mucosa only
I	T1 N0 T2 N0	T1: Tumor invades submucosa T2: Tumor invades muscularis propria
IIA	T3 N0	T3: Tumor invades through muscularis propria to subserosa (colon) or perirectal tissues (rectal)
IIB	T4a N0	T4a: Tumor invades surface of visceral peritoneum
IIC	T4b N0	T4b: Tumor directly invades adjacent structures
IIIA	T1-2, N1, M0 T1, N2a, M0	N1: Metastasis to 1–3 regional lymph nodes N2a: Metastasis to 4–6 regional lymph nodes
IIIB	T3-4, N1, M0 T2-3, N2a, M0 T1-2, N2b, M0	N2b: Metastases to ≥7 regional lymph nodes
IIIC	T4a, N2a, M0 T3-4a, N2b, M0 T4b, N1-2, M0	N3: Any node along major named vascular trunk
IVA IVB	Any T, any N, M1a Any T, any N, M1b	M1a: Distant metastasis confined to one organ or site M1b: Distant metastases in more than one organ/site or the peritoneum

Adapted from Edge, S. B., Byrd, D., Compton, C., et al. (Eds.). (2010). *AJCC cancer staging manual* (7th ed.). New York: Springer.

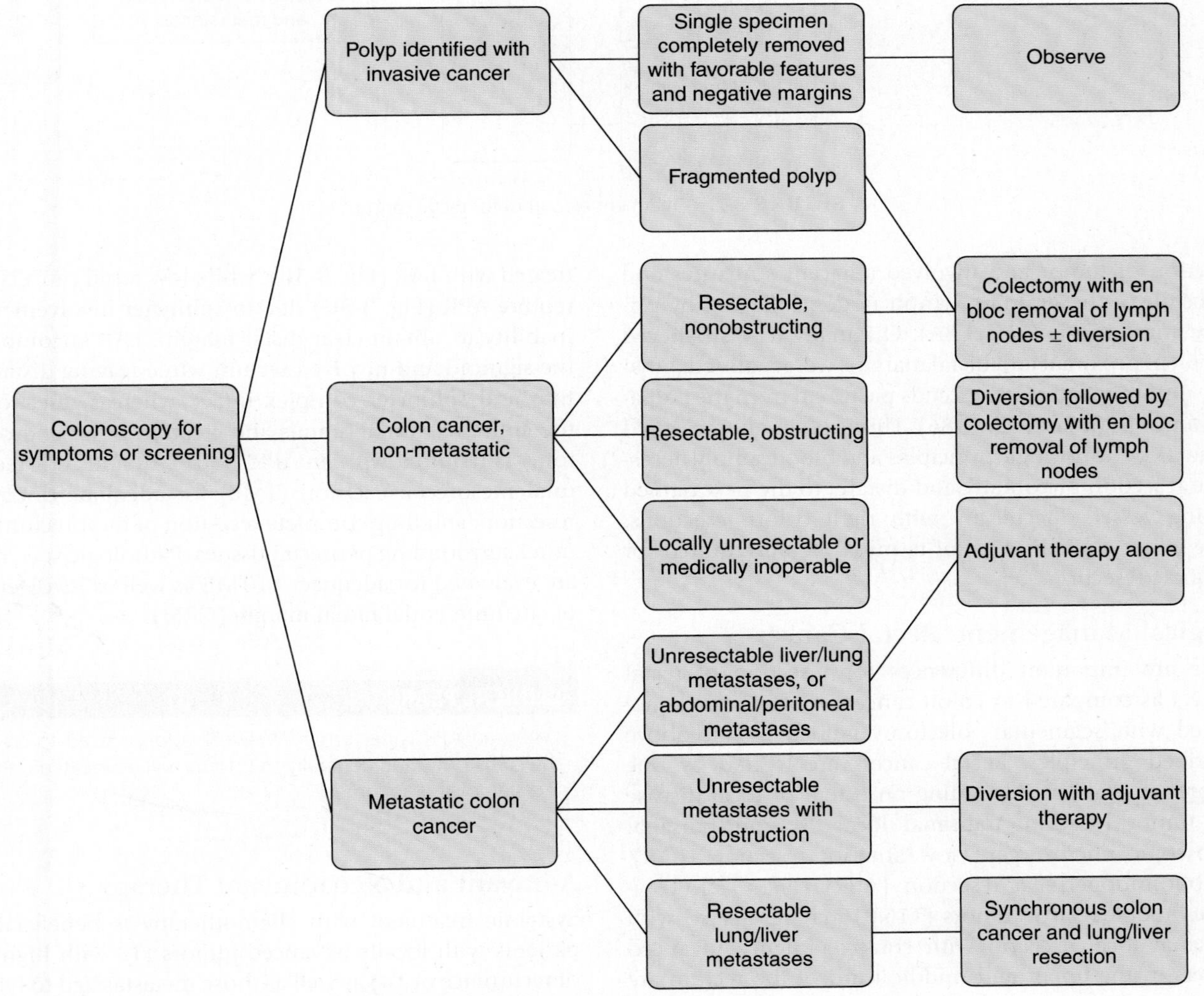

FIGURE 3-1. Treatment algorithm for colon cancer.

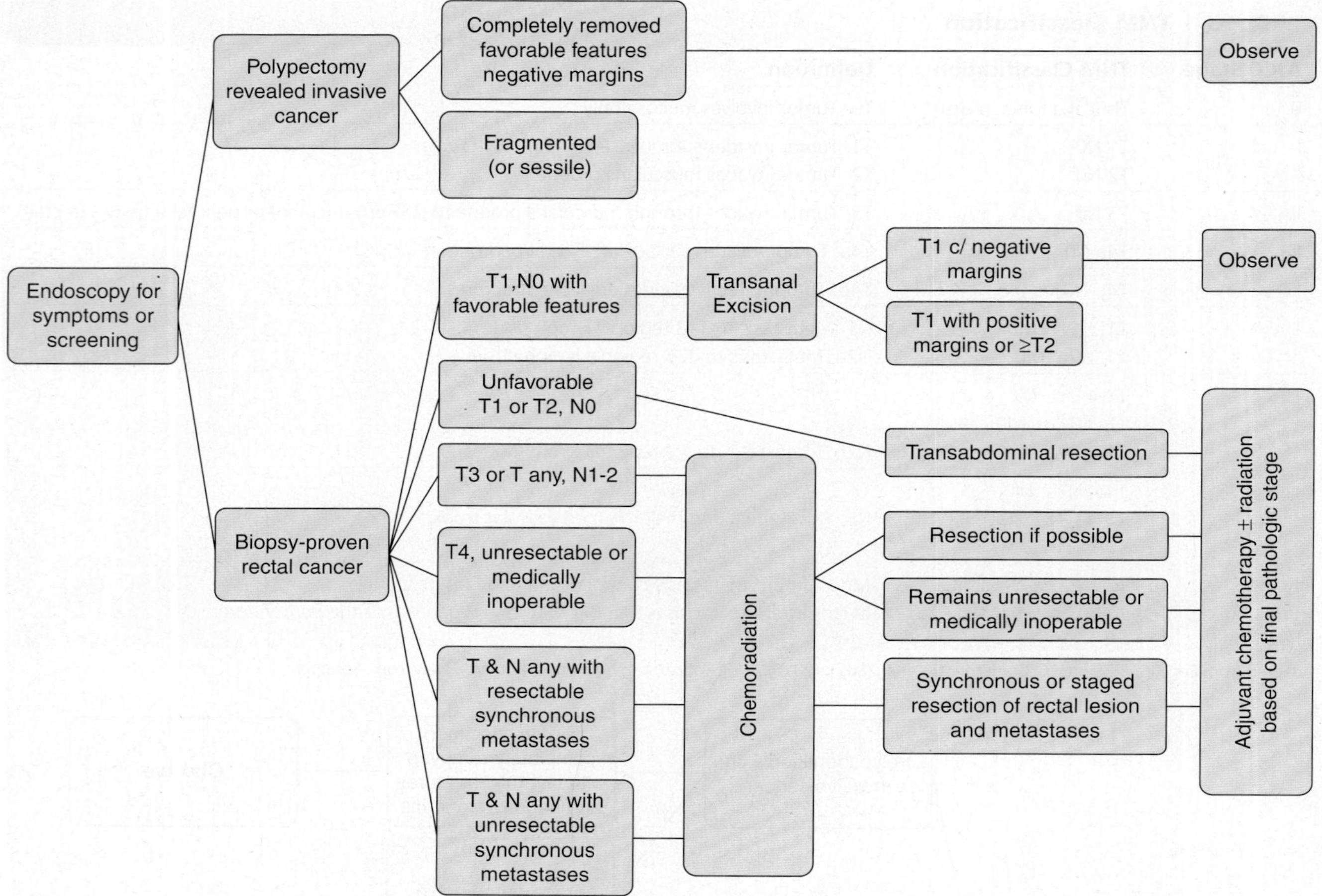

FIGURE 3-2. Treatment algorithm for rectal cancer.

resection of tumor and involved adjacent structures and inclusion of the draining lymph nodes, followed by primary anastomosis (Fig. 3-3A). Originally it was believed that 5-cm proximal and distal margins were required; however, mural spread rarely extends past 2 cm from the palpable tumor (Quirke et al., 1986). This is often not measured in practice as oncologic principles and blood supply necessitate resection proximally and distally to the next named feeding vessel. Specifically with right colon resections, there is not a set distance of terminal ileum required for adequate resection.

Surgical Management: Rectal Cancer

There are important differences for resection of rectal cancers as compared to colon cancers. Colon cancers are treated with segmental colectomy guided by the above described principles. Rectal cancers are treated by one of three operations depending on extent of local disease and tumor location: transanal local excision/transanal endoscopic microsurgery, low anterior resection (LAR), or abdominoperineal resection (APR) (Fig. 3-2). Low-grade, node-negative tumors (T1N0) may be treated with transanal local excision with curative intent. Advanced cancers in the upper and middle third of the rectum are treated with LAR (Fig. 3-3B), while low rectal cancers may require APR (Fig. 3-3C) due to sphincter involvement or inability to obtain clear distal margin. LAR encompasses the sigmoid and involved rectum while leaving distal rectum and sphincter complex intact, whereas resection of the entire rectum and anus and creation of an end colostomy is required with an APR. Both LAR and APR require total mesorectal excision (TME) for adequate oncologic resection, entailing complete resection of mesorectum and other surrounding perirectal tissues. Pathologic specimens are evaluated for adequacy of TME as well as involvement of circumferential radial margin (CRM).

CLINICAL PEARL

When an APR is performed, the left colon is used to create the colostomy, and generally the stoma will be located on the left side of the abdomen.

Adjuvant and Neoadjuvant Therapy

Systemic treatment with chemotherapy is beneficial for patients with locally advanced tumors (T3 with high risk of recurrence or T4) as well as those metastasized to lymph

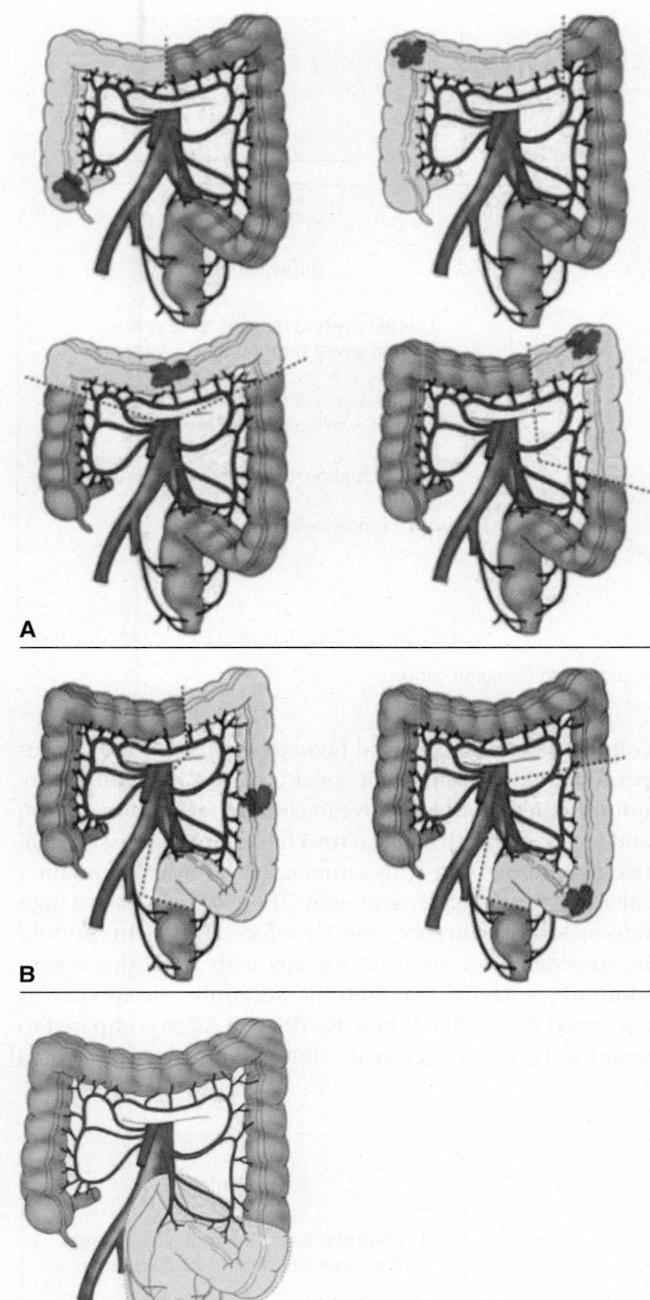

FIGURE 3-3. **A.** Segmental colon resection for colon cancer based on tumor location. **B.** LAR for distal colon or mid/upper rectal cancers. **C.** APR for distal rectal cancer.

nodes or distant sites (Fig. 3-4). Based on the results of the MOSAIC trial and the National Surgical Adjuvant Breast and Bowel Project (NSABP) C-07, the current adjuvant regimen consists of 5-FU, leucovorin, and oxaliplatin (FOLFOX) (André et al., 2009; Kuebler et al., 2007). Both overall survival and disease-free survival were improved on the order of 5% on the FOLFOX regimen.

Radiation therapy is recommended for rectal cancers with advanced local disease or lymph node involvement (Figs. 3-2 and 3-5). For these tumors, the incidence of local recurrence is decreased from 30% to 65% to 5% to 10% with adjuvant radiation (Colorectal Cancer Collaborative Group, 2001). Adjuvant radiation of the colon yields less benefit, as there is less overall risk of local recurrence as compared to rectal cancer. Additionally, it presents the risk of radiation toxicity to surrounding structures and organs that are difficult to exclude from the treatment field.

Other Cancers of the Colon and Rectum

Although adenocarcinoma is the predominant colorectal neoplasm, there are several other tumors of the colon and rectum that occur with less frequency but may require surgical management and possible stoma formation.

Carcinoid Tumors

Carcinoid tumors are a type of neuroendocrine tumor originating from the crypts of Lieberkühn. Approximately 65% of carcinoid tumors arise within the gastrointestinal tract, 30% of which arise in the colon and 20% in the rectum (Kulke & Mayer, 1999). These tumors are twice as common in individuals of African American descent and occur primarily in the fifth or sixth decades of life. Carcinoid syndrome is present in 10% to 18% of patients with symptoms including flushing, watery diarrhea, abdominal pain, wheezing, and right-sided heart failure. Unfortunately, 90% of symptomatic patients already have advanced or metastatic disease. Colorectal carcinoids are more commonly asymptomatic and identified on screening colonoscopy. Small (<2 cm) rectal carcinoids may be treated with transanal local excision alone. Rectal tumors >2 cm and all colon carcinoid tumors are treated with standard oncologic colorectal resection. Patients with carcinoid syndrome may be treated with somatostatin analogs for symptomatic control.

Melanoma: Primary and Metastatic

Melanoma of the gastrointestinal tract is most commonly metastatic from a different primary site and occurs in the small intestine. Approximately 15% of melanoma metastatic to the GI tract occurs in the colon (Allen & Cott, 2002; Rengtgen et al., 1984). Primary GI melanoma may occur in the rectum or anus with only case reports of primary colonic melanoma (Avital et al., 2004; Schuchter et al., 2000). Unfortunately, GI melanoma often carries a worse prognosis than does cutaneous melanoma, which many attribute to the later stage at diagnosis. Patients are often asymptomatic but may present with bleeding, obstruction, or pain. The only curative treatment modality is wide surgical excision; however, there is no survival benefit with radical excision with an APR, and therefore, this is reserved for those with intractable pain.

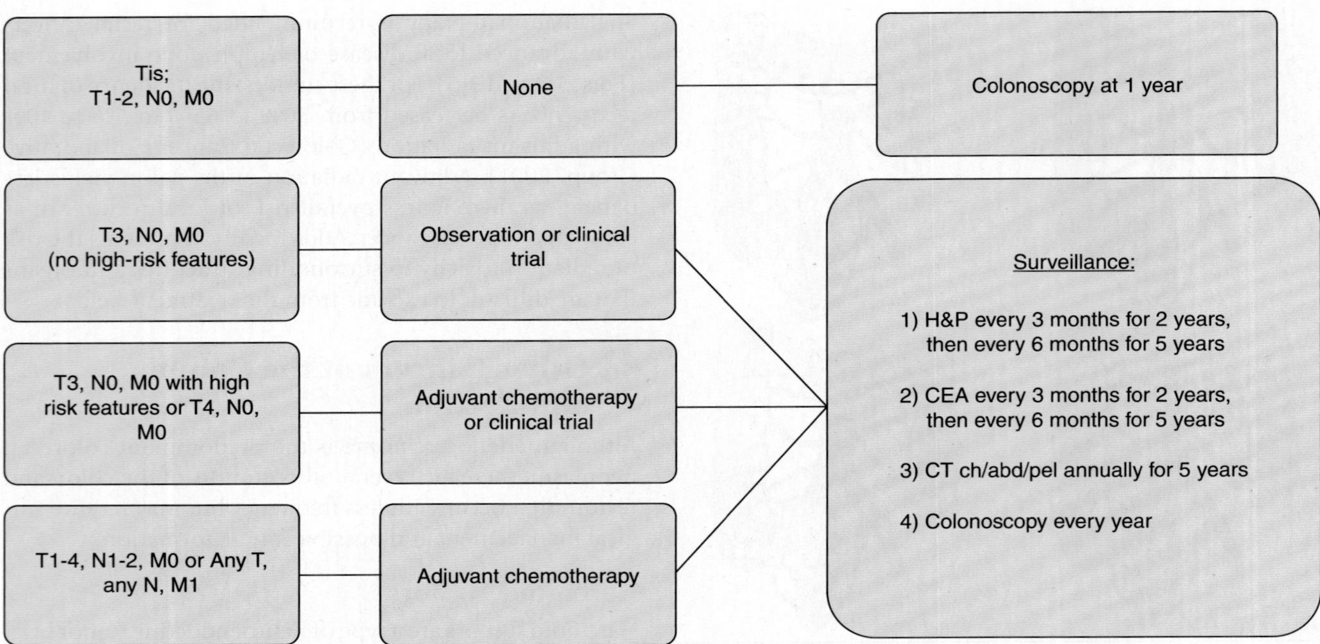

FIGURE 3-4. Adjuvant treatment algorithm for colon cancer.

Gastrointestinal Stromal Tumor

Gastrointestinal stromal tumors (GISTs) can occur anywhere in the GI tract and arise from the interstitial cells of Cajal. They are most commonly diagnosed in men in their fifth or sixth decades of life (Tryggvason et al., 2005). GISTs are slow growing and can grow to a very large size before causing symptoms. Median size at diagnosis for symptomatic patients was found to be 8.9 cm as compared to 2.7 cm in asymptomatic patients (Kingham & DeMatteo, 2009). They occur most commonly in the small intestine and may occur in the rectum, but are rarely present in the colon. These tumors spread hematogenously to the liver or peritoneum, and lymphatic spread is rare. These tumors are unfortunately not responsive to chemotherapy or radiation and are treated with surgical resection alone. A grossly negative margin of 1 cm is recommended in order to obtain a microscopically negative margin. These tumors have a high rate of local recurrence, and therefore all patients should be considered for adjuvant therapy with a tyrosine kinase inhibitor, such as imatinib or sunitinib. Recurrence is decreased for rectal GISTs with APR or LAR as compared to wide local excision (Yeh et al., 2000). If the tumor is deemed

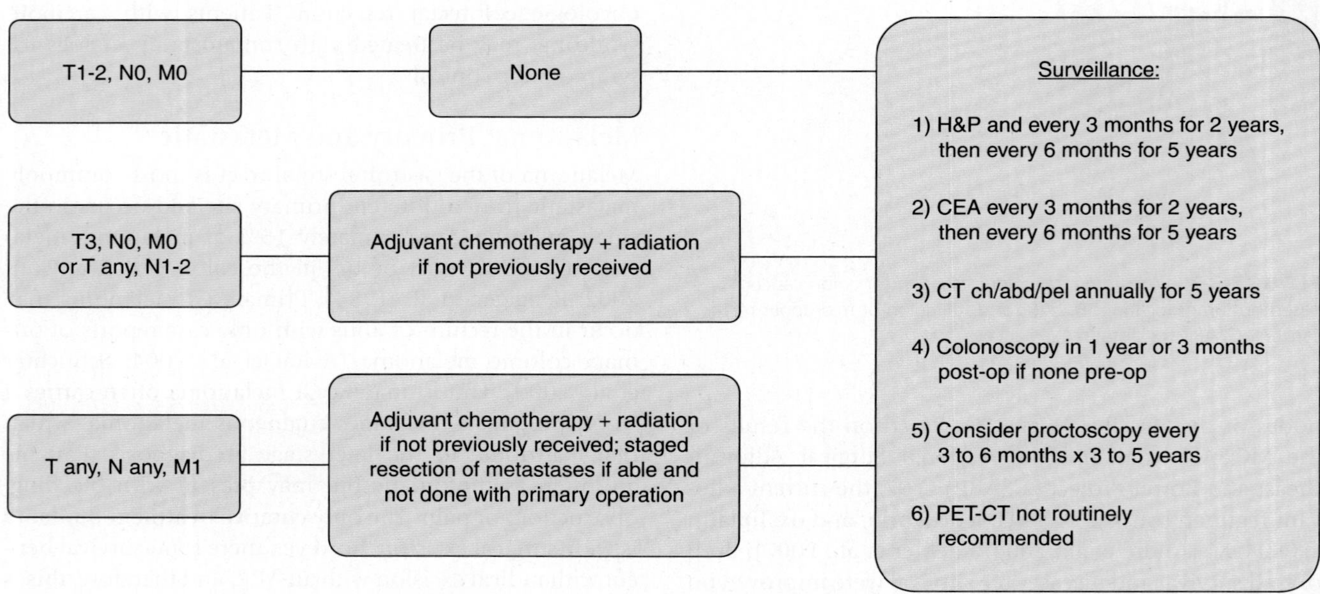

FIGURE 3-5. Adjuvant treatment algorithm for rectal cancer.

unresectable, consider neoadjuvant therapy to potentially decrease tumor burden and allow resection in the future.

Sarcoma

Sarcomas may involve the lower intestine either as a primary colorectal sarcoma or as direct extension from a surrounding sarcoma such as a retroperitoneal sarcoma. Primary colorectal sarcomas are rare and are usually of the subtype leiomyosarcoma. As with all sarcomas, tumor grade is the most significant prognostic indicator, and treatment includes radical en bloc resection of all tumor including adjacent structures if able.

Lymphoma

The gastrointestinal tract is the most common site of extranodal lymphoma with colorectal lymphoma accounting for 15% to 20% of GI lymphomas (Koch et al., 2001; Quayle & Lowney, 2006). Due to the increased concentration of lymphatic tissue, approximately 70% of colorectal lymphomas are located in the cecum and ascending colon. Patients most often present in the fifth to seventh decades of life with symptoms of abdominal pain or palpable abdominal mass. Lymphomas, including colorectal lymphoma, are generally considered to be widespread systemic processes and therefore are most often treated with radiation for locoregional control and adjuvant chemotherapy for intermediate or high-grade disease. Surgery may be considered for truly focal disease but is generally reserved for diagnostic purposes or to treat lymphoma-related complications such as perforation, bleeding, and obstruction.

Indications for Stoma Formation for Colorectal Neoplasia

Patients with colorectal tumors may require a stoma that can be categorized as permanent or temporary. Temporary stomas provide diversion of the fecal stream to either decompress proximal to an obstructing mass or protect a distal anastomosis. These are generally loop colostomies or loop ileostomies (Fig. 3-6) depending on the patient's anatomy, tumor location, and indication for diversion. Patients with obstructing CRC who are not candidates for immediate resection may benefit from a diverting stoma. This allows for continued GI function while the patient completes the workup or undergoes neoadjuvant treatment to reduce tumor burden, or for palliative intent for unresectable and/or metastatic disease.

A temporary stoma may be created at the time of surgical resection to "defunctionalize" or "protect" a distal anastomosis. Surgical management of colon and upper third rectal cancers includes resection of tumor with adequate proximal and distal margins including lymph nodes and blood supply, segmental colon resection (Fig. 3-3A), and LAR (Fig. 3-3B), respectively. Both are followed by primary anastomoses of the remaining segments. Anastomoses must be made with adequately perfused healthy tissue without tension and without evidence of leak. Loop diverting stomas may be created at this time to protect anastomoses that do not meet one or more of these criteria and are therefore at risk for future breakdown. An end ileostomy or colostomy (Fig. 3-7) may be created with temporary intent when patient-specific or tumor conditions deem it not appropriate to perform a primary anastomosis as in patients with severe comorbid conditions, sepsis, or malnutrition.

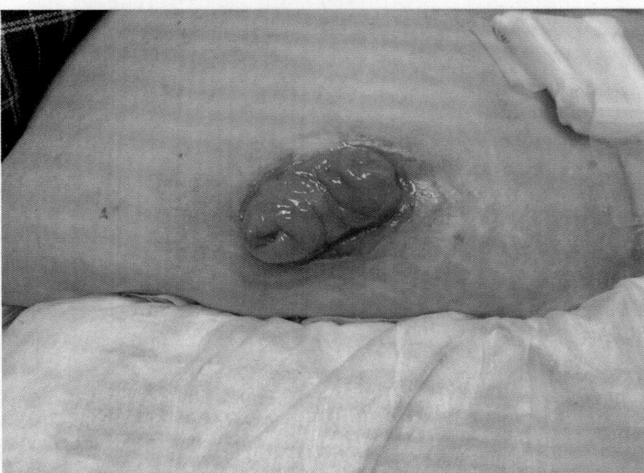

FIGURE 3-6. Diverting loop ileostomy in a patient with a distal rectal cancer and a low anastomosis.

CLINICAL PEARL

When marking a patient with colorectal cancer, consult the surgeon to determine if marking both sides of the abdomen might be prudent as the surgical procedure may depend upon intraoperative findings.

Permanent stomas generally take the form of an end colostomy or ileostomy. These may be created when reestablishment of intestinal continuity will not be achieved or when the disease process necessitates resection of the anal sphincter complex. Such operations include APR (Fig. 3-3C) and pelvic exenteration. Indications for APR

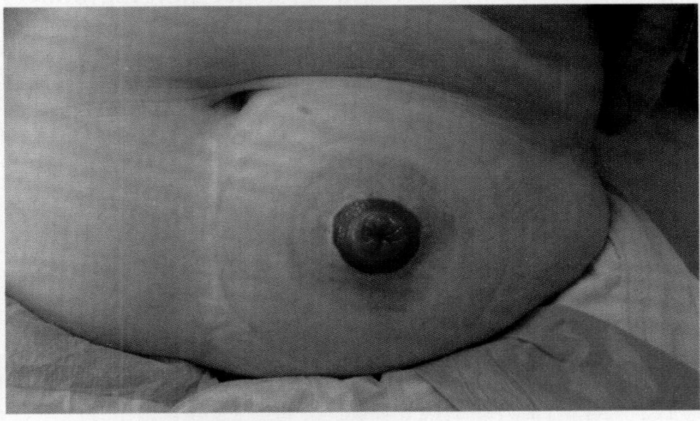

FIGURE 3-7. End colostomy after APR.

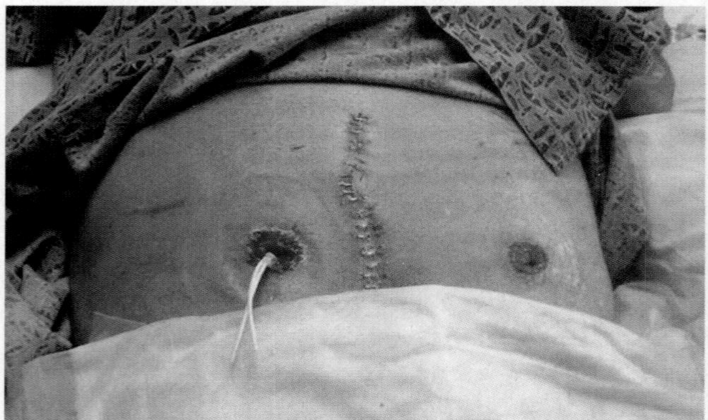

FIGURE 3-8. Urostomy **(right)** and end colostomy **(left)** in a patient with a locally advanced rectal cancer invading the bladder. (Courtesy of Mary Arnold Long, MSN,RN,CRN,CWOCN-AP, ACNS-BC.)

include cancers of the distal rectum in which distal negative margins cannot be achieved, those with direct extension into levator muscles, or patients with preoperative fecal incontinence. APR includes resection of the sigmoid colon, rectum, and anus; closure of the perineum; and creation of end colostomy. Total pelvic exenteration includes resection of other pelvic structures including the uterus, vagina, bladder, urethra, and rectum. This is indicated for rectal tumors with invasion to adjacent pelvic structures or gynecologic or urinary malignancies with involvement of the rectum. Depending on cancer location and extent of local invasion, patients may require an anterior, posterior, or total pelvic exenteration. Anterior exenteration includes only genitourinary and gynecologic structures, while posterior exenteration includes only GI and gynecologic structures. Given resection of both GI and GU structures with total pelvic exenteration, patients will have both a permanent colostomy and urostomy (**Fig. 3-8**). Both operations, APR and pelvic exenteration, are highly morbid and should be performed primarily for curative intent in patients fit to tolerate the operation as well as its possible complications.

Preoperative stoma site marking is essential for those either with a planned stoma creation or at high risk for requiring a stoma. Special attention must be taken for patients in whom an intraoperative decision will be made regarding type of stoma and for those needing both a colostomy and urostomy. This becomes more of an issue in patients who have already had a stoma reversed and now need a second diversion.

Conclusions

CRCs remain common in United States patient populations and are frequently managed with surgery as a component of a multidisciplinary approach. The majority of patients will not require fecal diversion as a part of their treatment; however, colostomies and ileostomies are often necessary for the reasons previously mentioned. Preoperative planning with site marking, patient counseling, precise operative technique, and postoperative patient follow-up and education are hallmarks of optimal outcomes.

REFERENCES

Allen, P. J., & Cott, D. G. (2002). The surgical management of metastatic melanoma. *Annals of Surgical Oncology, 9*(8), 762–770.

American Cancer Society. (2014). *Cancer facts and figures, 2014*. http://www.cancer.org/cancer/news/cancer-statistics-report-deaths-down-20-percent-in-2-decades

André, T., Boni, C., Navarro, M., et al. (2009). Improved overall survival with oxaliplatin, fluorouracil, and leucovorin as adjuvant treatment in stage II or III colon cancer in the MOSAIC trial. *Journal of Clinical Oncology, 27*, 3109–3116.

Avital, S., Romaguera, R. L., Sands, L., et al. (2004). Primary malignant melanoma of the right colon. *The American Surgeon, 70*, 649–651.

Bal, D. G. (1992). Cancer in African Americans. *CA: A Cancer Journal for Clinicians, 42*, 5–6.

Colorectal Cancer Collaborative Group. (2001). Adjuvant radiotherapy for rectal cancer: a systematic overview of 8,507 patients from 22 randomized trials. *Lancet, 358*(9290), 1291–1304.

Conlin, A., Smith, G., Carey, F. A., et al. (2005). The prognostic significance of K-ras, p53 and APC mutations in colorectal carcinoma. *Gut, 54*(9), 1283–1286.

Eaden, J. A., Abrams, K. R., & Mayberry, J. F. (2001). The risk of colorectal cancer in ulcerative colitis: a meta-analysis. *Gut, 48*(4), 526–535.

Edge, S. B., Byrd, D., Compton, C., et al. (Eds.) (2010). *AJCC cancer staging manual* (7th ed.). New York, NY: Springer.

Etzioni, D. A., Beart, R. W. Jr, Madoff, R. D., et al. (2009). Impact of the aging population on the demand for colorectal procedures. *Diseases of the Colon and Rectum, 52*, 583–590; discussion 590–591.

Hardcastle, J. D., Armitage, N. C., Chamberlain, J., et al. (1986). Fecal occult blood screening for colorectal cancer in the general population. Results of a controlled trial. *Cancer, 58*(2), 397–403.

Howlander, N., Noone, A. M., Krapcho, M., et al. (2014). SEER Cancer Statistics Review, 1975–2011, National Cancer Institute. Retrieved from: http://seer.cancer.gov/csr/1975_2011/; Accessed May 29, 2014.

Johns, L. E., & Houlston, R. S. (2001). A systematic review and meta-analysis of familial colorectal cancer risk. *The American Journal of Gastroenterology, 96*(10), 2992–3003.

Kingham, T. P., & DeMatteo, R. P. (2009). Multidisciplinary treatment of gastrointestinal stromal tumors. *Surgical Clinics of North America, 89*, 217–233.

Koch, P., del Valle, F., Berdel, W. E., et al. (2001). Primary gastrointestinal non-Hodgkin's lymphoma: I. Anatomic and histologic distribution, clinical features, and survival data of 371 patients registered in the German Multicenter Study GIT NHL 01/92. *Journal of Clinical Oncology, 19*(18), 3861–3873.

Kuebler, J. P., Wieand, H. S., O'Connell, M. J., et al. (2007). Oxaliplatin combined with weekly bolus fluorouracil and leucovorin as surgical adjuvant chemotherapy for stage II and III colon cancer: results from NSABP C-07. *Journal of Clinical Oncology, 25*, 2198–2204.

Kulke, M. H., & Mayer, R. J. (1999). Carcinoid tumours. *New England Journal of Medicine, 340*, 858–868.

National Comprehensive Cancer Network. (2014a). Clinical Practice Guidelines in Oncology: Colorectal Cancer Screening (Version 1.2014). Retrieved from: http://www.nccn.org/professionals/physician_gls/pdf/colorectal_screening.pdf, Accessed May 29, 2014.

National Comprehensive Cancer Network. (2014b). Clinical Practice Guidelines in Oncology: Colon Cancer (Version 3.2014). Retrieved from: http://www.nccn.org/professionals/physician_gls/pdf/colon.pdf; Accessed May 29, 2014.

National Comprehensive Cancer Network. (2014c). Clinical Practice Guidelines in Oncology: Rectal Cancer (Version 3.2014). Retrieved from: http://www.nccn.org/professionals/physician_gls/pdf/rectal.pdf; Accessed May 29, 2014.

National Cancer Institute. (2014). Surveillance, Epidemiology, and End Results Program; SEER Stat Fact Sheets: Colon and Rectum Cancer. Retrieved from: http://seer.cancer.gov/statfacts/html/colorect.html; Accessed May 29, 2014.

Quayle, F. J., & Lowney, J. K. (2006). Colorectal lymphoma. *Clinics in Colon and Rectal Surgery, 19*, 49–53.

Quirke, P., Dixon, M. F., Dundey, P., et al. (1986). Local recurrence of rectal adenocarcinoma due to inadequate surgical resection: histopathologic study of lateral tumor spread and surgical excision. *Lancet, 2*, 996–998.

Rengtgen, D. S., Thompson, W., Garbutt, J., et al. (1984). Radiologic, endoscopic and surgical considerations of melanoma metastatic to the GI tract. *Surgery, 95*, 635–639.

Schuchter, L. M., Green, R., & Fraker, D. (2000). Primary and metastatic diseases in malignant melanoma of the gastrointestinal tract. *Current Opinion in Oncology, 12*, 181–185.

Tryggvason, G., Gisalason, H. G., Magnusson, M. K., et al. (2005). Gastrointestinal stromal tumors in Iceland, 1990–2003: the Icelandic GIST study, a population based incidence and pathologic risk stratification study. *International Journal of Cancer, 117*, 289–293.

Umar, A., Boland, C. R., Terdiman, J. P., et al. (2004). Revised Bethesda Guidelines for hereditary nonpolyposis colorectal cancer (Lynch syndrome) and microsatellite instability. New clinical criteria for hereditary nonpolyposis colorectal cancer (HNPCC, Lynch syndrome) proposed by the International Collaborative group on HNPCC. *Journal of the National Cancer Institute, 96*(4), 261–268.

Umar, A., Boland, CR, Terdiman, J. P., et al. (2000). The effect of fecal occult-blood screening on the incidence of colorectal cancer. *New England Journal of Medicine, 343*(22), 1603–1607.

Yeh, C., Chen, H., Tang, R., et al. (2000). Surgical outcome after surgical resection of rectal leiomyosarcoma. *Diseases of the Colon and Rectum, 43*, 1517–1521.

QUESTIONS

1. Which intervention by a WOC nurse is directed at reducing a nonmodifiable risk factor for colorectal cancer development?
   A. Planning a diet for the patient that is high in fiber
   B. Instructing the patient to eat foods that are low in fat
   C. Investigating a family history of polyps
   D. Developing an exercise plan for the patient

2. The WOC nurse is providing teaching to a patient diagnosed with familial adenomatous polyposis (FAP). What information accurately describes this condition?
   A. FAP is inherited in an autosomal dominant pattern with a 100% risk of developing colon cancer by age 40 years.
   B. It is recommended that individuals with FAP undergo segmental resection rather than total colectomy or proctocolectomy for treatment.
   C. FAP is inherited by mutations in one of several mismatch repair genes leading to microsatellite instability.
   D. People with FAP are at risk for extracolonic cancers such as endometrial, ovarian, stomach, small bowel, and bladder.

3. A 55-year-old patient visits a gastroenterologist with complaints of anal bleeding upon defecation. Which test would most likely be ordered for this patient to perform diagnostic biopsies and/or therapeutic procedures?
   A. FOBT
   B. Sigmoidoscopy or colonoscopy
   C. CT colonography
   D. Virtual colonoscopy

4. Which symptom is NOT characteristic of colorectal cancer?
   A. Nonspecific abdominal pain
   B. Weight loss
   C. Fatigue
   D. Increased stool caliber

5. A patient is diagnosed with colon rectal cancer manifested by a tumor that invades to the submucosa. What stage of cancer would be documented?
   A. Stage 0
   B. Stage 1
   C. Stage II
   D. Stage III

6. A patient with a stage IVa TNM classification would need to meet which diagnostic requirement for this staging?
   A. Tumor invading surface of visceral peritoneum
   B. Metastasis to one to three regional lymph nodes
   C. Distant metastasis confined to one organ or site
   D. Distant metastases in more than one organ/site or the peritoneum

7. A patient undergoing a colonoscopy is diagnosed with nonmetastatic colon cancer that is resectable/obstructing. What is the recommended treatment for this patient?
   A. Diversion followed by colectomy with en bloc removal of lymph nodes
   B. Colectomy with en bloc removal of lymph nodes +/− diversion
   C. Adjuvant therapy alone
   D. Diversion with adjuvant therapy

8. A patient diagnosed with colon cancer is scheduled for synchronous colon cancer and lung/liver resection. For what type of cancer is this the recommended treatment?
   A. Polyp identified with invasive cancer
   B. Nonmetastatic colon cancer that is resectable/obstructing
   C. Nonmetastatic colon cancer that is resectable/unobstructing
   D. Metastatic colon cancer with resectable lung/liver metastases

9. A patient who is diagnosed with rectal cancer through an endoscopy presents with the following findings: T1, NO with favorable features. A transanal excision shows T1c/negative margins. What is the recommended treatment for this patient?
   A. Observation
   B. Chemoradiation alone
   C. Chemoradiation and resection if possible
   D. Synchronous or staged resection of rectal lesion and metastases

10. A patient is diagnosed with a very low rectal cancer. For what type of resection would the WOC nurse prepare the patient?
   A. Low anterior resection
   B. Abdominoperineal resection
   C. Segmental colectomy
   D. Total mesorectal excision

11. A 62-year-old male patient is diagnosed with a gastrointestinal stromal tumor in the small intestine. For what treatment would the WOC nurse prepare the patient?
   A. Chemotherapy
   B. Radiation
   C. Surgical resection alone
   D. Radiation and surgical resection

ANSWERS: 1.**C**, 2.**A**, 3.**B**, 4.**D**, 5.**B**, 6.**C**, 7.**A**, 8.**D**, 9.**A**, 10.**B**, 11.**C**

CHAPTER 4

Inflammatory Bowel Disease

Crohn's Disease and Ulcerative Colitis

Adam C. Stein, Russell D. Cohen, and Michele Rubin

OBJECTIVES

1. Describe medical management of inflammatory bowel disease that can lead to a fecal stoma or diversion.
2. Describe surgical management of inflammatory bowel disease that can lead to a fecal stoma or diversion.

Topic Outline

Part 1—Medical Management

- **Etiology**
- **Presentation**
  - Epidemiology
  - Overview and Differential Diagnosis
  - Ulcerative Colitis
  - Crohn's Disease
- **Medical Management**
  - Ulcerative Colitis
    - Mild to Moderate Disease
    - Moderate to Severe Disease
  - Crohn's Disease
    - Fistulizing Disease
    - Strictures
- **Extraintestinal Manifestations**
- **Diet in IBD**
- **Nutrition in IBD**
  - Protein and Caloric Malnutrition
  - Micronutrient Deficiencies
  - Wound Healing
  - Supportive Care
- **Conclusions**

Part 2—Surgical Management

- **Crohn's Disease**
  - Indications for Surgery
  - Laparoscopic Approach
  - Bowel Resection
  - Subtotal Colectomy
  - Proctocolectomy with Ileostomy
  - Potential Complications
    - Nonhealing Perineal Wound, Urinary and Sexual Function
  - Stricturoplasty
- **Ulcerative Colitis**
  - Indications for Surgery
  - Operative Management
    - Proctocolectomy with Ileostomy
    - Ileal Pouch Anal Anastomosis
    - Minimally Invasive Laparoscopic Technique
  - Management of the Patient with IPAA
    - Between Stages with a Diverting Loop Ileostomy
    - Measures to Reduce Stool Frequency and Perianal Skin Irritation with an IPAA
    - Ileal Pouch Anal Function and Expected Outcomes
    - Potential IPAA Complications
    - Pouchitis Management
  - Continent Ileostomy
    - Indications
    - Contraindications
    - Surgical Procedure
    - Complications with the Continent Ileostomy
    - Management of a Continent Ileostomy
    - Catheter Care
    - Diet
    - Stoma Care
    - Pregnancy and Childbirth
- **Conclusions**

Part 1—Medical Management

Adam C. Stein and Russell D. Cohen

Crohn's disease (CD) and ulcerative colitis (UC) are chronic inflammatory bowel diseases (IBD) characterized by relapsing and remitting inflammation in the gastrointestinal (GI) tract. Clinical presentation typically mirrors the location and severity of disease, which can range from bloody, loose stools due to rectal inflammation to obstructive-type symptoms caused by stricturing in the small bowel. The underlying etiology of these disorders remains elusive, and as such, traditional treatments such as steroids target the inflammatory cascade rather than the actual disease process. These treatments often fail to control the disease, leading to surgery and consequences of bowel resection including the chance of having a permanent ostomy. Recent advances in medical therapy, along with a paradigm shift in treatment goals, have led to glimpses of improved outcomes and potentially decreasing surgical rates (Bouguen et al., 2013; Laharie et al., 2013). This section focuses on the presentation and medical management of IBD, and the following section discusses surgical management.

Etiology

Accounts of IBD in the scientific literature date back to the 17th century, yet it was not until 1932 that a cohort of patients with "regional enteritis" was rigorously characterized and published in the medical literature, a disease later named Crohn's disease after the first author of the paper (Crohn et al., 1984). Efforts since have characterized many different clinical presentations of IBD, grouped into the two major types of IBD, CD and UC. Despite careful phenotypic characterization and rigorous scientific research, the mechanisms leading to disease onset and progression remain largely unknown.

Current leading concepts regarding the pathogenesis of both CD and UC involve a multifactorial process where genetically predisposed individuals have a dysregulated, inappropriate immune response to one or more of a variety of environmental insults, leading to bowel inflammation (Cho, 2008; Knights et al., 2013). Multiple genes have been identified in various populations with IBD; the best studied has been the Nod-2 gene, which is important in immune-mediated events, such as stimulation of the release of inflammatory cell signals (cytokines), the creation of proteins directed against microorganisms, as well as intracellular trafficking and killing of intracellular microbes (Abraham & Cho, 2006). Postulated environmental factors include but are not limited to infection, antibiotic use, tobacco use, tobacco cessation, and overall hygiene (Berg et al., 2013; Dam et al., 2013). More recently, emerging evidence suggests that environmental insults lead to alterations in the GI microbiota, which play a role in triggering or furthering this aberrant immune response (Kostic et al., 2014). As a result, virtually all of the prior and current therapies target the immune system, inflammatory cascade, and/or the microbes themselves.

Overall, however, the etiology remains a mystery. This impacts therapeutic approaches, as it is not clear what target(s) are the ultimate causes of disease in most patients. As a result, therapies to date have focused on curbing the immune system, rather than eliminating or arresting the actual cause of disease. Currently, no medical therapy has been found to be definitively disease modifying to the point of creating a reliable, long-term, disease-free state. Medications instead target the inflammatory cascade, which mechanistically is well characterized. Newer classes of drugs utilize antibodies targeted to biological targets such as proteins or cellular receptors. These have proven to be effective, yet less than half of patients achieved a disease-free state, and long-term safety and efficacy data are limited for the newest therapies (Allen & Peyrin-Biroulet, 2013).

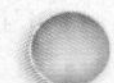

Presentation

Epidemiology

Once thought to be a disease of the "westernized" nations, IBD is now considered to be a worldwide disease, with patients increasingly diagnosed in developing countries that are becoming more industrialized (Duricova et al., 2014). This highlights the role of environmental influences on the development of IBD, including the hygiene hypothesis. Nonetheless, the highest annual incidence rates continue to be seen in Europe, North America, and Australia. The incidence is continuing to rise throughout the world, regardless of industrialization. In the United States, the incidence of UC and CD have been reported to be 8.8 and 7.9 per 100,000; the prevalence was 214 and 174 per 100,000 (figures are adjusted using data from Olmstead County, Minnesota) (Loftus et al., 2007). The highest annual incidence rates in the world have been reported for UC as 24.3 per 100,000 (Iceland) and for CD as 29.3 per 100,000 (Australia) (Duricova et al., 2014).

While patients can present at any age, both for CD and UC, the vast majority will present within the second to fourth decades of life (Duricova et al., 2014). For unknown reasons, patients with CD on average tend to be diagnosed earlier than do those with UC. A "second peak" of new UC cases in the fifth and sixth decades has been reported in many series and is attributed to individuals who have stopped smoking cigarettes (Regueiro et al., 2005). In fact, smoking seems to "protect against" developing UC; unfortunately, it is strongly linked to CD (especially aggressive disease) (Nunes et al., 2013). As these are chronic conditions that often require hospitalization and even surgery, these diseases especially at a young age can lead to significant emotional and financial burden.

CLINICAL PEARL

Smokers with Crohn's disease are more refractory to medical treatment, as are ex-smokers that develop ulcerative colitis.

Overview and Differential Diagnosis

CD and UC are chronic, relapsing, and remitting diseases, with periods of time without significant symptoms, called "remission," and times where they have symptoms of inflammation, called "active disease" or "flaring." Clinical presentations can vary widely and for the most part are dependent on the pathophysiologic inflammatory process, including the severity and histologic depth of inflammation as well as the location of disease (Table 4-1). Patients may often exhibit signs and symptoms for years prior to diagnosis; many patients ignore or overlook symptoms until they interfere with their life, or persist without resolution.

An initial step in patients who present with diarrhea, hematochezia (bloody stools), or other similar symptoms is to first rule out an infectious cause. Adequate patient history should be taken and stools tested for *Clostridium difficile*, other bacterial agents, *Giardia*, other parasites, and pathogens specific to the location or setting that the patient presents or visited.

It is important to differentiate IBD from other diseases and disorders of the GI tract. Symptoms of either UC or CD often overlap with other etiologies, including other inflammatory conditions such as celiac disease or autoimmune enteritis as well as noninflammatory or functional disorders such as irritable bowel syndrome ("IBS"). Symptoms of functional bowel disorders can be difficult to distinguish from those related to IBD, yet treatments differ substantially between the two. Additionally, functional bowel disorders are often present in patients with IBD, and distinguishing the etiology of symptoms will prevent overaggressive treatment of inflammation that may not be present.

TABLE 4-1 Distinguishing Features of Ulcerative Colitis Compared to Crohn's Disease

	Ulcerative Colitis	Crohn's Disease
Location	Colon only	Anywhere in the GI tract
Endoscopic appearance	Continuous	Patchy; skip areas
Mucosal penetration	Superficial	Full thickness
Histological inflammation	Continuous	Patchy
Granulomas	No	Yes
Extraintestinal manifestations	Yes	Yes
Fistulas	No	Yes
Perianal disease	No	Yes
Strictures	No	Yes
Smoking association	Nonsmokers or ex-smokers	Commonly smokers
Bleeding	Yes	Yes
Pain	Minimal (crampy)	Yes

Patients who are already diagnosed with IBD that subsequently present with active inflammatory symptoms should prompt workup into the trigger of their symptoms. Concurrent infection may worsen inflammation and prevent traditional treatments from optimally working. Patients should be assessed for more common enteric infections such as *Clostridium difficile* (*Cdiff*), *Giardia*, and *Cytomegalovirus* (*CMV*) and promptly treated if these are found. Many patients may flare due to noncompliance with their treatment regimens or major stressors (i.e., death, divorce, employment change, etc.).

CLINICAL PEARL

The clinical distinction between ulcerative colitis and Crohn's disease is vital, since the type of inflammatory bowel disease will direct the therapeutic approach.

Ulcerative Colitis

Inflammation in UC follows a characteristic pattern: the rectum is always involved, and it extends proximally to include part or all of the colon. Classically, the pattern of inflammation is broken down into three major categories: (1) proctitis (involving only the rectum); (2) left-sided colitis (involving the area of the colon distal to the splenic flexure, or 60 cm as measured from the anal verge on colonoscopy); and (3) extensive colitis (involving the colon proximal to the splenic flexure as well as the areas distal). Within this last category, the term "pancolitis" refers to the entire colon being involved. The additional category "proctosigmoiditis" is also used in some settings to describe disease involving the rectum and sigmoid colon (Table 4-2).

The pattern of inflammation is continuous and circumferential, which often differentiates UC from the often patchy and discontinuous inflammation seen in CD. Histologically, inflammation is limited to the superficial mucosal lining of the bowel but does not extend deeper into the submucosa, muscularis, or serosal surface of the colon (Table 4-1). Symptoms consist of frequent, bloody

TABLE 4-2 Major Classifications of Ulcerative Colitis

Disease Type	Disease Location	Distance Measured from Anal Verge
Proctitis	Rectum only	20 cm
Proctosigmoiditis	Rectum and sigmoid colon	~35–40 cm
Left-sided ulcerative colitis	From rectum extending up to the splenic flexure	60 cm
Extensive ulcerative colitis	From rectum extending beyond the splenic flexure	>60 cm
Pancolitis	Entire colon	Entire colon

stools associated with urgency to defecate, sometimes waking patients up from sleep to have a bowel movement. There may or may not be abdominal cramping, particularly around times of bowel movements. Otherwise, constant abdominal pain is not commonly seen because inflammation is limited to the mucosa lining where there is little nervous innervation. As the severity increases, patients may have fevers, night sweats, weight loss, and fatigue. Additionally, patients may have other symptoms outside of the colon; these extraintestinal manifestations include the joints (arthritis), skin (erythema nodosum, pyoderma gangrenosum), and eyes (iritis, uveitis, episcleritis).

Patients suspected of having UC typically undergo assessment of their colon via colonoscopy or flexible sigmoidoscopy. There is a characteristic inflammatory pattern on endoscopy, with inflammation starting in the rectum and extending proximally in a circumferential, continuous pattern. Inflammation may be limited to the rectum or extend the entire length of the colon. In rare cases, inflammation may continue into the last portion of the small bowel, the terminal ileum, but characteristically, the small bowel is not affected. Histologically, only the superficial layer of the colon, the mucosa, is involved.

CLINICAL PEARL

The person with ulcerative colitis will present with chronic persistent or intermittent diarrhea and/or rectal bleeding. The inflammation usually spares the small bowel, except in severe extensive disease when the terminal ileum may display inflammation called backwash ileitis.

Crohn's Disease

CD differs from UC in that inflammation may occur anywhere within the GI tract, from the mouth to the anus, and may be continuous or patchy, and symptoms are based on the area or areas of involvement. The most commonly affected area is the terminal ileum, and many of those patients have cecal and/or right colonic involvement as well. About 20% of patients have disease limited to the colon, and 5% have involvement of the mouth, esophagus, stomach, or upper small bowel. Symptoms of patients with distal colonic involvement, including the rectum and sigmoid, often include bloody, frequent stools, similar to UC. Isolated small bowel involvement usually presents as abdominal pain, loose but less frequent stools usually with minimal or no blood, and weight loss. Inflammation in the small bowel can lead to narrowing and even obstruction, and patients can present with obstructive symptoms. Upper GI involvement is variable, presenting as painful oral ulcerations, dysphagia, odynophagia, or upper abdominal pain. Regardless of location, patients may have weight loss and sometimes require parenteral nutrition (PN) depending on the severity of malnutrition and treatment plan.

CD differs also from UC in that inflammation can extend beyond the mucosal layer, penetrating deep into the submucosa, even extending the full thickness of the bowel wall. As inflammation progresses deep into the bowel, fluid collections outside of the bowel can form, known as abscesses. Additionally, inappropriate connections between the bowel and other organs, called fistulas, may form. Fistulas can occur between the bowel and adjacent organs, including other parts of the bowel, the bladder, the vagina, and the skin. When this involves the rectum or anal canal, characteristic abscess formation and even drainage can occur in the perianal area, commonly referred to as the phenotypic CD with perianal disease.

Ongoing deep bowel inflammation in CD can also lead to scar formation, causing narrowing, or stricturing, of the bowel. This mostly occurs in the small bowel. Over time, strictures can lead to blockages and surgery is required for treatment.

CD, like UC, can have extraintestinal manifestations. These are similar in nature to UC and often parallel underlying bowel inflammation. This is discussed later in the chapter.

Workup of CD should focus on characterizing the location and extent of inflammation, as well as fistulizing or perianal disease. This usually requires both endoscopic and radiologic assessments. The colon and terminal ileum are usually assessed by colonoscopy, which allows not only for assessment of disease activity but also for biopsy. The small bowel can be assessed either radiologically or endoscopically depending on the resources available. Classically, dynamic barium studies under x-ray were utilized; however, now, both computerized tomography (CT) and magnetic resonance (MR) enterography can be used to get detailed images of the small bowel and also evaluate for fistulas or perianal disease. Recent advances in endoscopy now allow imaging of the small bowel via either video capsule endoscopy (VCE) or deep enteroscopy. For VCE, the patient swallows a camera, which is the shape and size of a large pill, which takes several thousand pictures over a period of time and transmits them for viewing. A number of different techniques for deep enteroscopy allow for endoscopic assessment of the small bowel, with capability of visualization of the entire small bowel around 50% of the time. The danger of VCE in CD is capsule retention at an area of stricturing, which may require deep enteroscopy or surgery to remove.

Medical Management

Management of IBD is unique in that most patients are diagnosed at an early age and are otherwise healthy, yet despite medical therapy, many will require surgery at some point during their lifetime. Additionally, many of the medications, while for the most part are safe and well tolerated, have potential serious complications. As such, the decision regarding treatment, either medical or surgical, needs to be done in partnership with the patient.

In principle, management for all patients with IBD is based on location of inflammation as well as disease

TABLE 4-3 Medications Commonly Used in Ulcerative Colitis and Crohn's Disease

Medication Class	Ulcerative Colitis	Crohn's Disease
Aminosalicylate	Balsalazide, mesalamine, olsalazine, sulfasalazine	Balsalazide, mesalamine, olsalazine, sulfasalazine
Traditional corticosteroids	Hydrocortisone, prednisolone, prednisone	Hydrocortisone, prednisolone, prednisone
Corticosteroids with minimal systemic impact	Budesonide	Budesonide
Immunosuppressants	Azathioprine, 6-mercaptopurine, cyclosporine, tacrolimus	Azathioprine, 6-mercaptopurine, methotrexate
Anti-TNF	Adalimumab, infliximab, golimumab	Adalimumab, certolizumab, infliximab
Antiadhesion molecule	Vedolizumab	Natalizumab, vedolizumab

Anti-TNF, anti–tumor necrosis factor antibodies.

severity. The basic tenets of treatment for UC and CD are the same: get patients well ("induction") and keep them well ("maintenance"). Medications used for induction therapy often overlap with maintenance therapy, with some notable exceptions. Fortunately, the armamentarium of medical options for both UC and CD has substantially increased over the past several years (Table 4-3). Now, more than ever, patients have several reasonably effective medications to choose from. This is paramount as patients often lose response or fail to respond to medications; having alternate medications can often prevent surgery or needing to be on more toxic, induction-only medications as maintenance therapy. Additionally, based on disease severity, consideration for early, aggressive treatment that may potentially be disease modifying must be weighed against the more traditional approach of adding systemically acting medications as less potent medications fail to control inflammation.

Disease severity dictates not only treatment options but also if treatment can safely be provided at home or if hospitalization is required. This decision is primarily based on symptomatic severity, need for expedited workup, urgent surgical consultation, and ability to meet nutritional and hydration needs.

Ulcerative Colitis

Mild-to-Moderate Disease

Both induction and maintenance involve medications that act directly on the colonic mucosa with limited systemic absorption, including 5-aminosalicylicacid (5-ASA) and topical steroids such as budesonide and hydrocortisone (Marshall & Irvine, 1995; Marshall et al., 2010; Marshall et al., 2012; Ruddell et al., 1980). Systemically acting medications such as prednisone are usually not needed, but may be reserved for induction therapy only. The route of medication depends on the extent of inflammation as well as patient preference. Disease limited to the rectum responds well to topical therapy delivered per rectum, while disease extending beyond the distal sigmoid colon will respond to oral medication plus rectal topical therapy. Topical therapy includes hydrocortisone and 5-ASA and can be delivered via suppository, foam, or enema. Typically, patients with active rectal inflammation have difficulty retaining rectal therapy, so they are started on topical hydrocortisone twice a day as a fast-acting agent, with transition to 5-ASA therapy with improvement in inflammatory symptoms as well as ability to retain medication. As the extent of disease moves further into the colon, the addition of oral therapy is warranted. Oral therapy options include 5-ASA, sulfasalazine, and extended-release budesonide (Cohen et al., 2000; Travis et al., 2014). If using 5-ASA, combination of oral and topical rectal therapy is superior to oral therapy alone; however, patient preference can often dictate if rectal therapy is given (Safdi et al., 1997). Sulfasalazine, 5-ASA, and extended-release budesonide may be given as oral therapy alone.

Moderate-to-Severe Disease

With increasing disease burden, systemic therapy is required. The mainstay induction therapy is glucocorticoids, either oral or intravenous (IV); IV therapy is typically reserved for patients who are failing oral steroids or require hospitalization. Glucocorticoids have several short- and long-term side effects and should only be given for a limited period of time. As such, a treatment strategy allowing successful tapering of steroids is necessary and should be implemented as early as possible. Three non–steroid containing medical options are available as induction therapy: anti–tumor necrosis factor antibodies (anti-TNF) including infliximab, adalimumab, and golimumab; anti-integrin antibodies (vedolizumab); and the T-cell inhibitors cyclosporine and tacrolimus (Feagan et al., 2013; Lichtiger et al., 1994; Rutgeerts et al., 2005).

Anti-TNFs and vedolizumab carry the benefit of being effective for both induction and maintenance (Feagan et al., 2013; Rutgeerts et al., 2005; Sandborn et al., 2012). Cyclosporine and tacrolimus are only used as an induction agent, and a separate strategy is required for maintenance. If symptoms persist despite maximal medical therapy including steroids, or steroids are unable to be weaned, surgery should be considered. With symptomatic improvement, maintenance strategies beyond anti-TNF or vedolizumab include immunomodulators (azathioprine [AZA] and 6-mercaptopurine [6MP]) as well as 5-ASA (Miner et al., 1995; Timmer et al., 2012). Of note, immunomodulators are often added to anti-TNF or anti-integrin therapy, as evidence suggests that the combination of a monoclonal antibody and an immunomodulator is more efficacious in allowing patients to stop therapy than is either medication alone (Colombel et al., 2010).

Crohn's Disease

In general, most treatment options for CD are in line with that of UC. The role of sulfasalazine and 5-ASA is limited to mild disease. The immunomodulator methotrexate has been proven effective in CD, and it is an important part of the treatment regimen. The current anti-TNF antibodies approved by the FDA for use in CD are infliximab, adalimumab, and certolizumab. In the anti-integrin antibody category, both vedolizumab and natalizumab are effective in CD. The role of the cyclosporine and tacrolimus are less clear, as studies did not show as promising results as in UC. Due to the full-thickness and penetrating characteristics of CD, there are some other notable differences in treatment than for UC, which are discussed in detail below.

CLINICAL PEARL

Patients undergoing biologic therapy must be tested for tuberculosis because the drugs can increase the risk of reactiving TB for those who have been exposed.

Fistulizing Disease

Medical options for fistulizing disease are limited, and surgery is often required for drainage of abscesses or removal of the fistulous tract. The treatment approach is dictated by the location of the fistulas and the presence of infection. For patients with perianal disease, it is important to assess for the presence of an abscess. If there is concern for abscess, antibiotics with coverage of enteric flora (typically ciprofloxacin and metronidazole) should be initiated with surgical drainage and seton placement to prevent recurrence (Van Assche et al., 2010). Additionally, systemic anti-inflammatory medication should be initiated after active infection is treated. Thiopurines and the anti-TNFs infliximab and adalimumab have the most supporting evidence for efficacy in fistulizing disease (Van Assche et al., 2010).

For perianal fistulas without abscess, or fistulas outside the perianal area without associated infection, anti-inflammatory treatment with thiopurines or anti-TNFs should be utilized. Consideration should be placed on bowel rest with parenteral nutritional support to limit flow through the fistula. Surgical treatment should be considered if medical therapy fails or complex fistulizing disease is present.

Strictures

Prolonged inflammation can lead to scarring and over time luminal narrowing. This may lead to obstructive-type symptoms, which, depending on the location of the narrowing and grade of obstruction, can present as abdominal pain, distention, nausea, and vomiting. Treatment depends on the grade of obstruction, with complete obstruction often requiring prompt surgical resection, and lower-grade obstructions with carefully observed conservative nonoperative management in the hospital setting. There should be evaluation for an inflammatory component; inflammation in the area of a prior stricture may lead to worsening luminal narrowing causing symptoms. In this situation, treating inflammation can lead to symptomatic improvement, as can the implementation of antibiotics (classically ciprofloxacin or metronidazole) to decrease bacterial overgrowth, as well as other possible functions. Ultimately, surgery is usually needed to remove the narrowed area or areas.

Extraintestinal Manifestations

Patients with UC or CD can develop inflammatory-type involvement of areas outside of the GI tract (Vegh et al., 2014). These extraintestinal manifestations can involve a number of different areas, including joints, skin, eyes, and the liver. For the most part, these extraintestinal manifestations parallel the course of intestinal inflammation; patients with active extraintestinal manifestations are likely to also have active bowel inflammation.

For wound ostomy and continence nurses, a less common but serious extraintestinal manifestation of the skin is pyoderma gangrenosum. This is an ulcerating, inflammatory disorder of the skin, characterized by the progression of a single papule or pustule on the skin that turns into painful ulcerated, purulent wounds. It often is precipitated by mild trauma, including peristomal appliance maintenance. Peristomal pyoderma gangrenosum can be difficult to manage and requires close follow-up with the patient to ensure progress.

Once recognized, the initial treatment for peristomal pyoderma gangrenosum is a combination of wound care and medical therapy. Barrier protection as well as changing the fit of the appliance will promote healing as well as avoid further trauma to the peristomal area. Topical or systemic corticosteroids are normally used as first line to help decrease inflammation. If these measures fail to produce wound healing, the medical management is usually escalated by adding either an anti-TNF agent or a T-cell inhibitor (cyclosporine or tacrolimus) (see Chapter 15).

Diet in IBD

The link between diet and IBD remains an area of relative speculation and uncertainty. Given the increased incidence of IBD in more socioeconomically developed populations, the environment likely has some role in the pathogenesis of inflammation. Speculation exists that a more "westernized" diet influences the development of IBD, perhaps by changing the gut microbiota, or the increased fat content; however, this has yet to be fully elucidated (Wu et al., 2013).

Mixed evidence suggests that dietary modification may provide some limited benefit to symptomatic improvement, especially in CD. However, there is a paucity of evidence regarding dietary manipulation as an effective treatment of IBD. This is not surprising given both the uncertain role in the etiology of IBD and the difficulty in rigorously controlling the day-to-day food and drink consumption needed to produce scientifically sound results. There is some evidence in the pediatric population that a severely restrictive elemental diet with or without PN leads to some improvement in CD; however, this remains controversial and not universally accepted (Sigall-Boneh et al., 2014; Zachos et al., 2007). Overall, there is a lack of evidence at this time to suggest dietary modification as first-line therapy for IBD, especially in the adult population.

Nutrition in IBD

Malnutrition is common among patients with IBD, with manifestations based on severity and location of bowel inflammation. The most evident signs of malnutrition are loss of weight and muscle mass, and common symptoms include fatigue and decreased energy. Even in the absence of more obvious physical attributes of malnutrition, more subtle exam findings such as hair loss, rash, visual changes, and neuropathic-type symptoms such as numbness, tingling, and balance problems indicate the presence of micronutrient deficiencies. As such, nutritional assessments including measuring micronutrients should be performed periodically throughout the disease course, especially during periods of time with active disease. Abnormalities should be addressed promptly and interventions performed as appropriate. Specific recommendations for treatment are outside the scope of this chapter.

Protein and Caloric Malnutrition

There are a multitude of factors that lead to deficiencies in protein and calories in patients with IBD. The overall state of inflammation leads to a hypermetabolic rate, which given abdominal symptoms is nearly impossible to match via dietary intake. This caloric deficit leads to weight loss, which in turn is exacerbated by protein loss in the stool from luminal inflammation along with decreased protein intake. Prolonged inflammation leads to loss of weight and muscle mass. In the pediatric and young adult population, this can lead to major consequences with decreased growth and development, delayed puberty, and decreased peak bone mass.

Micronutrient Deficiencies

The source of most vitamins and minerals, at least in part, is dietary. Patients with IBD are at risk for deficiencies due to a multitude of potential processes, including decreased availability from poor oral intake and absorptive capacity, and losses coming from diarrhea and bleeding (Hwang et al., 2012). The specific types of deficiencies patients are at risk for depend on the nature and location of inflammation. Clinically, there are often subtle findings suggesting possible micronutrient deficiencies, with nonspecific skin changes and oral lesions that indicate a potential underlying problem (Kaminski & Drinane, 2014).

For the most part, vitamins and minerals are absorbed in the small bowel. Patients with CD who have either small bowel inflammation or small bowel resections are at risk for specific deficiencies based on involvement. At-risk patients should have levels routinely monitored and deficiencies repleted, and often taking a proactive approach of supplementation even prior to low levels is appropriate and encouraged. In CD, the most common location of inflammation and surgical resection is the terminal ileum, which is primarily responsible for vitamin B_{12} absorption.

Typically, patients at risk for vitamin B_{12} deficiency are given supplementation even prior to onset of deficiency. Aggressive repletion should be done if a deficiency is identified. Surgery to remove the terminal ileum often involves resecting the ileocecal valve and cecum. This can lead to loose stools even without inflammation due to rapid transit, bile salt wasting, or fat malabsorption. In this setting, deficiencies include fat-soluble vitamins and zinc. Repletion involves improvement in diarrhea by addressing the underlying cause and oral repletion. The use of bile acid sequestrants such as cholestyramine, colestipol, and colesevelam before meals can dramatically decrease diarrhea in many cases. Patients who have lost too much small bowel to surgery, disease, or both may end up with inadequate absorptive surface area and require PN.

While patients with UC do not have small bowel disease, they are still at risk for iron deficiency due to blood loss, and other vitamin/mineral deficiencies from decreased nutritional intake.

Wound Healing

A common belief is that malnutrition, including micronutrient deficiencies, contributes to both the potential for developing wounds and the degree and success of overall wound healing. The evidence is mixed, however. For example, trials looking at nutritional interventions in patients with pressure ulcers are split, with some showing benefit, while others showing little or no effect (Mechanick, 2004). These divergent results are likely multifactorial, including running the risk of relative undertreatment or overtreatment of nutritional deficiencies, with many micronutrients having deleterious effects on wound healing both at deficient and toxic levels. Despite the mixed evidence regarding wound healing, we recommend nutritional optimization for both prevention and promotion of wound healing as well as treatment of any other abnormal physiologic processes contributing to impaired wound healing such as elevated blood glucose levels and infection.

Supportive Care

If malnutrition is suspected, it is important that a comprehensive nutritional assessment be performed and any vitamin/mineral deficiencies be addressed. Certain situations make oral nutrition difficult or contraindicated, such as obstructive disease, fistulizing disease, or pending surgical treatment. In these situations, there should be consideration for PN (Nguyen et al., 2014).

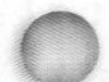 Conclusions

CD and UC are the two common categories of IBD. These chronic relapsing disorders possibly result from a misguided immune response stimulated by an environmental factor in a genetically susceptible host. Often striking the young, therapeutic approaches have centered on therapies with anti-inflammatory or immunosuppressive properties. CD can occur anywhere in the GI tract, often with skip areas, transmural inflammation, and sometimes with fistulas or other perianal disease. UC is limited to the mucosal layer of the colon, with a continuous pattern of inflammation from the rectum, extending proximally. Extraintestinal manifestations can be seen with both conditions; dietary implications are often more of an issue with CD, as the small intestine is important for maintaining proper nutritional state. Future breakthroughs in determining more predictably the epidemiology, disease course, and selection of therapeutic regimens are anticipated in the coming years.

Part 2—Surgical Management

Michele Rubin

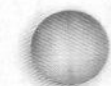 Crohn's Disease

CD is a panintestinal disease that may affect any part of the GI tract but is most often located at the terminal ileum. Although medical management is effective, surgical therapy will be required in at least one half of patients during their disease course. Operative management is reserved for patients who develop complications or have disease refractory to medical therapy and can alleviate symptoms, manage serious complications, or improve quality of life. If the disease is diagnosed and medically treated early, then the need for surgical intervention within the first 2 years of diagnosis has decreased in some settings (Nguyen et al., 2011). It remains to be seen whether more aggressive and newer medical therapies that are personalized to the individual patient will decrease the need for surgical intervention in the future (Bernstein et al., 2012). However, the need for surgery should not be perceived as a failure of medical management, rather that surgery is another treatment modality in addition to medical therapy and each is required at different times. In the surgical treatment of CD, a fecal stoma may be indicated as either a permanent or as a temporizing procedure until inflammation subsides or the healing of diseased tissue occurs.

Indications for Surgery

Because of the high rate of disease recurrence after segmental bowel resection, the guiding principle of surgical management of CD is preservation of intestinal length and function (Kornbluth et al., 1998). In some clinical settings, surgical resection may be the most efficient means to restore health and improve quality of life. Approximately 85% to 90% of patients develop disease recurrence within the first postoperative year (Rutgeerts et al., 1999). Therefore, every attempt at conserving the small bowel should be made in the surgical approach to CD. The recommended indications for surgical treatment of CD are outlined in Box 4-1.

BOX 4-1 Indications for Surgical Treatment in Crohn's Disease

- Unresponsive to medical management
- Perforation—may require diverting stoma, surgical drainage with or without resection
- Obstruction due to fibrotic stricture not amendable to medical treatments or that cannot be surveyed
- Hemorrhage that cannot or fails to be managed
- Cancer/neoplasia
- Growth retardation or extraintestinal manifestations with presence of significant growth retardation in perpetual patients despite appropriate medical treatment, presence of symptomatic dermatologic, oral, ophthalmologic, or joint disorders refractory to medical management

Laparoscopic Approach

CD is an ideal indication for the laparoscopic approach especially given the recurrent nature of the disease. The laparoscopic approach to CD has been shown to be feasible as well as safe (Liu et al., 1995; Sardini & Wexner, 1998). Studies have found that the need for conversion to an open procedure was predicted by the severity of disease; independent predictors of conversion included a history of recurrent medical episodes of CD and the presence of intra-abdominal abscesses or fistula at the time of laparoscopy (Bergamaschi et al., 2003; Maartense et al., 2006). In a long-term follow-up study, the recurrence rates in laparoscopic ileocolic resection compared favorably with those in conventional surgery (Chaudhary et al., 2011). The laparoscopic approach has been found to shorten the duration of postoperative ileus, decrease morbidity, shorten length of hospital stay, and reduce costs while decreasing the incidence of small bowel obstruction and incisional hernias due to fewer developments of adhesions and reduced incision size (Maartense et al., 2006; Tan & Tjandra, 2007; Young-Fadok et al., 2001). Patients who undergo laparoscopic abdominal surgery tend to experience a better quality of life than do those with an equivalent open approach. In addition, patients who undergo laparoscopic resection report that they are more satisfied with the physical appearance of their scars (Eshuis et al., 2008).

Bowel Resection

Resection of the diseased bowel is the most common surgical procedure performed for CD, especially ileal or ileocolonic disease. An ileocecectomy with removal of the terminal ileum and the cecum is the most common operation performed, as this is the most common site for the development of CD. Given the risk of recurrent disease after intestinal resection, surgical resection of diseased bowel should be conservative, resecting only sections causing symptomatic complications, such as obstruction, bleeding, or perforation. The two ends of bowel are brought together in a side-to-side or side-to-end anastomosis. With an ileocolonic resection, a side-to-side anastomosis is preferred by some surgeons as it is thought that the large width at the anastomosis leads to less fecal stasis, thereby impeding the development of symptomatic recurrence. A meta-analysis of eight comparative studies found that a side-to-side anastomosis was associated with fewer anastomotic leaks and postoperative complications, that is, need for a stoma, a shorter hospital stay, and lower perianastomotic recurrence rates compared with end-to-end anastomosis (Similus et al., 2007).

Decisions as to whether primary anastomosis should be performed will depend on whether the procedure is performed electively or as an emergency, the status of the patient including the nutritional status, whether the patient is on high doses of steroids and/or biologics and immunosuppressive agents, and the local condition of the bowel if obstructed or if there is presence of an abscess. The optimal procedure depends upon the extent of disease and the clinical setting.

A segmental colectomy may be adequate for isolated areas of colonic involvement, and an ileorectal anastomosis can be performed if the rectum has no disease involvement; however, one half of such cases require a subsequent proctectomy with removal of rectum and anus with an end ileostomy due to disease recurrence (Horgan & Dozois, 1999). In suboptimal conditions, it may be safest to perform a subtotal colectomy and bring out the proximal end of the bowel as an ileostomy or to perform an anastomosis and a diverting ileostomy with the plan to reanastomose the bowel at a later date. If surgery is performed in an emergency because of a free perforation, abscess, or obstruction, it may be too risky to perform an anastomosis because of the risk of developing an anastomotic leak. In this situation, the proximal end can be brought out as an ileostomy or colostomy or the anastomosis can be performed with a proximal diverting ileostomy.

Subtotal Colectomy

In patients with severe perianal disease and associated sepsis of the rectum and anus, it is recommended to initially perform a subtotal colectomy and ileostomy with a Hartmann's pouch. A Hartmann's pouch, named after the surgeon Hartmann who developed the procedure, consists of the anus and rectum that remain in place with the top of the rectum sewn closed as a defunctionalized segment. If initially a completion proctectomy is planned, a low short Hartmann's procedure is considered in the presence of severe anorectal disease and ongoing sepsis. Once the disease and sepsis subsides, the proctectomy can be performed using a perineal approach without going back through the abdomen, thereby reducing postoperative hospitalization and recovery time (Sher et al., 1992).

CLINICAL PEARL

It is important to remind patients with a Hartmann's pouch that they will have a discharge from the rectum and feel the urge to pass it like a bowel movement. This is normal, and it is a mucous discharge they pass once a day or even less frequently.

A diverting stoma is often indicated in patients who have severe perianal disease that is unresponsive to more conservative surgical therapy with drains, setons (Silastic bands placed through a fistula tract from the anus/rectum to the outside perianal skin), and medical therapy. The stoma allows the fecal stream to be diverted from the diseased portion of bowel in order to allow the perianal disease to go into remission. Placement of drains into an abscess cavity or setons into fistula tracts to decrease inflammation, in addition to a diverting stoma, is a frequently temporizing procedure to an eventual need for a permanent end stoma in perianal CD.

Often, it is not possible to take down the stoma in the future because of the risk of CD recurring once the fecal stream is returned. However, the diverting stoma often reduces the risk of perianal sepsis such that a proctectomy can be safely performed at a later time when the infection has subsided (Bauer et al., 1986). Initially, these patients may not be willing to have a permanent stoma, but may be more accepting knowing that there is a remote possibility of it being temporary (Smith et al., 2009; Thorpe et al., 2009). When severe perianal CD patients experience an improved quality of life with the diverting stoma and decreased perineal sepsis without pain, constant fistula drainage, and inability to sit or walk, many are much more accepting of having the completion of proctectomy for a permanent stoma.

Proctocolectomy with Ileostomy

Proctocolectomy with permanent end ileostomy is the procedure of choice for patients with pancolitis or extensive colorectal CD. The entire colon, rectum, and anus are removed and end ileostomy performed.

CLINICAL PEARL

An important factor in the initial acceptance of a permanent ileostomy is that the decision needs to be the patient's decision of choice and he or she needs to own it. This means the patient needs to have all the information necessary to make an informed choice and understand that a permanent ileostomy is the best option given his or her medical condition.

Often, this procedure is initially difficult for patients to accept as they do not want to wear a pouching system and have body image, quality of life, activity, relationship, and sexual concerns. However, with time, once patients begin to feel better, learn how to live with and manage the ileostomy, as well as regain an improved quality of life, most patients are very happy living with an ileostomy (Recalla et al., 2013).

It is also noted that patients with colonic CD who have had a proctocolectomy with end ileostomy have a decreased risk of a recurrence of CD in the small bowel (Leal-Valdivesio et al., 2012). However, when disease does recur, it occurs usually at the stoma site with complications of a stricture or fistulae or as a localized skin manifestation around the stoma such as pyoderma gangrenosum.

Potential Complications

Nonhealing Perineal Wound, Urinary and Sexual Function

An intersphincteric proctectomy is recommended to minimize the risk of a nonhealing wound and sexual or urinary dysfunction. The major complication, however, is the risk of a nonhealing perineal wound with a small sinus tract, which has been reported to occur in 20% of patients (Bauer et al., 1986; Leicester et al., 1984). Six months of healing time is given for the perianal wound or sinus tract to fully heal. If needed, an exam under anesthesia with curettage and debridement of the wound is performed to stimulate granulation tissue to close the wound (Bauer et al., 1986).

CLINICAL PEARL

Often, sitz baths and use of silver nitrate applied to the nonhealing tissue to stimulate tissue granulation are attempted prior to the need for additional surgery.

Patient education on the use of a pressure redistribution seat pad while sitting is important in order to decrease pressure on the perineal wound. Sitting from side to side from one buttock to the other may also help to relieve the pressure from sitting and the pulling tension put on the incisional wound. Patients need to be reminded not to use a donut cushion to sit on as it causes a pulling or spreading of the incisional wound and applies pressure on the outer buttocks, which impedes the blood flow to the area. In addition, very warm sitz baths or shower water concentrated in the perineum will help to cleanse and soothe the area as well as allow any excess serosanguinous fluid to drain so the wound can heal (Box 4-2).

The nerves related to urinary and sexual function lie close to the rectum in the pelvis, and if disturbed or irritated during the removal of the rectum, their function may be suboptimal or delayed until complete healing occurs. Pelvic nerve injury is rare but an important complication in which male patients may develop decreased erections or retrograde ejaculation. In female patients, dyspareunia (pain with intercourse) may occur due to scar tissue, which lessens over time as scar tissue softens and becomes more pliable. The ability to conceive may be compromised due to adhesions causing a blockage of the fallopian tubes (Cornish et al., 2007; Hahnloser et al., 2004; Leicester et al., 1984). Use of laparoscopic and robotic-assisted technique may cause less manipulation of tissue and scar tissue formation, decreasing the risk of nerve damage related to urinary and sexual function (Miller et al., 2012).

BOX 4-2 Perineal Wound Care

- Use a pressure redistribution pad; do not use a donut-shaped pad.
- Take warm sitz baths or concentrate the shower water daily to cleanse and soothe the wound; pat dry.
- Alternate sitting from one buttock cheek to the other to avoid pressure directly on the incision.
- Wear an anal leakage pad or butterfly pad to absorb any seepage from the wound.

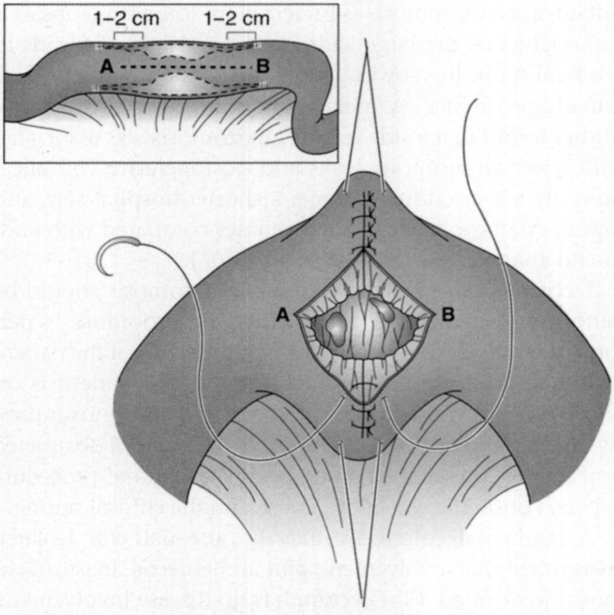

FIGURE 4-1. Heineke-Mikulicz stricturoplasty. This technique is limited to patient with short segment disease in close proximity.

Stricturoplasty

Stricturoplasty is used for the treatment of fibrotic strictures in CD. It has been used with increasing frequency, especially in patients who have multiple skip lesions or have had multiple resections in the past but should not be performed in acutely inflamed bowel. Stricturoplasty can relieve an obstruction and can be performed with or without a synchronous small bowel resection. It involves the creation of a longitudinal incision through the narrowed area while closing the incision transversely, which widens the intestinal lumen. The Heineke-Mikulicz is performed for short strictures up to 10 cm (Fig. 4-1), and the Finney stricturoplasty is performed for longer strictures up to 15 cm (Fig. 4-2). For extensive and/or strictures occurring

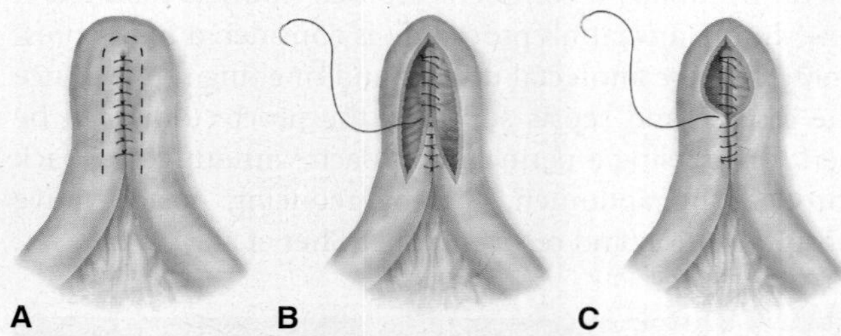

FIGURE 4-2. Finney stricturoplasty. **A.** After a row of interrupted sutures is placed between the two loops of bowel, a longitudinal enterotomy is created along the antimesenteric border of the strictured segment. **B.** The enterotomy is then closed using a running suture from the posterior wall of the stricturoplasty and then (**C**) on the anterior wall of the stricturoplasty.

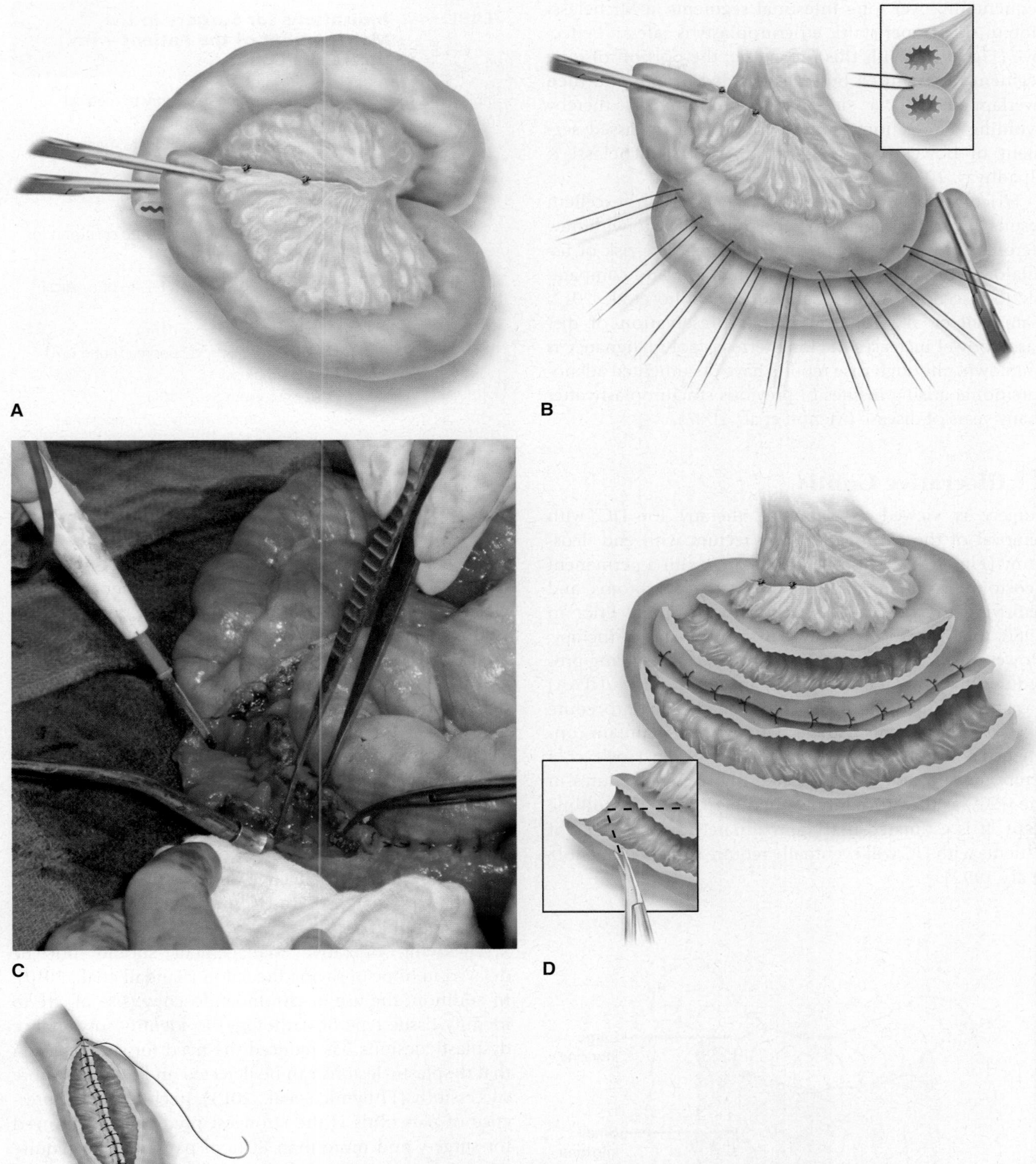

FIGURE 4-3. **A.** Michelassi stricturoplasty: the mesentery and bowel wall are transected at the midpoint. **B.** The loops of the small intestine are overlaid with dilated segments of the proximal loop aligned with stenotic segments of the distal segment. **C.** The ends of the stricturoplasty are tapered to prevent creation of the diverticula with stasis as the corners of the stricturoplasty. **D.** The inner layer is completed on the back wall and runs medially from the end of the stricturoplasty. **E.** The completed side-to-side isoperistaltic stricturoplasty.

sequentially over long intestinal segments, a Michelassi side-to-side isoperistaltic stricturoplasty is safe and effective (Fig. 4-3). With this procedure, the portion of long segment of strictured bowel is divided in half and then overlapped with a side-to-side anastomosis, thereby avoiding a resection, a blind loop, or a bypassed segment of bowel (Campbell et al., 2012; Michelassi & Upadhyay, 2004).

Stricturoplasty has been associated with excellent results, including relief of obstruction, ability to withdraw steroids, and improvement in symptoms. The risk of fistula or recurrent stricture formation is low and comparable to resection (Ambe et al., 2012; Bellolio et al., 2012; Campbell et al., 2012). Whether preservation of diseased bowel increases the long-term risk of malignancy is unknown, although case reports have documented adenocarcinoma arising in sites of previous stricturoplasty after many years of disease (Menon et al., 2007).

Ulcerative Colitis

Surgery is viewed as definitive therapy for UC with removal of the entire colon and rectum with end ileostomy (Fig. 4-4). Total proctocolectomy with a permanent ileostomy is often curative, alleviating symptoms and removing the risk of colonic adenocarcinoma. Prior to 1980, total proctocolectomy was the mainstay of therapy. However, since the late 1970s, continence-preserving procedures involving the ileal pouch anal anastomosis (IPAA) have been refined and the IPAA has become the procedure of choice for patients with UC who wish to maintain continence and not have a permanent ileostomy. However, a temporary ileostomy is indicated between procedures in the IPAA, as the procedure is often performed in multiple steps. It is estimated that approximately 20% to 30% of patients with UC will eventually require surgery (Langholz et al., 1992).

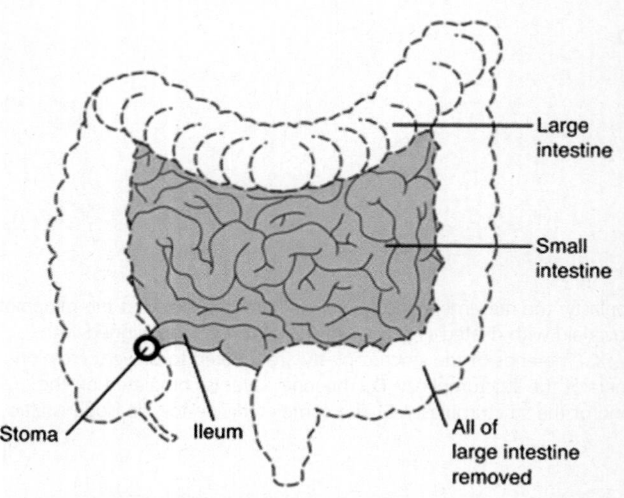

FIGURE 4-4. Proctocolectomy with end ileostomy.

TABLE 4-4 Indications for Surgery in the Management of the Patient with Ulcerative Colitis

Indications for urgent surgery	Toxic megacolon refractory to medical management Fulminant attack refractory to medical management Uncontrolled colonic bleeding Perforation (free or walled off) Obstruction and stricture with suspicion for cancer
Indications for elective surgery	Refractory disease with failure of medical management Chronic steroid dependency Dysplasia or adenocarcinoma found on screening biopsy Disease present for 7–10 y Systemic complications from medicine, particularly steroids Failure to thrive in children

Indications for Surgery

Indications for surgery in UC can be either urgent or elective (Table 4-4). Failure of medical management is the most common indication for surgery. An acute attack of UC that fails to respond to IV steroid therapy within 10 days warrants surgical intervention. Steroid dependency is a predictor for the need for surgery and is a marker for more severe disease (Becker & Stucchi, 2009). Advances in medical therapy, including the use of infliximab, have made it less likely that patients with toxic megacolon or fulminant colitis will require emergent colectomy (Cohen, 2009; Halverson & Jarnerot, 2009). However, a long duration of in-hospital medical therapy that is ineffective delays surgical therapy in patients with acute severe UC and thereby increases the risk of complications.

Lifesaving operative management should not be delayed in hope of saving the colon (Randall et al., 2010). In addition, the use of chromoendoscopy (use of dye to identify tissue type or pathology) to identify surveillance dysplastic lesions has reduced the need for surgery given that dysplastic lesions can be detected and removed more successfully (Efthymicu et al., 2013). In children, the presence of pancolitis is the strongest predictor of the need for surgery and more than 80% of patients who require surgery have total colonic involvement (Falcone et al., 2000). One major goal of management in children is the avoidance of growth retardation caused by long-term steroid use.

Operative Management

The choice of procedure is dependent on a number of factors that must be individualized to the patients' clinical

TABLE 4-5 Choice of Operations, Advantages and Disadvantages in the Management of the Patient with Ulcerative Colitis

Operation	Advantages	Disadvantages
Proctocolectomy with permanent ileostomy	Complete excision of large intestinal disease—curative One operation	Stoma Need for pouching system Risk of parastomal hernia
Ileal pouch anastomosis	**Hand-sewn Anal Anastomosis** Transanal defecation and fecal continence preserved Complete excision of large intestinal disease with decreased risk of rectal cancer—curative No permanent ileostomy	Staged multiple operations often required with ileostomy between stages Possible nighttime fecal incontinence up to around 9 mo Risk of pouchitis or other pouch complications
	Stapled Rectal Anastomosis Transanal defecation and fecal continence preserved Better nighttime fecal continence right away No permanent ileostomy Technically easier to perform	Staged multiple operations often required with ileostomy between stages Excision of large intestinal disease except 1–3 cm of rectal mucosa remains at risk for rectal cancer or cuffitis Risk of pouchitis or other pouch complications

condition. Three operative approaches in which a temporary or permanent stoma is often required are the proctocolectomy with end ileostomy, a staged restorative proctocolectomy with IPAA with an ileostomy between steps, and the proctocolectomy with continent ileostomy. These three surgical procedures can be performed either in a single stage or in multiple stages for patients with UC. Each technique can improve the quality of life and reduce the risk of colonic malignancy, and each has its own advantages and disadvantages (Hulten, 1998; McCLeod, 1999) (Table 4-5).

TABLE 4-6 Choice of Operative Procedure in the Management of the Patient with Ulcerative Colitis: Urgent versus Nonurgent

Patient Presentation	Preferred Procedure
Urgent Fulminate UC, toxic megacolon, perforation, hemorrhage, indeterminate colitis	Total abdominal colectomy, Hartmann's pouch with subsequent surgery
Nonurgent Chronic UC, nonemergent circumstances	Restorative proctocolectomy with IPAA and diverting ileostomy for patients in good health, continent, and <65 y of age Total proctocolectomy with end ileostomy or continent ileostomy in older patients or patients with poor continence
Chronic UC malignancy	Procedures same as above but oncologic considerations dictate operation selected For rectal cancers, mucosectomy is recommended with IPAA.

UC, ulcerative colitis.

Optimal surgical outcomes depend on surgical expertise, the clinical setting, and careful patient selection. The patient's age, previous intestinal or anal surgery, previous vaginal deliveries or history of anal incontinence, obesity, patient occupation, liver disease, and cancer risk should be considered. In general, the choice of operative procedure is dictated by the presentation of disease as urgent or nonurgent (Table 4-6). In the acute setting, a total abdominal colectomy is the operation of choice for management of acute fulminant UC with or without toxic megacolon or those patients who are in poor medical condition and on combination immunosuppressive therapy that includes IV or high-dose steroids, cyclosporin, and/or infliximab (Schluender et al., 2007; Selvaseker et al., 2007; Windsor et al., 2013).

Typically, in urgent clinical settings, the rectum is not removed but is managed as a mucous fistula or Hartmann's pouch and a temporary ileostomy is constructed. This approach is the safest procedure with less operative risk for the patient (Windsor et al., 2013). In the case of indeterminate colitis, when a definitive diagnosis of UC versus CD is not possible prior to surgery, an abdominal colectomy can be performed so that pathological review of the entire colectomy specimen may provide a more definitive diagnosis. Once the patient has recovered from the colectomy, the next choice of the surgical procedure can be made electively as to either an IPAA or completion proctectomy.

CLINICAL PEARL

By leaving the rectum in as a placeholder, the option remains available for the patient to later undergo an IPAA procedure or a completion proctectomy, if the patient so desires.

Proctocolectomy with Ileostomy

Proctocolectomy with ileostomy involves removing the entire colon, rectum, and anus with a permanent end ileostomy (Fig. 4-4). The procedure is curative for UC and can be performed laparoscopically as "scarless" or "incisionless" hand-assisted or robotic-assisted technique with removal of the rectum (Fichera et al., 2011; Miller et al., 2012). The indications for a total proctocolectomy with a permanent ileostomy include the following:

- Patient preference for one operation
- Medically unable to tolerate multiple operations (e.g., comorbidities, advanced age)
- Very low or ultralow rectal cancer, not amenable to sphincter-sparing procedures
- Poor anal sphincter function associated with fecal incontinence

An important factor in the acceptance of a permanent ileostomy is that the decision needs to be the patients' decision of choice and he or she needs to own it. This means the patient needs to have all the information necessary to make an informed choice and understand that a permanent stoma is the best option given his or her medical condition.

Telling a patient he or she needs a proctocolectomy with permanent ileostomy is often difficult, as most patients would prefer not to have a permanent ileostomy. The concerns are often related to body image, feeling dirty with stool in the pouching system, embarrassment related to accidental leaks of stool and smell, interpersonal relationships and their acceptance, and sexual relationships. These patients need a coordinated team approach with the gastroenterologist, surgeon, nurse, and ostomy nurse all working together to assist the patient in understanding and accepting the need for an ileostomy, its benefit to their overall health and quality of life, as well as education on stoma management and lifestyle concerns (Bass et al., 1997). Early discussions and providing the time needed for the patient and family to ask questions, express feelings, and verbalize their concerns in a supportive environment is the key to overall acceptance.

Ileal Pouch Anal Anastomosis

A restorative proctocolectomy with IPAA removes the entire colon and rectum while preserving the anal sphincter and hence normal bowel function and fecal continence (Fig. 4-5). The ileal pouch serves as an internal pelvic reservoir or "new rectum" for intestinal contents (Parks & Nicholls, 1978). Confirming a diagnosis of UC versus CD both clinically and by pathological review of tissue slides is important. The IPAA procedure is not routinely recommended in patients with CD due to the high incidence of pouch failure and pouch-related fistulas (Reese et al., 2007). However, with an indeterminate diagnosis without terminal ileal inflammation or perianal manifestations of abscess or fistulas, the IPAA may be considered but the potential risk of developing CD in the pouch needs to be clearly understood as these patients are at a higher risk.

The procedure can be performed in one, two, or three steps, with 3 months minimum between surgeries to allow the scar tissue to heal; however, most are done in two or three steps (Fig. 4-5). A one- or two-step procedure can be performed electively on a thin patient, who is not on immune suppressants, high-dose steroids, or infliximab and who has relatively quiescent disease. If at the time of surgery, the ileal pouch reaches down to the anus with minimal to no tension, the procedure can be performed without a diverting ileostomy as one step. On the other hand, if the ileal pouch reaches down to the anus with considerable tension and there is risk for an anastomotic dehiscence, then a diverting ileostomy would be required as the first step. After approximately 3 months of healing and radiologic confirmation that the pouch has healed, the diverting ileostomy can then be taken down as the second step and bowel continuity is restored.

A three-step procedure is often indicated in clinical settings such as pregnancy, acute fulminant colitis that is refractory to medical therapy, need for emergent operative management, obesity, narrow pelvis, and indeterminate colitis, or if a patient is in poor medical condition with immunosuppression and/or malnourished. These are all conditions of high risk for an ileal anal anastomotic leak and pouch failure (Pandey et al., 2011). Because of the trend toward more frequent postoperative complications associated with corticosteroids and infliximab, a three-staged procedure is typically performed (Schluender et al., 2007; Selvaseker et al., 2007; Windsor et al., 2013). A three-staged procedure (Table 4-7) consists of a total abdominal colectomy with a temporary end ileostomy and Hartmann's pouch as an initial interim first step as this allows the patient to get off all medications, recover nutritionally, and reduce the risk of infectious complications before moving forward to the second step. The second step is then removal of the rectum and formation of an ileal pouch from the distal segment of the ileum with a pouch anal anastomosis and diverting loop ileostomy. The third step is the takedown of the ileostomy, and bowel continuity is restored (Fig. 4-5).

The IPAA is performed using the stapled or hand-sewn technique (Fig. 4-6). Generally, a hand-sewn anastomosis removes all the rectal mucosa and is used in patients with biopsy-proven dysplasia or a colon cancer. A hand-sewn anastomosis may be performed to decrease the risk of dysplastic tissue developing in the retained cuff (Holder-Murray & Fichera, 2009; Remzi et al., 2003)

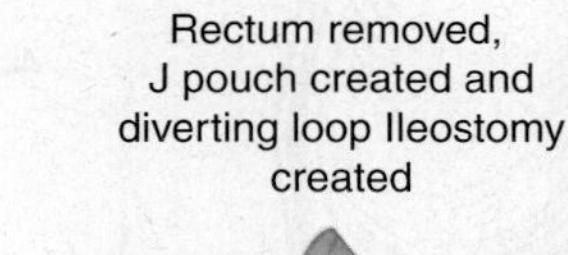

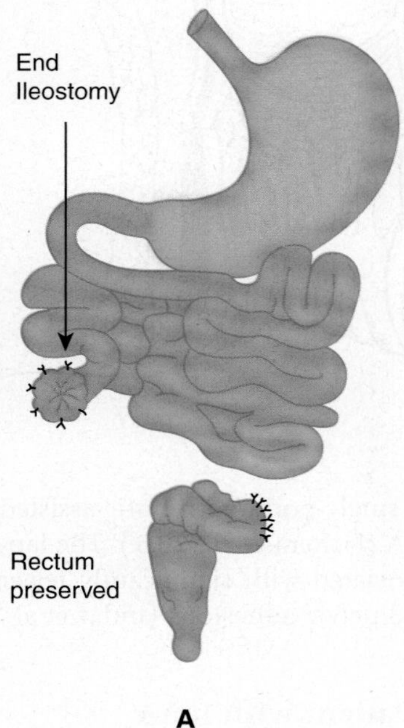

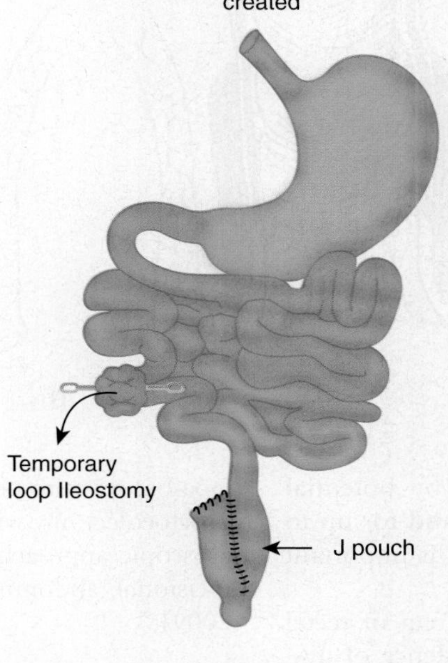

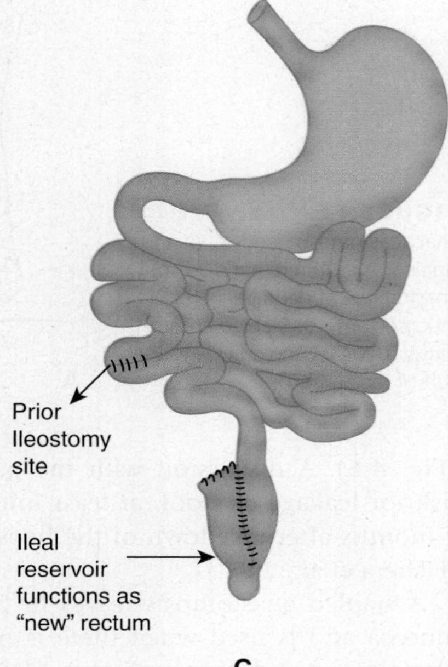

FIGURE 4-5. Ileal pouch anal anastomosis (IPAA).

TABLE 4-7 Ileal Pouch Anal Anastomosis: Three Stages with Management Considerations

Stage One	Management Considerations
Removal of the colon Creation of end ileostomy and Hartmann's pouch	The patient has end ileostomy Disease still present in retained rectum but usually goes into remission with no stool flow Expect a clear grayish mucous drainage per rectum, can be bloody while coming off anti-inflammatories Allows the patient to get off all medications Recovers nutritionally
Stage Two	**Management Considerations**
Removal of the rectum Formation of ileal pouch from distal segment of the ileum with pouch anal anastomosis Diverting loop ileostomy	Approximately 2 feet of small bowel is bypassed, and the patient can experience high stoma output and dehydration Loop stomas can be a management challenge due to lack of adequate protrusion High stoma output that is very liquid and frequent may at times pass into the blind loop and patients may report passing stool through the anus
Stage Three	**Management Considerations**
Ileostomy takedown, bowel continuity restored	Initially may have multiple loose stools Nighttime minor seepage of stool/wetness may occur initially Perianal dermatitis is common when stools are frequent, loose, or due to frequent wiping after bowel movements Annusitis (frequent bloody stools, urgency and tenesmus in the retained 1–2 cm of rectal cuff) could occur Pouchitis symptoms usually do not occur before 5–6 mo after takedown and only occur in 50% of all patients

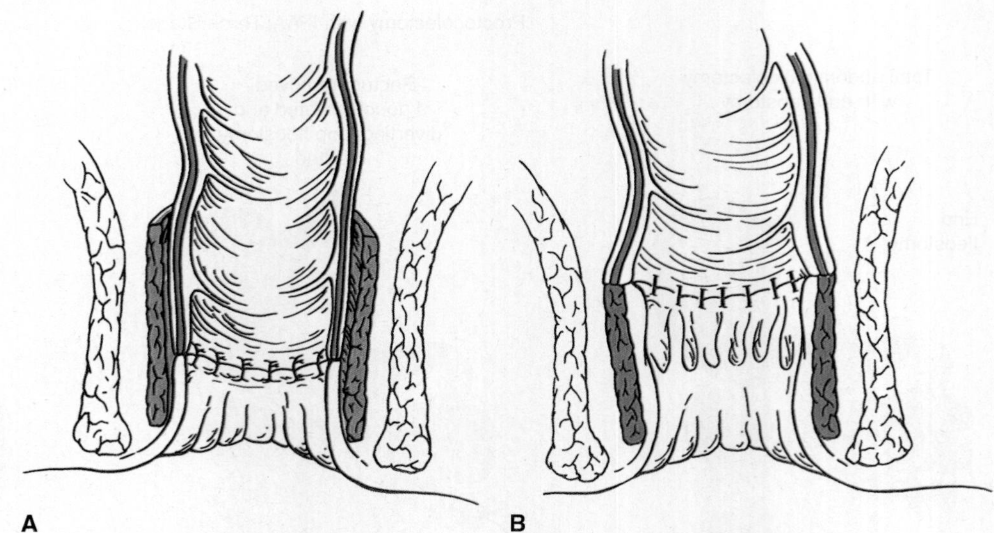

FIGURE 4-6. Ileal pouch anal anastomosis hand-sewn and stapled. **A.** Sutured (hand sewn) anastomosis at dentate line after mucosectomy. **B.** Stapled anastomosis. There is a residual 1- to 2-cm cuff of rectal mucosa.

(**Fig. 4-6**). A discussion with the patient on potential risk for leakage of stool, at least initially and for up to 9 months after takedown of the ileostomy, is important (Fichera et al., 2007).

A stapled anastomosis leaves in 2 to 3 cm of rectal mucosa and is used when there is no evidence of dysplasia or a colon cancer present. The stapled anastomosis is technically easier to perform and preserves the anal transition zone (ATZ), which is the area where the anal and rectal mucosa meet (**Fig. 4-6**). This 2 to 3 cm of ATZ is the area where sensations of passing gas or stool and the signals to the sphincter muscles to squeeze to hold stool and maintain stool continence (Fichera et al., 2007; Holder-Murray & Fichera, 2009). Dysplasia of the ATZ occurring after a stapled IPAA is infrequent and self-limiting. ATZ preservation has not led to the development of cancer with a minimum of 10 years of follow-up. There is speculation that if the patient has had UC for >10 years, the risk for developing a dysplasia or cancer may increase and long-term follow-up is recommended (Holder-Murray & Fichera, 2009).

Minimally Invasive Laparoscopic Technique

Laparoscopic-assisted restorative proctocolectomy has a positive impact on body image and cosmesis, particularly for women, and the laparoscopic approach is a safe and effective approach with short-term advantages in most clinical settings with fewer wound infections, lower rate of intra-abdominal abscesses, and shorter hospital stays (Dunkar et al., 2001; Larson et al., 2005; Polie et al., 2007). As experience with laparoscopic colorectal surgery increases, there are no absolute contraindications to laparoscopy and the decision is based upon surgeon judgment, skills, and experience. Laparoscopy can be performed electively as well as in the emergent setting of acute fulminant colitis. Technical advances have allowed skilled laparoscopists to perform single-port and robotic-assisted proctocolectomy with IPAA (Fichera et al., 2011). The laparoscopic approach is associated with significantly fewer incisional, abdominal, and pelvic adhesions (Indar et al., 2009).

Management of the Patient with IPAA

Between Stages with a Diverting Loop Ileostomy

With the formation of the ileal pouch, a loop ileostomy is created so that the final step to take down the stoma and reconnect the two ends of bowel is easily performed at the stoma site (**Fig. 4-5**). The patient with an end ileostomy that was performed in the initial step with removal of the colon and formation of Hartmann's pouch will need to be educated on the differences of an end stoma versus a temporary diverting loop stoma. It is important that he/she understands that the loop stoma will be in the same location on the abdomen as the end stoma and that it may not protrude out above the skin as the end stoma, but instead may be flush with the skin. In that setting, difficulty in managing a good seal to prevent leakage of stool may be more challenging and may require a convex system to bring out the stoma and close management surveillance by the ostomy nurse.

Dehydration is more common with a loop ileostomy than an end ileostomy. High output of 1,000 to 2,000 mL/24 hours is common with a loop ileostomy since it is more proximal in the small bowel and bypasses 20% or more of distal small bowel, which can lead to dehydration (Williams et al., 2007). Signs and symptoms of dehydration include fatigue, decreased energy, light-headedness and dizziness on standing, thirst, dark-colored urine, decrease in urination, and a high liquid ostomy output. Patients are advised to drink liquids with meals and snacks, but not on an empty stomach. Foods that will act like a sponge to soak up the liquids include starch-based products such as bread, pasta, crackers, pretzels or applesauce, and bananas.

CLINICAL PEARL

Education on the signs and symptoms of dehydration as well as measures to maintain hydration and a thickened output are key principles in patient education with a loop ileostomy (Recalla et al., 2013).

In addition, the use of antidiarrheal medications such as loperamide hydrochloride (Imodium) or diphenoxylate/atropine (Lomotil) before meals and at bedtime can thicken stool output and slow down the number of times the pouch needs to be emptied. Remind the patient to take the antidiarrheal medication on a consistent basis 30 minutes before meals and at bedtime, as needed. It is recommended to start out with one dose before breakfast and dinner and then increase doses as needed before lunch and bedtime until a thickened output is achieved at least 75% to 80% of the times the appliance is emptied in 24 hours. Maximum dosage is eight tablets of loperamide hydrochloride (Imodium) or diphenoxylate/atropine (Lomotil) per day.

CLINICAL PEARL

Patients best understand the concept of balancing liquid and solid intake by using the following example: "By eating and then drinking, the foods eaten will soak up the liquids we drink, thereby slowing down the transit time of both through our intestines so the fluids and nutrients have time to be absorbed. Drinking liquids without food often causes fluids to move rapidly through the intestines with minimal absorption, resulting in dehydration over time."

Assessing sexual and urinary function after the IPAA procedure is particularly important as most of the surgery is performed in the pelvis with removal of the rectum and placement of the ileal pouch (Zulkowski, 2012). The nerves related to urinary and sexual function may be manipulated or affected by swelling of tissues during the operation, and in males, the erections may initially be weak. The ability to urinate may also be affected where the urine stream is not as strong or difficulty in getting the urine flow started. Often, with time and healing of the pouch and pelvic tissues, these symptoms resolve (Cornish et al., 2007). If these problems continue after healing has occurred, the patient should be referred to a urologist for medical evaluation of urinary or sexual performance issues.

Measures to Reduce Stool Frequency and Perianal Skin Irritation with an IPAA

In the early postoperative phase when bowel continuity has been restored, patient's daily assessment of dietary intake, bowel function, and condition of the perianal skin is an important component to understanding and achieving successful outcomes with the ileal anal pouch (Michelassi et al., 2003; Perry-Woodford & McLaughlin, 2008). Initially, patients may experience a high number of loose bowel movements per day with some minor leaks of stool until they get into a pattern of eating foods to thicken their stool and to drink the bulk of liquids with meals.

CLINICAL PEARL

Keeping a diet and stool diary is most helpful in the beginning as patients quickly learn how dietary intake can influence their bowel function (Michelassi et al., 2003).

Use of antidiarrheal medications before meals and at bedtime and/or bulk-forming agents can be most helpful in decreasing the number of stools or leaks per day and night as well as increasing the stool consistency to pasty at least 75% to 80% per day. Patients often state that high-roughage foods such as raw vegetables or fruit, popcorn, or nuts as well as foods that are high in acid such as tomato sauce or fruit juices cause an increased number of stools and/or burning discomfort just inside the anus and near the anal opening. The burning discomfort may be due to bile salt diarrhea and can be treated with bile salt binding agents such as colestid (Colestipol) or cholestyramine (Questran) (Young & Vanderhoof, 2012). Patients either avoid these types of food or limit the frequency as to when and how often they include them in their diet. Eating a large meal late at night or after 7 PM can increase a patient's chance of having bowel movements at nighttime. One bowel movement during the night is often normal (Fichera et al., 2007; Michelassi et al., 2003).

It is important to note that most patients eventually do not avoid any foods and that each person is individually unique, and what bothers one person may not bother another. Each person needs to try food items one at a time to determine which foods increase symptoms and if symptoms are tolerable.

When a patient experiences 10 or more loose to watery stools per day, he or she is at risk for developing perianal skin irritation and breakdown and burning discomfort. Frequent wiping with toilet paper that can be rough and harsh also contributes to perianal skin irritation (Zulkowski, 2012). Use of moisturized cleansing pads as well as moisture barrier skin ointments is recommended to protect the skin, especially when stools are loose, with leakage of stool, or when experiencing an increased number of stools with frequent wiping. In addition, use of fecal incontinent pads or butterfly absorbing pads wicks away the wetness or seepage of stool to protect the skin. Moisture barrier ointments should be used when the patient is experiencing frequent, loose bowel movements or leakage of stool, as stool contains digestive enzymes that are irritating to the skin.

It is important to instruct the patient to be sure the skin is dry before applying the barrier ointment in order to not trap wetness on the skin. Skin that is exposed to continual wetness can appear denuded and has the potential for developing infections such as candidiasis (Gray, 2007; Zulkowski, 2012). Use of antifungal powder or an ointment is recommended after each bowel movement and at nighttime as needed until the rash subsides. Patients should carry wet wipes, a moisture barrier ointment, and an antifungal ointment with them whenever they have issues with bowel frequency or leaks of stool or when traveling distances from home. It is important to understand the cause of the skin irritation or breakdown of tissue such as high number of loose stools, leakage of stool, types of foods eaten which irritate, etc., so that steps can then be taken to minimize or eliminate the causes while treating the skin condition.

Ileal Pouch Anal Function and Expected Outcomes

Ileal anal pouch function continues to improve incrementally every 3 months the first year, and patients may see improvements for up to 2 years following restoration of bowel continuity. It is important to assess these patients every 3 months the first year as this is the adjustment phase in which pouch function improves as the pouch heals and the patient learns to live with an ileal pouch (Michelassi et al., 2003; Perry-Woodford & McLaughlin, 2008). The important factors to assess at each IPAA patient encounter in patients with an IPAA are outlined in Table 4-8.

TABLE 4-8 Assessment of Function in the Patient with an Ileal Anal Pouch

Bowel movements	Number per day, number during the night, percentage of consistency as watery, loose, pasty, or formed
Leakage of stool	Episodes during the day and night, actual stool or a wetness, requires wearing a pad to absorb stool day/night
Perianal skin integrity	Skin loss, erythema, denuded skin, fungal infection, etc.
Ileal anal anastomosis	Digital exam to assess patency or a stenosis, squeeze tone
Quality of life	Interferes with work, daily routines, sleep, diet, exercise, relationships, etc.
Sexual function	In women—dyspareunia, ability to reach orgasm, ability to get pregnant In men—erectile function, ability to reach orgasm, ejaculate present
Medications	Use of antidiarrheal medication, fiber preparations, and bile salt inhibitors Antibiotic use for pouchitis

Frequent assessment and monitoring the first year and then yearly thereafter unless issues arise will ensure the patient has a successful outcome and keeps the patient focused on what good functional results can be expected and measures to maintain good results. Often, these patients may revert back to losing their perspective over time if not followed, as to what good functional results are with a pouch. They forget to use stool-bulking agents or to call and speak to their health care provider as symptoms change with increased stools, perianal skin irritations, and breakdown or they develop pouchitis symptoms. Overall expected functional outcomes for patients after an IPAA are listed in Box 4-3.

Potential IPAA Complications

Complications of mechanical, inflammatory, functional, neoplastic, and metabolic conditions related to the pouch can occur postoperatively (Shen et al., 2008). Early and late complications include bowel obstruction, anastomotic dehiscence, pelvic abscess, wound infection, urinary tract infection, anastomotic stenosis requiring mechanical dilation, impotence, retrograde ejaculation, and dyspareunia (Farouk et al., 2000; Michelassi et al., 2003; Shen et al., 2008). Acute and chronic complications can lead to pouch failure such as recurrent pelvic sepsis, CD of the pouch with fistulas, chronic unrelenting pouchitis, or poor pouch function. Pelvic sepsis is a common early complication of IPAA and occurs in 6% to 16% of patients, and postoperative anastomotic leak with pelvic sepsis is associated with poor pouch function as well.

Pelvic contrast MRI or a dynamic proctography has proven to be invaluable for the diagnostic assessment of patients with clinically suspected pouch-related complications including leaks and fistulas. Pelvic sepsis

BOX 4-3 Expected Outcomes in a Patient with an Ileal Pouch anal Anastomosis

Average of 4 to 8 bowel movements per day.
70% to 80% of stools are thickened and NOT loose or watery.
At least 1 bowel movement at nighttime.
Can often delay bowel movements for a minimum of an hour or more.
No urgency to pass stool.
May or may not be able to pass gas without passing stool.
Rare blood in stool (runners may see blood when they run).
Most have no leakage of stool, but if occurs, usually at nighttime when in a deep sleep and is usually a wetness of stool.
Use perianal moisture barrier ointments as needed.
Can often eat most foods but may experience increased bowel movements with spicy, high-roughage raw fruits and vegetables, caffeine, or carbonated beverages.

is treated with antibiotics, and in some cases, a fluid collection may require drainage with interventional radiology drain placement. ATZ inflammation or cuffitis is an acute and chronic inflammation of the 1 to 2 cm of retained rectal mucosa in a stapled anastomosis (Andersson et al., 2011; Shen et al., 2008). Symptoms are severe tenesmus, urgency, bleeding, and frequent number of bowel movements with small amounts of stool. This can occur in a small number of patients and is treated with 5-ASA or steroid suppository or enema preparations. The development of dysplasia in the ATZ is infrequent and has not led to the development of cancer in a minimum of up to 10 years of follow-up. Biopsy of the ATZ is recommended every 3 to 5 years after an IPAA procedure, but if a patient experiences multiple episodes of pouchitis or ongoing inflammation, then surveillance of the pouch should occur yearly (Fichera et al., 2007; Holder-Murray & Fichera, 2009; Remzi et al., 2003).

Pouchitis Management

The most common late complication is inflammation of the ileal reservoir called pouchitis. It is an acute inflammatory process of the pouch that occurs in 25% to 40% of patients, which in a minority can become chronic (Hurst et al., 1996; Hurst et al., 1998; Pardi et al., 2009; Shen et al., 2008). Potential risk factors include extraintestinal manifestations such as primary sclerosing cholangitis, backwash ileitis, and extensive UC; use of nonsteroidal anti-inflammatory drugs (NSAIDS) over an extended period of days; as well as being a nonsmoker (Pardi et al., 2009; Shen et al., 2008). Pouchitis should be expected in any patients who experience abdominal cramps, increased stool frequency, watery diarrhea, urgency, and fatigue. Patients may or may not report blood in the stool, fever, leakage of stool, or a flare of joint or body aches. Patients commonly state "It feels like UC all over again or flu-like symptoms."

The exact cause of pouchitis is unclear, but it is often successfully treated with a 2-week course of antibiotics, particularly metrodiazole or ciprofloxin. If intolerant, other antibiotics such as augmentin, Levofloxacin, or sulfamethoxazole and trimethoprim can also be considered. Symptoms of pouchitis usually resolve within 24 to 48 hours but the patient needs to complete the 2 weeks of antibiotics. Around 30% of pouchitis patients develop a single episode, 60% develop two or more episodes, and about 10% develop chronic pouchitis (Hurst et al., 1996; Pardi et al., 2009; Shen et al., 2008). In chronic pouchitis, if the patient develops a prompt recurrence of symptoms within a week or two after stopping the antibiotic, then he or she needs to go back on a chronic antibiotic regimen and possibly a maintenance probiotic (VSL#3), which has been researched with some positive results in the treatment of pouchitis prevention. Attempts should be made to taper off the antibiotics when possible. VSL#3 is most effective in mild pouchitis symptoms but is not usually as effective for acute pouchitis and is often used as maintenance treatment (Pardi et al., 2009). Sometimes, a combination of antibiotics or cycling antibiotics may be effective when loss of response occurs.

When antibiotics are no longer effective, topical steroids, 5-ASA enemas, budesonide, and then immunomodulators may be utilized. Chronic treatment of pouchitis involves induction therapy as well as maintenance therapy, similar to the management of IBD. Chronic pouchitis may eventually turn into CD. These patients have a high risk of pouch excision. Many patients, however, are treated on the presence of clinical symptoms, but an accurate diagnosis requires endoscopic visualization of the pouch and histologic evaluation (Pardi et al., 2009; Shen et al., 2008).

IPAA may have long-term effects on female productive health. Some women experience increased dyspareunia, although the ability to experience orgasm and coital frequency remain unchanged. Female fertility and fecundity may be decreased due to pelvic adhesions, although successful pregnancies happen regularly (Cornish et al., 2007; Hahnloser et al., 2004; Pardi et al., 2009; Wax et al., 2003). It is still not clear whether use of laparoscopic and/or robotic-assisted techniques may improve these outcomes.

Pregnancy and delivery are safe in women with an IPAA. Women may experience a transient increase in stool frequency and incontinence during pregnancy as the fetus grows in size situated next to the pelvic pouch. Women should not be discouraged from childbearing because of the pouch. Whether vaginal or cesarean delivery is better for women remains controversial. The type of delivery should be influenced by obstetric considerations as well as the potential risk of sphincter injury (Cornish et al., 2007; Hahnloser et al., 2004).

Long-term functional results and quality of life with a pelvic ileal reservoir are typically superior to that of patients with a Brooke ileostomy, continent Kock ileostomy, or medically treated colitis (Andersson et al., 2011; Wasmuth et al., 2009; Pemberton et al., 1989). However, it is still unclear whether this complex procedure results in an improved quality of life because the disease was removed, or because they could control their stools. Other authors have shown that the quality of life improves no matter what procedure is performed and is due to eradication of the disease (Andersson et al., 2011; Jimmo & Hyman, 1998). In one study on ranking the impact of altered bowel emptying on quality of life and disability, the patients with pelvic pouches were found to rank altered bowel emptying as a significantly worse area than did those with stomas (O'Bichere et al., 2000). Although it is generally accepted that avoiding an abdominal stoma will improve quality of life by maintaining body image, it is unclear if the relative change in bowel emptying with a pouch causes enhanced quality of life relative to a stoma.

Continent Ileostomy

Continent ileostomy (Kock pouch) is an alternative to an end ileostomy for patients who have undergone total proctocolectomy (**Fig. 4-7**). The continent ileostomy introduced by Kock 1969a, 1969b improved patients' quality of life by eliminating the need for a protruding stoma and an external appliance (Kock 1969a, 1969b; Kock et al., 1977). Enthusiasm for the Kock pouch was initially strong but subsequently declined due to complexity of pouch construction and the valve that is associated with complications and the need for reoperation is high. In addition, Parks and Nicholls introduced an alternative in 1978, the restorative proctocolectomy or ileal–pouch–anal anastomosis (IPAA), which preserves the natural route of defecation by using the patient's own sphincters to maintain continence.

The IPAA has a relatively low reoperation rate for complications and high patient satisfaction and is thus currently the procedure of choice for most patients with UC. With the wide adoption of the procedure, the number of patients having a failed IPAA continues to increase over time, with pouch failure rates from 10% to 15% (McLaughlin et al., 2008). A continent ileostomy is currently an option for patients with a failed IPAA when repeat pelvic pouch surgery is not an option (Beart et al., 1979). In addition, the technical improvements to decrease the complication rates of a continent ileostomy in the last three decades have preserved a place for the procedure in the armamentarium of intestinal surgeons that is appropriate for some patients.

Indications

Currently, the continent ileostomy has increasingly become a rare commodity, but continues to have a role as a fallback and occasionally as the primary option for individuals who are not candidates due to poor sphincter tone, have low rectal cancer, or do not want an IPAA or in whom IPAA has failed and salvage surgery is not feasible, in a small select number of institutions (Behhrens et al., 1999; Nessar et al., 2006; Wasmuth et al., 2009). In the case of patients who have developed a septic complication leading to pelvic pouch failure due to an anastomotic leak and any abscess or fistula, the IPAA can be modified or converted for use as a continent ileostomy.

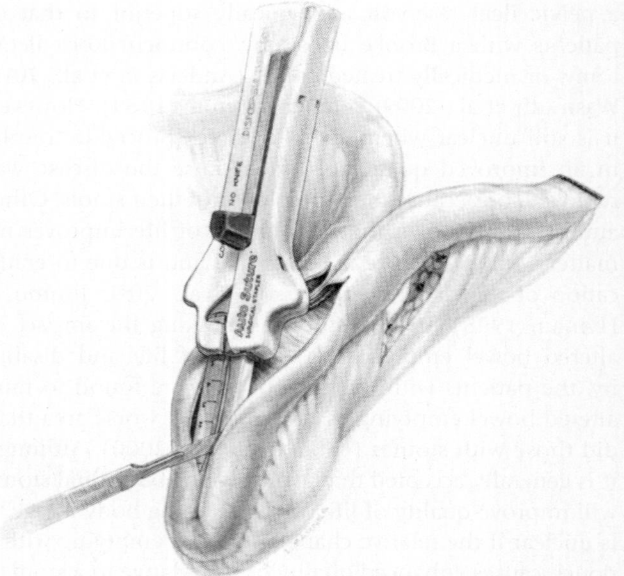

FIGURE 4-7. Continent ileostomy: Kock pouch.

Although the majority of patients with a conventional ileostomy live a near-normal life, some patients experience debilitating problems including hernia, prolapsed, fistula, recession, and leakage (Kock et al., 1977; Nessar et al., 2006). These patients are candidates for the continent ileostomy, especially if stoma revision and relocation have already failed and it is not possible to construct a pelvic reservoir. In addition, psychosocial maladjustment to an end ileostomy may also be a reason to convert to a continent ileostomy. A continent ileostomy provides little to no physiologic improvement but may significantly improve lifestyle and body image. Continence and the lack of an external appliance may enhance the individual's ability to engage in physical and social activities (Nessar et al., 2006).

Contraindications

Several IBD patients may not be considered for a continent ileostomy. Since the reservoir will not drain itself spontaneously, patients who are unlikely to master pouch intubation for mental, psychological, or physical limitations should not receive a continent ileostomy. Patients will not be eligible for the continent ileostomy if they are at risk for intestinal failure, have a diagnosis of CD of the small bowel and have a high risk for recurrence, or have inadequate small bowel such as in patients who have had an excision of a pelvic pouch, or if their body weight is excessive because excessive mesenteric fat increases the risk of valve dysfunction or slippage (Beart et al., 1979; Handelson et al., 1993; Nessar et al., 2006; Wu & Fazio, 2002).

Surgical Procedure

The continent ileostomy, or Kock pouch, first described by Nils Kock in 1969 as a high-volume, low-pressure intra-abdominal reservoir constructed from the terminal ileum using a double folding technique, was an alternative to an end ileostomy, which allowed patients to maintain continence of stool and flatus without the need for an external stoma appliance (Kock 1969a, 1969b). The original pouch had a high incidence of incontinence, and therefore, the "nipple valve," an intussuscepted segment of the efferent loop of the pouch, was introduced in 1973 and proved to be the key element in preservation of continence. The pouch consists of a reservoir made out of small bowel and a nipple segment that is created by intussuscepting the efferent 12 cm into itself, followed by the last 8 cm forming the exit conduit and ileostomy segment through the abdominal wall that is flush with the skin (**Fig. 4-7**) (Denoya et al., 2005). It is placed lower on the abdomen than the usual site for an ileostomy since it is not important to locate the stoma away from the incision or bony prominences because the use of an external appliance is not anticipated. The internal pouch is emptied by intermittent self-catheterization when increasing volume of intestinal contents causes the pouch to expand, giving the sensation of fullness to indicate it should be emptied.

Although most patients experience improved quality of life after the operation, the long-term pouch revision and excision rates are high and attributable to slippage of the nipple valve. Subsequent technical modifications included enlargement of the pouch with a third loop, use of mesh that caused fistula development, and stabilization of the nipple valve with staples or a collar segment introduced in 1979 as in the Barnett Continent Ileostomy Reservoir (BCIR) (Barnett, 1984; Denoya et al., 2005; Fazio & Tjandra, 1992; Nessar et al., 2006). Yet, the main problem has persisted, and the valve was predisposed to frequently pull apart, resulting in valve dysfunction with leakage and difficulty to intubate the pouch, stoma prolapse, or combinations thereof requiring reoperations (Fazio & Tjandra, 1992).

Nipple–valve slippage has been recognized as the major reason for operation or pouch failure in the conventional pouch technique. More recently in 2000, the T-pouch continent reservoir design with a nonintussuscepting valve was introduced. The reservoir features a serosal-lined antireflux mechanism instead of an intussuscepted valve. A recent study by Kaiser and associates in 2012 evaluating the first 10 years with 40 patients who had undergone the T-pouch continent ileostomy demonstrated that the valve was less likely to slip, but it is a very complex procedure with inherent surgical risks and requires good patient selection and meticulous surgical technique that still needs long-term results with significant numbers of patients (Kaiser, 2012). However, the study did show improved fecal control and decreased social, sexual, and work restrictions providing patients with a significant level of freedom and normality. While the nipple valve is the key to maintenance of continence, it is also the Achilles heel of the procedure because most complications are related to the valve. Currently, a continent 3-limbed S pouch, BCIR, or the T-pouch procedures are offered to patients in a select few centers as an alternative option to the permanent ileostomy (Beck, 2008; Kaiser, 2012).

Complications with the Continent Ileostomy

Similar postoperative complications that follow any intra-abdominal surgery also occur with this procedure. These include obstructions from adhesions, infections, blood clots, suture line leaks, bleeding, etc. Late complications include valve slippage, prolapsed, fistulas, volvulus, perforation hernia, valve stenosis, or pouchitis. There are very few anastomotic leaks and, with the modifications to the valve technique, very few fistulas through the nipple valve. Incontinence caused by nipple valve sliding is the major cause of failure in continent ileostomy and is the result of the unphysiologic construction of the nipple valve. Therefore, loss of continence is expected in the continent ileostomy after years of intubation. Valve slippage usually occurs in the first 3 months and is less common after 12 months. Symptoms of valve slippage are incontinence to gas or feces or difficulty in intubating the pouch. Weight gain continues to be an ongoing problem with slippage of the valve and needs to be cautioned in these patients with a continent ileostomy (Beck, 2008; Kaiser, 2012).

When a valve cannot be intubated but the pouch remains continent, the patient has a functionally complete bowel obstruction. A pediatric rigid or flexible endoscope can be inserted into the stoma and pouch; gas and pouch contents can be suctioned temporarily decompressing the functional obstruction. A catheter could also be placed to allow for continual drainage until the pouch can be revised surgically (Beck, 2008).

Fistulas and stenosis that threaten pouch function are less frequent. There is a small incidence of ileitis within the pouch (pouchitis), which varies from 10% to 30% and is manifested by an increase in volume of the effluent. The effluent becomes watery, foul smelling, and sometimes bloody. The patient may also develop abdominal pain, distension, fever, and nausea. The complication is thought to be secondary to bacterial overgrowth and is successfully treated with antibiotics (metronidazole and ciprofloxacin) or probiotics to help prevent recurrence. Continuous catheter drainage may be required to avoid stasis of effluent (Beck, 2008).

Revisions or reconstructions are frequent and expected. The revisions are usually successful, and most patients want reconstruction of the pouch to restore their function rather than a definitive conventional ileostomy. With the latest modifications in the creation of the valve, the recurrence rate has dropped from about 20% to 10% (Kaiser, 2012; Wasmuth et al., 2009).

Management of a Continent Ileostomy

Catheter Care

An indwelling Medina catheter (28 to 32 French) is placed in the pouch during surgery and left in to gravity drainage continuously for 2 weeks or more as needed for the pouch to heal (Beck, 2013). The patient should not experience pressure beneath the pouch, an absence of stool draining from the catheter, or stool leaking around the catheter. If any of these signs occur, the catheter may be kinked and need irrigation or need to be replaced. A split gauze dressing is placed around the indwelling catheter.

CLINICAL PEARL

The patient with a continent ileostomy should be taught how to gently irrigate the Medina Catheter (generally using no more than 30 ccs of fluid) to prevent an obstruction that can cause the pouch to retain stool.

It is important to avoid distension of the continent ileostomy pouch in the early postoperative period in order to avoid pressure on the suture line causing a dehiscence and leakage as well as to avoid any stress on the nipple valve resulting in slippage or a leak. The catheter will remain in place for at least 2 to 3 weeks to allow the pouch to heal and mature. After this, the catheter is removed during a postoperative visit and the patient is taught to reinsert the catheter through the stoma into the pouch through the valve. Initially, the catheter is inserted every 2 hours to drain the pouch and may be connected to gravity drainage at night until pouch capacity has increased. The catheter is inserted with decreasing frequency over the next few months as the pouch capacity increases to over 500 mL, and catheterizing will be down to between two and four times per day.

How often to drain the pouch varies from person to person and the patient learns to recognize a feeling of fullness that indicates a need for drainage. The patient is also taught on how to irrigate the pouch in case any undigested foods blocking the catheter can be removed and flushed through the catheter. If at any time the patient feels bloated or distended, he/she should drain the pouch. In addition, it is best to empty the continent ileostomy before engaging in physical activity and before bed. The stoma may be covered with a dry gauze dressing or stoma cap.

Diet

After surgery, a dietician should be consulted to give advice on eating and drinking. Immediately after the operation, the patient will start drinking sips of water and once gas and effluent passes through the catheter, the patient can begin to eat light low-fiber foods. The patient is usually instructed to add foods one at a time. High-fiber foods and those that cause gas formation are particularly likely to be problematic as the fiber may block the catheter. The patient is advised to chew his/her food very thoroughly as the waste will need to come through the drainage catheter. Foods that are best to avoid are sweet corn, mushrooms, skins and peels, nuts, etc., as these can block the catheter and make it difficult to drain. It is a good idea to drink grape or prune juice to keep the stool thin enough to drain easily. Thick secretions may be thinned by the injection of a little water into the pouch through the catheter. Eventually, patients are able to eat most foods in moderation.

Stoma Care

In the beginning, the stoma may be covered with a dry gauze dressing or stoma cap. It is important to teach the patient to recognize skin irritations as well as methods to prevent irritation of the skin around the stoma. The stoma may secrete a small amount of mucus, which helps with intubation with the catheter. The skin around the stoma should be washed with nonoily soap and water and patted dry as needed. Nonallergenic tape may be used to hold the pad in place. After healing in about 2 to 3 weeks, if there is no danger of a blow to the abdomen, a pad is often not necessary.

CLINICAL PEARL

Instruct the patient to carry at least two catheters and self-closure plastic bags with them in case they are unable to cleanse the catheter between pouch emptying, they can carry the soiled tube in the plastic bag.

Pregnancy and Childbirth

During pregnancy, it may be slightly more difficult to catheterize the continent ileostomy, especially during the third trimester, depending on the size of the baby and its position. If this happens, it may be necessary to leave the catheter in the stoma to gravity drainage during the third trimester.

Other helpful tips for patients with a continent ileostomy are outlined in Box 4-4. Patients with a continent ileostomy need yearly follow-up assessment and blood tests to assess for any nutritional deficiencies and pouch problems (Box 4-5). Patients should be strongly advised to get a Medic Alert Bracelet. This shows that the patient has a Kock pouch in case of an emergency and it should contain the following information:

- Internal pouch/continent ileostomy/Kock pouch
- Medena catheter to be inserted every 4 to 6 hours into the pouch

The continent ileostomy continues to be a useful alternative for selected patients who have undergone total proctocolectomy for whom IPAA and conventional end ileostomy are not possible or desirable. The continent ileostomy is also an alternative for patients when the IPAA fails and repeat pelvic pouch surgery is not an option. Continent ileostomy offers patients freedom from the

BOX 4-4 Helpful Tips for Patients with a Continent Ileostomy

Carry a catheter at all times.

Inspect stoma site daily for any changes. It should look shiny moist and red.

Inspect the catheter frequently to be sure drainage is flowing freely through the tube and for catheter breakdown and wear. Change the catheter every month.

Irrigate the catheter as instructed by your health care provider with 30 mL of tap water, and let it drain off if the catheter becomes clogged.

If stool becomes too thick and movement through the catheter appears slow or difficult, increase fluid intake to 10 to 12 eight-ounce glasses of fluid daily. Include water, juice, and other noncaffeinated beverages.

Do not take laxative preparations that can cause diarrhea and lead to dehydration.

Maintain a stable weight after the procedure to avoid valve slippage problems.

BOX 4-5 Follow-up Recommendations for a Patient with a Continent Ileostomy

Yearly outpatient visits with health care provider or APN-led pouch clinic
Annual blood tests
CBC
Urea and electrolytes
Liver function tests
Ferritin
Vitamin B_{12}
Folate
Iron and iron binding
Pouchoscopy with biopsy yearly or every 3 years to evaluate for inflammation or abnormalities per health care provider recommendations

need for a pouching system with continence provided by a small intestinal valve and unpleasant odors. The procedure needs to be performed by surgeons who are skilled in the procedure and is currently performed in only a few centers. The main drawback is that reoperation is still commonly required for valve-related problem.

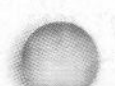

Conclusions

There are many surgical options in the management of patients with IBD. The type of surgical intervention is matched to the presenting symptoms as well as the patients' preference and overall health. It takes a coordinated team approach to help patients to understand the surgical procedure as well as the adjustments they will make following surgery to manage their disease.

REFERENCES

Abraham, C., & Cho, J. H. (2006). Functional consequences of NOD2 (CARD15) mutations. *Inflammatory Bowel Diseases, 12*, 641–650.

Allen, P. B., & Peyrin-Biroulet, L. (2013). Moving towards disease modification in inflammatory bowel disease therapy. *Current Opinion in Gastroenterology, 29*, 397–404.

Ambe, R., Campbell, L., & Cagir, B. (2012). A comprehensive review of stricturoplasty techniques in Crohn's disease: types, indications, comparisons, and safety. *Journal of Gastrointestinal Surgery, 16*, 209.

Andersson, T., Lunde, O. C., Johnson, E., et al. (2011). Long-term functional outcomes and quality of life after restorative proctocolectomy with ileo-anal anastomosis for colitis. *Colorectal Disease, 13*, 431–437.

Barnett, W. O. (1984). Modified techniques for improving the continent ileostomy. *Annals of Surgery, 50*, 66–69.

Bass, E. M., Del Pino, A., Tan, A., et al. (1997). Does preoperative stoma marking and education by the enterostomal therapist affect outcome? *Diseases of the Colon and Rectum, 40*, 440.

Bauer, J. J., Geiernt I. M., Salk, B. A., et al. (1986). Proctectomy for inflammatory bowel disease. *American Journal of Surgery, 151*, 157.

Beart, R. W., Jr., Beahrs, O. H., Kelly, K. A., et al. (1979). The continent ileostomy: A viable alternative. *Mayo Clinic Proceedings, 54*, 643–645.

Beck, D. E., (2008). Continent ileostomy: Current status. *Clinics in Colon and Rectal Surgery, 21*(1), 62–70. http://www.ncbi.nlm.nih.gov/pmc/articles/PMC2780187/

Beck, D. E.; Colorectal Health Center, WebMD updated. (2013). Continent Ileostomy; Beck, 2008, Cleveland Clinic Health Information Pack for Patients/Community, Kock Pouch Operation, Oxford Radcliff Hospital, Information for patients.

Becker, J. M., & Stucchi A. F. (2009). Treatment of choice for acute severe steroid-refractory ulcerative colitis is colectomy. *Inflammatory Bowel Diseases, 15*, 146.

Behhrens, D. T., Paris, M., & Luttrell, J. N. (1999). Conversion of failed ileal pouch-anal anastomosis to continent ileostomy. *Diseases of the Colon and Rectum, 42*, 490–495.

Bellolio, F., Cohen, Z., MacRae, H. M., et al. (2012). Stricturoplasty in selected Crohn's disease patients results in acceptable long-term outcome. *Diseases of the Colon and Rectum, 55*, 864.

Berg, A. M., Dam, A. N., & Farraye, F. A. (2013). Environmental influences on the onset and clinical course of Crohn's disease-part 2: Infections and medication use. *Gastroenterology and Hepatology (N Y), 9*, 803–810.

Bergamaschi, R., Pessaux, P., & Arnaud, J. P. (2003). Comparison of conventional and laparoscopic ileocolic resection for Crohn's disease. *Diseases of the Colon and Rectum, 46*, 1129.

Bernstein, C. N., Loftus, E. V., Jr., & Ng, S. C., et al. (2012). Hospitalizations and surgery in Crohn's disease. *Gut, 61*, 622.

Bouguen, G., Levesque, B. G., & Feagan, B. G., et al. (2013). Treat to target: A proposed new paradigm for the management of Crohn's disease. *Clinical Gastroenterology and Hepatology*, pii: S1542-3565(13)01301-3. doi: 10.1016/j.cgh.2013.09.006. [Epub ahead of print]

Campbell, L., Ambe, R., Weaver, J., et al. (2012). Comparison of conventional and nonconventional stricturoplasties in Crohn's disease: a systematic review and meta-analysis. *Diseases of the Colon and Rectum, 55*, 714.

Colorectal Health Center. (2012). Caring for a continent ileostomy or K-pouch. http://www.webmd.com/colorectal-cancer/guide/caring-continent-ileostomy

Chaudhary, B., Glancy, D., & Dixon, A. R. (2011). Laparoscopic surgery for recurrent ileocolic Crohn's disease is as safe and effective as primary resection. *Colorectal Disease, 13*, 1413.

Cho, J. H. (2008). The genetics and immunopathogenesis of inflammatory bowel disease. *Nature Reviews Immunology, 8*, 458–466.

Cohen, R. D. (2009). How should we treat severe acute steroid-refractory ulcerative colitis? *Inflammatory Bowel Diseases, 15*, 150.

Cohen, R. D., Woseth, D. M., & Thisted, R. A., et al. (2000). A meta-analysis and overview of the literature on treatment options for left-sided ulcerative colitis and ulcerative proctitis. *American Journal of Gastroenterology, 95*, 1263–1276.

Colombel, J. F., Sandborn, W. J., Reinisch, W., et al. (2010). Infliximab, azathioprine, or combination therapy for Crohn's disease. *New England Journal of Medicine, 362*, 1383–1395.

Cornish, J. A., Tan, E., Teare, J., et al. (2007). The effect of restorative proctocolectomy on sexual function, urinary function, fertility, pregnancy and delivery: a systematic review. *Diseases of the Colon and Rectum, 50*, 1128.

Crohn, B. B., Ginzburg, L., & Oppenheimer, G. D. (1984). Landmark article Oct 15, 1932. Regional ileitis. A pathological and clinical entity. By Burril B. Crohn, Leon Ginzburg, and Gordon D. Oppenheimer. *JAMA, 251*, 73–79.

Dam, A. N., Berg, A. M., & Farraye, F. A. (2013). Environmental influences on the onset and clinical course of Crohn's disease-part 1: An overview of external risk factors. *Gastroenterology and Hepatology (N Y), 9*, 711–717.

Denoya, P., Schuender, S., & Bub, D. (2005). Delayed Kock pouch nipple valve failure: Is revision indicated? *Diseases of Colon and Rectum, 51*, 1544–1547.

Dunkar, M. S., Bemelman, W. A., Slors, J. F., et al. (2001). Functional outcome, quality of life, body image, and cosmesis in patients after laparoscopic assisted and conventional restorative proctocolectomy: A comparative study. *Diseases of the Colon and Rectum, 44*, 1800.

Duricova, D., Burisch, J., Jess, T., et al. (2014). Age-related differences in presentation and course of inflammatory bowel disease: An update on the population-based literature. *Journal of Crohn's and Colitis, 8,* 1351–1361.

Dykes, S. L. Ostomies and stomal therapy. American Society of Colon and Rectal Surgeons (ASCRS). http://www.uptodate.com/contents/surgical-principles-of-ostomy-construction

Efthymicu, M., Allen, P. B., & Taylor, A. C., et al. (2013). Chromoendoscopy versus narrow band imaging for colonic surveillance in inflammatory bowel disease. *Inflammatory Bowel Diseases, 19,* 2132.

Eshuis, E. J., Polle, S. W., Slors, J. F., et al. (2008). Long-term surgical recurrence, morbidity, quality of life, and body image of laparoscopic-assisted vs. open ileocolic resection for Crohn's disease: A comparative study. *Diseases of Colon and Rectum, 51*(6), 858–867.

Falcone, R. A., Jr., Lewis, L. G., & Warner, B. W. (2000). Predicting the need for colectomy in pediatric patients with ulcerative colitis. *Journal of Gastrointestinal Surgery, 4*(2), 201–206.

Farouk, R., Pemberton, J. H., Wolff, B. G., et al. (2000). Functional outcomes after ileal pouch-anal anastomosis for chronic ulcerative colitis. *Annals of Surgery, 231,* 919.

Fazio, V. W., & Tjandra, J. J. (1992). Techniques for nipple valve fixation to prevent valve slippage in continent ileostomy. *Diseases of the Colon and Rectum, 35,* 1177–1179.

Feagan, B. G., Rutgeerts, P., Sands, B. E., et al. (2013). Vedolizumab as induction and maintenance therapy for ulcerative colitis. *New England Journal of Medicine, 369,* 699–710.

Fichera, A., Ragauskaite, L., Silvestri, M. T., et al. (2007). Preservation of the anal transition zone in ulcerative colitis. Long-term effects on defecatory function. *Journal of Gastrointestinal Surgery, 11,* 1647.

Fichera, A., Zoccali, M., & Gullo, R. (2011). Single incision ("scarless") laparoscopic total abdominal colectomy with end ileostomy for ulcerative colitis. *Journal of Gastrointestinal Surgery, 15,* 1247–1251.

Gray, M. (2007). Incontinence-related skin damage: Essential knowledge. *Ostomy Wound Management, 53,* 28–32.

Hahnloser, D., Pemberton, J. H., Wolff, B. G., et al. (2004). Pregnancy and delivery before and after ileal pouch-anal anastomosis for ulcerative colitis: Immediate and long-term consequences and outcomes. *Diseases of the Colon and Rectum, 47,* 1127.

Halverson, J., & Jarnerot, G. (2009). Treatment of choice for acute severe steroid-refractory ulcerative colitis is remicade. *Inflammatory Bowel Diseases, 15,* 143.

Handelson, J. C., Gottlieb, L. M., & Hamilton, S. R. (1993). Crohn's disease as a contraindication to Kock pouch. *Diseases of the Colon and Rectum, 35,* 840–843.

Holder-Murray, J., & Fichera, A. (2009). Anal transition zone in the surgical management of ulcerative colitis. *World Journal of Gastroenterology,* 15, 769.

Horgan, A. F., & Dozois, R. R. (1999). Management of colonic Crohn's disease. *Problems in General Surgery, 16,* 68.

Hull, T. L., Joyce, M. R., Geisler, D. P., et al. (2010). Adhesions after laparoscopic and open ileal pouch-anal anastomosis Surgery for ulcerative colitis. *British Journal of Surgery, 99,* 270.

Hulten, L. (1998). Proctocolectomy and ileostomy to pouch surgery for ulcerative colitis. *World Journal of Surgery, 22,* 335.

Hurst, R., Chung, T. P., Rubin, M., et al. (1998). The implications of acute pouchitis on the long term functional results after restorative proctocolectomy. *Inflammatory Bowel Diseases, 4,* 280.

Hurst, R. D., Molinari, M., Chung, T. P., et al. (1996). Prospective study of the incidence, timing and treatment of pouchitis in 104 consecutive patients after restorative proctocolectomy. *Archives of Surgery, 131,* 497.

Hwang, C., Ross, V., & Mahadevan, U. (2012). Micronutrient deficiencies in inflammatory bowel disease: From A to zinc. *Inflammatory Bowel Diseases, 18,* 1961–1981.

Indar, A. A., Efron, J. E., & Young-Fedorak, T. M. (2009). Laparoscopic ileal pouch-anal anastomosis reduces abdominal and pelvic adhesions. *Surgical Endoscopy, 23,* 174.

Jimmo, B., & Hyman, N. H. (1998). Is ileal pouch-anal anastomosis really the procedure of choice for patients with ulcerative colitis? *Diseases of the Colon and Rectum, 41,* 41–45.

Kaiser, A. (2012). T-Pouch: Results of the first year with a nonintussuscepting continent ileostomy. *Diseases of the Colon and Rectum, 55*(2), 155–167.

Kaminski, M. V., Jr., & Drinane, J. J. (2014). Learning the oral and cutaneous signs of micronutrient deficiencies. *Journal of Wound, Ostomy, and Continence Nursing, 41,* 127–135; quiz E1–2.

Knights, D., Lassen, K. G., & Xavier, R. J. (2013). Advances in inflammatory bowel disease pathogenesis: Linking host genetics and the microbiome. *Gut, 62,* 1505–1510.

Kock, N. G. (1969a). Intra-abdominal "reservoir" in patients with permanent ileostomy. Preliminary observations on a procedure resulting in fecal "continence" in five ileostomy patients. *Archives of Surgery, 14,* 1–52.

Kock, N. G. (1969b). Intraabdominal "reservoir" in patients with permanent ileostomy. Preliminary observation on a procedure resulting in fecal continence in 5 ileostomy patients. *Archives of Surgery, 99,* 223–231.

Kock, N. G., Darle, N., Hulten, L., et al. (1977). Ileostomy. *Current Problems in Surgery, 14,* 1–52.

Kock pouch operation, information for patients (2013). Colorectal Surgery, Oxford Radcliff Hospitals, Oxford, UK. (Reprint Reviewed 2013). www.uptodate.com

Kornbluth, A., Sachar, D. B., & Salomon, P. (1998). Crohn's disease. In M. Feldman, B. F. Scharschmidt, & M. H. Sleisenger (Eds.), *Sleisenger & Fordtran's Gastrointestinal and liver disease: Pathophysiology, diagnosis, and management. Vol 2.* (6th ed., pp. 1708–1734). Philadelphia, PA: WB Saunders Co.

Kostic, A. D., Xavier, R. J., & Gevers, D. (2014). The microbiome in inflammatory bowel disease: Current status and the future ahead. *Gastroenterology, 146,* 1489–1499.

Laharie, D., Filippi, J., Roblin, X., et al. (2013). Impact of mucosal healing on long-term outcomes in ulcerative colitis treated with infliximab: A multicenter experience. *Alimentary Pharmacology and Therapeutics, 37,* 998–1004.

Langholz, E., Munkholm, P., Davidsen, M., et al. (1992). Colorectal cancer risk and mortality in patients with ulcerative colitis. *Gastroenterology, 103,* 1444.

Larson, D. W., Dozois, E. J., Piotrowicz, K., et al. (2005). Laparoscopic-assisted vs open ileal pouch-anal anastomosis: Functional outcomes in a case-matched series. *Diseases of the Colon and Rectum, 48,* 1845.

Leal-Valdivesio, C., Marin, I., Manosa, M., et al. (2012). Should we monitor Crohn's disease patients for postoperative recurrence after permanent ileostomy? *Inflammatory Bowel Diseases, 18,* E196.

Leicester, R. J., Ritchie, J. K., Wadsworth, J., et al. (1984). Sexual function and perineal wound healing after intersphincteric excision of the rectum for inflammatory bowel disease. *Diseases of the Colon and Rectum, 27,* 244.

Lichtiger, S., Present, D. H., Kornbluth, A., et al. (1994). Cyclosporine in severe ulcerative colitis refractory to steroid therapy. *New England Journal of Medicine, 330,* 1841–1845.

Liu, C. D., Rolandelli, R., Ashley, S. W., et al. (1995). Laparoscopic surgery for inflammatory bowel disease. *American Surgeon, 61*(12), 1054–1056.

Loftus, C. G., Loftus, E. V., Jr., Harmsen, W. S., et al. (2007). Update on the incidence and prevalence of Crohn's disease and ulcerative colitis in Olmsted County, Minnesota, 1940–2000. *Inflammatory Bowel Diseases, 13,* 254–261.

Maartense, S., Dunkar, M. S., Slors, J. F., et al. (2006). Laparoscopic-assisted versus open ileocolic resection for Crohn's disease: A randomized trial. *Annals of Surgery, 243,* 143.

Marshall, J. K., & Irvine, E. J. (1995). Rectal aminosalicylate therapy for distal ulcerative colitis: A meta-analysis. *Alimentary Pharmacology and Therapeutics, 9*, 293–300.

Marshall, J. K., Thabane, M., Steinhart, A. H., et al. (2010). Rectal 5-aminosalicylic acid for induction of remission in ulcerative colitis. *Cochrane Database of Systematic Reviews, 20*, CD004115.

Marshall, J. K., Thabane, M., Steinhart, A. H., et al. (2012). Rectal 5-aminosalicylic acid for maintenance of remission in ulcerative colitis. *Cochrane Database of Systematic Reviews, 11*, CD004118.

McCLeod, R. S. (1999). Quality of life after surgery for ulcerative colitis. *Problems in General Surgery, 16*, 158.

McLaughlin, S. D., Clark, S. K., Tekkis, P. P., et al. (2008). Review article: Restorative proctocolectomy, indications, management of complications and follow-up: A guide for gastroenterologists. *Alimentary Pharmacology and Therapeutics, 27*, 10.

Mechanick, J. I. (2004). Practical aspects of nutritional support for wound-healing patients. *American Journal of Surgery, 188*, 52–56.

Menon, A. M., Mirza, A. H., Moolla, S., et al. (2007). Adenocarcinoma of the small bowel arising from a previous stricturoplasty for Crohn's disease report of a case. *Diseases of the Colon and Rectum, 50*, 257.

Michelassi, F., Lee, J., Rubin, M., et al. (2003). Long-term functional results after ileal pouch-anal restorative proctocolectomy for ulcerative colitis: A prospective observational study. *Annals of Surgery, 238*, 433.

Michelassi, F., & Upadhyay, G. A. (2004). Side-to-side isoperistaltic stricturoplasty in the treatment of extensive Crohn's disease. *Journal of Surgical Research, 117*, 71.

Miller, A., Berian, J., Rubin, M., et al. (2012). Robotic-assisted proctectomy for inflammatory bowel disease: A case-matched comparison of laparoscopic and robotic technique. *Journal of Gastrointestinal Surgery: Official Journal of the Society for Surgery of the Alimentary Tract, 16*(3), 587–594, doi: 10.1007/s11605-011-1692-6. [Epub Oct 1, 2011.]

Miner, P., Hanauer, S., Robinson, M., et al. (1995). Safety and efficacy of controlled-release mesalamine for maintenance of remission in ulcerative colitis. Pentasa UC Maintenance Study Group. *Digestive Diseases and Sciences, 40*, 296–304.

Nessar, G., Fazio, W., Tekkis, P., et al. (2006). Long-term outcome and quality of life after continent ileostomy. *Diseases of the Colon and Rectum, 49*, 336–344.

Nguyen, D. L., Parekh, N., Bechtold, M. L., et al. (2014). National trends and in-hospital outcomes of adult patients with inflammatory bowel disease receiving parenteral nutrition support. *Journal of Parenteral Enteral and Nutrition*.

Nguyen, G. C., Nugent, Z., Shaw, S., et al. (2011). Outcomes of patients with Crohn's disease improved from 1988 to 2008 and were associated with increased specialist care. *Gastroenterology, 141*, 90.

Nunes, T., Etchevers, M. J., Domenech, E., et al. (2013). Smoking does influence disease behaviour and impacts the need for therapy in Crohn's disease in the biologic era. *Alimentary Pharmacology and Therapeutics, 38*, 752–760.

O'Bichere, A, Wilkinson, K., Rumbles, S., et al. (2000). Functional outcomes after restorative panproctocolectomy for ulcerative colitis decreases an otherwise enhanced quality of life. *British Journal of Surgery, 87*, 802–807.

Pandey, S., Luther, G., Umanskiy, K., et al. (2011). Minimally invasive pouch surgery for Ulcerative Colitis: Is there a benefit in staging? *Diseases of the Colon and Rectum, 54*, 306–310.

Pardi, D. S., D'Haens, G., Shen, B., et al. (2009). Clinical guidelines for the management of pouchitis. *Inflammatory Bowel Diseases, 15*(9), 1424–1431.

Parks, A. J., & Nicholls, R. J. (1978). Proctocolectomy without ileostomy for ulcerative colitis. *BMJ, 2*, 85–88.

Pemberton, J. H., Phillip, S. F., Ready, R. R., et al. (1989). Quality of life after Brooke ileostomy and ileal pouch-anal anastomosis. Comparison of performance status. *Annals of Surgery, 209*, 620–628.

Perry-Woodford, Z., & McLaughlin, S. (2008). Recommended follow-up for the ileo-anal pouch patient. *British Journal of Nursing, 17*(4), 220–224.

Polie, S. W., Dunkar, M. S., Slors, J. F., et al. (2007). Body image, cosmesis, quality of life, and functional outcome of hand-assisted laparoscopic versus open restorative proctocolectomy, long term results of a randomized trial. *Surgical Endoscopy, 21*, 1301.

Randall, J., Singh, B., Warren, B. F., et al. (2010). Delayed surgery for acute severe colitis is associated with increased risk of postoperative complications. *British Journal of Surgery, 97*, 404.

Recalla, S., English, K., Nazaralli, R., et al. (2013). Ostomy care and management: A systematic review. *Journal of Wound, Ostomy, and Continence Nursing*, 40(5), 489–500; quiz E1-2, doi: 10.1097/WON.0b013e3182a219a1.

Reese, G. E., Lovegrove, R. E., Tilney, H. S., et al. (2007). The effect of Crohn's disease on outcomes after restorative proctocolectomy. *Diseases of the Colon and Rectum, 50*, 239.

Regueiro, M., Kip, K. E., Cheung, O., et al. (2005). Cigarette smoking and age at diagnosis of inflammatory bowel disease. *Inflammatory Bowel Diseases, 11*, 42–47.

Remzi, F. H., Fazio, V. W., Delaney, C. P., et al. (2003). Dysplasia of the anal transition zone after ileal pouch-anal anastomosis: Results of prospective evaluation after a minimum of ten years. *Diseases of the Colon and Rectum, 46*, 6.

Ruddell, W. S., Dickinson, R. J., Dixon, M. F., et al. (1980). Treatment of distal ulcerative colitis (proctosigmoiditis) in relapse: Comparison of hydrocortisone enemas and rectal hydrocortisone foam. *Gut, 21*, 885–889.

Rutgeerts, P., Sandborn, W. J., Feagan, B. G., et al. (2005). Infliximab for induction and maintenance therapy for ulcerative colitis. *New England Journal of Medicine, 353*, 2462–2476.

Rutgeerts, P., Geboes, K., Vantrappen, G., et al. (1999). Predictability of the postoperative course of Crohn's disease. *Gastroenterology, 99*, 956.

Safdi, M., DeMicco, M., Sninsky, C., et al. (1997). A double-blind comparison of oral versus rectal mesalamine versus combination therapy in the treatment of distal ulcerative colitis. *American Journal of Gastroenterology, 92*, 1867–1871.

Sandborn, W. J., van Assche, G., Reinisch, W., et al. (2012). Adalimumab induces and maintains clinical remission in patients with moderate-to-severe ulcerative colitis. *Gastroenterology, 142*, 257–265, e1–3.

Sardini, T. C., & Wexner, S. D. (1998). Laparoscopy for inflammatory bowel disease: Pros and cons. *World Journal of Surgery, 22*(4), 370–374.

Sigall-Boneh, R., Pfeffer-Gik, T., Segal, I., et al. (2014). Partial enteral nutrition with a Crohn's disease exclusion diet is effective for induction of remission in children and young adults with Crohn's disease. *Inflammatory Bowel Diseases, 20*, 1353–1360.

Schluender, S. J., Ippoliti, A., Dubinsky, M., et al. (2007). Does infliximab influence surgical morbidity of ileal pouch-anal anastomosis in patients with ulcerative colitis? *Diseases of the Colon and Rectum, 50*, 1747.

Selvaseker, C. R., Cima, R. R., Larson, D. W., et al. (2007). Effect of infliximab on short-term complications in patients undergoing operation for chronic ulcerative colitis. *Journal of the American College of Surgery, 204*, 956.

Shen, B., Remzi, F. H., Lavery, I. C., et al. (2008). A proposed classification of ileal pouch disorders and associated complications after restorative proctocolectomy. *Clinical Gastroenterology and Hepatology, 6*, 145.

Sher, M. E., Bauer, J. J., Gorphine, S., et al. (1992). Low Hartmann's procedure for severe anorectal Crohn's disease. *Diseases of the Colon and Rectum, 35*, 975.

Similus, C., Purkayastha, S., Yamamoto, T., et al. (2007). A meta-analysis comparing end-to-end anastomosis vs. other configurations after resection in Crohn's disease. *Diseases of the Colon and Rectum, 50*, 1674.

Smith, D. M., Lowenstein, G., Jankovic, A., et al. (2009). Happily hopeless: Adaptation to a permanent, but not to a temporary, disability. *Health Psychology, 28*(6), 787–791.

Tan, J. J., & Tjandra, J. J. (2007). Laparoscopic surgery for Crohn's disease: A meta-analysis. *Diseases of the Colon and Rectum, 50*, 576.

Thorpe, G., McArthur, M., & Richardson, B. (2009). Bodily change following fecal stoma formation:qualitative interpretive synthesis. *Journal of Advanced Nursing, 65*(9), 1778–1789.

Timmer, A., McDonald, J. W., Tsoulis, D. J., et al. (2012). Azathioprine and 6-mercaptopurine for maintenance of remission in ulcerative colitis. *Cochrane Database of Systematic Reviews, 9*, CD000478.

Travis, S. P., Danese, S., Kupcinskas, L., et al. 2014. Once-daily budesonide MMX in active, mild-to-moderate ulcerative colitis: Results from the randomised CORE II study. *Gut, 63*, 433–441.

Van Assche, G., Dignass, A., Reinisch, W., et al. (2010). The second European evidence-based Consensus on the diagnosis and management of Crohn's disease: Special situations. *Journal of Crohn's and Colitis, 4*, 63–101.

Vegh, Z., Burisch, J., Pedersen, N., et al. (2014). Incidence and initial disease course of inflammatory bowel diseases in 2011 in Europe and Australia: Results of the 2011 ECCO-EpiCom inception cohort. *Journal of Crohn's and Colitis, 8*, 1506–1515.

Wasmuth, H., Myrvold, H., & Helge, E. (2009). Durability of ileal pouch-anal anastomosis and continent ileostomy. *Diseases of the Colon and Rectum, 52*(7), 1285–1289.

Wax, J. R., Pinette, M. G., Cartin, A., et al. (2003). Female reproductive health after ileal pouch anal anastomosis for ulcerative colitis. *Obstetrical and Gynecological Survey, 58*, 270.

Williams, L., Armstrong, M. J., Finan, P., et al. (2007). The effect of fecal diversion on the human ileum. *Gut, 56*, 796.

Windsor, A., Michetti, P., Bemelman, W., et al. (2013). The positioning of colectomy in the treatment of ulcerative colitis in the era of biologic therapy. *Inflammatory Bowel Diseases, 19*, 2695.

Wu, G. D., Bushmanc, F. D., & Lewis, J. D. (2013). Diet, the human gut microbiota, and IBD. *Anaerobe, 24*, 117–120.

Wu, J. S., & Fazio, V. W. (2002). Continent ileostomy: Evolution of design. *Clinics in Colon and Rectal Surgery, 15*, 231–243.

Young-Fadok, T. M., HallLong, K., McConnell, E. J., et al. (2001). Advantages of laparoscopic resection for Crohn's disease. Improved outcomes and reduced costs. *Surgical Endoscopy, 15*, 450.

Young, R., & Vanderhoof, J. (2012). Pathophysiology of short bowel syndrome. Reprint www.uptodate.com

Zachos, M., Tondeur, M., & Griffiths, A. M. (2007). Enteral nutritional therapy for induction of remission in Crohn's disease. *Cochrane Database of Systematic Reviews*, CD000542.

Zulkowski, K. (2012). Diagnosing and treating moisture-associated skin damage. *Advances in Skin and Wound Care, 25*, 231–236.

QUESTIONS ON MEDICAL MANAGEMENT—PART 1

1. A WOC nurse is caring for a patient who is diagnosed with Crohn's disease. Which feature distinguishes this disease from ulcerative colitis?

A. Extraintestinal manifestations
B. Bleeding
C. Pain
D. Presence of granulomas

2. A patient is diagnosed with ulcerative colitis that is located in the rectum and extends up to the splenic flexure. This is an example of what disease type?

A. Proctitis
B. Proctosigmoiditis
C. Left-sided ulcerative colitis
D. Pancolitis

3. A WOC nurse has an order to administer an immunosuppressant to a patient who has Crohn's disease. Which drug would commonly be considered?

A. Balsalazide
B. Hydrocortisone
C. Budesonide
D. Azathioprine

4. The WOC nurse is explaining the progression of ulcerative colitis to a patient. Which statement accurately describes this disease?

A. The rectum may or may not be involved.
B. The disease extends proximally to include part or all of the colon.
C. The pattern of inflammation is patchy and discontinuous.
D. The inflammation extends into other layers of the surface of the colon.

5. A patient has ulcerative colitis that is limited to the rectum. What medication would be the first-line option for treatment?

A. Hydrocortisone enema, suppository or foam
B. Cyclosporin per IV administration
C. Adalimumab per IV administration
D. Vedolizumab per IV administration

6. Which therapy would the WOC nurse expect to initiate for a patient who manifests peristomal pyoderma gangrenosum related to UC or CD?

A. Surgical treatment
B. Wound care and medical therapy
C. Bowel rest with parental nutrition support
D. IV antibiotics

7. A WOC nurse helps a patient with IBD plan a diet to help alleviate symptoms. Which type of diet would the nurse promote?
   A. Low fat.
   B. High fiber.
   C. Low residue.
   D. No dietary modifications have been proven to be beneficial.

8. Which treatment would be considered for a perianal fistula without an abscess?
   A. Antibiotics IV
   B. Liquid diet
   C. Bowel rest and parenteral nutrition support
   D. Surgery to remove fistula tract

9. A patient is diagnosed with pancolitis. What is the amount of the colon involved?
   A. 20 cm
   B. 60 cm
   C. >60 cm
   D. The entire colon

10. What drug can be used in the treatment of ulcerative colitis that acts directly on the colonic mucosa with limited systematic absorption?
   A. Sulfasalazine
   B. Prednisolone
   C. Budesonide
   D. Golimumab

ANSWERS—PART 1 QUESTIONS: 1.**D**, 2.**C**, 3.**D**, 4.**B**, 5.**A**, 6.**B**, 7.**D**, 8.**C**, 9.**D**, 10.**C**

QUESTIONS ON SURGICAL MANAGEMENT—PART 2

1. A patient with Crohn's disease is scheduled for bowel resection. What is the guiding principle of surgical management for this condition?
   A. Preservation of intestinal length and function
   B. Removal of all necrotic intestinal tissue
   C. Providing surgical drainage without resection
   D. Avoidance of pharmaceutical treatment

2. A WOC nurse is explaining the procedure for laparoscopic ileocolic resection to a patient with Crohn's disease scheduled for surgery. What statement accurately describes an advantage/disadvantage of this procedure over open surgery?
   A. A longer hospital stay is required with the laparoscopic approach.
   B. The laparoscopic approach shortens the duration of postoperative ileus.
   C. The laparoscopic approach increases the incidence of small bowel obstruction.
   D. Recurrence rate is slightly higher with the laparoscopic approach.

3. A patient with Crohn's disease develops severe perianal disease and associated sepsis of the rectum and anus. What procedure would the WOC nurse expect to be scheduled for this patient?
   A. Segmental colectomy
   B. Subtotal colectomy
   C. Ileocecectomy
   D. Primary anastomosis

4. Which patient would be the most likely candidate for surgery for Crohn disease involving a proctocolectomy with a permanent end ileostomy?
   A. A patient with pancolitis
   B. A patient with isolated areas of colonic involvement
   C. A patient who undergoes emergency surgery for a free perforation
   D. A patient with a nonhealing wound and urinary dysfunction

5. What intervention would be one of the recommendations from the WOC nurse for a patient who has a nonhealing perineal wound?
   A. Use of a donut cushion when sitting
   B. Use of lukewarm sitz baths
   C. Use of a pressure redistribution seat pad when sitting
   D. Use of cold compresses on the perineum

6. A patient with Crohn's disease is diagnosed with a 12-cm stricture. What surgical procedure is recommended to correct this defect?
   A. Heineke-Mikulicz.
   B. Finney strictureplasty.
   C. Michelassi side-to-side isoperistaltic strictureplasty.
   D. This condition is inoperable.

7. What treatment is viewed as definitive therapy for ulcerative colitis (UC)?
A. Watch and see approach
B. Pharmaceutical management
C. Removal of the entire colon and rectum with end ileostomy
D. Stricturoplasty

8. A surgeon is creating an ileal anal pouch anastomosis using stapled technique. For what postsurgical complication would the WOC nurse monitor this patient?
A. Cuffitis
B. Parastomal hernia
C. Valve complications
D. Bowel perforation

9. A patient recovering from ileal pouch anal anastomosis (IPAA) surgery (post stoma closure) tells the WOC nurse: "I've been having cramping in my belly and a lot of watery stools." The patient also complains of being "tired all the time." What complication of surgery would the nurse expect?
A. Anastomotic stenosis
B. Anastomotic dehiscence
C. Pouchitis
D. Pelvic abscess

10. Which postsurgical complication is the major cause of failure in continent ileostomy?
A. Valve stenosis
B. Nipple valve sliding
C. Obstruction from adhesions
D. Volvulus

ANSWERS—PART 2 QUESTIONS: 1.**A**, 2.**B**, 3.**B**, 4.**A**, 5.**C**, 6.**B**, 7.**C**, 8.**A**, 9.**C**, 10.**B**

CHAPTER 5

Other Conditions that Lead to a Fecal Diversion

Janice Beitz

OBJECTIVE

Describe disease states and conditions that can lead to a fecal stoma.

Topic Outline

The formation of a fecal diversion is most frequently done for conditions such as colorectal cancer (CRC) or inflammatory bowel disease. However, several other disease states or patient conditions are associated with fecal ostomy formation. These conditions include intestinal polyposis syndromes, diverticular disease, radiation enteritis, abdominal trauma, and forms of intestinal obstruction (volvulus, intussusception, colonic inertia). Where the fecal diversion is located (colostomy vs. ileostomy) and the nature of its formation (temporary vs. permanent) are often related to the underlying pathology. CRC as an etiologic factor is discussed elsewhere; see Chapter 3.

Polyposis Syndromes

Several polyposis syndromes exist. The polyposis syndromes can usually be differentiated based on histologic and molecular characteristics of the polyps, involvement of different segments of the gastrointestinal (GI) tract, and alterations in other organs and tissues. Disease severity, cancer risks associated with the disorder, mode of inheritance, and underlying genetic aberration can also help distinguish the disorders (Lucci-Cordisco et al., 2013). However, some patients present with unexplained polyposis. A recent study of 38 patients in a polyposis registry demonstrated that only 17% (6 of 38) had their polyposis definitively identified. The challenge for optimal patient care is evident when geneticists, pathologists, and gastroenterologists cannot detect specific diagnostic criteria since care approaches differ for the various syndromes (Mongin et al., 2012). The focus of this discussion will be on more common conditions: familial adenomatous polyposis (FAP), Gardner's syndrome, and the less common Peutz-Jeghers syndrome (PJS).

CLINICAL PEARL

Polyposis syndromes although somewhat rare, it is important for the patient and his or her family to be aware of the existing health risks associated with these disorders.

Familial Adenomatous Polyposis Syndrome

Familial (or familiar) Adenomatous Polyposis (FAP) Syndrome was the first polyposis syndrome recognized and is the best investigated. It is one of the CRCs that are known to be associated with familial genetic passage of mutated genes. These disorders include hereditary nonpolyposis colorectal cancer (HNPCC), FAP, PJS, juvenile polyposis syndrome (JPS), and MYH-associated polyposis (Centelles, 2012, p. 6).

Etiology

FAP is an autosomal dominant disorder caused by a mutation in the APC (adenomatous polyposis coli) gene located on chromosome 5q21-22 (Shah et al., 2013). APC is a tumor suppressor gene. On monoallelic mutation analysis (a form of genetic testing), more than 95% of FAP patients display an identifiable mutation (Centelles, 2012, p. 7). Accurate classification of FAP and other CRC syndromes is imperative given the associated risks, management strategies, and consequent risk to family relatives. The histologic analyses of colorectal polyps in FAP are predominantly adenomatous polyps (Jasperson, 2012, p. 328). FAP is estimated to occur in about 1 in 10,000 individuals usually occurring between 20 and 40 years. FAP accounts for approximately 1% of all CRC cases (Kastrinos & Syngal, 2011).

Clinical Presentation

The classic clinical presentation of FAP includes the occurrence of hundreds to thousands of adenomatous polyps in the colon and rectum. The sheer number of polyps present in FAP results in nearly a 100% lifetime risk of CRC in untreated persons. Generally, colorectal polyps begin to develop around age 16 years with CRC developing anywhere from 5 to 30 years later (mean age of 39 years) (Shah et al., 2013). Other cancer syndromes have substantial extracolonic manifestations, but when they occur in FAP, the most common scenario is upper GI tract polyps (Jasperson, 2012).

These intestinal adenomatous polyps are usually discovered during endoscopic evaluation for symptoms such as GI bleeding. Conversely, they may be identified during routine screening in people with a known family history. Clinical diagnosis of FAP requires at least 100 colorectal adenomatous polyps (Lucci-Cordisco et al., 2013).

Extraintestinal malignancies can be associated with FAP. They include central nervous system tumors (e.g., medulloblastomas), papillary thyroid cancer, and duodenal cancer. The risk of duodenal or periampullary carcinoma in patients with FAP is estimated to be 100 to 330 times greater than that in the general population, but the absolute risk is below 5% (Jasperson, 2012). The most common extracolonic finding in individuals with FAP is upper GI tract polyps (Jasperson, 2012). The extracolonic manifestations of FAP can be benign including duodenal adenomas, gastric fundic gland polyps, and desmoids (Lucci-Cordisco et al., 2013).

Although malignancy can occur in childhood and adolescence, malignant degeneration occurs typically by 40 to 50 years of age. The most common age of cancer diagnosis in classic FAP patients is 39 years. The most common cancer location is the rectum followed by the sigmoid and other colon segments (Popek & Tsikitis, 2011). Cancers in other body locations also increase risk. Periampullary cancer (occurring in the duodenum near the ampulla of Vater) and desmoid tumors represent the most common cause of death in FAP patients (Popek & Tsikitis, 2011). Though benign, desmoid tumors cause serious damage by local invasion and compression of adjacent body structures.

Medical Management

Genetic testing and counseling are the standard of care for individuals with classic FAP and for at-risk family members. Genetic evaluation begins with the affected person with the polyposis phenotype and full gene sequencing looking for the APC gene mutation.

For known gene mutation carriers, colorectal screening with flexible sigmoidoscopy or colonoscopy should begin at 10 to 12 years of age. Once polyps are identified, colon screening must be annual. A recent systematic review supports that registration and screening of FAP patients resulted in a reduction of the CRC incidence and mortality in this hereditary registry of patients (Barrow et al., 2013).

Because of extraintestinal manifestations, screening of the stomach and duodenum is also necessary. Upper endoscopy is recommended every 1 to 3 years (Kastrinos & Syngal, 2011). Since thyroid cancer is a possibility, health care providers should perform thyroid palpation and possibly thyroid ultrasonography annually.

Some literature has suggested a role for chemoprevention against polyps. For example, sulindac, a nonsteroidal anti-inflammatory drug, has been shown to cause regression of colorectal adenomas. However, the long-term benefits have been inconsistent; therefore, chemoprevention is not considered a reasonable alternative to surgery (Kastrinos & Syngal, 2011).

Research has also addressed the psychological issues of requisite surveillance for cancer degeneration in persons with FAP and other polyposis syndromes. A systematic review in 2012 (Gopie et al., 2012) analyzed 32 studies looking at psychological burden of hereditary cancer surveillance (breast, colon, colorectum, melanoma, etc.). For most hereditary cancer syndromes, surveillance was associated with good psychological outcomes. However, distress levels increased in those persons who were at high risk for developing *multiple* tumors.

Surgical Management

Despite frequent colonoscopies and polypectomy, the tumor burden or sheer number of polyps may preclude the continuing use of endoscopy. Total proctocolectomy with ileal pouch anal anastomosis (IPAA) is the preferred surgery. Total colectomy with removal of the rectal mucosa is the goal of therapy (to remove potentially diseased tissue). Total colectomy with ileorectal anastomosis does not offer as clear a benefit as does total colectomy with IPAA since rectal mucosa remains. Annual colonoscopy would be required to follow this retained tissue for polyp development.

Gardner's Syndrome

At one time, Gardner's syndrome was considered a separate disease from FAP. Today, Gardner's syndrome is considered linked to FAP. Gardner's syndrome is an inherited polyposis syndrome that is also associated with germline APC mutation. Gardner's syndrome is thought to be a variation in the expressivity of APC mutations rather than being a distinct clinical entity from FAP (Jasperson, 2012). In fact, some authors suggest that Gardner's syndrome is the full-blown manifestation of the FAP spectrum of clinical features due to the APC gene mutation (Ponti et al., 2013; Popek & Tsikitis, 2011).

CLINICAL PEARL

Gardner's syndrome usually causes benign tumors to form in many different organs and causes a higher risk of developing CRC and other FAP-related cancers.

Etiology

Gardner's syndrome shares characteristics with FAP in that it is due to a mutation in the APC gene. Notably, Gardner's syndrome is also associated with formation of adenomatous polyps as opposed to hamartomas that occur in PJS (Omundsen & Lam, 2012). The APC gene of chromosome 5q21 is responsible for Gardner's syndrome too. The gene encodes a protein that plays a substantive role in cell adhesion and signal transduction. In Gardner's syndrome, the APC mutation goes beyond just effects on the colorectum and involves tissue growth in other body areas (hence the tumors and osteomas) (Ponti et al., 2013).

Clinical Presentation

Gardner's syndrome has a clinical presentation that is distinct from FAP. In addition to colonic polyposis, Gardner's syndrome is associated with osteomas, epidermoid cysts, soft tissue tumors, fibromas, and/or desmoid tumors (Jasperson, 2012; Ponti et al., 2013). In particular, skin manifestations of Gardner's syndrome include epidermoid cysts, trichilemmal hybrid, or pilomatricomas developing on the face, scalp, or limbs of patients; something called a nuchal fibroma (diffuse induration and swelling of the back of the neck); and a "Gardner fibroma" area of thick collagen bundles and interspersed fibroblasts located mostly on the trunk (Ponti et al., 2013, pp. 244–245). Osteomas can arise on the mandible and skull. Dental lesions occur in almost 1/5 of patients including odontomas, absent, excess, or rudimentary teeth, or multiple caries (Ponti et al., 2013). Desmoid tumors do not have a malignant potential since they are locally invasive fibromatoses but can be highly aggressive in growth (Shah et al., 2013). They are associated with a higher mortality and morbidity because they can cause local destruction or tissue blockade. Intra-abdominal desmoid tumors can cause intestinal obstruction, blockage of the ureters, intestinal hemorrhage, or enterocutaneous fistulae (Kastrinos & Syngal, 2011).

Medical Management

Like other polyposis syndromes, endoscopic surveillance is required in Gardner's syndrome. Panoramic dental radiographs may detect occult lesions in Gardner's syndrome patients.

Prophylaxis regimens for Gardner's syndrome have been proposed too. Celecoxib (a COX-2 NSAID) was recommended previously but is of questionable long-term safety due to associated cardiovascular events. Sulindac has also been tested but has a risk of adverse effects on the stomach. With appropriate medical management of GI toxicity (protective coating agents and use of H_2 blockers and proton pump inhibitors), sulindac may be more tolerable in longer usage (Ponti et al., 2013). It should be noted that osteoma formation may *precede* the formation of colon polyps in Gardner's syndrome. Persons with a family history should be screened for GI tract involvement if other extraintestinal lesions are identified (Ponti et al., 2013).

Surgical Management

Gardner's syndrome is associated with the potential for multiple extraintestinal tissue growth. Consequently, total colectomy is not "curative" therapy. However, surgery may be required if polyps or desmoid tumors obstruct the intestine or if desmoids obstruct the ureters, kidneys, or other vital body systems.

A notable finding in both Gardner's syndrome and FAP is the relationship of desmoid tumor formation and trauma. It is hypothesized that abdominal surgery can accelerate or precipitate desmoid formation and growth. The exact pathogenesis of this process is not understood (Popek & Tsikitis, 2011). When small bowel obstruction occurs related to desmoid tumors, several techniques are possible. Intestinal resection, bypass, and strictureplasty have all been used successfully (Xhaja & Church, 2013).

Peutz-Jeghers Syndrome

PJS is a polyposis syndrome characterized by the formation of hamartomatous polyps in the GI tract as opposed to adenomatous polyps. The hamartomatous syndromes like PJS are much less common than are adenomatous syndromes, approximately 1/10 the frequency (Omundsen & Lam, 2012).

PJS is a rare disease that has an autosomal dominant inheritance pattern. In addition, to the occurrence of hamartomatous polyps in the GI tract, there is usually a family history of PJS and a classical pigmentation finding. The hamartomatous polyps occur most frequently in the small bowel. The characteristic extraintestinal manifestation is mucocutaneous pigmentation (i.e., freckles) of the lips and buccal mucosa (Kastrinos & Syngal, 2011).

Etiology

Most PJS cases are due to a germ line mutation in the nuclear serine threonine kinase gene LKBI/STKII that regulates cell polarization, metabolism, and cell growth and is likely a tumor suppressor gene. The result of the mutation is a truncated protein with no kinase activity (Omundsen & Lam, 2012).

The hamartomas that occur in PJS are macroscopically large and pedunculated. The main histologic characteristic of Peutz-Jeghers polyps is the presence of a central core of bands of smooth muscle covered by mucosa similar to the body region with normal or hyperplastic glandular epithelium. A histologic description of a polyp with these characteristics can assist (along with demonstrable genetic findings) with the diagnosis of PJS (Lucci-Cordisco et al., 2013). They most commonly occur in the small bowel (jejunum most common) but can also occur in the stomach, colon, and, with much less frequency, in the bladder and lungs. They can also occur in the nose, uterus, and gallbladder. While polyps occur most commonly in the small intestine in PJS, the colon is the most frequent site for GI malignancy (Lucci-Cordisco et al., 2013; Omundsen & Lam, 2012).

Clinical Presentation

PJS usually presents around a median age of 11 years. Classic appearance is altered pigmentation in the form of dark blue to brown macules around the mouth, eyes, nostrils, buccal mucosa, palmar surface of the hands, and genitalia and perianally. It is from mucocutaneous melanin pigmentation (Jasperson, 2012). Notably, some patients have no pigmentary changes, but 95% of PJS patients have mucocutaneous pigmented lesions (Shah et al., 2013). When these pigmentary changes do occur, they usually start fading from the third decade onward (Omundsen & Lam, 2012).

Affected patients usually enter the health care system and begin surveillance after they present with an acute complication. The complications may include abdominal pain due to bowel obstruction, intussusception, volvulus, and rectal bleeding. Once identified, family members should be assessed as well. A definite diagnosis of PJS includes at least two of the following characteristics: (1) hyperpigmentation of the lips or buccal mucosa, (2) two or more hamartomatous polyps in the small bowel, or (3) a PJS family history (Kastrinos & Syngal, 2011).

Medical Management

Medical therapy involves ongoing intestinal endoscopic surveillance plus continuous screening for extraintestinal cancer (mammogram, PAP test, testicular ultrasound, etc.) (Kastrinos & Syngal, 2011). Endoscopy of both the upper and lower GI tract is recommended. Given PJS's predilection for the small bowel, a small bowel series or capsule endoscopy is usually recommended starting around 8 years of age. Polyps can be removed endoscopically depending on the number of polyps. Surveillance endoscopy should be done every 2 to 3 years (Kastrinos & Syngal, 2011). Notably, the cancer risks associated with PJS are more significant after 30 years with GI tract cancers having the highest cumulative risk (Jasperson, 2012). Ideally, PJS is best managed by specialist centers with expert providers (Omundsen & Lam, 2012).

Surgical Management

Acute surgical intervention is sometimes required for intussusception, volvulus, and small bowel obstruction. CRCs associated with PJS should be managed like other CRCs with segmental resection. Prophylactic colectomy is *not* recommended for PJS given its location in multiple body sites (Omundsen & Lam, 2012). If polyps are above 1.5 cm in size or are suspicious for malignancy, they should be removed endoscopically or, if necessary, surgically (Omundsen & Lam, 2012).

Diverticular Disease

Diverticular disease is a disorder that represents a spectrum of clinical presentation varying from totally asymptomatic and uncomplicated to acute situations requiring emergency surgery with a diversion of fecal stream. Diverticulosis is the term used to describe the presence of colonic diverticula, that is, small sac-like outpouchings of the intestinal wall. Diverticulitis describes when one or more of these diverticula become inflamed. Diverticular disease includes both diverticulosis and diverticulitis. For most people, diverticulosis is discovered only incidentally at colonoscopy or barium enema testing. Diverticular disease is a very common GI disorder in the developed world with highest rates in the United States and Europe. By age 80, about 70% of Americans have diverticulosis (Boynton & Floch, 2013). Acute diverticulitis is the most common complication of diverticular disease affecting 10% to 25% of patients (Lahat et al., 2013).

Etiology

Diverticular disease has been noted to be a disease of aging, that is, acquired over time (Boynton & Floch, 2013; Gardiner, 2013) and is likely linked to diet. Specifically, diverticulosis is thought to be a "deficiency" disease of western civilization based on low intake of fiber (McQuaid, 2014). Painter and Burkitt (1971) originally hypothesized that low-fiber diets resulted in small-volume dry stools that required higher pressures for colonic transit.

Low fiber theoretically creates the higher luminal pressures that are thought to encourage the mucosa and submucosa to herniate through the bowel wall muscle at the sites where blood vessels perforate the muscle layer (points of greater weakness). Diverticula may develop more in the sigmoid colon because intraluminal pressures are highest in this region (McQuaid, 2014). The theory provides a logical explanation of why diverticulosis increases with age (Burgell et al., 2013; Peery & Sandler, 2013). Note that this etiologic fiber hypothesis has persisted for over 40 years largely without proof. A recent study by Peery et al. (2012) demonstrated that a high-fiber diet was associated with a *higher* prevalence of diverticula. Conversely, there is some evidence that a high-fiber diet may protect against diverticular disease (i.e., diverticulitis) (Burgell et al., 2013; Peery & Sandler, 2013).

In a cross-sectional colonoscopy-based study of 539 people with diverticulosis and 1,569 without it, neither constipation nor a low-fiber diet was associated with an increased risk of diverticulosis (Peery et al., 2013). So findings continue to be mutually contradictory.

Another etiologic perspective relates to the effect of aging on colon tissue. Age-related changes in the connective tissue of the large bowel include an increase in collagen cross-linking and increased elastin; both may contribute to increased colon rigidity (Boynton & Floch, 2013).

Interestingly, when diverticulosis occurs in persons younger than 40 years of age, they tend to be obese and the cases are less likely to be complicated, however emergency operation rates are higher. The diagnosis of diverticulitis should be included in the differential diagnosis of younger obese patients with lower abdominal pain (Pilgrim et al., 2013). A cross-sectional study of 23 patients <50 years old demonstrated that risk factors for acute diverticulosis included obesity, male gender, and consumption of alcohol (Pisanu et al., 2013).

Notably, research has demonstrated that nuts and seeds do not increase the risk of diverticulitis or a diverticular bleed (Peery & Sandler, 2013). Though it was thought that nuts and seeds could obstruct the diverticula and cause a perforation, Strate and colleagues (2008) found no association.

Clinical Presentation

Diverticulosis remains asymptomatic in the majority of patients. However, about 20% will experience complications (Boynton & Floch, 2013). The two major recognized complications are acute episodes of bleeding and diverticulitis.

The symptom presentation in diverticulosis may be subtle and then more pronounced. Patients may report chronic vague GI symptoms including mild abdominal pain, bloating, constipation, and diarrhea or fluctuating bowel habits. Physical examination at this point is usually normal.

When acute diverticulitis strikes, the patient reports abdominal pain in the left lower abdominal quadrant. This presentation occurs because in almost all patients with diverticulosis the sigmoid and descending colon are involved (McQuaid, 2014).

Medical Management

Symptom management and medical management depend on the state of diverticular disease: diverticulosis versus diverticulitis. Though the fiber hypothesis is not fully supported by research, contemporary diverticulosis medical therapy still targets fiber. In asymptomatic disease that is discovered incidentally, the patient should be counseled to eat a high-fiber diet. Fiber supplements such psyllium or methylcellulose may also assist with less constipated stool movements.

Most diverticulitis patients can be managed conservatively. For those with mild symptoms and no signs of abdominal complications (e.g., peritoneal signs), they can be treated as outpatients via a clear liquid diet and broad-spectrum antibiotics covering anaerobes, for example, metronidazole 500 mg three times daily or amoxicillin/clavulanate 875/125 mg twice daily plus either ciprofloxacin 500 mg twice daily or trimethoprim–sulfamethoxazole 160/800 mg twice daily for 7 to 10 days or until the patient is afebrile for 72 hours (McQuaid, 2014). A recent retrospective review supported that outpatient treatment for acute uncomplicated diverticulitis was feasible and safe in 118 patients (Unlu et al., 2013).

If symptoms worsen (increasing pain, high fevers, increased white blood cell counts, or peritoneal signs e.g., rebound tenderness), patients should be hospitalized. Patients should be NPO, be placed on IV fluids, and be given antibiotics covering anaerobic and gram-negative bacteria usually for 5 to 7 days before converting to oral therapy. Commonly used agents include cefoxitin, piperacillin–tazobactam, or ticarcillin–clavulanate (McQuaid, 2014).

The degree of complexity of diverticulitis can be described using something called the modified Hinchey classification. Based on diagnostic testing and operative findings, the diverticulitis complexity can be placed into one of four stages: stage 1, pericolonic abscess; stage 2, pelvic abscess; stage 3, purulent peritonitis; and stage 4, fecal peritonitis (Hinchey et al., 1978; Wexner & Moscovitz, 2000). The higher the stage, the more likely a multistage surgery will be used and the higher the associated morbidities (Turley et al., 2013). If an abscess is developed related to the diverticulitis, a higher risk of surgical intervention is noted (Van De Wall et al., 2013).

Surgical Management

Surgical management is usually reserved for those individuals who have had diverticulitis with complications. For persons who have had multiple episodes of diverticulitis, an elective bowel resection of the worst affected parts may be done to ameliorate the likelihood of future attacks. However, prophylactic bowel resection is being questioned for its efficacy in prevention (Lutwak & Dill, 2013). Elective surgery for uncomplicated diverticulitis should be done on a case by case basis considering patient-specific factors like age, computed tomography (CT)-graded severity, and patients' medical condition (Turley et al., 2013).

For persons who develop acute diverticulitis with complications (e.g., peritonitis, abscess), emergency surgery will be performed. Most commonly, a temporary colostomy and a Hartmann's procedure will be done. This approach leaves the anus and rectal stump inside the body closed over with surgical staples. The proximal part of the bowel exits the body in the left lower quadrant as a stoma. When the sepsis resolves (usually 12 to 16 weeks later), the two segments can be reconnected. This approach is usually reserved for patients who are more severely toxic.

Some surgeons do not use the two-step Hartmann's surgery but rather complete it in one step. The diseased segment is removed, the two open bowel ends are cleansed with irrigation, and a primary anastomosis is completed. Both one-stage and Hartmann's procedures can be done laparoscopically (Turley et al., 2013). A recent systematic review by Gaertner et al. (2013) suggests that elective laparoscopic colon resection for diverticular disease is associated with better outcomes and less complications than open colectomy.

Radiation Enteritis

Radiation enteritis, sometimes called radiation enteropathy, is a rare complication of radiation therapy for pelvic malignancy, mainly prostate, rectal, and gynecological cancers. Tissue injury to the GI tract especially the small intestine may occur during treatment or at a variable time following therapy. As more patients survive cancer and radiation is included in multiple cancer care pathways, the incidence of radiation-related GI complications continues to increase. Recently, "pelvic radiation disease" has been suggested as the preferred nomenclature for the disorder (Hogan et al., 2013; Li et al., 2013).

CLINICAL PEARLS

Due to the nature of the treatment, radiotherapy can affect tissue and other organs in the pelvic region. Although they may be called "late effects," some symptoms may occur at anytime from during treatment to many years later.

The effects of radiation enteritis can be profound. Over half of patients so affected report that the disorder detrimentally affects their quality of life (Andreyev et al., 2013).

Etiology

The relationship of radiation enteritis or damage to the intestinal tissue from radiation effects is clear. The radiation damages tissue usually in a dose-dependent fashion. At higher doses, up to 50% of patients may experience radiation enteritis especially in its chronic form (Hogan et al., 2013). With radiation exposure, transient mucosal atrophy occurs with stem cell loss and reduced crypt mitoses causing epithelial denudation and dysfunction. Notably, a spectrum of disease exists with some individuals affected more potentially determined by genomic susceptibility to ionizing radiation (Hogan et al., 2013).

Radiation enteritis can develop acutely (usually within 2 weeks of radiation exposure). Tissue damage occurs, and nutrient and fluid loss ensue. Usually, symptoms are self-limiting.

Chronic radiation enteritis most commonly occurs within 18 to 80 months of treatment. However, cases have occurred up to two to three decades following exposure (Hogan et al., 2013; Stacey & Green, 2014). The damage underlying chronic radiation enteritis seems to be mostly related to fibrosis (Table 5-1). The intestinal tissue may appear pale, mottled, or telangiectatic. Vascular insufficiency may be present. In its severe form, chronic radiation enteritis may lead to intestinal obstruction or fistula formation (Li et al., 2013).

Patient risk factors may determine susceptibility to intestinal radiation injury. Medical comorbidities such as hypertension, diabetes mellitus, atherosclerosis, inflammatory bowel disease, collagen vascular disorders, and human immunodeficiency virus (HIV) infection may impact individual susceptibility to radiation toxicity. Genetic variations (a patient's genotype) may also play a role in radiotherapy susceptibility (Shadad et al., 2013a; Theis et al., 2010).

TABLE 5-1 Intestinal Tissue Changes Related to Radiation Enteritis

Acute	Chronic
Crypt micro-abscesses	Submucosal fibrosis
Inflammatory cell infiltrate	Lymphatic dilatation
Decreased crypt mitoses	Obliterative endarteritis
Epithelial ulceration and denudation	Tissue ischemia
	Tissue necrosis

Data from Hogan, N. M., Kerin, M. J., & Joyce, M. R. (2013). Gastrointestinal complications of pelvic radiotherapy: Medical and surgical management strategies. *Current Problems in Surgery*, *50*, 395–407; Shadad, Sullivan, Martin, & Egan (2013a); Stacey, R., & Green, J. T. (2014). Radiation-induced small bowel disease: Latest developments and clinical guidance. *Therapeutic Advances in Chronic Disease*, *5*(1), 15–29; and Theis, V. S., Sripadam, R., Ramani, V., & Lal, S. (2010). Chronic radiation enteritis. *Clinical Oncology*, *22*, 70–83.

Clinical Presentation

Clinical manifestations of GI radiation injury can be acute or delayed. Acute symptoms are related to acute mucosal injury and inflammation. Chronic symptoms derive from fibrosis and vascular sclerosis. Clinical symptoms are also dependent upon the degree and extent of tissue damage plus the location of injury (Stacey & Green, 2014).

Symptoms of acute and chronic GI radiation injury may include nausea, vomiting, abdominal pain, diarrhea, rectal pain, urgency, fecal incontinence, and bleeding. Chronic radiation enteritis may also be associated with malabsorption, bacterial overgrowth, rapid intestinal transit, and lactose intolerance. Bowel obstruction and fistulization can also occur. Constipation may alternate with diarrhea, and fecal incontinence may occur due to loss of anorectal compliance (Shadad et al., 2013b; Stacey & Green, 2014).

Medical Management

The evidence base for radiation enteritis medical treatment is limited. Approaches include nutrition therapy, medications (anti-diarrheals, anti-inflammatory agents, probiotics, antibiotics, cholestyramine, pentoxifylline, and tocopherol), hyperbaric oxygen therapy (HBOT), and endoscopic management (Theis et al., 2010).

Anti-diarrheal drugs like loperamide (preferred) or codeine phosphate can be used to slow diarrhea and transit time, thereby improving bile salt absorption. While these control symptoms, they do not target the etiology (Theis et al., 2010).

Anti-inflammatory agents like sulphasalazine and selected steroids (e.g., methylprednisolone), probiotics (VSL#3, a combination of live lactic acid bacteria, and bifidobacteria) (Stacey & Green, 2014), and antibiotics (e.g., metronidazole and doxycycline) have also been tried with limited success. No studies have addressed clinical efficacy with larger samples. Their use therefore may be empirical and based on individual response (Theis et al., 2010).

Many symptoms of chronic radiation enteritis are related to bile salt malabsorption. Cholestyramine has been used in selected patients with some success. The drug is not very palatable, and many patients discontinue usage (Theis et al., 2010).

Pentoxifylline and tocopherol have been used to help ameliorate radiation-induced fibrosis via a proposed antioxidant effect. Some patients have responded with symptom reduction, but further studies are required (Theis et al., 2010). Many other pharmacological agents have been raised as putative intestinal radioprotectants. These include things like captopril, rofecoxib, clopidogrel, thalidomide, octreotide, and prostaglandin. No formal trials of large sample size are available describing their efficacy (Shadad et al., 2013a).

HBOT has been used in small numbers of patients with some success since it is theorized to facilitate angiogenesis and possibly have an antibacterial effect. However, much research needs to be done to ascertain its true effectiveness (Stacey & Green, 2014; Theis et al., 2010).

Endoscopic laser therapy (e.g., argon plasma coagulation) has been used to help symptoms by treating radiation-induced colon telangiectasia and hemorrhages (Theis et al., 2010). It has to be used with great care given the risk of perforation in abnormal GI tissue (Stacey & Green, 2014).

Current research is investigating the possibility of *preventing* radiation enteritis. Medical approaches like nutrition (diets high in glutamine, arginine, vitamins) and pharmacological therapies like statins (e.g., simvastatin) and angiotensin-converting enzyme (ACE) inhibitors (Stacey & Green, 2014) are being conducted and show some promise (Theis et al., 2010). An interesting approach is use of circadian rhythm. Less cellular activity occurs in the GI tract during evening hours. Animal models are being used to test if evening radiotherapy is less damaging (Stacey & Green, 2014).

An interesting study in the United Kingdom described the use of an algorithm for management of GI symptoms in 218 patients who had pelvic radiation treatment. The researchers developed treatments based on assessments inherent in the algorithm. Though they were for new-onset (acute) GI symptoms after the radiotherapy, the algorithm demonstrated better symptom management than did the control group, and the study also showed that an educated nurse could use it as effectively as a gastroenterologist. The findings suggest that radiation-induced bowel injury is treatable in the acute phase offering hope for chronic radiation enteritis care (Andreyev et al., 2013).

Surgical Management

Up to one third of affected patients will require surgery. Owing to the challenges presented by these operations, surgery is usually used only for those with refractory, complicated disease (Hogan et al., 2013). Chronic radiation enteritis may generate strictures or adhesions requiring removal. In the past, bowel resection was more frequently used but often resulted in intestinal failure. Contemporary approaches are more conservative. Strictureplasty offers an intestine-preserving method that decreases mortality and morbidity. In the case of chronic radiation enteritis with small bowel obstruction, resection of the blockage is preferred (Li et al., 2013). The best "surgical" treatment is preventing radiation enteritis from occurring. The choice of incision for the surgery is also an area requiring careful thought. Many surgeons will choose a lower transverse incision to avoid irradiated areas. Laparoscopy would be a logical choice, but dense adhesions may preclude use. Due to the risk of poor wound healing and infection, many surgeons will avoid a large vertical incision (Hogan et al., 2013). If severe malnutrition due to chronic radiation enteritis does not respond to dietary manipulation, antimotility agents, electrolyte correction, probiotics or parenteral nutrition, surgical resection, or small bowel transplantation may be necessary (Webb et al., 2013).

Prevention of radiation enteritis has been attempted by surgical placement of intestinal slings to keep the bowel away from radiation. Other approaches include physical positioning during exposure so that small bowel segments are not exposed. Another approach is bladder distention during treatment to push small intestine away from the treatment field (Theis et al., 2010). Whatever the approach used, a resounding theme pervades the literature on radiation enteritis. *Preventing* damage is optimal treatment though how to best achieve this outcome is unclear. For those people affected, the key is early recognition and referral to a GI specialist.

Abdominal Trauma

Abdominal trauma is usually characterized or divided into two categories: blunt and penetrating. Both forms can cause serious damage to the GI tract and surrounding structures. In general, penetrating trauma is more likely to result in a fecal diversion especially if the trauma involves the rectum. Fecal diversion remains the mainstay of treatment for rectal trauma to prevent further pelvic contamination and limit sepsis.

Etiology

The abdomen is divided into three different anatomic sites: the peritoneal space, the retroperitoneal space, and the pelvis (Eckert, 2005). Any of these areas can be traumatized due to gunshot wounds, stabbing penetrating wounds, or blunt injuries due to seat belts, blast injuries of higher or lower velocity, or rapid deceleration damage. However, penetrating trauma is much more commonly related to intestinal and rectal injuries than blunt (Govender & Madiba, 2010).

Clinical Presentation

Patient presentation of abdominal trauma can vary widely depending on etiology and severity of injury. For example, a patient with a gunshot wound (or several) may display loss of consciousness and signs of hypovolemic shock. Conversely, a stab wound victim with a shallow depth injury may display less altered vital signs and be awake and cooperative.

Blunt abdominal trauma may present as bruising and pain or minimal apparent damage. Pieces of equipment like seat belts may leave distinctive marks on the skin. Attention to vital signs is critical in blunt trauma as well. Blunt trauma to the liver, intestine, and other vital structures can become life threatening.

Quality expeditious physical assessment is mandatory as abdominal trauma can affect blood and nerve supply to the extremities. In addition, more hidden injuries to the pelvic area may also be present. Diagnostic imaging will be used to assess the nature and severity of the damage as well.

Medical Management

Nonoperative management of abdominal trauma is more commonly associated with blunt or nonpenetrating trauma. However, the literature is also describing nonoperative management of penetrating abdominal gunshot wounds (Varga et al., 2013).

Since World War II, mandatory exploration of the abdomen was the customary approach. As imaging technology has evolved, CT scanning has permitted selective nonoperative management. However, appropriate patient selection is critical to outcomes success (Varga et al., 2013). Several contraindications are noted for nonoperative management. They include presence of hemodynamic instability, diffuse abdominal pain, peritonitis, or evisceration. In addition, patients who cannot have serial abdominal examinations (e.g., concomitant head or spinal injury) are not good candidates.

Medical management of abdominal trauma includes monitoring of vital signs, appropriate fluid resuscitation as necessary, CT scanning, and vigilance for signs of clinical deterioration (e.g., hemodynamic instability, discharge from peritoneum, febrile status) (Varga et al., 2013).

Surgical Management

Modern surgical management of abdominal trauma generally includes the concept of damage control. This process is a staged or stepped approach in which a shortened surgery is used to control immediate life-threatening issues of coagulopathy and hemorrhage, hypothermia, and metabolic acidosis. Physiological restoration then occurs in the intensive care unit with eventual return to the OR for definitive surgery (Georgoff et al., 2013). For abdominal trauma, damage control laparotomy (DCL) is considered standard of care.

In the case of intestinal especially colon injury, the trauma surgeon is left with a choice upon return to the OR for definitive repair. The surgeon can do a primary repair of colon discontinuity or create an ostomy for fecal diversion (Georgoff et al., 2013). While ostomy was considered the gold standard of treatment for decades following World War II, some surgeons decided to try primary repair instead. A recent analysis of the U.S. National Trauma Data Bank shows that there is a definite move away from mandatory fecal diversion to primary colon repair (Hatch et al., 2013). The analysis showed that the overall fecal diversion rate was 9% in the 6,817 patients from 2007 to 2009 who sustained primary colon injuries. Selected factors were associated with diversion: older age, higher injury severity scores, and especially sigmoid colon injury. In addition, US military and worldwide combat operations have demonstrated a change from mandatory fecal diversion or injury exteriorization to the current recommendation of primary repair or resection and reanastomosis (Johnson & Steele, 2013).

Recent surgical research has added another dimension to when surgeons will or won't divert the fecal stream in colonic injury. Sharpe et al. (2012) reported on the use of a management algorithm in penetrating colon injuries over 15 years in 252 patients with full-thickness colon injuries. More severe destructive injuries associated with pre- or intraoperative transfusion requirements of more than 6 units of packed red blood cells and/or significant morbidities were best managed with fecal diversion.

Another retrospective study examining the years 2000 to 2010 for surgical patients with colonic injuries and the use of DCL looked at the use of fecal diversion or primary anastomosis (Georgoff et al., 2013). The complication rate in both primary anastomosis patients ($N = 28$) versus diversion patients ($N = 33$) was similar. The authors supported that "a strategy of diversion over anastomosis cannot be strongly recommended" (Georgoff et al., 2013, p. 293).

One factor that can complicate postoperative recovery is the use of open abdomen management of abdominal trauma care whether a diversion is used or not. In a recent retrospective study of 120 open abdomen patients (35 for hemorrhagic situations), with mean follow-up at 21 months, 30 patients (25%) developed a ventral hernia, 13 patients (11%) experienced an enterocutaneous fistula, and 2 patients experienced bowel obstruction. If trauma care involved use of open abdomen therapy, a high incidence of complications can accompany long-term recovery (Frazee et al., 2013).

An instance in which abdominal trauma will likely involve a fecal diversion is rectal trauma. If the rectal trauma is below the peritoneal reflection, direct repair is usually impossible and the mainstay of treatment is fecal diversion to avoid further contamination (Barkley et al., 2012; Johnson & Steele, 2013).

Other Indications

Obstruction

Intestinal obstruction is a generic phrase that covers multiple pathologies both inherent to the GI tract and external to it in the peritoneal cavity. Given available space, only three disorders will be addressed: volvulus, intussusception, and colonic inertia. The former two are issues related to mechanical or structural forces, while inertia is more functional in nature.

CLINICAL PEARL

Tumors, scar tissue (adhesions), or twisting or narrowing of the intestines are mechanical bowel obstructions, and hernias, Crohn's disease, and tumors can also block the intestine.

Volvulus

Volvulus (from the Latin for "to roll") refers to torsion or twisting of the bowel around its own mesentery. It can affect any area of the GI tract, but colonic volvulus is more common with small bowel volvulus being rare (Jack, 2013). When volvulus does occur in the colon, it usually affects the sigmoid or cecal segments and less frequently the transverse colon and splenic flexure (Kulkarni et al., 2009). Colonic volvulus accounts for about 3% to 4% of bowel obstruction cases in the United States. However, higher areas of endemicity (prevalent in or peculiar to a particular locality, region, or people) occur across the globe. Africa, the Middle East, and South American rates are much higher; 10% to 50% of bowel obstructions in these regions are due to colonic volvulus. Variations may be due to dietary anatomical, cultural, or infection-related differences (Halabi et al., 2014). When colon volvulus, especially cecal volvulus, occurs in developed countries, adhesions, gynecologic operations, pelvic masses, poor muscle tone, and distal obstruction may be possible causes (Kulkarni et al., 2009).

Intussusception

Intussusception also generates bowel obstruction but in a different way. Intussusception, a disorder that is more common in children (Lochhead et al., 2013), is the process in which the intestine telescopes back on itself. Ileocolic intussusception represents 90% of all intussusceptions (Mandeville et al., 2012).

The etiology of intussusception is unknown, but the incidence peaks between 3 months and 5 years (Sachs & Hsieh, 2013). It is suggested to be due to lymphoid hyperplasia or uncoordinated peristalsis of the intestine. Other possibilities include viral infections especially adenovirus (Sachs & Hsieh, 2013). The blockage can result in bowel necrosis if left untreated (Mandeville et al., 2012). Intussusception is the most common cause of intestinal obstruction in the first 2 years of life (Mendez et al., 2012).

Volvulus and intussusception both present with abdominal pain and vomiting, and a palpable abdominal mass is usually present. In intussusception, bloody stool ("red currant jelly stool") (Mandeville et al., 2012, p. 842) may also be present. However, in intussusception, the four classic signs and symptoms just mentioned present in less than half of patients with the disorder (Mendez et al., 2012).

Medical and Surgical Management

Both medical and surgical interventions may be needed for volvulus and intussusception. Required surgery is dependent upon response to medical intervention and diagnostic studies.

Pillars of management for children with suspected volvulus are initial stabilization with aggressive fluid resuscitation, stomach decompression with a nasogastric tube, and immediate referral to a surgeon (Saliakellis et al., 2013).

Diagnostic studies (e.g., CT scan) are performed on both clinical situations. If obstruction is identified and associated with volvulus, a diagnostic laparoscopy may be considered. If adhesions are noted to be twisting and obstructing the GI tract, then removal of the adhesions and possible bowel resection may be needed, depending on bowel viability (Jack, 2013).

In intussusception, patients, mostly children, in this situation can have an abdominal ultrasound scan (the method of choice) (Sachs & Hsieh, 2013), or much less commonly, a CT scan can be used. Abdominal radiograph is also possible.

A retrospective study (Mendez et al., 2012) looked at the effectiveness of abdominal radiographs versus abdominal ultrasound in 6,314 children younger than 3 years from October 1999 to October 2004 who presented to the emergency department with suspected intussusception. Of the sample, 201 underwent radiographic evaluation. Of the 201 study patients, 171 had an abdominal radiograph and 65 had ultrasound, while 145 underwent air enema. The researchers found that RUQ mass, vomiting, and abdominal pain accompanied by a highly suggestive abdominal radiograph were significantly associated with intussusception. The highly suggestive findings included soft tissue mass, bowel obstruction, visible intussusception, and sparse large bowel gas pattern.

Medical management can include watchful waiting (Van Oudheusden et al, 2013) to see if the intussusception will resolve spontaneously (more in small bowel intussusception) or nonsurgical management with air enema reductions to reexpand the bowel. In a recent retrospective study of 152 children brought to the emergency room for intussusception from March 2005 to March 2007, air enema reductions were attempted in 102 of 114 children with large bowel intussusception. The success rate was 91% ($N = 93$). Nineteen children required surgery for air enema failure or bowel ischemia (Lochhead et al., 2013). When the patient fails air enema reduction or has signs of bowel necrosis, surgical intervention is used. Surgery may also be used if the patient displays signs of perforation, shock, or peritonitis (Sachs & Hsieh, 2013).

Colonic Inertia

Colonic inertia is a functional disorder of the intestine. That is, there is no clear structural abnormality or objective evidence of an underlying pathology but rather a dysfunctional enteric nervous system. Suggested causes include alterations in neurochemistry, neuronal loss, hypoganglionosis, and less numbers of colonic interstitial cells. Colonic inertia can create such poor bowel function that it mimics bowel obstruction. It can be so severe that colectomy is performed though it is considered a controversial treatment (Bratten & Jones, 2007).

The mechanism for colonic inertia may be related to an increased level of serotonin or distribution of serotonin in the colonic mucosa. Colonic inertia is associated with altered electrical activity contributing to dysmotility (Bratten & Jones, 2007; Cohen-Lewe, 2013).

Clinically, colonic inertia is usually characterized by severe functional constipation with abdominal pain and distention and possibly nausea. Other diagnostic criteria include lack of identified outlet obstruction, delayed colonic transit time identified by the use of radiopaque markers, and manometric demonstrated absent or severely diminished colonic motor activity (Cohen-Lewe, 2013). Diagnosis for colonic inertia may involve a variety of tests, but the most helpful is the transit time test that determines the speed at which the food moves through the digestive tract.

Both medical and surgical approaches are used in the disorder. Dietary changes like high-fiber diet, increasing water intake, avoiding fatty foods, and dairy product avoidance may help some persons that are affected.

Surgical therapy involved colectomy with the small intestine directly attached to the rectum (ileorectal anastomosis). Though the idea of shortening the colon seems to logically make sense, in some patient's symptoms can persist (Bratten & Jones, 2007). Though ileorectal anastomosis does not require the use of a diversion that is permanent, some surgeons may consider a temporary diversion to allow healing of anastomoses.

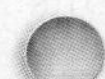

Summary

A variety of conditions can result in a fecal diversion. A review of common disease states that are etiologies for a stoma was presented. Clinical presentation and medical/surgical management were discussed.

REFERENCES

Andreyev, H., Benton, B. E., Lalji, A., et al. (2013). Algorithm-based management of patients with gastrointestinal symptoms in patients after pelvic radiation treatment (ORBIT): A randomized controlled trial. *Lancet, 382*, 2084–2092.

Barkley, S., Khan, M., & Garner, J. (2012). Rectal trauma in adults. *Trauma, 15*(1), 3–15.

Barrow, P., Khan, M., Lalloo, F., et al. (2013). Systematic review of the impact of registration and screening on colorectal cancer incidence and mortality in familial adenomatous polyposis and Lynch syndrome. *British Journal of Surgery, 100*, 1719–1731.

Boynton, W., & Floch, M. (2013). New strategies for the management of diverticular disease: Insights for the clinician. *Therapeutic Advances in Gastroenterology, 6*(3), 205–213.

Bratten, J. R., & Jones, M. P. (2007). Small intestinal motility. *Current Opinion in Gastroenterology, 23*, 127–133.

Burgell, R. E., Muir, J. G., & Gibson, P. R. (2013). Pathogenesis of colonic diverticulosis: Repainting the picture. *Clinical Gastroenterology and Hepatology*, 11, 1628–1630.

Centelles, J. J. (2012). General aspects of colorectal cancer. *International Scholarly Research Network*, Article ID 139268, 19 pages, doi: 10.5402/2012/139268

Cohen-Lewe, A. (2013). Osteopathic manipulative treatment for colonic inertia. *Journal of the American Osteopathic Association, 113*, 216–220.

Eckert, K. L. (2005). Penetrating and blunt abdominal trauma. *Critical Care Nursing Quarterly, 28*(1), 41–59.

Frazee, R. C., Abernathy, S., Jupiter, D., et al. (2013). Long-term consequences of open abdomen management. *Trauma, 16*(1), 37–40.

Gaertner, W. B., Kwaan, M. R., Madoff, R. D., et al. (2013). The evolving role of laparoscopy in colonic diverticular disease: A systematic review. *World Journal of Surgery, 37*, 629–638.

Gardiner, A. B. (2013). The effects of ageing on the gastrointestinal system. *Nursing & Residential Care, 15*(1), 30–33.

Georgoff, P., Perales, P., Laguna, B., et al. (2013). Colonic injuries and the damage control abdomen: Does management strategy matter? *Journal of Surgical Research, 181*, 293–299.

Gopie, J. P., Vasen, H. F., & Tibben, A. (2012). Surveillance for hereditary cancer: Does the benefit outweigh the psychological burden? A systematic review. *Critical Reviews in Oncology/Hematology, 83*, 329–340.

Govender, M., & Madiba, T. E. (2010). Current management of large bowel injuries and factors influencing outcome. *Injury, 41*, 58–63.

Halabi, W. J., Jafari, M. D., Kange, C. Y., et al. (2014). Colonic volvulus in the United States—trends, outcomes, and predictors of mortality. *Annals of Surgery, 259*(2), 293–301.

Hatch, Q., Causey, M., Martin, M., et al. (2013). Outcomes after colon trauma in the 21st century: An analysis of the U.S. National Trauma Data Bank. *Surgery, 154*, 397–403.

Hinchey, E. J., Schaal, P. G., & Richards, G. K. (1978). Treatment of perforated diverticular disease of the colon. *Advances in Surgery, 12*, 85–109.

Hogan, N. M., Kerin, M. J., & Joyce, M. R. (2013). Gastrointestinal complications of pelvic radiotherapy: Medical and surgical management strategies. *Current Problems in Surgery, 50*, 395–407.

Jack, L. A. (2013). Malrotation with volvulus: "Twisted guts" and a Dennis tube. *World Council of Enterostomal Therapists Journal, 33*(3), 17–21.

Jasperson, K. W. (2012). Genetic testing by cancer site: Colon (polyposis syndromes). *Cancer Journal, 18*(4), 328–333.

Johnson, E., & Steele, S. R. (2013). Evidence-based management of colorectal trauma. *Journal of Gastrointestinal Surgery, 17*, 1712–1719.

Kastrinos, F., & Syngal, S. (2011). Inherited colorectal cancer syndromes. *Cancer Journal, 17*(6), 405–415.

Kulkarni, D., Magee, D., & McGrory, D. (2009). Caecal volvulus-case report. *International Journal of Clinical Practice, 63*(4), 673.

Lahat, A., Avidan, B., Sakhnini, E., et al. (2013). Acute diverticulitis—A decade of prospective follow-up. *Journal of Clinical Gastroenterology, 47*(5), 415–419.

Li, N., Zhu, W., Gong, J., et al. (2013). Ileal or ileocecal resection for chronic radiation enteritis with small bowel obstruction: Outcome and risk factors. *American Journal of Surgery, 206*, 739–747.

Lochhead, A., Jamjoom, R., & Ratnapalan, S. (2013). Intussusception in children presenting to the emergency department. *Clinical Pediatrics, 52*(11), 1029–1033.

Lucci-Cordisco, E., Risio, M., Venesio, T., et al. (2013). The growing complexity of the intestinal polyposis syndromes. *American Journal of Medical Genetics Part A, 161*, 2777–2787.

Lutwak, N., & Dill, C. (2013). Mild to moderate diverticulitis: What's new on diagnostic approach, treatment, and prevention of recurrence? *Clinical Geriatrics, 21*(7), 6 pages. Retrieved from: www.clinicalgeriatrics.com/articles/mild-moderate-diverticulitis-whats-new

Mandeville, K., Chien, M., Willyerd, A., et al. (2012). Intussusception-clinical presentations and imaging characteristics. *Pediatric Emergency Care, 28*(9), 842–844.

McQuaid, K. (2014). Symptoms and signs of gastrointestinal disease. In M. Papadakis., S. J. McPhee, & M. W. Rabow (Eds.). *Current medical diagnosis and treatment 2014* (53rd ed.). New York, NY: McGraw-Hill Lange Publishers. Retrieved from www.accessmedicine.mhmedical.com/content.aspx?bookid=330

Mendez, D., Caviness, C., Ma, L., et al. (2012). The diagnostic accuracy of an abdominal radiograph with signs and symptoms of intussusception. *American Journal of Emergency Medicine, 30*, 426–431.

Mongin, C., Coulet, F., Lefevre, J., et al. (2012). Unexplained polyposis: A challenge for geneticists, pathologists, and gastroenterologists. *Clinical Genetics, 81*, 38–46.

Omundsen, M., & Lam, F. F. (2012). The other colonic polyposis syndromes. *ANZ Journal of Surgery, 82*, 675–681.

Painter, N. J., & Burkitt, L. P. (1971). Diverticular disease of the colon: A deficiency disease of western civilization. *British Medical Journal, 2*, 450–454.

Peery, A. F., & Sandler, R. S. (2013). Perspectives in clinical gastroenterology and hepatology: Diverticular disease: Reconsidering conventional wisdom. *Clinical Gastroenterology and Hepatology, 11*, 1532–1537.

Peery, A. F., Barrett, P. R., Park, D., et al. (2012). A high-fiber diet does not protect against symptomatic diverticulosis. *Gastroenterology, 142*, 266–272.

Peery, A. F., Sandler, R. S., Ahnew, D., et al. (2013). Constipation and a low-fiber diet are not associated with diverticulosis. *Clinical Gastroenterology and Hepatology, 11*, 1622–1627.

Pilgrim, S. M., Hart, A. R., & Speakman, C. T. (2013). Diverticular disease in younger patients—Is it clinically more complicated and related to obesity? *Colorectal Disease, 15*, 1205–1210.

Pisanu, A., Vacca, V., Reccia, I., et al. (2013). Clinical study—Acute diverticulitis in the young: The same disease in a different patient. *Gastroenterology Research and Practice*, ID 867961, 6 pages. Retrieved from: http://dx.doi.org/10.1155/2013/867961

Ponti, G., Pellacani, G., Seidenari, S., et al. (2013). Cancer-associated genodermatoses: Skin neoplasms as clues to hereditary tumor syndromes. *Critical Reviews in Oncology/Hematology, 85*, 239–256.

Popek, S., & Tsikitis, V. L. (2011). Epidemiology of inherited colon cancer. *Seminars in Colon & Rectal Surgery, 22*, 77–81.

Sachs, C., & Hsieh, T. (2013). Abdominal pain: A rational approach, part 2. *Consultant, 53*(2), 82–88.

Saliakellis, E., Borrelli, O., & Thapar, N. (2013). Pediatric GI emergencies. *Best Practice & Research Clinical Gastroenterology, 27*, 799–817.

Shadad, A. K., Sullivan, F. J., Martin, J. D., et al. (2013a). Gastrointestinal radiation injury: Symptoms, risk factors, and mechanisms. *World Journal of Gastroenterology, 19*(2), 185–198.

Shadad, A. K., Sullivan, F. J., Martin, J., et al. (2013b). Gastrointestinal radiation injury: Prevention and treatment. *World Journal of Gastroenterology, 19*(2), 199–208.

Shah, K. R., Boland, R., Patel, M., et al. (2013). Cutaneous manifestations of gastrointestinal disease: Part I. *Journal of American Academy of Dermatology, 68*(2), 189EI–189E21.

Sharpe, J. P., Magnotti, L. J., Weiberg, J. A., et al. (2012). Adherence to a simplified management algorithm reduces morbidity and mortality after penetrating colon injuries: A 15-year experience. *Journal of American College of Surgeons, 214*, 591–598.

Stacey, R., & Green, J. T. (2014). Radiation-induced small bowel disease: Latest developments and clinical guidance. *Therapeutic Advances in Chronic Disease, 5*(1), 15–29.

Strate, L. L., Liu, Y. L., Syngal, S., et al. (2008). Nut, corn, and popcorn consumption and the incidence of diverticular disease. *JAMA, 300*, 907–914.

Theis, V. S., Sripadam, R., Ramani, V., et al. (2010). Chronic radiation enteritis. *Clinical Oncology, 22*, 70–83.

Turley, R. S., Mantyh, C., & Migaly, J. (2013). Minimally invasive surgery for diverticulitis. *Techniques in Coloproctology, 17*(Suppl 1), S11–S22.

Unlu, C., Gunadi, P. M., Gerhards, M. F., et al. (2013). Outpatient treatment for acute uncomplicated diverticulitis. *European Journal of Gastroenterology and Hepatology, 25*, 1038–1043.

Van de Wall, B., Draaisma, W., Consten, E., et al. (2013). Does the presence of abscesses in diverticular disease prelude surgery? *Journal of Gastrointestinal Surgery, 17*, 540–547.

Van Oudheusden, T. R., Herts, B. A. C., DeHingh, I., et al. (2013). Challenges in diagnosing adhesive small bowel obstruction. *World Journal of Gastroenterology, 19*(43), 7489–7493.

Varga, S., Zakaluzny, S., & Inaba, K. (2013). Non-operative management of abdominal gunshot wounds. *Trauma, 15*(4), 271–278.

Webb, G. J., Brooke, R., & DeSilva, A. (2013). Chronic radiation enteritis and malnutrition. *Journal of Digestive Disease, 14*, 350–357.

Wexner, S., & Moscovitz, I. D. (2000). Laparoscopic colectomy in diverticular and Crohn's disease. *Surgical Clinics of North America, 80*, 1299–1319.

Xhaja, X., & Church, J. (2013). Small bowel obstruction in patients with familial adenomatous polyposis related desmoid disease. *Colorectal Disease, 15*, 1489–1492.

QUESTIONS

1. The WOC nurse is counseling the parents of a 5-year-old male patient about their family history of familial adenomatous polyposis (FAP) syndrome. What would the nurse include in the care plan for this family?

A. Begin colorectal screening with colonoscopy at age 10.
B. Once polyps are identified, colon screening should be done every 5 years.
C. Upper endoscopy should be performed every 5 years.
D. Thyroid ultrasonography should be performed every 2 years.

2. A 13-year-old male patient presents with dark blue macules around his mouth, eyes, nostrils, buccal mucosa, hands, and genitalia. What disease state would the WOC nurse suspect?

A. Familial adenomatous polyposis (FAP) syndrome
B. Gardner's syndrome
C. Peutz-Jeghers syndrome (PJS)
D. Diverticular disease

3. A WOC nurse is explaining the etiology of diverticular disease to a recently diagnosed patient. What would the nurse list as a possible cause of this disease?

A. Formation of hamartomatous polyps in the gastrointestinal tract
B. Mutation in the APC gene
C. Damage to the intestinal tissue from radiation
D. Low-fiber diet

4. A patient presents with pain in the left lower abdominal quadrant, bloating, and diarrhea. No abdominal masses are found on palpitation. What possible GI disorder is present?

A. Intussusception
B. Volvulus
C. Diverticulitis
D. Colonic inertia

5. The WOC nurse is developing a care plan for a patient diagnosed with radiation enteritis. What is a recommended first-line treatment modality for this disease?

A. Bowel resection
B. Use of anti-inflammatory agents
C. Strictureplasty
D. Fiber supplementation

6. What is considered the standard of care for a patient with abdominal trauma related to an automobile accident?

A. Damage control laparotomy.
B. Ostomy for fecal diversion.
C. Open abdominal surgery.
D. Surgery is not usually warranted.

7. What is a common cause of volvulus occurring in developed countries?

A. Diverticulitis
B. Pancreatitis
C. Radiation enteritis
D. Pelvic masses

8. A 10-year-old girl presents in the emergency department with abdominal pain, vomiting, palpable abdominal mass, and bloody stool. What condition may be present?

A. Volvulus
B. Intussusception
C. Colonic inertia
D. Diverticulosis

9. What medical management technique for intussusception is recommended prior to initiating surgery?

A. High-fiber diet
B. Dairy product avoidance
C. Air enema reduction
D. Antidiarrheal drugs

10. The WOC nurse is counseling a patient diagnosed with colonic inertia. What intervention would the nurse include in a care plan for this patient?

A. Avoiding fatty foods
B. Low-fiber diet
C. Restricting fluids
D. Encouraging consumption of dairy products

ANSWERS: 1.**A**, 2.**C**, 3.**D**, 4.**C**, 5.**B**, 6.**A**, 7.**D**, 8.**B**, 9.**C**, 10.**A**

CHAPTER 6

Urinary Stomas

Disease States That Lead to the Creation of a Urinary Stoma and the Use of Intestinal Segments in Urinary Diversion

Sanjay G. Patel, Joseph J. Pariser, and Gary D. Steinberg

OBJECTIVES

1. Describe disease states and conditions that can lead to a urinary diversion.
2. Discuss incontinent and continent urinary diversions and urinary sphincter saving procedures.

Topic Outline

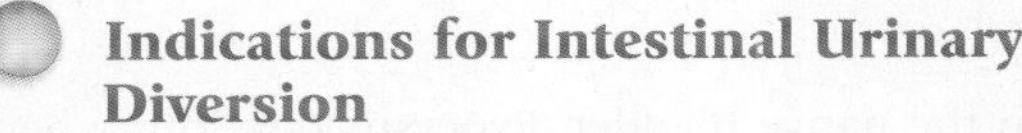

Indications for Intestinal Urinary Diversion

- Bladder Cancer
  - Risk Factors
  - Presentation
  - Histopathology
  - Diagnostic Considerations
  - Management
- Other Malignancies
- Benign Indications for Urinary Diversion
  - Neurogenic Bladder
  - Radiation Cystitis
  - Interstitial Cystitis
  - Trauma

Surgical Procedures

- Incontinent Urinary Diversions
  - Ileal Conduit
  - Colon Conduit
- Continent Urinary Diversions
  - Cutaneous Catheterizable Urinary Diversion
    - Indiana Pouch
    - Other Catheterizable Urinary Diversion
  - Orthotopic Urinary Diversion

Conclusions

Intestinal urinary diversion is a general term used to describe the elimination of urine from the body through a surgically reconstructed intestinal segment. The name of the diversion type typically describes the particular intestinal segment utilized or the name of the institution at which it was developed (e.g., ileal conduit or Indiana pouch). The surgically reconstructed reservoir or channel allows for passage of urine through the urethra, a continent catheterizable channel on the skin, or an incontinent stoma on the skin. A wide variety of diversions have been developed to utilize bowel segments since the late 1800s, and the techniques have evolved with time.

Early urinary diversions involved bringing the ureters or bladder directly to the skin, which oftentimes resulted in stenosis at the skin level. Ureterosigmoidostomy whereby the ureters were anastomosed to the sigmoid colon and the anal sphincter provided continence, many times resulted in increased pyelonephritis and colon cancer, and has largely been abandoned as a diversion choice. In the 1950s, Bricker popularized and developed the ileal conduit in which urine drained from a budded stoma that was constructed on the patient's abdomen. The ileal conduit resulted in improved patient quality of life and reduced

TABLE 6-1 Common Incontinent and Continent Urinary Diversion

Type	Procedure	Indications	Advantages	Contraindications/ Disadvantages
Incontinent				
Ileal conduit	Segment of small intestine isolated. Proximal end closed, ureters implanted into segment, and distal end to skin	Need for urinary diversion Bladder cancer, urinary fistula, neurogenic bladder, refractory cystitis Inability to manage continent reservoir	Simplest segment of bowel to use Familiar to urologists Lowest complication rate	Large body habitus may limit ability of stoma to reach skin level Prior radiation to the bowel Renal deterioration Hyperchloremic hypokalemic metabolic acidosis Need to wear pouching system for urine collection
Colon conduit	Same as ileal conduit but colon used in place of small bowel	Same as ileal conduit, but favored if small bowel disease present or in history of pelvic radiation	Less risk of stomal stenosis	Renal deterioration Hyperchloremic hypokalemic metabolic acidosis Need to wear pouching system for urine collection Larger stoma
Continent				
Orthotopic neobladder	Isolated, detubularized segment of ileum is used. Ureters implanted, and distal portion is connected to urethra to allow voiding	Same as ileal conduit, but patient selection is critical Cancer-free urethra Functional sphincter	Improved cosmesis: No stoma Voiding per urethra	Renal deterioration Must have urethra uninvolved with cancer Risk of: Incomplete emptying requiring catheterization Incontinence
Indiana pouch	Isolated, detubularized segment of ileocecal region used. Ureters implanted. Ileocecal valve used as continence mechanism. The patient will catheterize through abdominal wall stoma	Same as ileal conduit, but patient selection is critical	No pouching system needed Smaller stoma, which can be covered with dressing	Renal deterioration Patient must be capable of intermittent, self-catheterization Inability to catheterize is urologic emergency

stomal stenosis. More recently, continent diversions have improved the cosmesis of urinary diversion as patients eliminate their urine via small catheterizable channels on their abdomen or void via their native urethra (Pannek & Senge, 1998). Table 6-1 summarizes the most common incontinent and continent urinary diversions, which will be discussed further in this chapter.

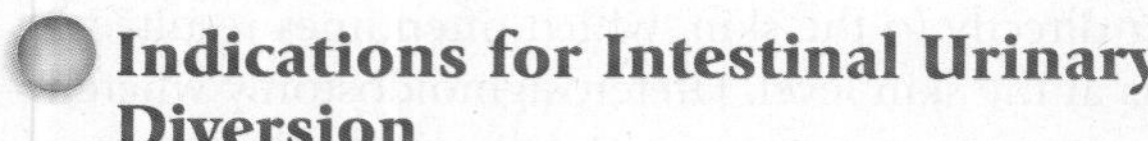

Indications for Intestinal Urinary Diversion

There are both benign and malignant indications for intestinal urinary diversion. Urinary diversion is most commonly utilized when the bladder has to be removed due to malignancy. Less commonly, urinary diversion is utilized to divert urine from the bladder for benign indications due to severe bladder dysfunction, incontinence, bladder pain, or bleeding. In instances of benign urinary diversion, consideration must be taken to remove the bladder as some patients may develop pyocystis or infection in the native bladder. Pyocystis develops when the secretions of the native bladder accumulate and develop into an infection because there is no flow of urine through the bladder to eliminate these secretions. Pediatric conditions leading to a urinary diversion will be covered in Chapter 14.

Bladder Cancer

Bladder cancer is the fourth most common cause of cancer death in men in the United States with a 3:1 male-to-female ratio (Bladder Cancer Support Society, 2014). The average age at diagnosis is approximately 70 years. The most common histologic subtype of bladder cancer is urothelial carcinoma of the bladder. Bladder cancer requiring removal of the bladder is the predominant indication for performing an intestinal urinary diversion.

Risk Factors

Several risk factors for bladder cancer have been implicated. The most common cause is cigarette smoking, which is a potent source for carcinogens that concentrate in the urine. Environmental exposure to chemicals (blue aniline dyes, chemicals in dye, paint, petroleum, rubber, and textile industries) has been implicated in the development of bladder cancer. Patients with chronic indwelling catheters or exposure to *Bilharzia* (parasite) have an increased risk of developing squamous cell carcinoma of the bladder.

Presentation

More than 80% to 90% of cases of bladder cancer present with gross hematuria, which is typically painless and intermittent. Twenty to thirty percent of patients present with irritative voiding symptoms such as urgency/frequency and dysuria (pain with urination). Diagnosis of bladder cancer is often delayed, as patients are commonly misdiagnosed as having routine urinary tract infections, which oftentimes contributes to many patients presenting with advanced disease.

Histopathology

Bladder cancer arises from the inner lining of the bladder known as the mucosa. Bladder cancers have a spectrum of aggressiveness, which can be described by their grade (microscopic appearance of their cancer) and their invasiveness (depth of penetration into the bladder). The bladder has several layers from innermost to outmost: mucosa → submucosa → muscle → perivesical fat (fat surrounding the bladder). On one end, low-grade superficial tumors stay limited to the mucosal layer and have low risk of invasion to the deeper layer of the bladder. On the other end, higher-grade tumors can infiltrate the layers of the bladder typically in a stepwise manner resulting in patient morbidity and mortality (mucosa → submucosa → muscle → perivesical fat → lymph nodes → distant metastases).

Diagnostic Considerations

Patients who present with gross or microscopic hematuria typically undergo a standard urologic evaluation with imaging (contrast-enhanced CT scan of the kidneys, ureter, and bladder), urine cytology, and endoscopic evaluation of the urethra and bladder using a cystoscope. Once a bladder tumor is identified, patients are taken to the operating room where the bladder tumor is resected using a cystoscope that is placed through the patient's urethra into the bladder. The resection allows for the microscopic determination of the histology (cell type), grade, and depth of penetration of the tumor into the bladder wall. Resection of the tumor is diagnostic, as well as prognostic, and therapeutic.

Management

Patients with lower-grade and noninvasive bladder tumors are good candidates for minimally invasive management, which includes administration of intravesical chemotherapy such as Bacille Calmette-Guerin (BCG) and cystoscopic resection. After complete resection, these patients undergo close surveillance with frequent (every 3 to 6 months) cystoscopic evaluation of their bladder to identify recurrent tumors.

Patients with high-grade, recurrent, or invasive bladder cancer are recommended to undergo radical cystectomy if suitable operative candidates. In male patients, the bladder, prostate, and pelvic lymph nodes are removed; in female patients, the bladder, uterus, fallopian tubes, ovaries, and anterior vagina are removed.

Alternative management strategies in patients who meet indications for radical cystectomy include administration of radiation and chemotherapy or partial resection of the bladder; however, these strategies are not a definitive or effective as is radical cystectomy.

Other Malignancies

Less common oncologic indications for removal of the bladder include gynecologic malignancy (vagina and uterus) and rectal malignancy, which locally invades the bladder necessitating cystectomy in appropriately selected patients.

Benign Indications for Urinary Diversion

Neurogenic Bladder

Neurogenic bladder is a generalized term describing bladder dysfunction caused by neurologic impairment of the central and peripheral nervous system, which innervates the bladder. Several conditions can result in neurogenic bladder and include stroke, multiple sclerosis, spinal cord trauma, diabetes, and postsurgical injury (radical hysterectomy, rectal surgery, spine surgery). These patients can have several bladder manifestations, namely, urinary incontinence, urinary retention, detrusor overactivity (irritable bladder), or high-pressure storage of urine. In a majority of cases, conservative medical and surgical management is adequate to treat neurogenic bladder; however, in severe cases, urinary diversion can be utilized as a last resort.

Radiation Cystitis

Patients who undergo radiation to their pelvis for treatment of malignancy (prostate, rectum, cervix/uterus) may develop incapacitating symptoms as a result of radiation-induced damage to the bladder and sphincter. This bladder damage can result in urinary incontinence, refractory bleeding, poorly compliant bladder, or painful bladder sensations with filling (Ratner, 2001). In cases refractory to medical management, urinary diversion is employed to divert the urine away from the bladder. These patients typically undergo ileal conduit diversions, since complication rates are higher in more complex continent diversions, especially in patients who have undergone radiation.

Interstitial Cystitis

Interstitial cystitis is a painful disorder of the bladder with unknown etiology. Patients typically present with pelvic/bladder pain with associated bladder symptoms (urgency, frequency, nocturia). These patients have negative findings in laboratory and urine studies and oftentimes have small ulcerations or petechial hemorrhage on cystoscopy. Only in refractory cases do these patients undergo urinary diversion and are good candidates for both incontinent and continent urinary diversions. After surgery, some patients continue to experience pelvic pain, and it is of paramount importance that these patients have appropriate preoperative counseling.

Trauma

Severe pelvic trauma resulting in partial or complete disruption of the urethra from the bladder may cause scarring and subsequent stricturing or the urethra. Patients with a severely strictured urethra who fail attempts to reconstruct the urethra typically drain their bladder with indwelling suprapubic catheters, which must be changed every 4 weeks to minimize infection and clogging. Some patients opt to have urinary diversion to avoid the use of an indwelling catheter.

Trauma involving the urinary sphincter can result in severe incontinence, which can be quite distressing to patients and negatively affect their quality of life. Furthermore, continuous leakage of urine results in perineal and sacral tissue breakdown and can negatively impair healing of sacral decubitus ulcers in patients with limited mobility and confined to their beds. Continent and incontinent urinary diversions are often performed depending on the patient's preferences and physical limitations.

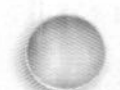

Surgical Procedures

Incontinent Urinary Diversions

Ileal Conduit

Incontinent urinary conduit in the form of an enterocutaneous stoma is a mainstay of urinary diversion. The ileum remains the most common segment of intestine used to create a conduit as it has the lowest complication rate and is most familiar to urologists. The ileal conduit may be the least cumbersome urinary diversion to manage from a patient perspective, as it only requires minor care of the stomal site and changing of the ostomy pouching system every 3 to 4 days. From a surgical perspective, the ileal conduit is the easiest to construct and requires shorter operative times.

Physician Considerations

Several factors are considered preoperatively when deciding what type of urinary diversion to construct for a patient. For patients with diseased intestine or multiple previous bowel resections, it is often preferred to maintain as much intestinal length as possible. Incontinent diversion requires shorter lengths of bowel (approximately 10 to 12 cm) compared to continent diversion (50 to 60 cm). Continent diversions are more technically challenging and may increase operative time, complication rate, and reoperation rate, compared to ileal conduits.

A history of prior pelvic radiation is a consideration when choosing the segment of bowel to use, as the ileum and sigmoid colon may have been included in the radiation field. A transverse colon conduit might be constructed in this circumstance.

Patient Considerations

Patient-specific factors are also important to consider. Undergoing urinary diversion can drastically alter body image. Patients who have ileal conduits must be willing to accept having a stoma on their abdomen and wearing pouching system to collect their urine. For continent cutaneous diversions, a minimal dressing is often placed over the small catheterizable stoma allowing patients to conceal their stoma. Patients with orthotopic urinary diversion or neobladders void via their urethra and do not have disfigurement of their abdomen with a stoma.

Patients who undergo continent diversion need to have sufficient general health, manual dexterity (i.e., ability to perform self-catheterization), motivation, and understanding to reliably manage their diversions. Patients who lack these qualities are better candidates for ileal conduit diversion, which is significantly easier to manage.

Regardless of continent or incontinent diversion choice, multiple studies have been performed without clear consensus of superior quality of life in patients with continent or incontinent urinary diversions (Gerharz et al., 2005).

Preoperative Considerations

Preoperative medical and cardiac clearance is performed to ensure that patient comorbidities are optimized before undergoing any intestinal urinary diversion. Specifically to urinary diversion, a preoperative consultation by the WOC nurse is critical for an optimal outcome. The visit is important for patient education, choice of preferred diversion type, and determination and marking of stoma site.

Some urologists choose to employ a mechanical and/or antibiotic preoperative bowel regimen. The goal is to decrease intestinal bacterial load in an effort to limit infectious complications. Mechanical preparations may include GoLytely, Fleet, Miralax, or magnesium citrate. All patients receive preoperative intravenous antibiotics immediately before surgery, which are usually stopped within 24 hours.

Surgical Procedure

The most distal 12- to 15-cm segment of ileum just proximal to the ileocecal valve is typically spared given its importance for bile salt and vitamin B_{12} absorption. A 10- to 12-cm segment of ileum proximal to this is identified. Transillumination of the mesentery is performed to ensure adequate blood supply to the segment. Surgical staplers are used to transect the bowel at each end of the conduit to isolate segment, and an anastomosis is performed to reestablish continuity of the bowel. It is important to maintain orientation of the conduit so that peristalsis is in the direction of urine flow.

Ureterointestinal anastomosis is performed in a refluxing manner near the proximal portion of the conduit over a stent, which aids in healing. There is some controversy over refluxing versus nonrefluxing anastomosis with some favoring nonrefluxing in an attempt to limit transmission of pressure and bacteria to the upper urinary tracts. While the nonrefluxing type is more technically challenging, it also has a higher stricture rate. There is no clear consensus as to an overall benefit of one method over the other (Kristjánsson et al., 1995).

There are a variety of methods to manage the proximal end of the conduit. Some surgeons suture and/or excise the staple line in order to prevent urine from contacting the staples in an effort to prevent future stone formation. The distal portion of the conduit is delivered through the skin, and the staple line is excised. The stoma is matured with multiple sutures to form a rosebud appearance (**Fig. 6-1**). This elevated rosebud-shaped stoma limits the amount of urine that directly contacts the skin when an external stoma appliance is applied.

Particularly in obese patients with a thick, short mesentery, a loop end ileostomy (Turnbull) can be performed. This allows creation of an ileal conduit with less tension, which may be required in these patients. If performed, a small rod is left in place temporarily through the mesentery at the skin level to prevent stomal retraction.

CLINICAL PEARL

A loop end (sometimes called an end loop) stoma will have a rod or support bridge under the bowel for support until healing takes place. The removal of the rod will depend upon the patient's potential to heal and the amount of tension over the rod. The time the rod remains in place can vary from 5 days to 3 weeks after surgery.

Postoperative Care

The ureterointestinal anastomoses are performed over ureteral stents in order to maintain patency and allow proper healing. The distal aspect of a stent exits the stoma and can be a variety of colors or sizes. They may be sutured into place and empty directly into the pouching system. The stents are typically left in place anywhere from 5 days to 2 weeks after surgery depending upon the surgeon's preference. Care must be taken with initial appliance changes

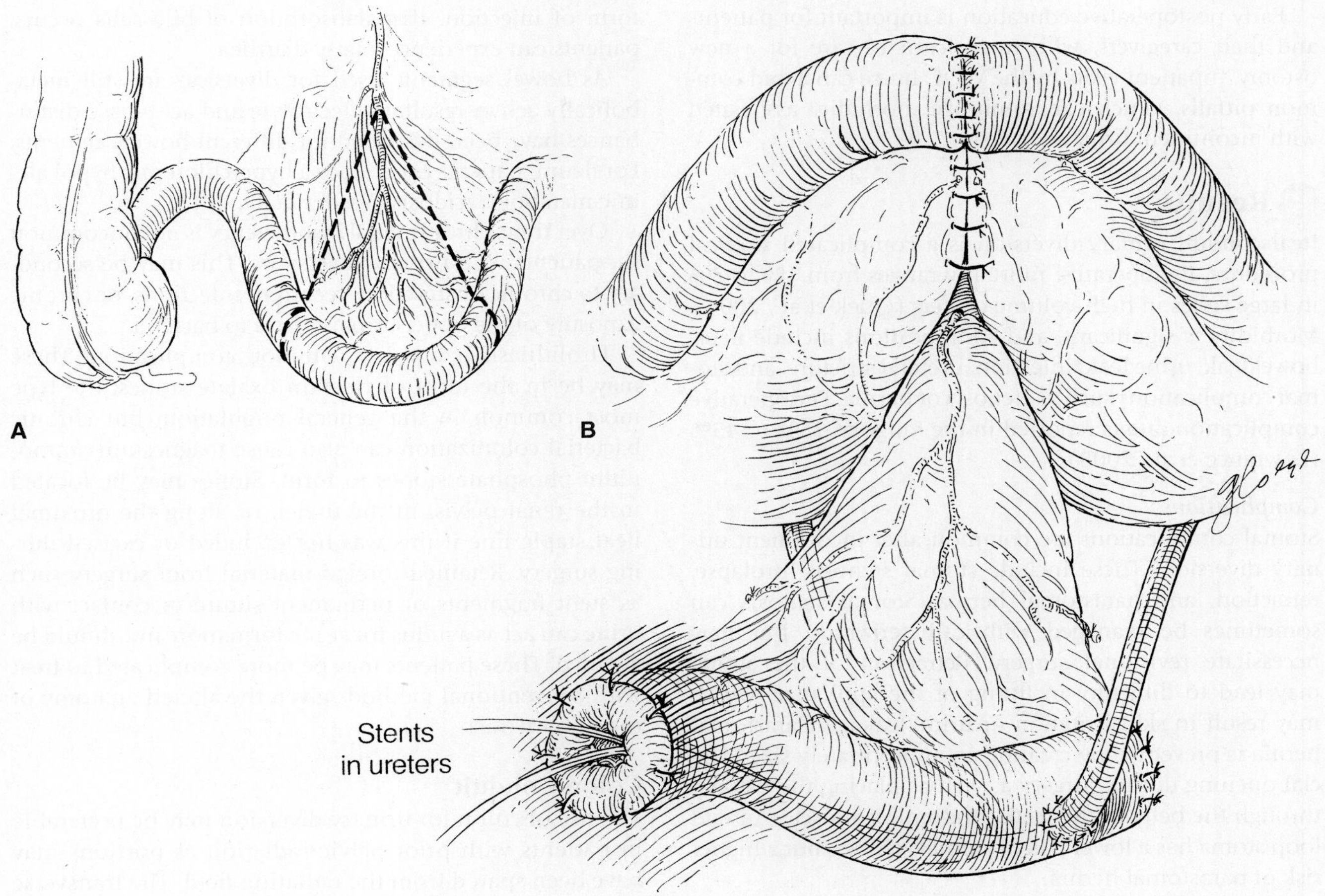

FIGURE 6-1. Ileal urinary conduit. **A.** A segment of nonirradiated ileum is used for the conduit. **B.** The ileum is reanastomosed, and the ureters are sewn into the "butt" end of the conduit. Note that ureters are stented individually.

not to dislodge the stents. Some surgeons choose to leave a catheter in the stoma to ensure adequate healing and drainage during the first initial days after surgery.

CLINICAL PEARL

Many surgeons will cut at least on stent on an angle to designate the right or left ureter. If the stents require shortening, a close examination of the stents should be performed prior to shortening (be sure to keep the cut on an angle).

Additionally, a closed suction, Jackson-Pratt or Blake drain is typically placed during surgery near the ureteroileal anastomosis and attached to bulb suction. This acts to diagnose and drain any urine leakage. This drain is typically removed before discharge as long as no significant leak is identified.

Some surgeons leave a nasogastric tube in place after surgery, which is removed at some point before initiating diet. Most practitioners await return of bowel function before starting any substantial oral intake. Early ambulation is critical in the prevention of deep vein thrombosis. A typical uncomplicated postoperative stay is between 5 and 10 days.

Early postoperative education is important for patients and their caregivers, who must learn to care for a new ostomy. Inpatient visits by the WOC nurse can avoid common pitfalls, which can minimize morbidity associated with incontinent urinary diversion.

Results

Ileal conduit urinary diversion is a complicated surgical procedure. Perioperative mortality ranges from 1% to 3% in large series in high-volume centers (Quek et al., 2006). Morbidity is significant, and complications include ileus, bowel leak, urine leak, infection, ureteral stricture, and stomal complications such as stenosis or hernia. Perioperative complication rate is reported in the range of 25% to 45% (Lowrance et al., 2008).

Complications

Stomal complications are common after incontinent urinary diversion. These include stomal stenosis, prolapse, retraction, and parastomal hernia. Stomal stenosis can sometimes be managed with catheterization but may necessitate revisional surgery. Retraction of the stoma may lead to difficulty in fitting of the appliance, which may result in skin irritation or urine leakage. Parastomal hernia is prevented by creating an appropriately sized fascial opening during surgery as well as placing the ostomy through the belly of the rectus abdominis muscle. An end loop stoma has a lower risk of stomal stenosis but a higher risk of parastomal hernia.

The ureterointestinal anastomoses may also be the source of complication, predominantly stricture or leak. Due to the more extensive mobilization of the left ureter, the left side is more commonly affected. Management of ureterointestinal stricture can be performed endoscopically with dilation/incision of the stricture with placement of ureteral stent; however, the most definitive and successful management strategy is open surgical revision. A fraction of these strictures may represent urothelial cancer as the ureteral margin may be a site of disease recurrence (Fichtner, 1999).

Infectious complications are common, especially in the initial period after urinary diversion. These may be in the form of abdominal abscess, urine leak, bowel leak, pyelonephritis, or wound infection. Treatment includes antibiotics and adequate drainage of any infectious collection. Patients with incontinent bowel diversion will commonly have chronic bacteriuria, and a majority of asymptomatic patients will have positive urine cultures. These patients are oftentimes treated inappropriately with repeated rounds of antibiotics resulting in multidrug-resistant organisms. Antibiotics should be reserved for patients with other clinical signs of infection.

The distal ileum is active in the absorption of vitamin B_{12} and bile salts. Vitamin B_{12} deficiency can potentially develop years after urinary diversion. Some practitioners routinely monitor and replace it as needed, often in the form of injection. If malabsorption of bile salts occurs, patients can experience a fatty diarrhea.

As bowel segments used for diversion are still metabolically active, resultant electrolyte and acid–base disturbances have been described for different bowel segments. For ileum, patients experience a hyperchloremic hypokalemic metabolic acidosis (Vasdev et al., 2013).

Over time, chronic renal insufficiency is not uncommon for patients with urinary diversions. This may be secondary to chronic obstruction, recurrent infections, or chronic exposure of the upper urinary tracts to bacteria.

Urolithiasis is another common complication. These may be in the form of calcium oxalate stones, the type most common in the general population, but chronic bacterial colonization can also cause magnesium ammonium phosphate stones to form. Stones may be located in the renal pelvis, in the ureter, or along the proximal ileal staple line if this was not excluded or excised during surgery. Retained foreign material from surgery such as stent fragments or permanent suture in contact with urine can act as a nidus for stone formation and should be avoided. These patients may be more complicated to treat with conventional methods given the altered anatomy of the urinary tract.

Colon Conduit

The use of colon for urinary diversion may be preferable in patients with prior pelvic radiation as portions may have been spared from the radiation field. The transverse colon is outside most radiation templates and is appropriate for use. A colon conduit urinary diversion may also be preferable in a patient with an existing colostomy for stool as it can obviate the need for bowel anastomosis and its associated morbidity.

Surgical Procedure

Sigmoid or transverse colon is most commonly used for creation of a colon urinary conduit. The steps are similar to creation of an ileal conduit. Directionality is maintained, and identification of adequate blood supply is critical. The segment of colon is taken out of continuity, and a bowel anastomosis is performed as previously described.

Postoperative Care

Immediate postoperative care is similar to an ileal conduit.

Complications

The stoma is slightly larger secondary to the caliber of colon, and therefore, stomal stenosis is less common. Otherwise, complications are similar. Patients with colonic urinary diversion also may experience a hyperchloremic hypokalemic metabolic acidosis.

Continent Urinary Diversions

Cutaneous Catheterizable Urinary Diversion

Cutaneous catheterizable urinary diversions involve the creation of an intestinal reservoir with an intestinal channel (catheterizable channel) that is brought from the reservoir to the skin. A variety of bowel segments can be used to create the reservoir (colon, ileum) as well as the catheterizable channel (colon, ileum, appendix). Generally, the continence between the reservoir and catheterizable channel is provided by either anatomic (i.e., ileocecal valve) or surgically constructed valves. The catheterizable channel must be catheterized several times during the day to empty the reservoir. It is imperative that any patient undergoing catheterizable continent urinary diversions has adequate mental capacity and hand–eye coordination to perform catheterizations multiple times per day.

Indiana Pouch

The Indiana pouch has become the predominant urinary diversion for patients who desire a continent catheterizable urinary diversion. Compared to orthotopic neobladders, patients do not need to have a patent urethra or a functional urinary sphincter. Indiana pouches can be performed in instances where the small intestinal segments are unable to reach the urethra in patients planned to undergo orthotopic neobladders; Indiana pouches are used as second-line continent urinary diversion in these instances (Rowland, 1996).

Contraindications for continent catheterizable channels include hepatic dysfunction, compromised intestinal function (i.e., previous surgery, radiation, inflammatory bowel disease), and renal failure (serum creatinine >1.7).

Physician Considerations

Indiana pouches are constructed from the terminal ileum, ileocecal valve, and right colon, and thus, these segments must be present (no prior resection, no significant disease burden, i.e., Crohn's disease) in order to perform this diversion. Furthermore, the ileocecal valve must be functional as incompetence of this valve may result in leakage of urine from the valve (incontinence).

Patient Considerations

With any continent catheterizable diversion, patients must have both the mental capacity and motivation to maintain their urinary diversion, which requires frequent self-catheterizations and occasional irrigation of mucus from the reservoir of the Indiana pouch. Sufficient manual dexterity to perform self-catheterization is also critical. From a cosmetic standpoint, patients must accept the appearance of the catheterizable channel; however, the small stoma of the catheterizable channel can be easily concealed with a dressing (Lee et al., 2014).

Preoperative Considerations

Patients should undergo evaluation and stoma marking by the WOC nurse. This is an opportunity to determine the patient's motivation, manual dexterity, and mental capacity. Selection of stoma site is determined on the right lower quadrant with consideration of belt line, skin folds, and ease of visualization by the patient.

Similar to patients undergoing ileal conduits, some urologists choose to employ a mechanical and/or antibiotic preoperative bowel regimen. All patients receive preoperative intravenous antibiotics immediately before surgery, which are usually stopped within 24 hours.

Surgical Procedure

The Indiana pouch is created from 10 to 12 cm of ileum (catheterizable channel), the ileocecal valve (continence mechanisms), and the right colon (reservoir). This segment of bowel is mobilized and discontinued from the remaining small and large bowel. Bowel continuity is reestablished by anastomosis of the ileum to the transverse colon using surgical staplers.

Next, the right colon is detubularized by incising it along its length to disrupt the muscular connections of the bowel (**Fig. 6-2**). Care is taken to avoid incising the ileocecal valve and terminal ileum. The ureters are passed through the posterior wall of the detubularized right colon and are secured to the inside of the pouch. These ureteral anastomoses are refluxing. Lastly, ureteral catheters or stents are placed into the ureters to protect the anastomoses and aid in their healing.

The detubularized right colon is folded over in a clamshell fashion and sutured closed, thus forming the reservoir for urine. Once closed, a 24-Fr Malecot catheter is placed into the reservoir thru a stab wound, and the ureteral stents are passed out of the reservoir.

The distal ileum forms the catheterizable channel and is tapered over a 14- to 16-Fr catheter by stapling on the antimesenteric side of the bowel to remove excess bowel. The reservoir is filled with normal saline via the Malecot catheter to make sure that ileocecal valve maintains continence preventing urine leaking from the reservoir.

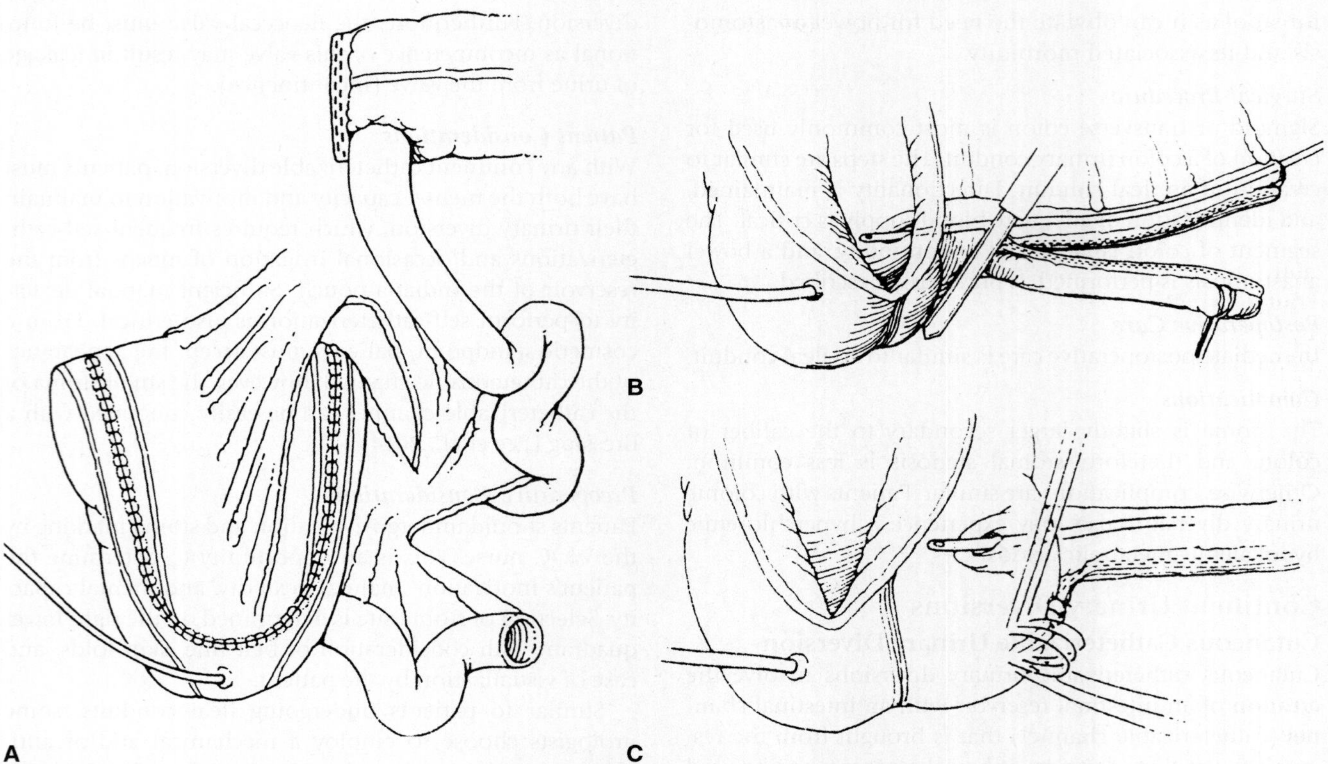

FIGURE 6-2. Indiana pouch. The entire right colon and 10 cm of distal ileum are isolated. The colon is incised along its antimesenteric border (making sure to preserve the ileocecal valve) and then folded upon itself in a Heineke-Mikulicz configuration. **A.** Prior to this step, however, the ureters are tunneled along the teniae in order to prevent reflux. The efferent ileal limb is tapered by imbrication over a 14-Fr catheter or, as performed by the authors, using a GIA stapler to remove excess ileum. **B.** The technique of ileocecal buttressing can be accomplished in several ways, including by taking purse-string sutures around the valve and apposing Lembert along the terminal ileum **(C)**.

The tapered ileum is then brought to the skin and secured while maintaining a straight path for catheterization.

Postoperative Care

The ureterointestinal anastomoses are performed over ureteral stents in order to maintain patency and allow proper healing. These stents are externalized and drain to gravity and are typically left for 1 to 2 weeks after which time they are pulled out if there is no evidence of urinary leak. A Jackson-Pratt or Blake drain is placed near the reservoir to drain excess fluid and monitor for urinary leak. The Jackson-Pratt or Blake drain is typically removed prior to discharge from the hospital if there is no evidence of urinary leak.

The 24-Fr Malecot catheter is used to drain the reservoir of the Indiana pouch during the immediate postoperative period. Irrigation of the reservoir is performed intermittently during the first several days after surgery to clear mucous and is titrated to a frequency that makes the mucus manageable. Initially, irrigation is with 30 to 60 mL of normal saline three times or more until irrigant is clear. This process should be performed four times per day and can be spaced out accordingly. The irrigant is introduced into the pouch and allowed to flow out without suction from the syringe.

CLINICAL PEARL

The patient and a family member should be taught how to irrigate the pouch prior to discharge. The patient should be discharged with a dependent drainage collector to use at night and a leg bag to use during the day.

A 16-Fr Foley is placed through the catheterizable channel into the reservoir and capped. This catheter maintains the patency of the catheterizable channel and is kept in place for at least 2 to 3 weeks after surgery.

Once the patient is ready to perform self-catheterization (2 to 3 weeks after the operation), the patient is taught to use sterile technique and catheterize the pouch every 2 to 4 hours. The patient starts with self-catheterization every 2 hours for 1 week, then every 3 hours for week 2 to 3, and then every 4 hours for week four and onward. The patient can increase catheterization if he/she has an increase in fluid intake. During this initial learning period, the Malecot catheter is capped, but it can be uncapped and drained should the patient encounter difficulty in catheterizing.

Once the patient has proven the ability to perform intermittent catheterization, the Malecot catheter is removed. Some urologists choose to perform a pouchogram whereby the reservoir is filled with contrast and x-ray imaging is performed to ensure there is no urinary leak prior to removal of the Malecot catheter.

A small dressing or Band-Aid can be placed over the catheterizable site for protection. With time, the reservoir will expand between 300 and 500 mL. The patient will achieve increased independence as the frequency between catheterization increases.

Early postoperative education is important for patients and their caregivers, who must learn to care for the new continent catheterizable urinary diversion. Inpatient visits by the WOC nurse can avoid common pitfalls, which can minimize morbidity associated with continent catheterizable urinary diversion.

CLINICAL PEARL

The patient should be instructed to carry at least two catheters with him or her at all times along with self-closing plastic bags in which he or she can place the used catheters if he or she is unable to cleanse the tube after using.

Lastly, patients should obtain medical alert bracelets to inform other caregivers of the catheterizable channel in the event of an emergency.

Results

The primary objective of a continent urinary diversion is to maintain continence, with a low-pressure, high-volume reservoir, which allows urine to exit via catheterization at reasonable intervals. With time, the capacity of the Indiana pouch increases to 300 to 500 mL, and the incidence of urinary incontinence at 1 year is <2% (Rowland, 1996).

Complications

Similar to patients undergoing ileal conduit diversion, morbidity is significant, and complications include ileus, bowel leak, parastomal hernia, urine leak, infection/pouchitis, urinary stone formation, metabolic alterations (metabolic acidosis, B_{12} deficiency), and ureteral stricture (Kouba et al., 2007; Vasdev et al., 2013). Strictures of the stoma or catheterizable channel can make catheterization difficult and often requires endoscopic incision or dilation. Rupture of the pouch can occur in patients due to poor compliance with catheterization and can be life threatening.

Other Catheterizable Urinary Diversion

While the Indiana pouch is the most predominantly utilized catheterizable urinary diversion, several other catheterizable urinary diversions have been developed over the years. In a Miami pouch, the bowel segments used are the same as the Indiana pouch; however, cutting the ascending colon and folding it into a U shape and construct the reservoir. The Koch pouch is constructed by folding 60 cm of ileum into a U shape and creating proximal and distal nipple valves. The ureters are anastomosed to the proximal valve, and the distal valve is brought to the skin as a catheterizable stoma. In a Mitrofanoff procedure, the appendix is used as the catheterizable channel. The proximal end is tunneled into the mucosa of the reservoir, which serves as the continence mechanism, and the distal end of the appendix is brought to the skin.

Orthotopic Urinary Diversion

Orthotopic urinary diversion, also called a neobladder, involves the creation of a low-pressure, high-volume reservoir that is anastomosed to the urethra. Patients rely on their urinary sphincter for continence and void by relaxing their sphincter and pelvic floor in combination with increasing intra-abdominal pressure by performing Valsalva or Credé maneuver. A minority of patients will develop hypercontinence (inability to empty) and will need to perform intermittent self-catheterization to adequately empty their neobladder.

Orthotopic urinary diversion is created in patients who want improved cosmesis (no stoma) and wish to void per urethra. Neobladder diversions are occasionally performed on patients with a large body habitus where bringing a conduit or continent catheterizable channel to the skin is technically difficult.

Similar to continent catheterizable diversion, absolute contraindications for orthotopic urinary diversions include hepatic dysfunction, compromised intestinal function (e.g., previous surgery, radiation, inflammatory bowel disease), and renal failure (serum creatinine >1.7). Specific to orthotopic urinary diversion, patients should have a competent urinary sphincter and no evidence of urethral obstruction (Lee et al., 2014).

Physician Considerations

Orthotopic urinary diversions typically are constructed from 50 to 60 cm of ileum, and thus, these segments must be present (no prior resection) and healthy (no inflammatory bowel disease, no radiation damage) in order to perform this diversion. In oncologic cases, patients must have no disease at the bladder neck or urethra and have a low risk of cancer recurrence. Having a history of prior pelvic radiation significantly increases the complexity of the surgery and the complication rate postoperatively and must be considered prior to performing a neobladder diversion.

Patient Considerations

Patients must be motivated and mentally capable of performing the more rigorous maintenance of their neobladder compared to ileal conduit diversion. Maintenance includes scheduled voiding every 2 to 3 hours and performing self-catheterizations if needed to empty their reservoir or irrigate mucus that may accumulate within the reservoir. Patients with poor mental capacity, social support, and general health should undergo ileal conduit diversion.

Preoperative Consideration

In the event that during the surgical procedure it is determined an orthotopic urinary diversion cannot be created, patients should undergo evaluation and stoma siting by the WOC nurse to mark for either a continent catheterizable channel or ileal conduit. This is another opportunity to determine the patient's motivation, manual dexterity, and mental capacity.

Similar to patients undergoing ileal conduits and continent catheterizable channels, some urologists choose to employ a mechanical and/or antibiotic preoperative bowel regimen. All patients receive preoperative intravenous antibiotics immediately before surgery, which are typically stopped within 24 hours.

Surgical Procedure

In male patients, the bladder and prostate are removed, while in female patients, the bladder, anterior vagina, uterus, fallopian tubes, and ovaries are removed. In both instances, care is taken to perform meticulous dissection near the urethra and urinary sphincter to preserve continence.

Reservoirs are typically created from 50 to 60 cm of ileum, which is mobilized and discontinued from the remaining bowel. Continuity of the bowel is reestablished using bowel staplers. Next, the bowel is detubularized by incising it on the antimesenteric side.

There are two main types of orthotopic neobladders that are commonly performed: the Studer and Hautmann neobladders. The main differences between these diversions are the shape the bowel is folded when constructing the reservoir. In a Studer diversion, the bowel is folded over in a U configuration (**Fig. 6-3**), while in a Hautmann diversion, the bowel is folded to create an M or W configuration (**Fig. 6-4**).

After the posterior plate of the reservoir is sutured, the ureters are anastomosed to the neobladder in an end-to-side fashion over a stent, which is placed up the ureter to protect the anastomosis and aids in healing. The anterior plate of the reservoir is next closed with suture. The ureteral stents are brought out of the neobladder, and a 24-Fr Malecot catheter is placed through the skin into the neobladder and secured.

Lastly, a small buttonhole opening is created in the most dependent portion of the neobladder, which is used as the anastomosis to the urethra.

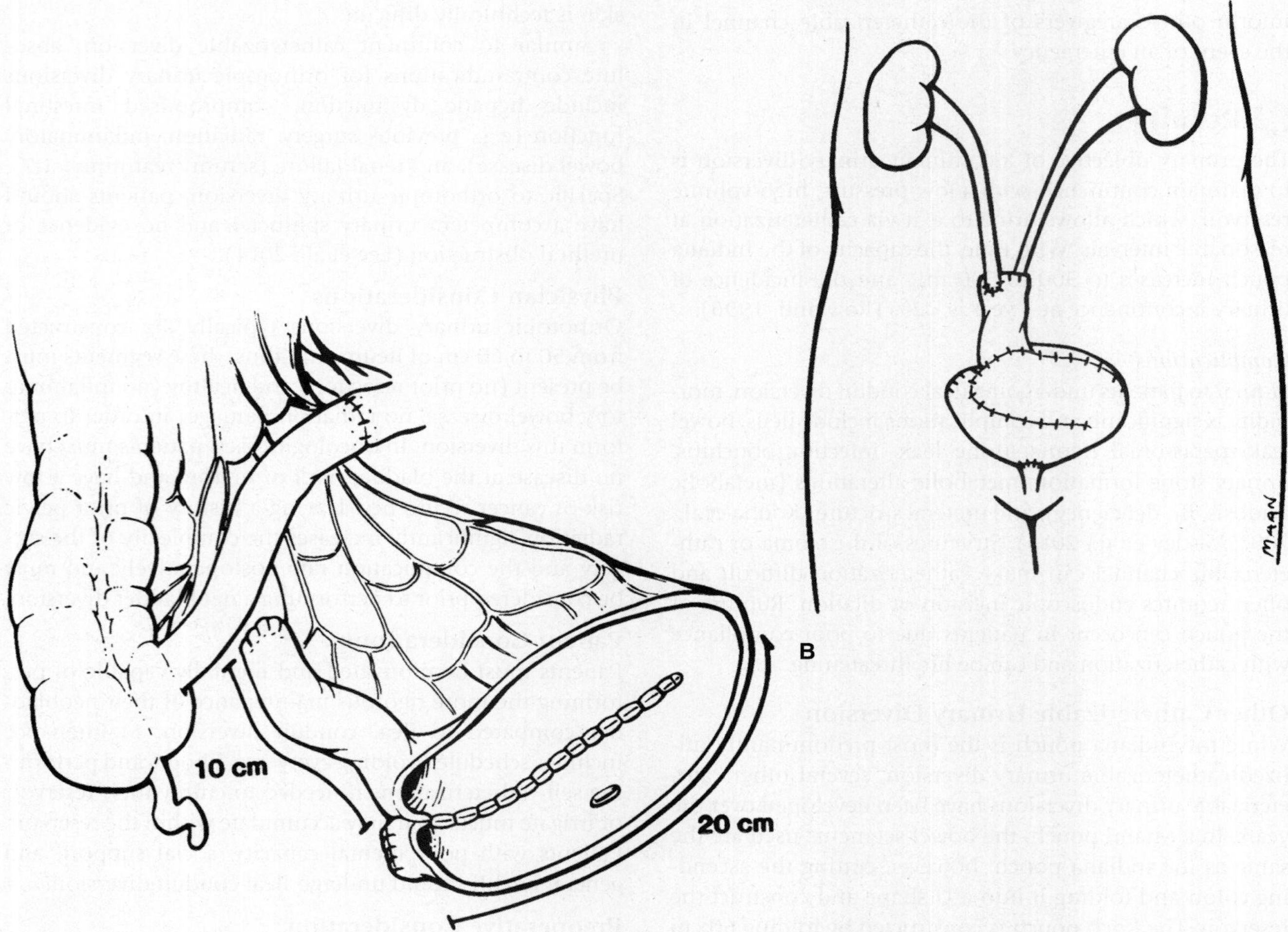

FIGURE 6-3. Studer neobladder. **A.** A U-shaped pouch is created from 40 cm of ileum while sparing the terminal 15 cm. Another proximal 15-cm segment of ileum acts as the "chimney" into which the ureters are reimplanted. **B.** The bottom of the pouch is closed up, but not before the most dependent portion is brought down and anastomosed to the urethra.

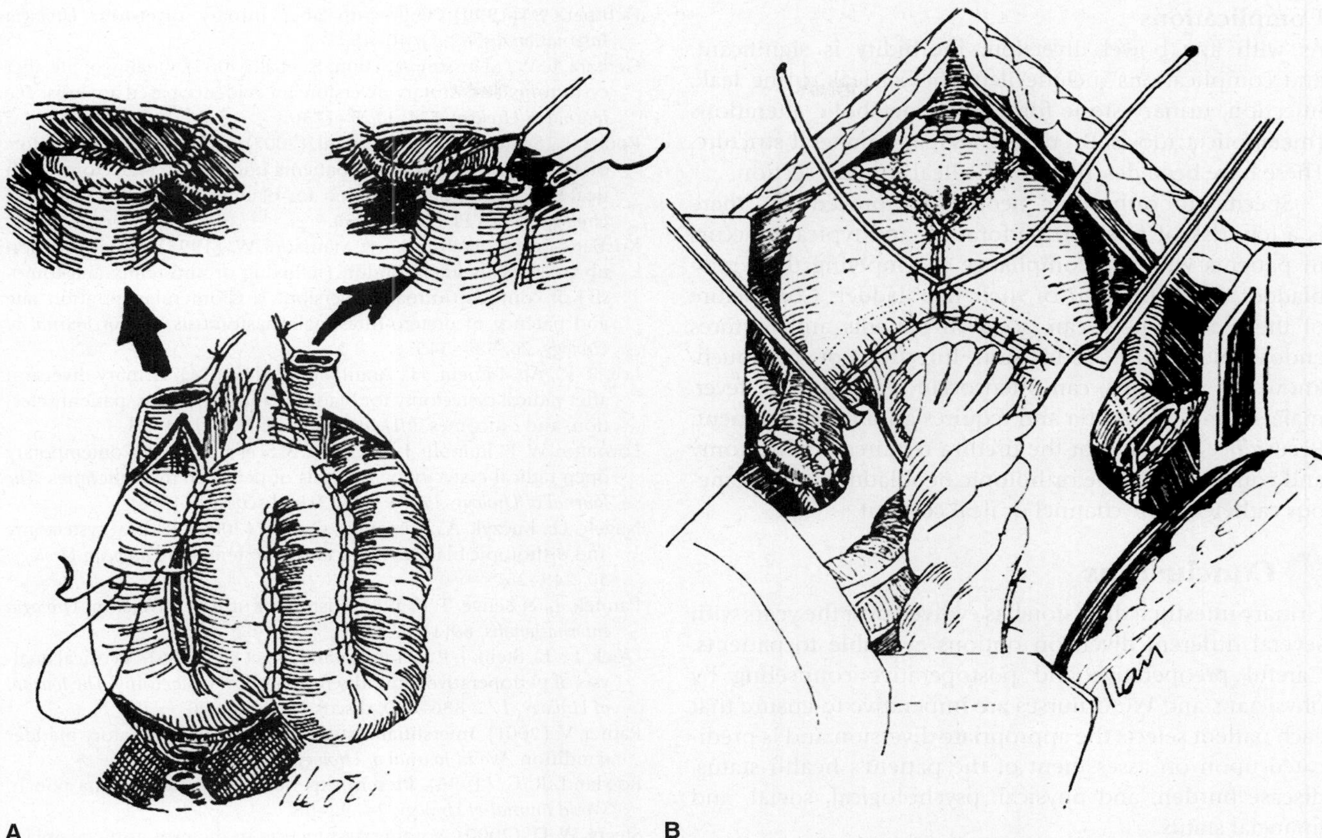

A B

FIGURE 6-4. **A.** The modified Hautmann neobladder technique with refluxing ileoureteral anastomosis using chimneys of 3- to 5-cm afferent limb on each side. **B.** Final aspect of neobladder, ileourethral, and ileoureteral anastomoses.

Postoperative Care

The ureteral stents are externalized and allowed to drain to gravity. They are typically left for 1 to 2 weeks after which time if there is no evidence of urinary leak they are removed. A Jackson-Pratt or Blake drain is placed near the reservoir to drain excess fluid and is typically removed prior to discharge from the hospital if there is no evidence of urinary leak.

The 24-Fr Malecot catheter is externalized and is used to drain and irrigate the reservoir of the neobladder during the immediate postoperative period. Irrigation of the reservoir is performed intermittently during the first several days after surgery and is titrated to a frequency that makes the mucus manageable.

A 22-Fr Foley is placed through the urethra into the reservoir and is also used to drain and irrigate the neobladder. The catheter aids in the healing of the anastomosis between the neobladder and urethra. It is kept in place for at least 2 to 3 weeks after surgery.

Once the patient is ready to start voiding, the urethral Foley is removed and the 24-Fr Malecot catheter is capped. During this initial learning period, the Malecot catheter can be uncapped and drained should the patient encounter difficulty in emptying the neobladder. The 24-Fr Malecot catheter is removed once the patient is comfortable and proficient at emptying their neobladder per the urethra.

Emptying of the neobladder relies on relaxation of the urethral sphincter and pelvic floor in combination with increasing intra-abdominal pressure by performing Valsalva or Credé maneuver. Patients should be taught how to perform self-intermittent catheterization if they are unable to completely empty their neobladder or need to irrigate accumulated mucus. Patients should also perform pelvic floor exercises to aid in strengthening their urinary sphincter and pelvic floor. Patients often develop nighttime incontinence and need to set an alarm clock to one to two times per night to empty their neobladder and prevent overflow incontinence.

As with continent catheterizable urinary diversion, patients with neobladders should wear medical alert bracelets stating that they have a "continent internal urinary diversion."

Results

There is a general improvement with continence from 6 to 12 months when the neobladder increases in capacity to around 300 to 500 mL. Daytime continence rates are generally >90% based on results from pooled series with nighttime continence rates of 80% to 90% (Steers, 2000). Failure to empty the neobladder has been reported to be 4% to 25% necessitating intermittent self-catheterization (Nagele et al., 2006; Steers, 2000).

Complications

As with any bowel diversion, morbidity is significant, and complications include ileus, bowel leak, urine leak, infection, urinary stone formation, metabolic alterations (metabolic acidosis, B_{12} deficiency), and ureteral stricture. These have been described in the ileal conduit section.

Specific to orthotopic neobladder procedures, there is a low risk of reservoir perforation and typically occurs in patients with noncompliance in emptying their neobladder or obstruction of their neobladder. Contracture of the bladder neck can occur in patients and requires endoscopic dilation or incision. Infections of the pouch, known as pouchitis, can often occur causing pain, fever, malaise, and hematuria and requires antibiotic treatment. Recurrence of cancer at the urethra requires urethrectomy and conversion of the orthotopic neobladder to a cutaneous catheterizable channel or ileal conduit.

Conclusions

Urinary intestinal diversion has evolved over the years with several different diversion options available to patients. Careful preoperative and postoperative counseling by physicians and WOC nurses are imperative to ensure that each patient selects the appropriate diversion and is predicated upon on assessment of the patient's health status, disease burden, and physical, psychological, social, and financial status.

REFERENCES

Bladder Cancer Support Society. (2014). Accessed August 8-18, 2014. Retrieved from: http://bladdercancersupport.org/bladder-cancer-help/bladder-cancer-facts/statistics?gclid=CN_qhJyEnsACFYk7MgodTywAMA

Fichtner, J. (1999). Follow-up after urinary diversion. *Urologia Internationalis, 63*(1), 40–45.

Gerharz, E. W., Månsson, A., Hunt, S., et al. (2005). Quality of life after cystectomy and urinary diversion: an evidence based analysis. *The Journal of Urology, 174*, 1729–1736.

Kouba, E., Sands, M., Lentz, A., et al. (2007). Incidence and risk factors of stomal complications in patients undergoing cystectomy with ileal conduit urinary diversion for bladder cancer. *The Journal of Urology, 178*(3 Pt 1), 950–954.

Kristjánsson, A., Wallin, L., & Månsson, W. (1995). Renal function up to 16 years after conduit (refluxing or anti-reflux anastomosis) or continent urinary diversion. 1. Glomerular filtration rate and patency of uretero-intestinal anastomosis. *British Journal of Urology, 76*, 539–545.

Lee, R. K., Abol-Enein, H., Arani, W., et al. (2014). Urinary diversion after radical cystectomy for bladder cancer: Options, patient selection, and outcomes. *BJU International, 113(1)*, 11–23.

Lowrance, W. T., Rumohr, J. A., Chang, S. S, et al. (2008). Contemporary open radical cystectomy: Analysis of perioperative outcomes. *The Journal of Urology, 179*, 1313–1318; discussion 1318.

Nagele, U., Kuczyk, A., Aristotelis, G., et al (2006). Radical cystectomy and orthotopic bladder replacement in females. *European Urology, 50*, 249–257.

Pannek, J., & Senge, T. (1998). History of urinary diversion. *Urologia Internationalis, 60*(1), 1–10.

Quek, M. L., Stein, J. P., Daneshmand, S., et al. (2006). A critical analysis of perioperative mortality from radical cystectomy. *The Journal of Urology, 175*, 886–889; discussion 889–890.

Ratner, V. (2001). Interstitial cystitis: a chronic inflammatory bladder condition. *World Journal of Urology, 19(3)*, 157–159.

Rowland, R. G. (1996). Present experience with the Indiana pouch. *World Journal of Urology, 14*, 92–98.

Steers, W. D. (2000). Voiding dysfunction in the orthotopic neobladder. *World Journal of Urology, 18(5)*, 330–337.

Vasdev, N., Moon, A., & Thorpe, A. C. (2013). Metabolic complications of urinary intestinal diversion. *Indian Journal of Urology, 29(4)*, 310–315.

QUESTIONS

1. A patient with refractory cystitis is scheduled for surgery for a urinary diversion. Which diversion is a good choice for this patient as it involves the simplest segment of bowel and has the lowest complication rate?
   A. Ileal conduit
   B. Colon conduit
   C. Orthotopic neobladder
   D. Indiana pouch

2. Which disease state is the most predominant indication for performing an intestinal urinary diversion?
   A. Neurogenic bladder
   B. Refractory cystitis
   C. Bladder cancer
   D. Urinary fistula

3. Which patient would the WOC nurse place at greatest risk for bladder cancer?
   A. A patient who has diabetes mellitus
   B. A patient who smokes two packs of cigarettes a day
   C. A patient who drinks a six pack of beer a day
   D. A patient who has experienced trauma involving the urinary sphincter

4. A patient who presents with gross hematuria, which is typically painless and intermittent, should be screened for:
   A. Urinary tract infection
   B. Prostatitis
   C. Interstitial cystitis
   D. Bladder cancer

5. A patient with an identified bladder tumor would most likely undergo which diagnostic procedure to formulate a prognosis and manage the tumor therapeutically?
A. Contrast-enhanced CT scan of the kidneys
B. Bladder tumor resection
C. Endoscopic evaluation of the urethra and bladder
D. Urine cytology

6. A continence nurse is evaluating patients with bladder dysfunction in a urologist's office. Which patient would the nurse place at risk for neurogenic bladder?
A. A patient who has multiple sclerosis
B. A patient who has undergone radiation to the pelvis for a malignancy
C. A patient who presents with bladder pain, urgency, and nocturia
D. A patient who experienced trauma to the bladder

7. A WOC nurse evaluating the urine studies of a patient notes that the patient has petechial hemorrhage as a finding of cystoscopy. Which bladder disorder would the nurse suspect?
A. Bladder cancer
B. Neurogenic bladder
C. Interstitial cystitis
D. Trauma to the bladder

8. A surgeon is performing a continent diversion for a patient who has bladder cancer. What amount of bowel length would be required to create this type of diversion?
A. 10 to 15 cm
B. 15 to 30 cm
C. 40 to 50 cm
D. 50 to 60 cm

9. The most distal 12- to 15-cm segment of ileum just proximal to the ileocecal valve is typically spared during the surgical procedure for an ileal conduit given its importance for bile salt and:
A. Vitamin B_{12} absorption
B. Calcium absorption
C. Vitamin C absorption
D. Protein absorption

10. Which complication of an incontinent urinary diversion can sometimes be managed with catheterization, but may necessitate revisional surgery?
A. Prolapse
B. Retraction
C. Parastomal hernia
D. Stomal stenosis

11. Which urinary diversion is the predominant urinary diversion for patients who desire a continent catheterizable urinary diversion?
A. Indiana pouch
B. Colon conduit
C. Orthotopic urinary diversion
D. Mitrofanoff procedure

12. The WOC nurse is evaluating a patient for an orthotopic urinary diversion. What is a major patient consideration for creating this type of diversion?
A. Ease of maintenance
B. Improved cosmesis
C. No need for self-intermittent catheterization
D. Low risk of infection of the pouch

ANSWERS: 1.**A**, 2.**C**, 3.**B**, 4.**D**, 5.**B**, 6.**A**, 7.**C**, 8.**D**, 9.**A**, 10.**D**, 11.**A**, 12.**B**

CHAPTER 7

Fecal and Urinary Stoma Construction

Linda Stricker, Barbara Hocevar, and Jean Asburn

OBJECTIVE

Discuss construction of fecal and urinary stomas.

Topic Outline

- **Fecal Stoma Construction**
  - Stoma Maturation
  - Stoma Construction Types
    - End Stoma
    - Loop Stoma
    - Loop–End Stoma
  - Anatomic Classification
    - Duodenostomy
    - Jejunostomy
    - Ileostomy
    - Cecostomy
    - Colostomy
    - Mucous Fistula
- **Urinary Stoma Construction**
  - Types
    - Ureterostomy
    - Ileal Conduit
    - Jejunal Conduit
- **Conclusions**

A stoma is a surgically created opening in the gastrointestinal tract or within the urinary system. The word stoma comes from the Greek word for mouth. Writings about spontaneous stomas occur throughout history, and many of these stomas were originally the result of battle-related wounds or disease. Over the years, surgical techniques improved as did techniques for stoma construction. These advancements enhanced a surgeon's ability to treat disease or repair and minimize the effects of trauma, thereby saving lives (Wu, 2012). Optimizing quality of life and maintaining good health are now primary goals for a person with an ostomy. Preoperative stoma site marking, ideal stoma construction, and the promotion of self-care through postoperative fitting of ostomy system and management contribute to enhanced quality of life for the individual with a stoma.

There are a variety of classifications of stomas, including by level of permanence (temporary or lifelong), by anatomic name, or by surgical construction (Table 7-1). Temporary stomas usually remain in place for 3 to 6 months but may become permanent for 20% to 50% of individuals (Forgoine & Cataldo, 2003; Pine & Stevenson, 2014; Wexner et al., 1993; Kairaluoma et al., 2002). An example would be a patient with an ostomy after bowel resection that chooses to keep the stoma rather than undergoing another operation to restore bowel continuity.

There are two broad anatomic categories of abdominal stomas: fecal and urinary. Stomas are further anatomically categorized by construction as end, loop, and loop–end. The concept of maturation is important when discussing stomal construction and will be addressed first.

Fecal Stoma Construction

Stoma Maturation

Initially, stomas were created flush to skin level. This technique resulted in severe tissue destruction as stomas were very difficult to manage due to leaking of the pouching system. The concept of a spouted (non–skin level) stoma was introduced in 1913; however, this exposed the serosal layer of the intestine to the air, resulting in inflammation called serositis. As a result of serositis, there is massive edema of the stoma with a risk for partial or complete obstruction, diarrhea, fluid and electrolyte imbalances, and dehydration (Kaidar-Person et al., 2005; Martin & Vogel, 2012; Wu, 2012). Eventually, these stomas would self-mature.

TABLE 7-1 Stoma Classifications

Length of Time	Construction Type	Anatomic Location	
Temporary	End	Fecal	Urinary
Permanent	Loop	Colon	Conduit + bowel segment used
	Loop–end	Ileum	Ileum
	Continent	Jejunum	Sigmoid colon
		Duodenum	Jejunum
			Continent diversion

TABLE 7-2 Stoma Construction Types

Type of Stoma*	Features
End	One stoma with one opening
Loop	One stoma with two openings Proximal or functioning opening Distal or nonfunctioning opening
Loop–end	One stoma with two openings Used in patients with thick abdominal walls and possible vascular compromise if created as an end stoma

*Anatomic location dictates type, amount, and quality of effluent.

Maturation refers to the eversion of the bowel segment to expose the mucosa. Stomas not matured at surgery undergo self-maturation, a process that occurs when the inflamed and gummy serosal surfaces adhere to each other, causing a gradual eventual eversion of the stoma (Doughty, 2004).

Eversion of the bowel is a gradual process taking approximately 4 to 6 weeks. The stoma will look the same at the end of this process as a matured stoma. An unmatured stoma is difficult for patients to deal with due to the large size and dramatic appearance. The concept of eversion or primary maturation introduced by Dr. Bryan Brooke in 1952 paved the way for increased survival for the majority of individuals requiring ostomy surgery; this technique is referred to as a Brooke stoma (Kaidar-Person et al., 2005; Martin & Vogel, 2012; Wu, 2012). In primary maturation, the intestinal segment is brought through the predesignated site and everted, similar to cuffing a sleeve. The matured stoma will expose the inner mucosal lining of the bowel with a beefy red, shiny, and moist surface. There are stretch receptors, so patients may sometimes feel a stretch as the bowel content exits the stoma, particularly if a large, formed stool passes through similar to bowel motions encountered with a sigmoid colostomy.

CLINICAL PEARL

There are no sensory nerve endings in the stoma.

Stoma Construction Types

There are three anatomic stoma construction types: end, loop, and loop–end (Table 7-2).

CLINICAL PEARL

End stoma construction results in one stoma with one opening.

End Stoma

To create the end stoma, the surgeon, after surgical management of the disease process or traumatic event, prepares and mobilizes the bowel segment needed for the stoma. The well-vascularized bowel segment is then brought through a predetermined abdominal aperture to create the stoma (Fig. 7-1). This aperture is two fingerbreadths in size in order to minimize the risk of herniation or prolapse (Forgione & Cataldo, 2003; Garofalo, 2012; Martin & Vogel, 2012; Pine & Stevenson, 2014; Saunders & Hemingway, 2008; Stocchi, 2012). The application of sterile dressings or drapes protects the incision from possible fecal contamination; maturation of the stoma follows. The edge of this intestinal segment is everted using four equidistant sutures placed through the entire bowel wall followed by suturing through the subcuticular (dermal) layer of the adjacent skin (Fig. 7-2). This is done to prevent seeding of the epidermis with mucosal cells, which can result in peristomal mucosal implants.

It is important to bring a well-vascularized bowel segment through the abdominal wall without tension or twisting (Martin & Vogel, 2012; Saunders & Hemingway, 2008; Wu, 2003). Once full eversion is accomplished, additional sutures are added to complete the process, and the newly created stoma is ready for the appropriate pouching system (Garofalo, 2012). End ileostomies

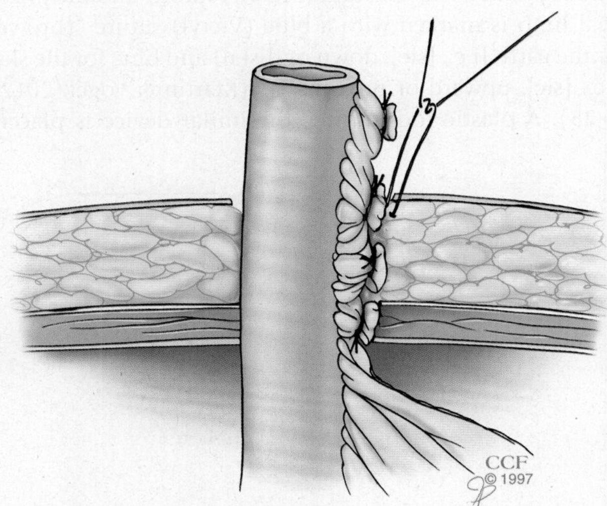

FIGURE 7-1. End ileostomy. The end of the ileum is brought through the preselected stoma site.

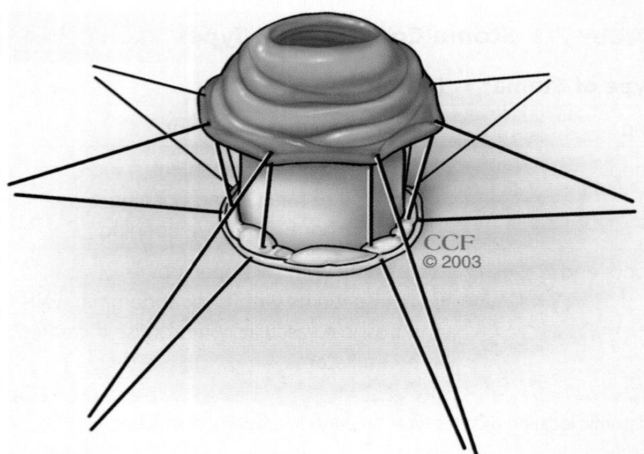

FIGURE 7-2. Stoma maturation. Absorbable sutures are placed through the full thickness of the bowel wall and secured to the subcuticular (dermal) layer of skin only. Full-thickness suturing of the skin (through the epidermis) can result in tracking of mucosal cells through the epidermis, resulting in mucosal implants.

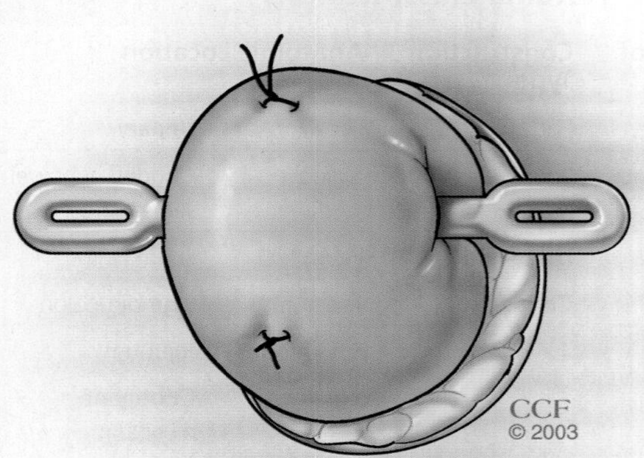

FIGURE 7-4. Loop ileostomy construction. Note the placement of sutures (each would be in a different color) that help maintain appropriate orientation of the proximal and distal portions of the intestine. The loop of the small bowel is brought out through the predetermined stoma site, and a rod is placed underneath the intestine and on top of the skin in order to provide support to the intestinal loop.

should protrude from the skin approximately 2 to 3 cm (Martin & Vogel, 2012; Stocchi, 2012). The formation of a spout should prohibit the effluent from going beneath the pouching system (Fig. 7-3). End colostomies should protrude, but flush construction may also occur (Forgione & Cataldo, 2003; Garofalo, 2012; Martin & Vogel, 2005; Saunders & Hemingway, 2008).

Loop Stoma

In general, loop stoma construction usually protects a distal anastomosis or diverts from a downstream obstruction. After completion of the surgery on the distal intestinal anastomosis, the surgeon brings a loop of intestine, usually located 12 to 15 cm from the ileocecal valve for an ileostomy (Martin & Vogel, 2012), through a predetermined site on the abdomen. It is important that the proximal and distal ends of the intestine are properly identified in order to maintain appropriate anatomic orientation. The distal limb is marked with a catgut (brown) suture, and the proximal limb is marked with a blue (Vicryl) suture "(brown for the earth [i.e., [sic], down or distal] and blue for the sky [i.e., [sic], upward or proximal])" (Martin & Vogel, 2012, p. 25). A plastic rod, tubing, or similar device is placed under the loop of intestine to provide support in order to prevent early retraction of the stoma (Fig. 7-4).

After closing the abdominal wounds, sterile dressings or towels protect the incision from contamination when opening the bowel. The intestine is then cut open about 5/8ths of its circumference. The intestine remains joined along its mesenteric or inside edge, and maturation of the two cut edges creates one stoma with two openings (Figs. 7-5 and 7-6). The proximal opening is the functional lumen through which effluent will pass. The distal lumen leads to the lower intestine; a small quantity of mucus will occasionally pass from the distal lumen or anus. The proximal

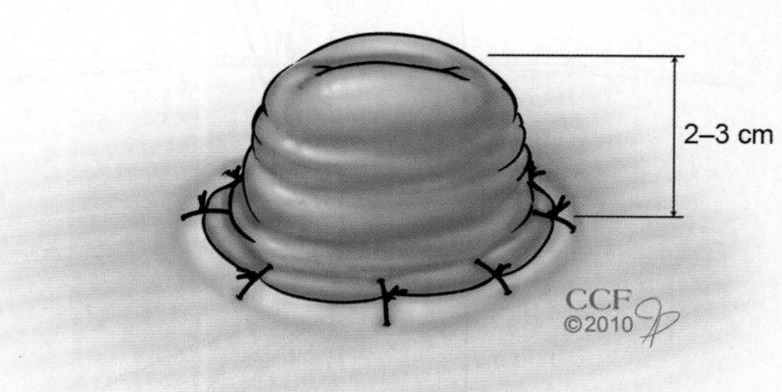

FIGURE 7-3. Matured end ileostomy. The stoma ideally protrudes 2 to 3 cm above skin level. This helps to protect the skin from stomal output and makes for easier pouching.

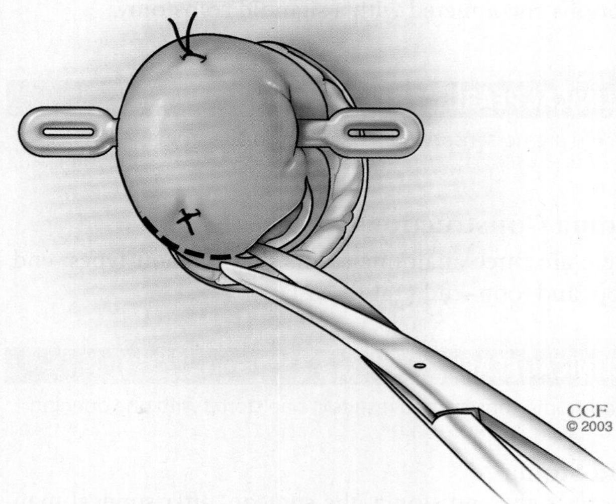

FIGURE 7-5. Loop ileostomy construction. The appropriate area of the intestine is opened from one side to the other, leaving intact intestine on the underside.

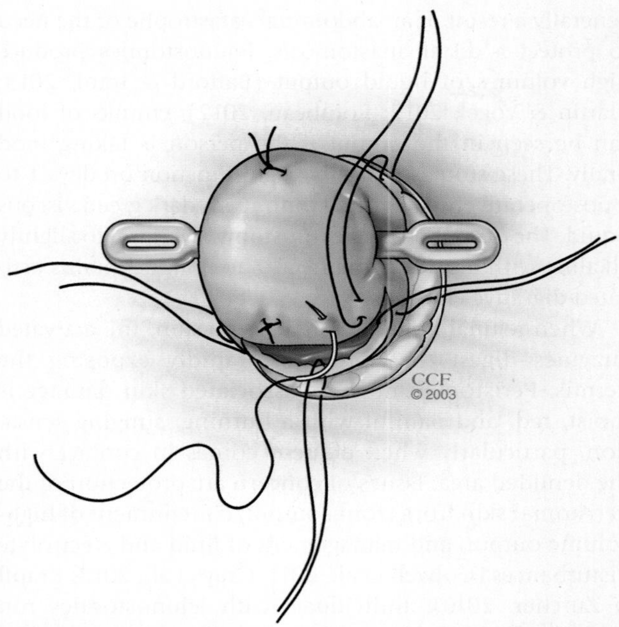

FIGURE 7-6. Loop ileostomy construction. Maturation of the stoma: Note the placement of the sutures through full thickness of the intestinal wall and the subcuticular (dermal) layer of the skin.

lumen usually protrudes more from the abdomen than the distal lumen (Fig. 7-7).

The rod under the stoma stays in place for 2 to 7 days depending on whether the case is laparoscopic or open, the amount of tension present on the rod, and surgeon preference (Garofalo, 2012; Martin & Vogel, 2012; Pine & Stevenson, 2014; Stocchi, 2012). For example, the rod remains in place for 2 days following a laparoscopic creation of the stoma and 3 days following conventional surgery. As with an end stoma, it is important to bring the intestine used to create the stoma through the abdominal opening with as little tension as possible, a good blood supply, and with normal orientation of the mesentery.

CLINICAL PEARL

The loop stoma is one stoma with two openings, proximal and distal. The loop stoma protects a distal anastomosis.

Loop–End Stoma

With loop–end construction, the intestine is transected from the lower bowel. After closing this end with a stapler, a loop of intestine approximately 10 cm proximal to this stapled end is brought to the abdominal surface through the premarked stoma site. Loop type construction is then used to create the stoma (Martin & Vogel, 2012; Stocchi, 2012; Wu, 2003). Externally, there is no difference in how a loop or loop–end stoma looks. With loop–end construction, the distal lumen leads to a blind pouch. The blind segment is usually not very long and will produce mucus as the bowel is viable. A loop–end ileal conduit uses this type of construction, which is discussed in more detail under ileal conduits. The rod under this type of urinary stoma is generally kept in place for 5 days versus the 2 to 3 days for a bowel stoma. Loop–end construction is used in bowel stomas when the person has a thick abdominal wall, shortened mesentery, or a combination, and there is concern about adequate blood supply to the distal end of the stoma (**Figs. 7-8** and **7-9**). Additionally, when there is a need for a permanent stoma and a loop stoma is already present, the distal limb can be transected and the stoma converted to loop–end construction (Martin & Vogel, 2012; Stocchi, 2012; Wu, 2003).

CLINICAL PEARL

Loop-end stoma is sometimes called Turnbull loop-end stoma.

Double-barrel ostomy construction is seen rarely; when it is, it usually occurs with colostomies. Two stomas are created in proximity to each other, resembling the end

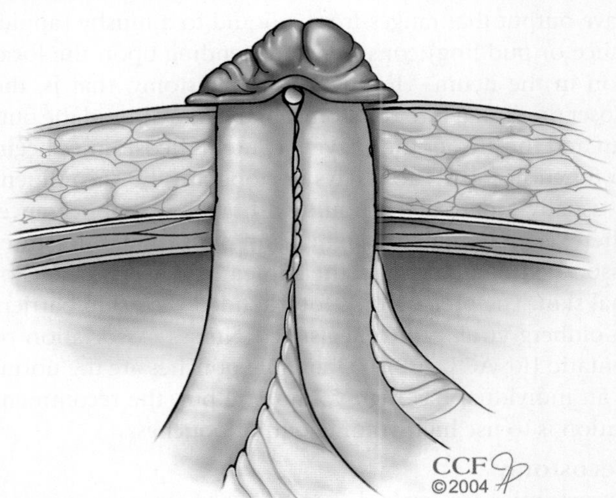

FIGURE 7-7. Matured loop ileostomy: The proximal (afferent) limb of the stoma is the protruding end, and the distal (efferent) limb is flush to skin level.

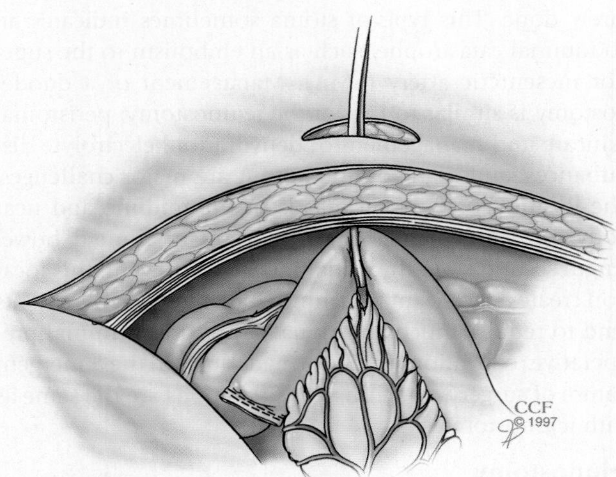

FIGURE 7-8. Loop–end ileostomy construction: Distal intestine is removed or left dormant. The proximal end of the intestine is stapled closed. The vascular arcade is protected with this technique.

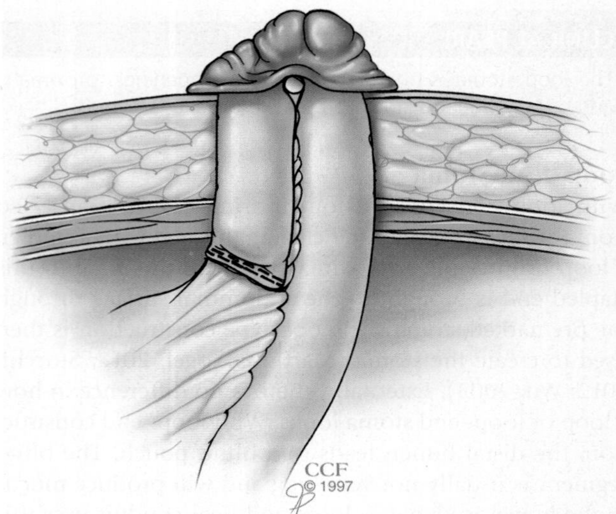

FIGURE 7-9. Loop–end ileostomy construction: A loop of intestine above this staple line is brought through the premarked site, and a loop of ileum is matured. This creates one stoma with a proximal, functioning lumen and a short distal segment.

of a double-barrel shotgun, hence the name. The proximal stoma is functional, and the distal stoma serves as a mucous fistula (Saunders & Hemingway, 2008). Double-barrel construction prevents any effluent from flowing into the distal stoma (mucous fistula). Indications for this type of stoma construction include massive infection and situations of distal obstruction where the bowel above the obstruction needs venting. Leaving a blind loop in the abdomen increases the risk for perforated viscus; there needs to be a way for the mucus to exit the bowel. Pouching can be difficult with double-barrel ostomies depending on how far apart the stomas are.

Anatomic Classification

Duodenostomy

Duodenostomies, that is, stomas in the duodenum, are rarely done. This type of stoma sometimes indicates an abdominal catastrophe, such as an embolism to the superior mesenteric artery (SMA). Management of a duodenostomy is similar to that of the jejunostomy; peristomal skincare and management of dehydration, electrolyte disturbances, and high-volume output are major challenges. The location of these stomas is in the midline and near body creases, which is a direct result of limited bowel length secondary to the initial catastrophic event; this location creates significant pouching challenges. These patients tend to require much emotional support as minimal preoperative education is performed due to the emergent nature of surgery. Pouching considerations are the same as with jejunostomies.

Jejunostomy

The location of jejunostomies is usually in the left upper quadrant of the abdomen. Creation of this stoma type is generally a result of an abdominal catastrophe or the need to protect a distal anastomosis. Jejunostomies produce high volumes of liquid output (Bafford & Irani, 2013; Martin & Vogel, 2012; Rombeau, 2012); chunks of food can be seen in the output if the person is taking food orally. These stomas typically begin function on days 1 to 3 postoperatively. The initial output is a dark green viscous liquid. The output from a jejunostomy is neutral to slightly alkaline with a pH ranging from 7 to 9 and contains activated digestive enzymes.

When jejunal effluent contacts the skin, the activated enzymes digest the epidermis, rapidly exposing the dermis. Peristomal moisture-associated skin damage is moist, red, and painful with a burning, stinging sensation, particularly when effluent comes in contact with the denuded area. Issues of concern are protection of the peristomal skin from stoma output, containment of high-volume output, and management of fluid and electrolyte disturbances (Colwell et al., 2011; Gray et al., 2013; Krapfl & Zurcher, 2010). Individuals with jejunostomies run the risk of dehydration and may require total parenteral nutrition to maintain proper nutrition and fluid intake; use of medication to slow intestinal motility is common (Parekh & Seidner, 2012). Suggested for use with liquid output are pouching systems with extended wear barriers, which have components that withstand liquid output better than do standard wear barriers (Goldberg et al., 2010). High-volume output pouches are standard. The output has minimal odor.

CLINICAL PEARL

Duodenostomy and jejunostomy are rare and usually done following a catastrophic event.

Ileostomy

Ileostomies, usually located in the right lower quadrant, have output that ranges from a liquid to a mushy (applesauce or pudding) consistency depending upon the location in the ileum. The higher the ileostomy, that is, the closer the stoma is to the stomach, the more liquid the output and the greater the enzyme content. Ileostomies begin to function from 1 to 3 days postoperatively. The effluent is usually a dark green liquid with a viscous appearance. There is potential for significant peristomal moisture-associated skin damage if the effluent contacts the peristomal skin. The preference is for extended wear skin barriers (Goldberg et al., 2010; Registered Nurses' Association of Ontario [RNAO], 2009). Drainable pouches are the norm; if an individual has high-volume output, the recommendation is to use high-volume output pouches.

Cecostomy

Cecostomies are rarely done, and when they are, it is as a tube cecostomy. The tube cecostomy acts to decompress the colon, treat cecal volvulus, or manage perforation of the cecum when resection is not an option (Garofalo, 2012; Saunders & Hemingway, 2008). A large-bore tube or catheter is inserted into the cecum, secured to the skin, and connected to gravity drainage. The output is liquid with particles, is malodorous, and frequently clogs the drainage tubing even with irrigation (Garofalo, 2012). Leakage around the catheter or tube is very common, and peritubular moisture-associated skin damage can occur.

Colostomy

Ascending colostomies are another rare type of stoma. They have output similar to cecostomies in that it is semiliquid with a strong odor secondary to the effects of colonic bacteria (Martin & Vogel, 2012). The effluent can cause considerable tissue destruction to the peristomal skin. Fluid and electrolyte imbalances are also a concern.

Transverse colostomies may be in the right upper quadrant, midabdomen, or left upper quadrant depending upon where in the transverse colon the stoma creation occurs. The stool is a liquid to a pasty consistency and usually malodorous. They are generally created for protection of an anastomosis or to relieve a distal obstruction and are often constructed as part of an emergent surgery (Garofalo, 2012). Stomal prolapse, particularly of the distal lumen in loop transverse colostomies, and hernia formation are common problems seen in transverse colostomies. Pouching can be problematic, should these problems occur.

The location of a descending or sigmoid colostomy is usually in the left lower quadrant. The stool is a pasty to a formed consistency; the stool is not as irritating to the skin as ileostomy effluent but can still cause peristomal moisture-associated skin damage (Fig. 7-10). Depending upon how often the stoma functions, an individual will use either a drainable pouch or closed-end pouch. A closed-end pouch is recommended if the stoma functions once to twice a day. Individuals with a descending or sigmoid colostomy may choose to irrigate the stoma to control its activity. Irrigation entails instilling water into the bowel at the same time every day in order to stimulate the bowel to function. This procedure is discussed in more detail in Chapter 12.

Odor and gas are a concern for the individual with a colostomy (Goldberg et al., 2010; Registered Nurses' Association of Ontario [RNAO], 2009). Use of filtered pouches; pouch deodorant; or oral, intestinal deodorizing medications can assist in odor and gas control. Dietary measures also are used to deal with gas and odor (see Chapters 9 and 12 for more information).

Mucous Fistula

The mucous fistula is formed when the end of a section of defunctionalized bowel is brought through the abdominal wall and a stoma is created (Pine & Stevenson, 2014). The output from a mucous fistula is mucus, sometimes mixed with small amounts of blood depending on the reason for its formation. A classic example of a mucous fistula occurs when someone has toxic megacolon. The surgery initially performed is a subtotal colectomy, also known as total abdominal colectomy. In this surgery, the colon is removed, and the rectum remains in place; it is known as the rectal stump.

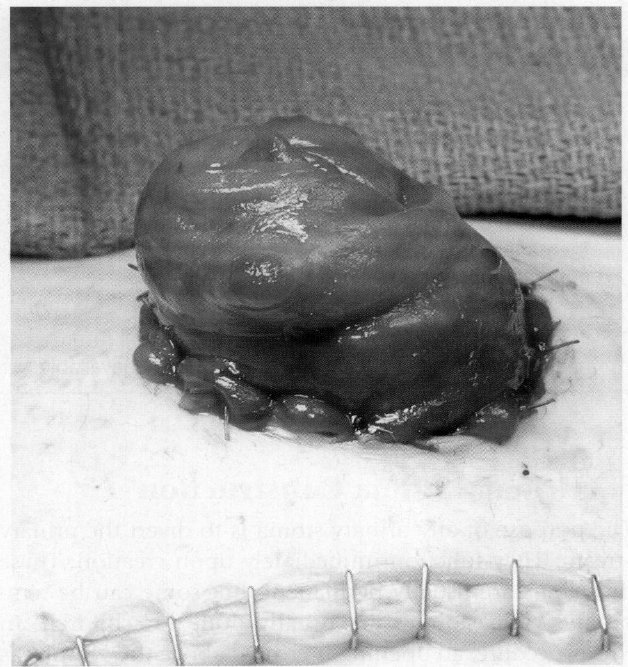

FIGURE 7-10. Matured end colostomy. Note the degree of stomal eversion and presence of sutures to secure mucocutaneous junction.

The method used to manage the top of the rectum depends on the integrity of the rectal tissues. Sometimes, stapling or suturing the top of the rectum closed and placing it immediately under the skin with incisional closure occurs when rectal tissues are relatively healthy. In this way, finding the top of the rectal stump is easy when a person undergoes further surgery. Additionally, if the top of the rectum opens, the drainage becomes a nuisance rather than a crisis, as the pus and blood drain onto the abdomen and not into the peritoneal cavity. Alternately, if tissue integrity is poor, formation of a stoma from the top of the rectal stump serves as an exit point for the pus and blood of the retained rectum. This stoma is the mucous fistula, which tends to produce small amounts of drainage. Initially, a pouch is applied over a mucous fistula and consideration of use of absorbent dressings occurs as drainage decreases. It is normal for the individual to feel the need to have a bowel action or pass mucus and a small amount of blood through the anus. Education on this point needs to occur, so individuals are not frightened or confused when it happens. Some points the patient should know about their stoma are listed in Box 7-1.

BOX 7-1 Points about the Stoma, the Patient Needs to Know

Patients need to know:

The number and location of openings in the stoma (one or two) to prevent worry when openings are visualized after edema resolves. Gently inserting a cotton-tipped applicator about 0.5 cm into the lumen(s) of the stoma helps the patient remember. Before inserting the applicator, let patients know they will not feel any pain.

The type of stoma they have—such as descending colostomy, ileal conduit, or ileostomy—so that they can tell future health care providers if the medical record is unavailable.

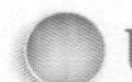

Urinary Stoma Construction

The purpose of any urinary stoma is to divert the urinary stream. They function immediately upon creation. These diversions are usually permanent, but some can be temporary. Vesicostomies are usually done for children. In this procedure, an opening is created above the symphysis pubis, the bladder opened, and the bladder mucosa approximated to the skin (Patel & Fergany, 2012). Containment of the urine is commonly done with diapering if the child is at an age where this is acceptable. Protecting the peristomal skin is needed to prevent peristomal moisture-associated skin damage (Gray et al., 2011). Products used to protect the skin include non–water-soluble skin sealants, cyanoacrylate-based monomer, or petrolatum-based products. It is difficult to obtain a predictable seal with pouching, so it is not usually a management option.

CLINICAL PEARL

Vesicostomy is a temporary urinary diversion that is usually closed before toilet-training age.

Types

Ureterostomy

The role of the ureterostomy is limited. In this procedure, the ends of the ureters are brought onto the abdomen or flank and sutured to the skin. These stomas are very tiny, less than 7/8″, and tend to become stenotic. Ureterostomies are also freely refluxing, so there is a danger of increased urinary tract infections and hydronephrosis. Indication for this procedure would be if the patient is not a candidate for an intestinal diversion.

Ileal Conduit

The most common urinary diversion is the ileal conduit (Colombo & Naspro, 2010). The right lower quadrant is the usual location for ileal conduits. In ileal conduit surgery, if removal of the bladder is necessary, the cystectomy is completed first. Resection of a 12- to 18-cm segment of

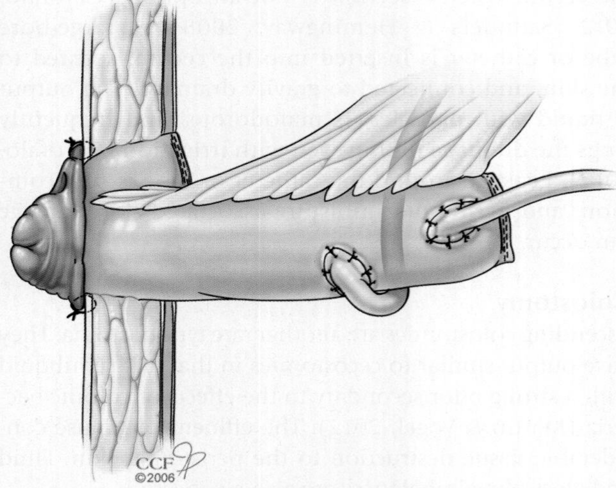

FIGURE 7-11. Loop–end ileal conduit. A short segment of ileum is resected from the gastrointestinal tract along with its mesentery. A loop of ileum is brought through the premarked stoma site and matured in the usual manner. The ureters are implanted at the proximal end of this segment.

ileum, which remains attached to the mesentery preserving its blood and nerve supply, follows the cystectomy. Gastrointestinal continuity is then restored through an ileal to ileal anastomosis. The proximal end of the resected ileal segment is sutured closed, and the distal end is used to create a stoma. Ileal conduits can have either end or loop–end construction; the details of these construction methods are detailed earlier in this section. After fashioning the stoma, the ureters are anastomosed into the ileal segment (Colombo & Naspro, 2010; Patel & Fergany, 2012) (Fig. 7-11).

It is important to keep adequate blood supply to the distal ureters, prevent ureteral kinking or twisting, have clear ureteral margins if cancer is the underlying reason for surgery, and maintain a tension-free ureteroileal anastomosis (Patel & Fergany, 2012). Placed at the time of surgery are ureteral stents, which remain in situ for 8 to 12 days postoperatively (Colombo & Naspro, 2010). Urine freely refluxes back into the kidney, leaving the individual at increased risk for urinary tract infections and hydronephrosis. Urine flows almost continuously from these stomas (Registered Nurses' Association of Ontario [RNAO], 2009). Urostomy pouches with urinary drainage spouts are used, allowing ease of drainage and the ability to connect to leg or bedside urinary drainage bags.

CLINICAL PEARL

An extended wear skin barrier is recommended for an ileal conduit pouching system. Extended wear barrier is recommended for ileal conduit pouching system.

Jejunal Conduit

When it is not feasible to use ileum as a conduit, jejunum or a segment of colon may be used. Jejunal conduits lead to electrolyte disturbances that are characterized by hyponatremia, hypochloremia, hyperkalemia, acidosis, and azotemia. Clinically, individuals present with nausea, vomiting, dehydration, anorexia, lethargy, and muscle weakness. Treatment of electrolyte disturbances includes hydration and salt and bicarbonate replacement. In colon conduits, the ureters are able to be implanted in a nonrefluxing manner secondary to the thicker musculature of the colon (Patel & Fergany, 2012).

Conclusions

Surgical creation of a stoma is often as important to patient survival and quality of life as managing the disease process or traumatic event. The ability for a person (or caregiver) to self-manage his or her ostomy care is directly dependent on many factors, including preoperative site selection and the quality of stoma construction. These factors will provide a mechanism for a reliable and predictable pouch seal that contains effluent and odor and minimizes the chances for stomal and peristomal skin complications (Erwin-Toth et al., 2012). Stoma construction types include end, loop, and loop–end. Determining the type of stoma construction depends on the intestinal anatomic location used, abdominal wall thickness, whether the stoma is temporary or permanent, and the disease process involved.

REFERENCES

Bafford, A., & Irani, J. (2013). Management and complications of stomas. *Surgical Clinics of North America, 93*(1), 145–166. doi: 10.1016/j.suc.2012.09.015

Colombo, R., & Naspro, R. (2010). Ileal conduit as the standard for urinary diversion after radical cystectomy for bladder cancer. *European Urology Supplements, 9*(10), 736–744. doi:10.1016/j.eursup.2010.09.001

Colwell, J., Ratliff, C., Goldberg, M., et al. (2011). MASD part 3: Peristomal moisture-associated dermatitis and periwound moisture-associated dermatitis. A consensus. *Journal of Wound, Ostomy and Continence Nursing, 38*(5), 541–553. doi: 10.1097/WON.0b013e31822acd95

Doughty, D. (2004). History of stoma creation and surgical advances. In J. Colwell, M. Goldberg, & J. Carmel (Eds.), *Fecal & urinary diversions. Management principles* (pp. 3–17). St. Louis, MO: Mosby.

Erwin-Toth, P., Hocevar, B., & Stricker, L. (2012). Wound, ostomy, and continence/enterostomal therapy (WOC/ET) nursing. In V. Fazio, J. Church, & J. Wu (Eds.), *Atlas of intestinal stomas* (pp. 75–84). New York, NY: Springer.

Forgione, P., & Cataldo, P. (2003). Colostomy. *Operative Techniques in General Surgery, 5*(4), 264–272. doi: 10.1053/j.optechgensurg.2003.10.004

Garofalo, T. (2012). Colostomy: Types, indications, formation, and reversal. In V. Fazio, J. Church, & J. Wu (Eds.), *Atlas of intestinal stomas* (pp. 127–145). New York, NY: Springer.

Goldberg, M., Aukett, L., Carmel, J., et al. (2010). *Management of the patient with a fecal ostomy: Best practice guideline for clinicians*. Mount Laurel, NJ: Wound, Ostomy and Continence Nurses Society.

Gray, M., Black, J., Baharestani, M., et al. (2011). Moisture-associated skin damage: Overview and pathophysiology. *Journal of Wound, Ostomy, and Continence Nursing, 38*(3), 233–241. doi: 10.1097/WON.0b013e318215f798

Gray, M., Colwell, J., Doughty, D., et al. (2013). Peristomal moisture-associated skin damage in adults with fecal ostomies. A comprehensive review and consensus. *Journal of Wound, Ostomy, and Continence Nursing, 40*(4), 389–399. doi: 10.1097/WOCN,0b013e3182944340

Kaidar-Person, O., Person, B., & Wexner, S. (2005). Complications of construction and closure of temporary loop ileostomy. *Journal of the American College of Surgeons, 201*(5), 759–773. doi: 10.1016/j.jamcollsurg.2005.06.002

Kairaluoma, M., Rissanen, H., Kultti, V., et al. (2002). Outcome of temporary stomas. A prospective study of temporary intestinal stomas constructed between 1989–1996. *Digestive Surgery, 19*(1), 45–51. doi: 10.1159/000052005

Krapfl, L., & Zurcher, S. (2010). High volume output from a jejunostomy. *Journal of Wound, Ostomy, and Continence Nursing, 37*(6), 662–664. doi: 10.1097/WON.0b013e3181fac09e

Martin, S., & Vogel, J. (2012). Intestinal stomas. Indications, management, and complications. *Advances in Surgery, 46*(1), 19–49. doi:10.1016/jyasu.2012.04.005

Patel, A., & Fergany, A. (2012). Urinary stomas. In V. Fazio, J. Church, & J. Wu (Eds.), *Atlas of intestinal stomas* (pp. 213–229). New York, NY: Springer.

Parekh, N., & Seidner, D. (2012). Medical management of the high-output enterostomy and enterocutaneous fistula. In V. Fazio, J. Church, & J. Wu (Eds.), *Atlas of intestinal stomas* (pp. 97–109). New York, NY: Springer.

Pine, J., & Stevenson, L. (2014). Ileostomy and colostomy. *Surgery (Oxford), 32*(4), 212–217. doi: 10.10161/j.mpsur.2014.01.007

Registered Nurses' Association of Ontario (RNAO). (2009). Ostomy care and management. *US National Guideline Clearing House.* Retrieved from https://search.ebscohost.com/login.aspx?direct=true&db=nrc&AN=5000013298&site=ede-live

Rombeau, J. (2012). Physiologic and metabolic effects of intestinal stomas. In V. Fazio, J. Church, & J. Wu (Eds.), *Atlas of intestinal stomas* (pp. 59–67). New York, NY: Springer.

Saunders, R., & Hemingway, D. (2008). Intestinal stomas. *Surgery (Oxford), 26*(8), 347–351. doi: 10.1016/j.mpsur.2008.05.001

Stocchi, L. (2012). Ileostomy. In V. Fazio, J. Church, & J. Wu (Eds.), *Atlas of intestinal stomas* (pp. 85–95). New York, NY: Springer.

Wexner, S., Taranow, D., Johansen, O., et al. (1993). Loop ileostomy is a safe option for fecal diversion. *Diseases of the Colon & Rectum, 36*(4), 349–354. doi: 10.1007/BF02043937

Wu, J. (2003). Ileostomy. *Operative Techniques in General Surgery, 5*(4), 257–263. doi: 10.1053/j.optechgensurg.2003.10.003

Wu, J. (2012). Intestinal stomas: Historical overview. In V. Fazio, J. Church, & J. Wu (Eds.), *Atlas of intestinal stomas* (pp. 1–37). New York, NY: Springer.

QUESTIONS

1. A patient is scheduled for surgery for the creation of an end ileostomy. What technique would the surgeon perform to prevent seeding of the epidermis with mucosal cells resulting in mucosal implants?

A. A plastic rod, tubing, or similar device is placed under the loop of intestine to provide support.
B. Two stomas are created in proximity to each other, resembling the end of a double-barrel shotgun.
C. The well-vascularized bowel segment is brought through a predetermined three-fingerbreadth abdominal aperture to create the stoma.
D. Eversion is performed using four equidistant sutures through the entire bowel wall and suturing through the subcuticular (dermal) layer of the adjacent skin.

2. What type of stoma construction would the surgeon most likely choose for a patient scheduled for ileal conduit who has a thick abdominal wall with a shortened mesentery?

A. Loop–end stoma
B. Double-barrel stoma
C. End stoma
D. Loop stoma

3. In the emergency department, a patient is diagnosed with an embolism to the superior mesenteric artery (SMA). If needed, what type of diversion may be created following this type of catastrophic event?

A. Jejunostomy
B. Ileostomy
C. Duodenostomy
D. Cecostomy

4. The WOC nurse is describing the ileostomy to a patient scheduled for the surgery. What statement accurately describes an aspect of this diversion?

A. The stoma is usually located in the left lower quadrant.
B. The higher the ileostomy, the more liquid the output.
C. Ileostomies begin to function within 1 week postoperatively.
D. The effluent is usually a light yellow liquid with viscous appearance.

5. What is a common complication when a loop transverse colostomy is created?

A. Stomal prolapse
B. Leakage around the catheter or tube
C. Tissue destruction to the peristomal skin
D. Fluid and electrolyte imbalances

6. The creation of a fecal stoma with a mucous fistula may be indicated in which of the following conditions?

A. A patient with rectal polyps
B. A patient with stomal prolapse
C. A patient with stomal hernia
D. A patient who has been diagnosed with toxic megacolon

7. What complication would the WOC nurse assess for in a patient with a ureterostomy?

A. Hydronephrosis
B. Kidney infection
C. Dehydration
D. Septicemia

8. Which procedure is the most common urinary diversion?

A. Vesicostomy
B. Ureterostomy
C. Ileal conduit
D. Cystectomy

9. The WOC nurse is explaining the procedure for constructing an ileal conduit to a patient scheduled for the surgery. Which statement by the nurse adequately describes a step in this procedure?

A. Resection of an 8- to 10-cm segment of ileum occurs.
B. Gastrointestinal continuity is restored through an ileal to ileal anastomosis.
C. The distal end of the resected ileal segment is sutured closed.
D. Ileal conduits must end in a loop–end construction to allow free flow of urine.

10. A support rod is placed under a loop stoma to prevent which of the following stoma complications?

A. Prolapse
B. Retraction
C. Stenosis
D. Necrosis

ANSWERS: 1.**D**, 2.**A**, 3.**C**, 4.**B**, 5.**A**, 6.**D**, 7.**A**, 8.**C**, 9.**B**, 10.**B**

CHAPTER 8

Preoperative Preparation of Patients Undergoing a Fecal or Urinary Diversion

Mary F. Mahoney

OBJECTIVE

Demonstrate preoperative preparation of a patient undergoing a fecal and/or urinary diversion including stoma site marking.

Topic Outline

Evidence indicates that patients who receive preoperative ostomy education experience better recovery, possibly a shorter hospital stay, and fewer postoperative complications (Goldberg et al., 2010). Preoperative education can assist in alleviating the patients' fears and anxieties associated with surgery and help them understand the adjustments that they will need to make for living with a stoma. The United Ostomy Associations of America's (UOAA) Bill of Rights adopted in 1977 outlines 11 elements of care that should be the expectation of the person undergoing ostomy surgery (see Box 8-1). The elements include the right to have a preoperative counseling session, to receive emotional support, and to have an appropriately positioned stoma site. This chapter covers the development of a plan of care for preoperative education for the person anticipating ostomy surgery and the principles of stoma site marking.

BOX 8-1 Ostomate Bill of Rights

The ostomate shall:

1. Be given pre-op counseling
2. Have an appropriately positioned stoma site
3. Have a well-constructed stoma
4. Have skilled postoperative nursing care
5. Have emotional support
6. Have individual instruction
7. Be informed on the availability of supplies
8. Be provided with information on community resources
9. Have posthospital follow-up and lifelong supervision
10. Benefit from team efforts of health care professionals
11. Be provided with information and counsel from the ostomy association and its members

Adopted by the United Ostomy Association House of Delegates at the UOA Annual Conference 1977.

CLINICAL PEARL

Support and education in the preoperative is effective in improving recovery after ostomy surgery.

 Patient Assessment

The development of a plan of care for the preoperative education of the patient undergoing ostomy surgery will include the diagnosis that necessitated the surgical procedure, the type and date of surgical procedure, the patient's understanding of the upcoming procedure, any limitations to learning such as inability to read, physical limitations, and the presence or absence of a support system. Other important assessments include religious affiliation, culture, family, employment status, and medical/surgical history.

Planned Procedure, Diagnosis, Prognosis, and Treatment Plan

Prior to the preoperative educational session, the wound ostomy continence (WOC) nurse should determine the reason for the surgical procedure and the type of surgical procedure that will be performed (Table 8-1). Reinforce with the surgeon that the stoma construction should protrude 2 to 3 cm above the abdominal plane to direct the effluent into the pouch and promote a good seal of the ostomy appliance system (Cottam et al., 2007). A panel of experts agreed that the ideal stoma should protrude approximately 2.5 cm to prevent peristomal skin irritation (Gray et al., 2013).

Review general postoperative care with the patient and include the probable location of the incision or incisions and the type of tubes they may have such as IVs, abdominal drains, and a urinary catheter. Describe how pain will be managed and the importance of early ambulation. Be sure that the patient understands that he or she will be NPO until bowel function has returned as indicated by the presence of gas in the pouch.

TABLE 8-1 Surgical Procedure, Type of Ostomy, Typical Location

Surgical Procedure	Type of Ostomy	Typical Stoma Site Location
Abdominal perineal resection	Permanent end colostomy Rectum removed Perineal surgical incision	Left side
Hartmann's procedure	Temporary (in certain situations may be permanent) end colostomy or ileostomy Rectum is retained.	Left or right side
Ileal pouch anal anastomosis	Stage one: temporary end ileostomy Stage two: temporary loop ileostomy	Right side
Proctocolectomy	Permanent end ileostomy Rectum removed, perineal surgical incision	Right side
Low anterior resection (LAR)	Temporary loop ileostomy	Right side
Subtotal colectomy	Temporary end or loop ileostomy	Right side
Sigmoid colectomy	Temporary loop ileostomy	Right side
Continent ileostomy (Kock pouch)	Continent stoma	Right side
Cystectomy (ileal conduit or colon conduit)	Urostomy	Right side if ileal conduit, left side if colonic conduit
Continent urine reservoir (Indiana reservoir)	Continent intestinal stoma	Right side

Use the teach-back method to evaluate the patient's understanding. Suggested examples to ask the patient are as follows: "I want to be sure that I explained your ostomy surgery correctly. Can you tell me what your stoma will look like and how it will function?" or "We covered a lot of information about ostomy surgery today. Can you tell me three things that you learned about your ostomy surgery?"

Many manufacturers of ostomy equipment provide kits for ostomy education to WOC nurses, or are available online. See Appendix C resources for a list of manufacturers.

CLINICAL PEARL

Patients who feel well prepared for ostomy surgery experience better post-operative adjustment to ostomy.

Major Concerns of Patient and Family/ Significant Others

Ask the patient and support person to describe their understanding of the surgical procedure, since Weiss (2003) has demonstrated that 40% to 80% of the medical information patients receive is forgotten immediately and nearly half of the information retained is incorrect. Establishing what information the patient knows helps to gain an understanding of his or her grasp of the upcoming procedure and identifies the educational gaps to be addressed during the preoperative session.

The patient and family should be asked what, if anything, they know about ostomy surgery. Encourage them to share concerns they have regarding the upcoming surgery and describe anyone they may have known with an ostomy. This question facilitates the conversation regarding the patient's worries and possible misconceptions of ostomy care. The patient may have a relative or friend who had a bad experience with an ostomy, and this is a good time to allay any unnecessary fears.

For example, it is not uncommon that an elderly grandparent may have had an ostomy and the pouching system was not effective, causing odor or leakage. This can provide the nurse with the opportunity to explain that the ostomy equipment available today is much improved from the past. Describe that the patient may have been unknowingly in the presence of someone with an ostomy, but since there are no visible signs (odor, bulging under the clothes), the ostomy is not apparent. Many times, people will discover a friend or acquaintance who has an ostomy that they didn't discuss. Patients who are anxious about a certain aspect of the ostomy will have difficulty learning at the preoperative session. In addition to facing ostomy surgery, many patients are simultaneously faced with a potentially terminal diagnosis or life-changing disease. Patients facing emergency surgery are often in pain, and there may be limited time for the WOC nurse to provide preoperative education.

Barriers to Self-Care

Psychological

There is a good deal of psychological stress when a patient has been diagnosed and told about the need for surgery. Patients should be encouraged to express fears, concerns, worries, disgust, and potential embarrassment regarding the upcoming surgery that will result in the creation of an ostomy (Dorman, 2009). Patients' fears can be unfounded and may be easily dealt with calmly. For instance, some patients think their diets will change greatly in the presence of an ostomy, and this is not necessarily true. Other people think their clothing must be loose to accommodate the pouching system and that everyone will know they have an ostomy. Alleviating these fears can help the patients cope with all of the changes they will be facing. A visit from a person with an ostomy might be beneficial and an option to talk with a trained ostomy visitor can be obtained by contacting the UOAA.

Physical

Evaluate the patient's physical abilities. Note if the patient has physical conditions such as arthritis or stroke that could affect his or her ability for self-care. Does the patient have visual limitations that will need to be considered when teaching the patient how to manage his or her stoma? Inadequate coordination and function as seen in Parkinson disease and poststroke weakness are also barriers to self-care (Dorman, 2009). Reinforce to the patient that self-care can be awkward and frustrating in the beginning, but confidence is gained with experience as patients develop new skills to perform the task of emptying and changing the pouching system.

Dorman (2009) indicates that the physical and emotional disabilities of the surgery may have an impact on the ability to perform ostomy care. If there are disabilities that render self-care difficult or impossible, a caregiver must be identified and included in the pre- and postoperative teaching sessions.

Cognitive

Many people have difficulty reading and understanding medical information. Reinforce that the patient and family can call the ostomy nurse with questions after surgery and discharge. Suggest that the patient start a notebook to write down questions in order to remember to ask the nurse or the doctor. The patient can keep all notes regarding the surgery, phone numbers, Web sites, and other information gathered in this special notebook. For the person who may have problems grasping all of the preoperative information, the family member or support person should be included. People with low literacy skills tend to use family or friends to assist the interpretation of the medical information shared (Weiss, 2003).

Understanding Fears

According to the UOAA, odor control and leakage are two major concerns of the ostomy patients, and these need to be addressed during the preoperative education. An explanation of how odor is managed should be provided in a manner that the patient's fears are alleviated. Describe to the patient how his or her fear of leakage will be addressed, by instructing the patient in how a pouch seal is maintained. Dietary, clothing, and sexual issues can all be discussed and the patient helped to understand that these challenges are normal and fairly easily managed.

Learning Style/Learning Level

Patients should be asked if they are comfortable with learning by reading or if they prefer another way of learning such as photos, video, or audio instruction. Asking in a shame-free manner will more likely elicit an honest response (Weiss, 2003). If reading is not their preferred manner of learning, offer other methods, for example, watching a demonstration video, practicing on a model, or working with the nurse on changing their pouch as many times as possible. See Box 8-2 for teaching methods.

BOX 8-2 Teaching Strategies and Methods

Verbal instruction

Printed instructional sheets or booklets (many ostomy manufacturers provide comprehensive instruction booklets, the United Ostomy Associations of the America [UOAA] has printed information, or the place of nurse's employment may provide instruction sheets)

Photos

Illustrations or diagrams

Plain paper with pen to draw diagrams

Models made by the nurse or manufactured models such as VATA anatomical healthcare models (http://www.vatainc.com) or The Anatomical Apron by Joy (http://www.apronsbyjoy.com)

Actual pouch system demonstrations

Videos of people changing the ostomy pouch or sharing testimonials

Valid Web sites (such as manufacturer or UOAA Web sites)

Patient's Support System

The WOC nurse should determine the patient's emotional support system. This would be a person who can be available during the preoperative visit and at several postoperative sessions as well as follow-ups and someone the person can call when he or she needs to talk. It is important to include the patient's support system in the preoperative as well as the postoperative education sessions. When patients are in crisis, specifically facing ostomy surgery, absence of social support may result in poor coping and adapting behaviors (Nichols, 2011).

While it is ideal to meet with the patient several weeks prior to surgery, time may be limited and the appointment may be the same day as the surgery. Factor this timing into the amount of education shared with the patient as you might need to limit the provision of information to addressing the patient's greatest fears and providing basic information on the skills the patient will need to acquire after surgery. Educational materials regarding the specific type of ostomy planned should be provided. This may include printed instructional sheets or booklets, photos, illustrations, models, pouches, and/or videos (see Chapter 11 for patient education resources).

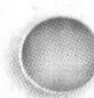

Guidelines for Preoperative Education

CLINICAL PEARL

Preoperative education should include (1) Brief discussion of anatomy and physiology of affected area, (2) Procedure, (3) Briefly describe lifestyle adjustment, (4) Focus on psychological preparation, (5) Introduction to ostomy equipment (WOCN 2010).

Explanation of Planned Procedure

Anatomy and Physiology

Begin with a simple review of the anatomy and bodily functions. Take time for this review because patients often do not have a clear understanding of how their bodies work or how organs are positioned in the abdomen. Explain the physiology of the abdominal organs, particularly the roles of the gastrointestinal and genitourinary systems. Use a diagram or a model to illustrate the changes associated with the planned surgery. A 3D model helps to reinforce the concepts of the anatomy inside the abdomen. Explain that the actual stoma does not come off or have the ability to move around like the model.

The effect of the surgery on other organs inside the abdomen needs to be explained; many individuals need to be assured that the body can continue to function despite the loss of a portion of the intestinal tract or the bladder. For example, the nurse must be very clear that the patient undergoing urostomy surgery will have a section of the intestine used for urine drainage, but the intestine will be reconnected to function as the normal passageway for stool.

The WOC nurse should identify any other education the patient will need. For example, the patient undergoing a temporary ileostomy for ileal pouch anal anastomosis (IPAA) may be ready to have information regarding diet, sphincter exercises, and skin care.

Bowel Prep

Review the bowel preparation prior to surgery. Be sure to check with the surgeon regarding the current methods to prepare for surgery. Some surgeons require mechanical bowel preparation (MBP); however, according to a Cochrane Review done by Guenaga et al. (2011), the need for MBP prior to elective colorectal surgery is optional. The review did state that colon cleansing preparation is necessary for patients with small tumors or the need to determine the precise location of a lesion. Some surgeons consider MBP potentially harmful (Yang et al., 2013). The solutions do not clean out the colon completely, and leave a watery residue. Studies have indicated that infection rate for operations without MBP is equal to or in some cases less than operations done with the bowel preparation (Ellis, 2010). The authors and researchers unanimously agreed that the use of prophylactic antibiotics is universally accepted as one of the most important steps to prevent infections and complications in colorectal surgery (Guenaga et al., 2011).

Since the type of bowel preps used will depend upon the surgical team, it is important to determine their preferred type of prep. There are many different types of MBP, and some are used alone and some used in combination.

The bowel preparation involves dietary restriction and mechanical cleansing of the gastrointestinal tract with the use of a bowel preparation. Typically, the patient is on clear liquids for one to two days before surgery and begins the mechanical bowel prep the day before surgery. Examples of MBPs are as follows: polyethylene glycol (PEG) electrolyte solution; laxatives (mineral oil, agar, and phenolphthalein); mannitol; glycerin enemas (900-mL water containing 100-mL glycerin); sodium phosphate (NaP) solution; bisacodyl (10 mg) and enemas; diets, low residue, nonresidue, and with clear liquids; and saline enema per rectum (Guenaga et al., 2011).

The most common solutions used prior to colorectal surgery are the PEG solution and the NaP solution. The PEG solution is an osmotic laxative. The large-volume solution causes watery diarrhea to cleanse the stool out of the colon. The PEG laxative solution also contains electrolytes to prevent dehydration and other serious side effects that may be caused by fluid loss as the colon is emptied. Patients complain of the salty taste, nausea, abdominal fullness, discomfort, and vomiting that may be associated with this preparation. The NaP solution is a low-volume, hyperosmotic liquid. The effectiveness of oral NaP solution is generally similar to or significantly better than PEG solution in patients preparing for colorectal surgery. Typically, oral NaP solution is significantly more acceptable to patients than is the PEG solution due to the low volume, but may cause electrolyte imbalances and dehydration (Ellis, 2010; WOCN Bowel Prep for Patients with a Colostomy, 2008).

Stoma Appearance and Function

The WOC nurse should describe how the stoma is created, the appearance of the stoma, and expectations of the stoma output. It is important that the patient understand that the stoma will be red and moist and will have no sensation. Many patients express that since the stoma is red, they associated red with pain or infection. Diagrams or models help to demonstrate the surgical creation of the stoma. An easily accessible method to describe the maturation of a stoma is to suggest that the stoma is matured much like a turtleneck that is everted. Explain the lining of the mouth is much like the appearance of the stoma: red, moist, and soft. The use of analogies is helpful to describe the expected output from the stoma (e.g., ileostomy output is similar to pudding consistency).

Overview of Management

CLINICAL PEARL

Technical difficulties of managing the ostomy is negatively correlated with psychosocial adjustment.

Pouching System Management

Demonstrate the type of pouching system that will be used following surgery. While indicating the features of the pouching system, be sure not to overload the patient with unnecessary information. It is best to only demonstrate one pouch system. Explain that the WOC nurse will help direct the patient to the most appropriate pouching system after surgery.

BOX 8-3 Pouching Overview

Pouches are available in different sizes, shapes, and materials.
Features include one- and two-piece systems.
Pouching systems are odor proof.
Usual wear time is four days (Richbourg et al., 2007).
Follow-up with the ostomy nurse should be done on a routine visit and as needed.

Emptying

Instruct the patient that the first skill the patient or a caregiver will need to acquire before discharge is to learn how to empty the pouch. Let the patient know approximately how many times in 24 hours he or she will need to check the pouch to see if it needs to be emptied. Describe that most people sit on the toilet and direct the pouch contents into the toilet. If the patient has a urostomy, the pouch may be connected to large capacity drainage system at night. If this is a fecal stoma, the patient may wipe the inside of the pouch tail spout with toilet tissue, apply deodorant (if used), and reseal or clamp pouch closed. Help the patient to visualize how to accommodate for these changes in the home setting.

Changing

Provide the patient with an overview on changing the pouching system (Box 8-3). Patients should understand that they will plan a pouching system change on a routine scheduled basis. They will practice changing the pouch while in the hospital but may not acquire the skills prior to discharge and in most cases will have home care nursing to continue to work toward independence in stoma care. Be sure the patients understand that they will go home with ostomy supplies and written instructions to use as they work toward acquiring the necessary skills.

Importance of Peristomal Skin Management

Be sure the patient understands that the skin around the stoma should not be reddened or sore and must be maintained intact to avoid problems with the pouch seal. Patients need to understand the principles of ostomy care to prevent skin irritation or redness and to apply a pouch system securely. The skin around the stoma should be healthy, and the appliance should not leak between planned changes. Several studies have shown that some patients do not seek assistance for signs of peristomal skin breakdown. Erwin-Toth et al. (2012) revealed that 61% of participants had signs of peristomal skin disorder upon inspection by the WOC nurse. Reinforce the availability of the WOC nurse for follow-up care; one method is to provide a discharge packet with a follow-up appointment after discharge with the ostomy outpatient clinic.

Obtaining and Paying for Supplies

Instruct the patient that most insurances cover the majority of the cost of ostomy supplies. Since insurance coverage varies, the patient should check with the insurance provider to verify coverage of the ostomy supplies and to determine if there is a preferred vendor. The patient also needs to know that he or she may need a prescription to obtain ostomy supplies.

CLINICAL PEARL

Important considerations in pouching system selection include stoma type and location, abdominal contours, lifestyle, personal preference, visual acuity and manual dexterity.

Attention to Sexual Concerns/Explanation of Potential Sexual Dysfunction

Chapter 13 describes the potential impact of an ostomy on body image and sexual function. The topic of sexuality may be difficult for the patient to broach but is usually a concern, and it is important that the nurse assess the patient's need to learn about sexuality with an ostomy and to help identify the need for further counseling. The PLISSIT counseling model (described in Chapter 13) highlights the four levels of sexual counseling, Permission, Understanding-Limited Information, Specific Suggestions, and Intensive Therapy (Anon, 1987), and the WOC nurse is encouraged to intervene at the permission and limited information level. This is where the patient is given permission to acknowledge the need for the discussion, and in the simple explanation phase, some simple suggestions for initial sexual encounters after surgery such as emptying the pouch and checking the seal, clothing options, for example, and the patient should be encouraged to ask specific questions.

Patients and their significant others need reassurance that sexual enjoyment can still be a part of their lives, despite the alteration in physical changes (Junkin & Beitz, 2005). The stoma itself should not be used for sexual intimacy, as it is easily damaged and is not an erogenous area.

Basic Explanations Regarding Lifestyle Issues

Diet

Many patients assume that they will need to alter their diet following ostomy surgery. Let the patient know that he or she may have a restricted diet after surgery up to approximately 6 weeks. Most people with ostomies will not have to follow a diet once surgical healing has taken place.

Activity

Determine whether the patient is concerned about resuming normal activity after surgery. Explain that the pouch system should not interfere with activity, and give specific examples of how the patient can integrate the ostomy into his or her lifestyle. Patients often wonder if the pouch can get wet. Assure the patient that typically a daily shower is acceptable, and in some cases, submersion under water for a length of time such as swimming or hot tub may require extra waterproof tape, applied around the barrier edges. Prior to bathing, the seal should be checked, and many people use tape to "picture frame" the four edges of pouch adhesive to further protect from leakage; tape may be paper or waterproof.

Clothing

Discuss the patient's current clothing and determine if there are any challenges the patient will encounter. Most people are able to return to their former clothing styles after surgery.

Medications

Some medications or nutritional supplements may change the color, odor, or consistency of the stool or urine. Certain medications may not be completely absorbed (see Chapter 12 for more information). For example, in a patient with an ileostomy, time release capsules are not recommended as they may pass through the stoma without breaking down. Medications may need to be converted to liquid form to get the full benefit of the medicine.

Travel

Be sure the patient knows that there are no limitations to travel with the ostomy. Patients should carry ample amount of supplies with them when they travel and to be aware that certain screening processes, when flying, may note the presence of a pouch. Some airport screening systems will detect the presence of a pouching system and require a personal screening. These screenings are usually very professional, in private with two of the same sex officers, and the TSA staff will be discreet to limit embarrassment. This is done for everyone's safety and is conducted as efficiently and quickly as possible. The UOAA has a travel card that can be carried while traveling that explains some of the conditions associated with an ostomy; copies can be obtained from http://www.ostomy.org/uploaded/files/travel_card/Travel_Card_2011b.pdf.

Acknowledgment of Normal Stages of Adjustment

Adjustment to a new stoma requires a period of time to incorporate the stoma into the patients' life and to acquire the necessary skills to manage the stoma. Chapter 13 describes the stages of adjustment. Patients should understand that adjustment to an altered body image and function takes time and energy. They should also be aware that the WOC nurse will be available for consultation after discharge for any challenges that arise.

Determination of Need for Referrals

Ostomy Visitor

Patients facing ostomy surgery are at all levels of acceptance. Patients may be ready to accept the upcoming changes, but most patients need further assistance. One suggestion is to refer the patient to a trained visitor who has an ostomy or to refer the patient to an ostomy support before the ostomy surgery. There are local and national ostomy support groups affiliated with the UOAA. The people in these groups have experienced the physical and emotional stressors associated with disease, surgery, body image changes, and lifestyle changes associated with an ostomy. Some local chapters or groups offer Ostomy Education Days to provide all patients with ostomies the opportunity to learn more about having an ostomy, receive encouragement, and see new supplies at a vendor fair. Despite advances in ostomy system technology, many patients still experience problems with psychosocial adjustment.

CLINICAL PEARL

Many patients relate that the personal turning point in learning to accept the ostomy was the moment he or she met another person with a similar ostomy.

Seeing the trained visitor or another person with an ostomy in regular clothing, sharing experiences, and hearing the recovery stories can help patients and families to move toward acceptance. Another method to connect with people with an ostomy is to seek information on qualified Web sites. The UOAA has videos sharing patients' stories. The ostomy manufacturers also have education and tools for patients and families (see resource list in Appendix C). Many patients eventually learn to live a healthy lifestyle with an ostomy.

Counseling Professional

There are times when a patient is unable to cope with an ostomy in a healthy manner. The patient's primary care provider may be able to offer assistance in the form of counseling, but it may be necessary to refer the patient and/or family to a clinical psychologist or psychiatrist for expert consultation regarding issues with coping. Patients may be reluctant to make an appointment with a specialist due to the stigma of mental illness. The nurse should help the patient and/or family understand that people need help to overcome the barriers of healthy recovery. It is not a failure for the patient to see the specialist; it is a negative outcome if the patient fails to follow up with a professional and does not learn to live with the ostomy in a healthy manner. Assessment and identification of psychosocial issues the patient faces is a challenge for the nurse and primary care provider. Patients in this situation feel alone and may not reach out for help. Nichols (2011) provides evidence that some adults with ostomies become socially isolated and this can lead to decreased satisfaction and emotional support. The author states that in some patients, the ostomy has a negative impact on life satisfaction and health care clinicians need to ensure the patient has access to follow-up after leaving the hospital.

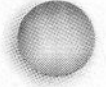

Stoma Siting

The term *stoma siting* refers to identification and marking the optimal location for the stoma on the patient's abdomen. Stoma siting is vital to the patient's quality of life with an ostomy. Marking the proposed stoma site prior to surgical intervention was introduced by Turnbull and Gill in the 1950s (Doughty, 2008) and quickly emerged as best practice in the medical and nursing fields. Stoma siting is also an expectation of the person about to undergo planned or potential ostomy surgery.

CLINICAL PEARL

Stoma site marking may reduce the incidence of complications and improve self care.

Rationale

Stoma site marking should be performed for all patients who are scheduled for surgery that may result in a stoma. Bass et al. (1997) studied the relationship of stoma site marking and preoperative education to the outcomes of ostomy surgery. The study demonstrated that patients who were educated and marked by a WOC nurse experienced fewer ostomy-related difficulties. Selection of the stoma site during surgery cannot take into account the contours and abdominal plane; skin folds and creases while the patient is lying flat are not obvious during the surgical procedure. Marking the stoma site before surgery is vital for all patients to improve quality of life, promote independence, and decrease postoperative complications associated with the ostomy surgery (Person, et al., 2012). Chaudri and Brown et al., in a 2005 report, note that stoma site marking decreases the time to learn the skills to care for the ostomy, decreases length of hospital stay, and reduces the need for pouching system troubleshooting after discharge. Clinical expert opinion maintains that patients who receive preoperative education and marking experience less complications and pouching problems (Goldberg, et al., 2010). Even though there is strong evidence that stoma site marking should be done for every patient who may have ostomy surgery, not all ostomy patients receive stoma site marking. Richbourg et al. (2007), in an ostomy patient survey, noted that less than 50% of respondents had been seen by an ostomy nurse prior to surgery. Pittman et al., (2008) found 71% of stoma complications were related to location and in a separate study noted that less than 67% of patients were marked preoperatively (Pittman, 2011).

According to the World Council of Enterostomal Therapists (WCET) (2014), preoperative education for the patient should include explanation of the surgical procedure, stoma site marking, and postoperative management. "The ideal stoma site is located below the umbilicus, within the rectus muscle, away from scars, creases, bony prominences, umbilicus, and belt line, on the summit of the infraumbilical fat mound, and visible to the patient" (WCET, 2014, p. 13) (**Fig. 8-1**).

The choice of the proposed stoma site is a guide for the surgeon, as the location of the stoma may need adjustment if issues are encountered during surgery. The patient should understand that this is a proposed stoma site and the actual site may be in a different location depending upon the findings at the time of surgery.

Procedure Guidelines

The physical planes of abdomens are affected by age, previous surgeries, and treatments. Knowing the patient's background helps to anticipate abdominal plane issues such as habitus of the abdomen, scars from previous surgeries, or radiation treatments that may alter the area that can be used as a stoma site. Understanding the patient's disease process will help to determine if the patient may gain weight (possible in the case of Crohn's disease or ulcerative

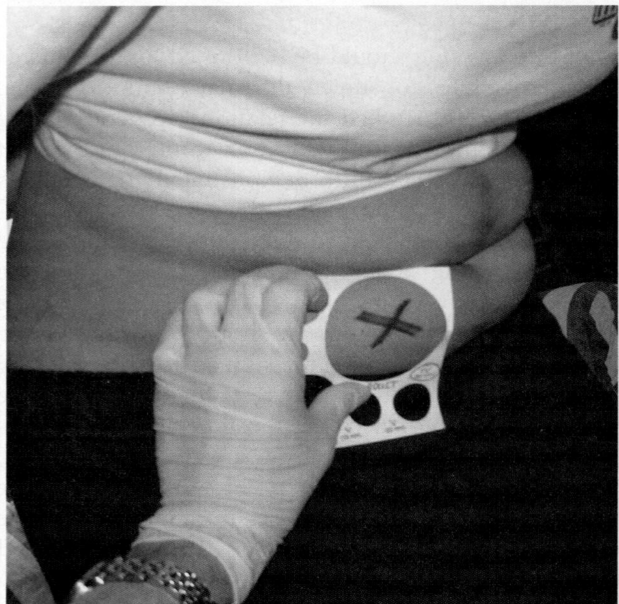

FIGURE 8-1. The stoma site is located below the umbilicus, within the rectus muscle, away from scars, creases, bony prominences, umbilicus, and belt line, on the summit of the infraumbilical fat mound, and visible to the patient.

colitis) or lose weight (possible in the case of cancer) after surgery.

After the information is gathered, schedule an appointment with the patient. Explain that the surgeon has asked the patient to meet with a WOC nurse before the procedure to learn about the surgery, the expectations of the surgery, the care after surgery, and the stoma site marking. Allow an hour or sometimes longer based on the patient's needs for the education and marking.

The information the ostomy nurse teaches during the preoperative session regarding the anatomy, physiology, and bowel preparation should coincide with the information the surgeon shared. The nurse needs to notice nonverbal cues that the information is too much or at too high level for the patient to understand. The nurse also needs to be attentive to the patient's emotional needs as the patient may need to stop to cry or gather composure to be ready to learn more. The focus is not to dole out copious information; the goal is to help the patient understand the implications of the surgery at the level he or she is ready to understand. If possible, scheduling multiple, short sessions will help the patient to absorb the information being given.

Stoma Site Marking Procedure

Begin by explaining the procedure and obtain verbal consent or written consent, based on institutional policy.

1. Gather items needed for the procedure: surgical marker, transparent film dressing, and flat skin barrier. If a preoperative kit is used, open kit and lay out all supplies.
2. Explain the stoma marking procedure to the patient, and encourage patient participation and input.
3. In a warm, private room, carefully examine the patient's abdominal surface. Begin with the patient fully clothed in sitting position with feet on the floor. Observe for the presence of belts, braces, and any other ostomy appliances. Ask patients if they are employed in an industry in which they wear clothing in or around the waist area such as a carpenter with a tool belt.
4. Examine the patient's exposed abdomen in various positions (standing, lying, sitting, and bending forward) to observe for creases, valleys, scars, folds, skin turgor, and contour.
5. With the patient lying on the back, identify the rectus muscle. This can be done by asking the patient to do a modified sit-up (raise the head up off the bed). Placement within the rectus muscle can help to prevent peristomal hernia formation.
6. Choose an area that is visible to the patient, a flat area of at least three inches and if possible below the belt line to conceal the pouch. In many cases, this is the apex of the infraumbilical bulge (Fig. 8-2). Rationale: This area usually does not crease as the person's weight may shift.

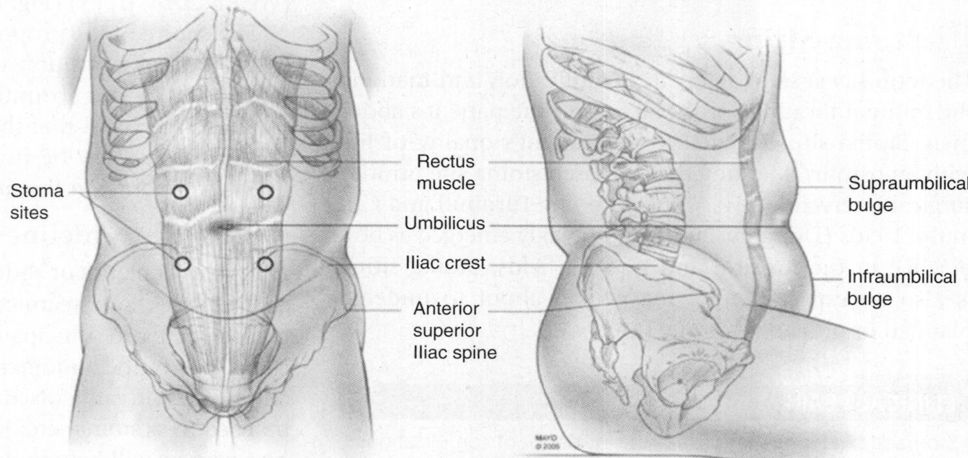

FIGURE 8-2. Supra- and infraumbilical bulges.

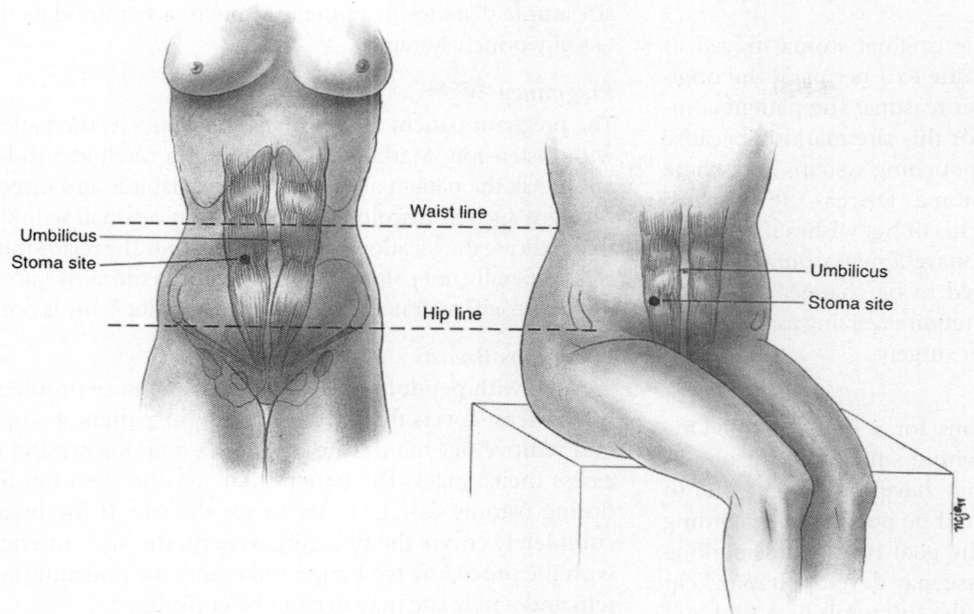

FIGURE 8-3. Stoma site marking.

7. If the abdomen is obese, consider the placement high in the upper abdominal quadrants to allow the patient to visualize the stoma. The patient with soft obesity needs special attention to locate the stoma on the outer curve of the fold and not in a crease. Consider that the obese patient may also develop a retracted stoma and possibly require a belt. Attempt to place the stoma mark in an area that will be supported by the ostomy belt. The mark is ideally placed on the infraumbilical bulge, but the patient may see the stoma better and have better access on the supraumbilical bulge (Fig. 8-2).

   For the patient with a soft protuberant belly, the belt line is typically well below the lower abdominal fold. Marking the site below the fold will result in the inability of the patient to visualize the stoma and lack the flat surface area needed for a secure seal of the pouching system. If the rectus muscle cannot be seen because of obesity, use the nipple line to determine the outer edge of the rectus muscle. Mark the stoma site in an upper quadrant on a flat surface, where it is visible to the patient and on a smooth plane for better pouch adhesion (Fig. 8-3).
8. Once the mark is chosen, ask the patient to place a finger on the mark to indicate that he or she can visualize the stoma to provide self-care. Ensure the patient agrees with the stoma mark. The patient may want to fasten shirt and trousers to check the site in relation to clothing.
9. Clean the desired site with alcohol and allow to dry. Mark the selected site with a surgical marker/pen. Cover with transparent film dressing (ASCRS and WOCN, 2007; AUA and WOCN, 2009).

Considerations in Stoma Site Marking

If there are two locations for the stoma placement, consider marking both and numbering by preference. Chart in the patient's medical record the reason for choosing the two sites, and if possible, have a conversation with the surgeon before surgery. Watt (1986) suggested that marking several sites with a preferential ranking on the abdomen gave the surgeon more than one option to use during the surgery with the best option ranked first. Colwell and Folkedahl (2001) concurred with this guidance to mark several stoma sites.

For some patients with abdomens that have many creases and folds that will not be visible to the surgeon in a flat position (as when the patient is on the operating table), consider noting areas that would be inadvisable to place the stoma. This can be done by marking the word "no" in creases or skin folds that would make pouching a stoma difficult or impossible.

Unique Stoma Marking Considerations

Patients who have spinal deformities, obesity, or excessive uneven scar tissue may have special needs for stoma site marking.

Marking for Two Stomas

Occasionally, a patient may need to be marked for two stomas, typically a urinary stoma and a fecal stoma. The goal of marking two stomas on the same abdomen is to mark the stomas at different abdominal heights. If one of the pouching systems needs an ostomy belt, the variation in height will allow the use of the belt without interfering with the other ostomy pouch. When marking the two stomas at the same time, it is preferable to mark the urostomy at least one inch higher.

For individuals who already have a stoma and now need to be marked for another stoma, use the general principles of stoma siting and allow ample surface area for the ostomy pouch barrier in relation to the other stoma and offset the height of the stoma sites in the event that one of the stoma sites would require a belt.

Moving the Stoma

Patients may need to have the original stoma moved to another site. Typically, this is due to a hernia at the original site, but there may be other reasons. The patient commonly is more participative for this site marking because he or she is familiar with the pouching systems and where he or she likes to have the stoma. Discuss the site with the patient and accommodate his or her wishes if possible. Explain that the new site will have a new stoma and that the pouching system may need to be changed. The new stoma will be edematous and require resizing as the stoma changes in shape and size after surgery.

Thin Patient

There are several considerations for a thin patient. One consideration is the patient with a small amount of adipose tissue. A thin patient may have lost weight due to lengthy illness. The mark should be positioned according to anticipated weight gain. The goal is to avoid marking the site in an area where a crease may develop. It may help to gently squeeze the skin of the infraumbilical fold and mark away from the crease of the fold.

Another consideration is the patient who is thin and has loose, wrinkly skin over a firm abdomen. This is a challenge because the mark may be placed but the loose skin moves easily and the mark will move with the skin. In this case, the nurse must contact the surgeon and be very clear on the placement of the stoma site in relation to the skin's integrity. It may help to assess the patient with the surgeon.

Creases and Folds

People of all body types have creases and folds to take into consideration. It is imperative to watch the patient's abdomen as the patient moves from standing to sitting to lying and as the patient bends over. Mark the site on the outer curve of a crease to avoid placement in a location that would be difficult to get a pouch to seal.

Scars

Note any scars and the texture of the scar. Some scars are soft, and the stoma location may be safely placed near the scar. However, scars may also be firm or sinewy and may cause uneven pouching surface or tension on the pouching surface. The firm, sinewy scars should be avoided in the peristomal plane.

Distension

Patients with distension are often seen prior to emergent surgical situations, for example, bowel blockage. Ask the patient to describe what his or her abdomen generally looks like. Inspect carefully for signs of creases that are not currently present due to the distension, such as discolored skin tones or light wrinkles. Take these areas into account when selecting a site. If the outer edge of the rectus muscle cannot easily be determined, use the nipple lines as a marker for the edge of the rectus muscle. Keep in mind the abdomen distension will decrease and the mark will become more midline as the swelling recedes. Mark the site ample distance from the midline to accommodate the ostomy pouch system.

Pregnancy

The pregnant patient faces similar challenges as the patient with distension. Marking the site requires careful consideration. Ask the patient about her normal habitus and inspect for signs such as discoloration of the skin or small wrinkles that indicate the location of a crease to avoid. The rectus muscle is generally not palpable. Mark the stoma site fairly lateral, as the site will migrate toward midline after the baby is born.

Pendulous Breasts

Women with pendulous breasts may experience problems if the breast covers the stoma site. Ask the patient to apply and remove her bra during the stoma marking session to assess the changes. The patient may need to wear her bra during ostomy care in order to see the site. If the breast completely covers the pouching system, this may interfere with the procedure to change and empty the pouching system and a new site may need to be considered.

Tattoos

Patients may have tattoos on their abdomen. When choosing the site, be sure to explain to the patient that you are choosing the best site based on obtaining a secure pouch seal. When the patient has a tattoo, do not hesitate to mark on the tattoo if it is in the best interest of the patient. Be sure the mark is visible and contact the surgeon to explain the situation and the patient's response to the mark. Piercings should be avoided and the jewelry for them should be worn so it can be considered when marking the site. The patient will be instructed to remove the pierced jewelry before surgery.

Contractures, Kyphosis, or Scoliosis

Patients with bony structural changes such as contractures, kyphosis, or scoliosis pose unique problems for stoma siting because the body alignment distorts the abdominal plane and may limit the space for an ostomy pouch. The goals are to select a site where a pouch will adhere and where the patient can perform the self-care. While visualization is optimal, the patient may need to learn techniques to adjust to lack of seeing the stoma. It may benefit the patient to wear an ostomy pouch after the stoma marking to confirm the stoma site.

Spiritual Beliefs

Patients may have strong spiritual beliefs that require the stoma site to be in a specific location. For example, patients of the Muslim faith may request the stoma located on the left side. In a letter to the Journal of Wound Ostomy Continence Nursing Editor, Iqbal et al. (2013) explain that Muslim patients report that the left-sided stoma is more compliant with their spiritual beliefs and is easier to manage during the ritual of sacred washing (refer to Chapter 12). The nurse should discuss the implications with the patient and consult with the surgeon regarding the patient's wishes and the safety to have the stoma placed on the left side. Consider marking several sites with the preferences numbered.

Difficult Stoma Siting Using Computed Tomography

Craig et al. (2007) share an excellent case study that involved team work to determine the site marking in a difficult case. The team reported the patient had undergone multiple abdominal procedures. The standard surgical procedure is to perform a laparotomy to identify the bowel segment that is mobile enough to reach the skin surface. The laparotomy often requires extensive adhesiolysis (the process of cutting adhesions between two abdominal structures), and the stoma site is often at the mercy of the length of the bowel. In this case study, the patient was assessed by the WOC nurse and marked with several potential sites away from scars. The patient then had a computed tomography (CT) examination with the medical team present. Areas in the abdomen were identified with radiopaque markers and rescanned to confirm the positions over the bowel. The final stoma site was then chosen by the WOC nurse based on the available sites. The patient had successful construction of a loop colostomy.

Continent Stoma Marking

Verify the type of continent stoma the surgeon will perform. Mark the continent stoma site in a location that follows the guidelines of general stoma site marking. Be sure the site is visible to the patient and in a location that the patient is able to manage the stoma drainage procedure. Ideally, mark the location on a smooth abdominal plane. In the event the patient would need to pouch the stoma, it is ideal to have a location that allows pouch adherence.

Wheelchair

Assess the patient in his or her own wheelchair. Sitting on the exam table is not the same posture the patient will assume in his or her own wheelchair. Discuss activities and watch the patient use the chair to note any changes in abdomen contour. The site chosen for a person in a wheelchair is slightly higher than normal. This allows better visualization and usually a better abdominal plane. The person may have a large abdomen because of the lack of strength of the abdominal muscle, and the abdomen may rest directly on the thigh (Colwell & Folkedahl, 2001).

Brace or Leg Prosthesis

Assess the patient wearing the brace. Determine if the brace will cause undue pressure or shearing of the pouching system. Consult with the surgeon if the site may interfere with the brace in order to choose a location that will allow the patient to be independent with care.

Pain/Limited Mobility

The patient may be in too much pain or be unable to assume the positions required for stoma siting. Sitting may be simulated with raising the head of the bed.

Special Equipment/Work Belts

Patients may have careers or hobbies that require the use of belts or other apparatus that may need to be considered as the stoma is marked. Ask the patient to bring the belt or apparatus to the stoma siting appointment to show the nurse where the item comes in contact with the abdomen. The patient should also perform movements that mimic the activity necessary while wearing the item. For example, police and carpenters need to wear thick, heavy leather belts and the stoma mark may be better sited above this belt to avoid compression and possible dislodgement of the pouch.

Radiation

Areas treated with radiation should be avoided for stoma marking if possible. Radiation treatments cause narrowing of the capillaries and can increase the risk of mucocutaneous separation as the ostomy heals after surgery. Radiation causes skin changes in the epidermis to be dry and fragile and easily traumatized by the adhesives of the pouch barrier (Erwin-Toth & Barrett, 1997).

Marking during Surgery

Even in emergent situations prior to surgery, the patient is usually able to sit up to visualize the abdominal planes and detect skin creases or folds. However, there are occasions the surgeon is faced with stoma creation without a preoperative site mark. If the nurse has the opportunity to help surgeons or surgical residents during a surgical case, or help the surgeon to use stoma siting principles during surgery, there are suggestions in Box 8-4.

Infants and Children

Babies have special needs due to the small abdomen. Newborns often have a large umbilical cord area and the baby may have tubes or access sites also on the abdomen. Avoid marking close to the umbilical cord, because once the cord falls off, the surface will be uneven (Boarini, 1988). It

BOX 8-4 Tips for Stoma Site Marking during Surgery

Most abdomens appear flat when body is supine.

The main goals are to avoid placing the stoma in a crease and to place the stoma high enough for the patient to see the stoma.

The abdomen can be gently squeezed to identify the natural infraumbilical and supraumbilical folds.

Look for signs of belt lines or creases by skin discoloration and small wrinkles in the skin. Avoid placing the stoma along these lines.

The ideal placement is on the infraumbilical bulge, but in more obese patients, the supraumbilical bulge may be more appropriate (**Fig. 8-4**).

Use the nipple lines as guidance for lateral placement.

Allow ample room between the midline incision and the stoma site for the barrier adhesive.

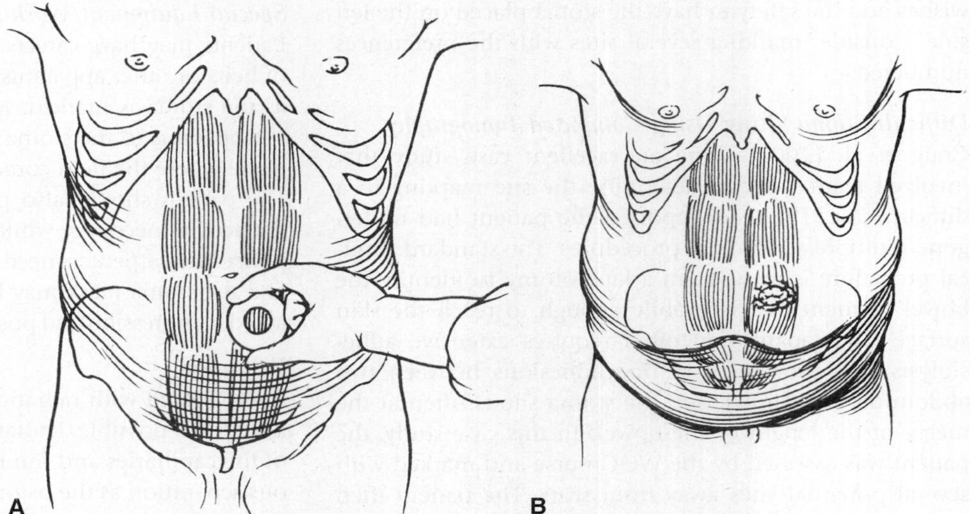

FIGURE 8-4. Stoma site through rectus muscle. **A.** The usual site for a stoma is on the apex of the infraumbilical bulge. **B.** In obese patients, the stoma is located on the upper abdomen, where it is visible and on flat skin.

is important to choose a site that has enough surface for a pouch barrier and avoid these other obstacles. Discuss the site with the surgeon if necessary. Explain the requirement of space needed to accommodate the barrier of the pouching system. See Chapter 14 for pediatric ostomy.

Teenagers

Teenagers have many different styles of body type. The guidelines followed for adults can be followed for teenagers. Consider that the teen will grow and develop over the years and that the stoma will need to be placed accordingly. The teen may want the mark as low as possible, but the nurse must place the mark in the best interest of the teen for the future years. Teens may have a narrow abdomen, and it will be difficult for the mark to avoid the midline, iliac crest, and costal margin. Belt line and style of clothing can be a challenge to meet their needs for ideal stoma siting

Documentation

Document the preoperative educational session thoroughly. Include ostomy teaching information covered, tools for education, the consent of the patient to mark for the stoma, and the stoma site marking procedure. Document the measurement using anatomic markings such as the umbilicus in the event the stoma mark fades and surgeon is unable to locate during surgery. Document patient teach-back, that a pouch was sent home with patient, and note the patient's response to teaching. It is important to document the patient's agreement on the stoma site marking. Note referrals for further education or counseling if the patient has time for these interactions before surgery.

Conclusions

The preoperative counseling session(s) should include physical and emotional assessment and help to determine sources of ongoing support for the patient. This preoperative education helps to alleviate the patient's fears and anxieties associated with the potential surgery. In addition, stoma site marking prior to surgery has been found to prevent problems associated with poor ostomy appliance fitting. The WOCN Best Practice Guidelines (2010) conclude that the person who is well prepared for the challenges that the new ostomy brings will have a less protracted period of adjustment.

REFERENCES

American Society of Colon and Rectal Surgeons Committee Members; Wound Ostomy Continence Nurses Society Committee Members. (2007). ASCRS and WOCN joint position statement on the value of preoperative stoma marking for patients undergoing fecal ostomy surgery. *Journal of Wound, Ostomy and Continence Nursing, 34*(6), 627–628.

Anon, J. S. (1976). The PLISSIT model: A proposed conceptual scheme for the behavioral treatment of sexual problems. *Journal of Sex Education Therapy, 2*(2), 1–15.

AUA and WOCN. (2009). AUA and WOCN Society Joint Position Statement on the Value of Preoperative Stoma Marking for Patients Undergoing Creation of an Incontinent Urostomy. *Journal of Wound, Ostomy and Continence Nursing, 36*(3), 267–268.

Bass, E., Del Pino, A., Tan, A., et al. (1997). Does preoperative stoma marking and education by the enterostomal therapist affect outcome? *Diseases of the Colon & Rectum, 40*(4), 440–442.

Boarini, J. H. (1988). Principles of stoma care for infants. *Journal of Enterostomal Therapy, 16*(1), 21–25.

Chaudhri, S., Brown, L., Hassan, I., et al. (2005). Preoperative intensive, community based vs. traditional stoma education: A randomized, controlled trial. *Diseases of the Colon and Rectum, 48*, 504–509.

Colwell, J. C., & Folkedahl, B. (2001). Stoma site selection in a patient with multiple enterocutaneous fistulae. *Journal of Wound, Ostomy and Continence Nursing, 28*(2), 113–115.

Cottam, J., Richards, K., Hasted, A., et al. (2007). Results of a nationwide prospective audit of stoma complications within 3 weeks of surgery. *Colorectal Disease, 9*(9), 834–838.

Dorman, C. (2009). *Ostomy basics: The nurse's personal feelings toward ostomies play a role in patient outcomes*. www.rnweb.com [RN], 22–27.

Doughty, D. (2008). History of ostomy surgery. *Journal of Wound Ostomy and Continence Nursing, 35*(1), 34–38.

Ellis, C. N. (2010). Bowel preparation before elective colorectal surgery: What is the evidence? *Seminars in Colon and Rectal Surgery 21*(3), 144–147.

Fellows, J. (June, 2013). Highways, byways, and detours of stoma siting. Wound Ostomy Continence Nursing Society National Conference Lecture.

Erwin-Toth, P., & Barrett, P. (1997). Stoma site marking: A primer. *Ostomy/Wound Management, 43*(4), 18–22.

Erwin-Toth, P., Thompson, S., & Davis, J. (2012). Factors impacting the quality of life of people with an ostomy in North America: Results from the Dialogue Study. *Journal of Wound Ostomy and Continence Nursing, 39*(4), 417–422.

Goldberg, M., Aukett, L. K., Carmel, J., et al. (2010). Management of the patient with a fecal ostomy: Best practice guideline for clinicians. *Journal of Wound Ostomy and Continence Nursing, 37*(6), 596–598.

Gray, M., Colwell, J., Doughty, D., et al. (2013). Peristomal moisture–associated skin damage in adults with fecal ostomies: A comprehensive review and consensus. *Journal of Wound Ostomy and Continence Nursing, 40*(4), 389–399.

Guenaga, K. F., Matos, D., & Wille-Jorgensen, P. (2011). Mechanical bowel preparation for elective colorectal surgery. *Cochrane Database Systematic Review*, (9):CD001544. doi: 10.1002/14651858.CD001544.pub4.

Iqbal, F., Zaman, S., & Bowley, D. M. (2013). Stoma location requires special consideration in selected patients. *Journal of Wound Ostomy and Continence Nursing, 40*(6), 565–566.

Junkin, J., & Beitz, J. (2005). Sexuality and the person with a stoma implications for comprehensive WOC nursing practice. *Journal of Wound Ostomy Continence Nursing, 32*(2), 121–128.

Nichols, T. R. (2011). Social connectivity in those 24 months or less postsurgery. *Journal of Wound Ostomy and Continence Nursing, 38*(1), 63–68.

Person, B., Ifargan, R., Lachter, J., et al. (2012). The impact of preoperative stoma site marking on the incidence of complications, quality of life, and patient's independence. *Diseases of the Colon and Rectum, 55*(7), 783–787.

Pittman, J. (2011). Characteristics of the patient with an ostomy. *Journal of Wound Ostomy and Continence Nursing, 38*(3), 271.

Pittman, J., Rawl, S., Schmidt, C., et al. (2008). Demographic and clinical factors related to ostomy complications and quality of life in veterans with an ostomy. *Journal of Wound Ostomy and Continence Nursing, 35*(5), 493–503.

Richbourg, L., Thorpe, J. M., & Rapp, C. G. (2007). Difficulties experienced by the ostomate after hospital discharge. *Journal of Wound Ostomy and Continence Nursing, 34*(1), 70–79.

United Ostomy Associations of America (UOAA). (2008). *Controlling odor*. Columbus Discovery. http://www.ostomy.org

Watt, K. (1982). Stoma placement. In D. Broadwell, & B. Jackson (Eds.), *Principles of ostomy care*. St. Louis, MO: Mosby.

Weiss, B. (2003). *Health literacy. A manual for clinicians* (2nd Ed.). Chicago, IL: American Medical Association Foundation and American Medical Association.

WCET (2014). Zulkowski, K. (Ed.). *WCET International Ostomy Guideline*. Osborne Park, Australia: WCET.

WOCN (2008). *White Paper: Wear time of a fecal or urinary pouching system. Mount Laurel, NJ: WOCN. www.wocn.org*

WOCN (2010). *Management of the patient with a fecal ostomy: Best practice guidelines for clinicians*. Mount Laurel, NJ: WOCN. www.wocn.org

WOCN (2011). *Bowel prep for patients with a colostomy*. Mount Laurel, NJ: WOCN. www.wocn.org

WOCN (2013). *Colostomy and ileostomy products and tips: Best practice for clinicians*. Mount Laurel, NJ: WOCN. www.wocn.org

Yang L., Chen H., Welk B., et al. (2013). Does using comprehensive preoperative bowel preparation offer any advantage for urinary diversion using ileum? A meta-analysis. *International Urology and Nephrology, 45*(1), 25–31.

QUESTIONS

1. A patient is scheduled for surgery for an abdominal perineal resection. What type of ostomy will be created during this procedure?
   A. Temporary end colostomy or ileostomy
   B. Permanent end colostomy
   C. Permanent end ileostomy
   D. Temporary loop ileostomy

2. There are many ways a WOC nurse can help patients with their fears and concerns as they face surgery for an ostomy. These include which of the following?
   A. Tell them the ostomy isn't so bad and could be a lot worse.
   B. Advise them to keep quiet about their fears and they will feel better soon.
   C. Discuss the opportunity for them to meet with an ostomy visitor, someone who has an ostomy and can describe ways to manage ostomy issues.
   D. Nurses can deliver stoma care so the patient doesn't have to.

3. The WOC nurse is teaching a patient with a new stoma about pouching systems. Which teaching point accurately describes an important aspect of using a pouching system?
   A. There are two- and three-piece pouching systems available.
   B. Pouching systems are not odor proof and may have an odor.
   C. Follow-up with an ostomy nurse is usually scheduled on an emergency basis.
   D. The usual wear time for a pouch is 4 days.

4. If the surgeon is siting the stoma in the OR, what advice would you give for general information for stoma site marking?
   A. Ideally, the stoma should be placed on the infraumbilical bulge.
   B. If possible, the stoma should be placed in a crease.
   C. The stoma should be placed over wrinkles if possible for more available skin.
   D. Placement in the incision line allows for ease of pouching.

5. The patient with ulcerative colitis who is being prepared for a surgical procedure to create a permanent end ileostomy should receive preoperative education that includes:
   A. Instructing patients they will need to change their clothing style after this surgery
   B. Assuming that 25% of information provided will be forgotten by the patient
   C. Telling patients they will be NPO until bowel function has returned
   D. Reinforcing to the patient that self-care is simple with few steps to follow

6. The WOC nurse helps prepare the patient for ostomy surgery by:
   A. Determining the patient's emotional support system
   B. Meeting with the patient undergoing elective surgery 5 weeks prior to surgery
   C. Administering mechanical bowel prep prior to surgery
   D. Explaining that the stoma will be red and dry and will have minimal sensation

7. Which aspect of self-care for a stoma should a WOC nurse teach preoperatively?
   A. Explain the patient will perform a pouching system change on an as-needed basis.
   B. Describe that most people sit on the toilet and direct the pouch contents into the toilet when emptying it.
   C. Note that the patient will acquire the skills necessary to change the pouching system prior to discharge.
   D. Explain that the skin around the stoma normally will be reddened, but should not be sore.

8. The WOC nurse counsels patients regarding lifestyle issues following stoma surgery. What statement accurately describes an important teaching tip?
   A. Patients with an ostomy should take a tub bath instead of a shower.
   B. Most patients will not have to follow a special diet once healing takes place.
   C. Most patients need to modify their clothing to accommodate the pouch.
   D. Travel on airplanes is prohibited with an ostomy appliance.

9. Which of the following should be considered for stoma site marking in special populations?
   A. The goal of marking two stomas on the same abdomen is to mark the stomas at the same abdominal heights.
   B. When marking two stomas at the same time, it is preferable to mark the urostomy at least one inch lower.
   C. For a thin patient, the nurse should gently squeeze the skin of the infraumbilical fold and mark within the crease of the fold.
   D. The nurse should choose a site for a person in a wheelchair that is slightly higher than normal.

10. Which statement accurately represents a recommended guideline for marking the stoma site of patients with special needs?
   A. Assess a patient who is in a wheelchair while he or she is sitting on the examination table.
   B. Have the patient lie flat to better assess the creases and fold in his or her abdomen.
   C. For an infant, avoid marking the stoma site close to the umbilical cord as this area will be uneven when it falls off.
   D. Mark the stoma site of an adolescent as low as possible in order to honor their wishes for belt line and current clothing styles.

ANSWERS: 1.**B**, 2.**C**, 3.**D**, 4.**A**, 5.**C**, 6.**A**, 7.**B**, 8.**B**, 9.**D**, 10.**C**

CHAPTER 9

Postoperative Nursing Assessment Management

Janice C. Colwell

OBJECTIVE

Plan for postoperative nursing assessment and management following surgical procedures that result in a fecal and/or urinary diversion.

Topic Outline

Postoperative Assessment

Following the surgical procedure to create an intestinal stoma, a thorough patient assessment and understanding of the surgical procedure must be completed in order to plan care. The surgical report should be read to determine the type of surgical procedure performed as well as any intraoperative findings such as the type of stoma created, presence of advanced disease, existence of adhesions, and/or unusual findings not anticipated before the surgical event (Sonia, 2013). This information will be necessary to support the patient after surgery. The immediate postoperative notes should be read to understand the patient's first 24 hours after surgery, noting pain management and participation in ambulation, coughing, and deep breathing. Self-care ostomy management will need to be started as soon as the patient can concentrate on the acquisition of new skills; understanding his or her response to pain management as well as his or her ability to participate in routine postoperative activities may help in knowing when teaching can begin. It is more than likely that the first postoperative teaching session will start within 24 hours after surgery.

Postoperative patient assessment includes the following:

- *Incisional integrity* noting the type of closure (primary, left open to heal by secondary intention, staples, stitches, liquid bonding agent). If the wound has been approximated and closed, examine the incision and if present the dressing for drainage. Wearing gloves, gently palpate either side of the incision noting the firmness or lack of firmness of the tissue, the temperature of the skin as well as any oozing that might be present while examining the area. Note the color of the skin at the incision and compare to the area outside of the surgical area. If the wound is healing by secondary intention, note the approximate size of the wound, the depth, the quality of the tissue as well as the type of dressing, and the presence of wound drainage (color, amount, presence of odor).

CLINICAL PEARL

Examine the periwound skin and determine the amount of space between the wound and the outer footprint of the ostomy pouching system. This information will help in determining the appropriate pouching system to avoid injury to the new surgical wound/incision.

- *Presence of abdominal drains* noting the insertion site for drainage at the skin/drain interface, the amount of drainage (number of gauze pads used and how often changed), and quality of drainage. Assess how the drain is secured (with or without sutures). Assure that the drainage tube has the suction source intact and that the container is emptied when at least three fourths full and that the amount emptied is captured in the intake and output record.
- Note the amount and frequency of *pain medication* and the patient's response to pain medications.
- Assessment of the presence or absence of *bowel sounds*. Using a stethoscope, listen in the four abdominal quadrants for the presence of bowel activity. Examine the ostomy pouch for the presence of gas; trapped air in the pouch is one sign that bowel activity has returned.
- Gently *palpate the abdomen* noting firmness and excessive tenderness as indicated by the patient's response.
- Assess the *respiratory status* by listening to breath sounds and encourage the use of the incentive spirometer, deep breathing, and coughing.
- Patient's *overall response* to the surgery and recovery. It is important to determine the patient's understanding of his/her role in the postoperative recovery and to educate the patient on meeting goals to help move toward recovery. The patient should be ambulating several times in 24 hours and spending time out of bed to decrease the incidence of postoperative complications and increase strength and endurance. Remind the patient that he or she will need to learn how to empty his or her pouch prior to discharge as well as have a good understanding of how the pouching system will be changed.
- Review of the daily *intake* (IV fluids and when started oral intake) and *output* (urinary, stool and, if present, drainage collected in drainage collectors).

Diet: Once bowel activity has returned, the diet is resumed. For most patients, a clear liquid diet is ordered and the patient instructed to sip a small amount of fluid to determine if he or she can tolerate fluid. Since gas is an issue after abdominal surgery, avoiding a straw is suggested as well as encouraging ambulation to help peristalsis. Once a liquid diet is tolerated, a low-residue diet is ordered; suggest to the patient to eat small frequent meals and to chew all foods well. A fecal stoma will be edematous after surgery, and a low-residue diet will allow the stool to pass through the stoma. The patient with a colon or ileal conduit has a bowel anastomosis (where the conduit was excised) and because of potential edema at the anastomosis, a low-residue diet is preferred.

CLINICAL PEARL

As the patient resumes oral intake, discourage the use of a straw as using a straw can increase the intake of air causing blotting and excessive gas.

Stoma Assessment

Although the surgical report should describe the type of stoma constructed, a thorough assessment of the stoma should be performed. Assessments will include the anatomic location of the stoma (where in the GI or urinary system), the function of the stoma (volume and consistency), and the type of stoma (the configuration-end, loop or end loop) (Tables 9-1 and 9-2).

Anatomic Location and Function

Review the operative report, the history and physical, and other pertinent notes to understand from what section of the intestine the stoma was created. The function of the fecal stoma will depend upon the location in the GI tract; closer to the end of the colon the output will be less in volume and thicker in consistency. A fecal stoma will generally start to function 1 to 3 days after surgery, commonly earlier when the patient undergoes a laparoscopic surgical procedure. Gas followed by liquid is the initial output of both a small and large bowel fecal stoma. A urostomy will begin to function immediately with the presence of mucus and blood-tinged urine.

A jejunostomy, an opening into the jejunum, will have liquid stoma output, and the volume can be as high as 2,400 mL in 24 hours. An ileostomy is an opening into

TABLE 9-1 Patient with a New Fecal Stoma: Assessment Parameters

Anatomic location (most likely obtained from OR report/chart)	Small intestine: jejunum, ileum Large intestine: ascending, transverse, descending, sigmoid Amount (cm) of bowel above stoma
Function	Presence of gas: note pouch inflation Volume, color, and consistency of effluent
Construction	End: single lumen (opening) Loop or end loop: double lumens (openings) Note presence of support bridge. If possible determine which opening is the proximal end w/mucous fistula
Stoma assessment	Stoma mucosa: Color: deep red Edema: lack of normal folds, creases, taut tissue firm to touch Protrusion: above skin, at skin, below skin Lumen location: center, off center, even with skin Mucocutaneous junction: Junction of stoma/skin: intact Junction of stoma/skin: not intact—separation between stoma and skin Percentage of junction that is separated Approximate depth of approximation Type of tissue in separation (see Chapter 16)

TABLE 9-2 Patient with a New Urinary Stoma: Assessment Parameters

Anatomic location (most likely obtained from OR report/chart)	Small intestine: ileal conduit Large intestine: colonic conduit
Function	Volume and color of urine, presence of mucus in urine
Construction	End: single lumen (opening) End loop: observe presence of support bridge Stents: check end of each, note cut (even or slanted) and presence/location of sutures around stents into stoma
Stoma assessment	Stoma mucosa: Color: deep red Edema: lack of normal folds, creases, taut tissue firm to touch Protrusion: above skin, at skin, below skin Lumen location: center, off center, even with skin Mucocutaneous junction: Junction of stoma/skin: intact Junction of stoma/skin: not intact—separation between stoma and skin Percentage of junction that is separated Approximate depth of approximation Type of tissue in separation (see Chapter 16)

the last portion of the small intestine, the ileum. The output will vary but is generally about 1,200 mL in 24 hours (Orkin & Cataldo, 2007), and while dietary choices can influence the output, it should vary between a thick liquid to a semi-pasty consistency (like oatmeal). A colostomy is an opening into any section of the colon, and the activity of the colostomy will depend upon the location of the stoma in the colon; closer to the rectum, the output will be pasty to almost formed because the stool has had time to sit in the colon, more fluid is absorbed, and the stool is more formed. Thus, a right-sided colostomy (ascending) will have stoma output similar to that of an ileostomy, a transverse colostomy will have pasty to semisolid stool, and a left-sided colostomy (descending and sigmoid) will have a semisolid to formed stool depending on how close the stoma is to the end of the colon. Colostomy volume will vary from 600 to 1,000 mL in 24 hours depending on the anatomic location. However, after surgery each of the above-noted stomas will have variable function, starting liquid and moving toward "normal" depending on oral intake, medications, and past medical/surgical history. A person who has lost some of the small bowel from other surgeries will have an alteration in the type and volume of stoma output. Examples of diagnoses that can alter stoma function can include Crohn's disease, previous radiation to the abdomen, ischemic disease, medications, and concurrent treatment such as chemotherapy.

A high-output fecal stoma, usually a jejunostomy or ileostomy, can cause dehydration, slow the rehabilitative process, and in severe cases cause metabolic issues. It is important that ostomy output be carefully measured during the postoperative period, and if the volume of output exceeds what is considered to be the normal amount, a plan of care will need to be worked out that will include ruling out a partial or intermittent bowel obstruction, abdominal sepsis, enteritis (such as *Clostridium difficile*), or sudden drug withdrawal (opiates or corticosteroids). The plan of care may include the following: the use of isotonic fluids, restriction of hypo- and hypertonic fluids, dietary restrictions of high-sugar foods and fluids, dietary inclusions of starch-based foods, and/or the use of antidiarrheal medications (Baker et al., 2011).

A urostomy can be created from a segment of the colon or ileum. The most common approach is to use the terminal ileum (ileal conduit), but in some cases, the colon is used (colon conduit). The function of a urostomy depends upon kidney function and hydration, but minimal output should be 800 mL/24 hours. It is important to remember that since the intestine is used to make a conduit, there will be at least initially a large amount of mucus expelled from the stoma. The intestinal mucosa secretes mucus to lubricate the intestinal contents and continues to secrete mucus when diverted. For most people with a urostomy, the volume of mucus is high for the first few months and is reported to decrease over time.

An ileal or colon conduit will have stents that are placed at the time of the ureter/conduit anastomosis, the purpose of which is to protect the anastomosis (**Fig. 9-1**). The length of time that the stents remain in place will depend upon the integrity of the anastomosis, the patient's ability to heal, and the surgeon's preference. Note the number of stents (one for each ureter) and the securement device (sutures from the stents to the stoma). Should a stent push out of the stoma before the planned removal, notify the urology team.

It is important not to rely on the location of the stoma on the abdominal wall to indicate the type of stoma. While it is likely in many cases if the ileum is used the stoma should be on the right side of the abdomen, the physical location of the stoma should be correlated with the medical record/operative report and consultation with the surgical team to verify the anatomic location of the stoma.

Stoma Construction/Type

The type of stoma constructed by the surgeon will depend on the etiology of the medical or surgical problem and the patient's anatomy. The type of stoma needs to be assessed, as the structure of the stoma will impact the choice of management system.

An *end stoma* is created by dividing the intestine, bringing the proximal end of the intestine through the abdominal wall, maturing the stoma once outside of the abdominal

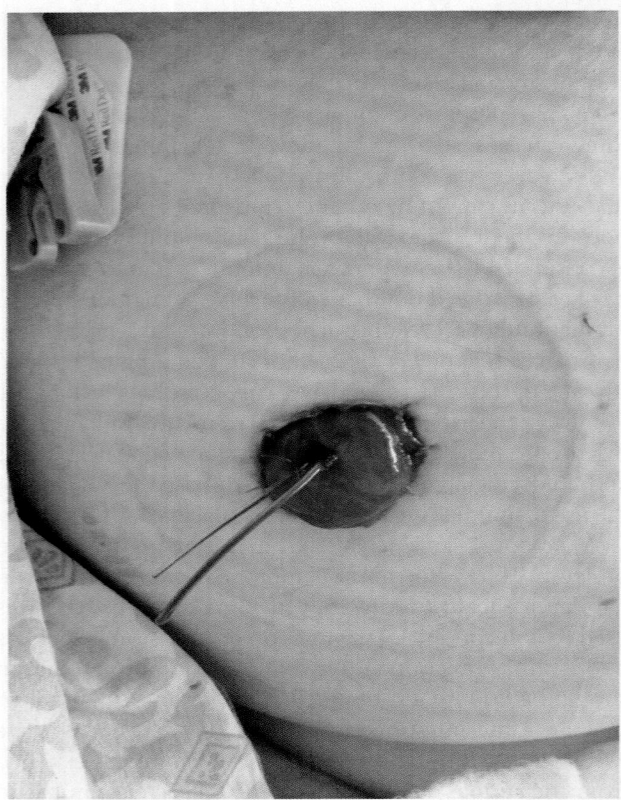

FIGURE 9-1. Urostomy with stents.

wall to attach to the skin (see Chapter 7). Any portion of the GI tract can be used to create an end stoma. The distal end of the intestine can be removed or closed off. Surgical interventions that create an end stoma include the abdominal perineal resection (see Chapter 3), proctocolectomy (see Chapter 4), or a bowel resection and the creation of a Hartmann's pouch. A Hartmann's pouch is the resection of a portion of the colon, creation of a colostomy, and the oversewing of the remaining colon, and creating a Hartmann's pouch or also referred to as the Hartmann's procedure.

CLINICAL PEARL

The patient with a Hartmann's pouch may pass old stool from the rectum if their bowel was not cleansed prior to the operation. Advise the patient that they may feel pressure at the rectum and they should sit on the commode to pass any old stool.

A *loop stoma* is created in the small or large intestine by mobilizing the side of the intestine up through the abdominal wall, making a transverse incision on the intestine and maturing the mucosa (see Chapter 7). A support bridge is placed under and in many cases around the stoma, and the intestine is attached to the abdominal wall. Surgical indications for creation of a loop stoma include protection of a distal anastomosis, diversion of an obstruction below the stoma, and diversion of an anastomotic leak. Most loop stomas are created as a temporary stoma but can become permanent depending upon the patient's condition.

Support bridges are left in place until the stoma heals to the abdominal skin, and the time frame can vary depending upon the surgical technique, the reason for creation, and the amount of tension of the support bridge on the skin and the ability of the patient to heal. The support bridge should be removed when there is little tension of the stoma on the abdominal wall and when the stoma has healed to the abdominal wall. The time frame for use of the support bridge can be as little as 5 days and as long as a month. The decision for removal should be a joint decision between the surgeon and the WOC nurse. After explaining the procedure to the patient, the support bridge is removed by clipping the sutures that were placed during surgery and the suture location will vary by surgeon. After the sutures are removed, the bridge is slipped out from under/around the stoma. If there are openings in the skin where the bridge or sutures were located, skin barrier powder can fill the defect until healing takes place.

In infrequent cases, when the intestine is resected, both ends of the intestine are brought to the skin, the proximal or functioning stoma as well as the distal or nonfunctioning stoma. The distal end is considered a *mucous fistula* as there will be no active stool from this opening, yet mucus on occasion may be present. One indication for this type of diversion may be a distal obstruction, and the mucous fistula can allow any drainage to be expelled since nothing can get beyond the obstruction. Care of the mucous fistula depends on the type and amount of drainage. If the colon was not cleaned out prior to the surgical intervention, old stool may drain for a short time period and the use of a pouch would be indicated. Once the segment is no longer passing stool, a dry dressing can be placed over the stoma to protect the patient's clothes from mucus.

An *end loop ileostomy*, sometimes referred to as a Turnbull end loop (see Chapter 7), is an option when the thickness of the abdominal wall does not allow for an easy passage of an end ileostomy such as in the obese patient. The end section of the small bowel is closed, and a loop of the segment is then used to make the stoma. A support bridge is placed under the stoma until healing takes place.

A urostomy can be constructed from the small or large intestine (see Chapter 6). The term urostomy defines that there is an opening that drains urine; the type of stoma will be an ileal or colon conduit, or a ureterostomy. An ileal or colon conduit uses the ileum or colon to make a passage for the urine to exit the body. A ureterostomy uses the ureters, either each brought to the skin in two separate stomas or one ureter anastomosed to the other and a single ureter brought out as a stoma. The ureterostomy is rarely created but if used is generally performed as a temporary diversion (Rhee et al., 2012).

The *end loop urinary stoma (also called a Turnbull loop urostomy)* can be used to create a urostomy in an obese patient with short mesentery as described above for a fecal diversion.

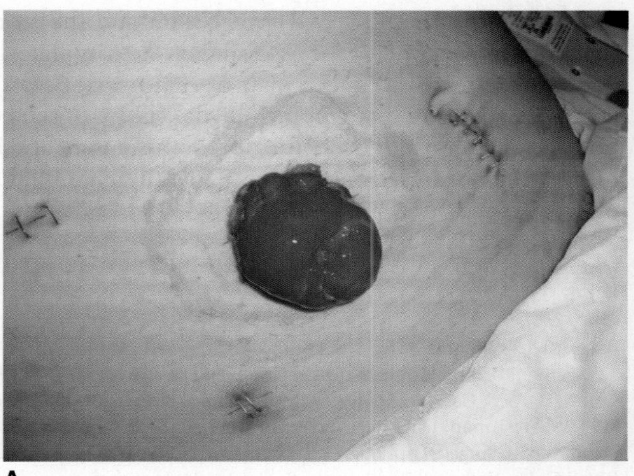

A

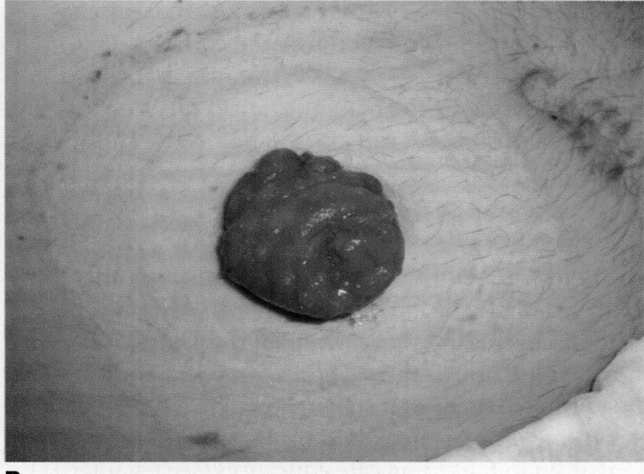

B

FIGURE 9-2. Edematous stoma. **A.** Postoperative edema. **B.** Two-week postoperative resolving edema.

Stoma Assessment

The following variables are included when assessing a stoma:

- *Stoma mucosa*: color, presence of edema, and texture
- *Stoma structure*: size, shape, protrusion, location of the lumen, and mucocutaneous junction
- *Peristomal skin*: integrity and abdominal contours: creases and folds

Stoma Mucosa

A newly created stoma will be red, moist, and edematous, and the mucosa will be shiny and taut with fluid (Fig. 9-2). As the stoma heals, there will be a texture to the stoma and creases and folds will be visible. Most stomas are a deep red with the exception of a ureterostomy that generally is a pale pink. If the stoma is a dark red to purple or there is dark nonvascular tissue present, this can indicate a blood flow problem and the surgical team should be consulted.

CLINICAL PEARL

Advise the patient with a new fecal diversion that because of the post-operative edema they may hear noise as stool and gas pass from the stoma.

Stoma Structure

The stoma should be assessed and reevaluated periodically during the postoperative period for the *size and shape as well as protrusion*, because stoma edema will reduce slowly for the first 6 weeks after creation. The size and shape will help to determine the size of the opening in the skin barrier of the pouching system (see Chapter 10). Preferably, all stomas should protrude at least 2 cm above the skin to allow the stool or urine to drain into the pouching system. When there is inadequate stoma protrusion or if the stoma is flush to the skin or retracted, there may be effluent leakage under the seal and a specific pouching system should be considered (see Chapter 10). Ideally, the *stoma lumen* (Fig. 9-3) would be at the top apex of the stoma to allow the urine or stool to exit the stoma and drain directly into the pouching system; determine the location of lumen by looking at the stoma in a sitting and lying position as the lumen may change as the body contours change. A lumen that is even with the skin will need special consideration in choosing the pouching system (see Chapter 10). Evaluate the *mucocutaneous junction* (skin–stoma junction) for presence and type of sutures as well as note any gaps between the stoma and skin that can indicate delayed or poor healing (see Chapter 16).

Peristomal Skin

The peristomal skin should be evaluated for any alterations in the skin integrity. Ideally, the skin should be intact, free from any injury. When a pouching system is first removed, the peristomal skin maybe pink, but this should resolve quickly. Examine the skin in good lighting to determine if there is a partial or full skin loss, papules or pustules, or other alterations in the skin integrity. Skin loss can indicate a poor pouching system seal, prolonged wear time, inappropriate use of product or sensitivity to a product (see Chapter 10). The abdominal contours are examined with the patient standing, lying flat, and sitting. The area around the stoma can change in each position,

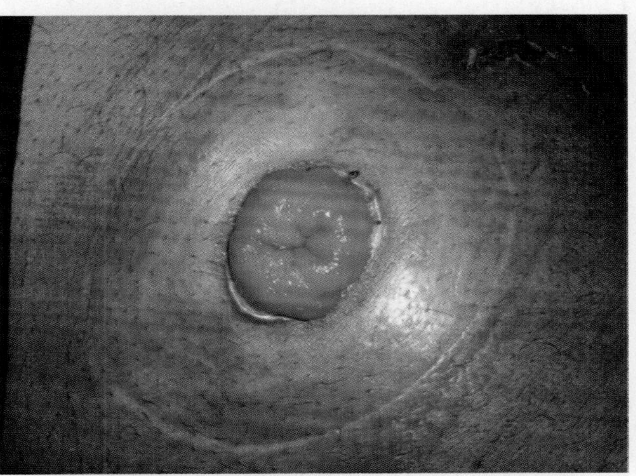

FIGURE 9-3. Stoma with lumen in center, top of stoma.

and knowing the presence of creases or folds in each of these positions can help determine the correct skin barrier shape or the use of accessories (see Chapter 10). The stoma should be assessed as the patient changes positions, as the stoma shape or size that can also change as the abdominal contours change.

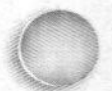

Postoperative Planning

The patient (or a family member or significant other) will need to acquire the skill of emptying the ostomy pouch prior to discharge, and the teaching of this skill should start within 24 hours after surgery. The teaching session should be planned immediately after surgery working with the patient to determine if he or she would like or needs a second person involved in the stoma care education (see Chapter 11).

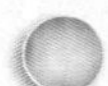

Conclusions

Postoperative management of the patient undergoing a fecal and/or urinary diversion will include a thorough assessment of the patient's overall status as well as a special focus on the stoma, the peristomal skin, and the stoma functioning. Once all of the assessments are complete, the data can be reviewed and a plan of care developed. The goal is to plan care that will include the choice of the best pouching system and the instruction of the patient and his or her designee in self-care and a successful rehabilitation of the person with a stoma.

REFERENCES

Baker, M. L., Williams, R. N., & Nightingale, J. M. (2011). Causes and management of a high output stoma. *Colorectal Disease, 13*(2), 191–197.

Orkin, B. A., & Cataldo, P. A. (2007). Intestinal stomas. In B. G. Wolf, J. W. Fleshman, D. E. Beck, et al. (Eds.), *The ASCRS textbook of colon and rectal surgery* (pp. 622–630). New York, NY: Springer.

Rhee, C. H., Yerkes, E. B., & Rink, R. C. (2012). Incontinent and continent urinary diversions. In A. G. Coran, A. Caldamone, N. Scott Adzick, et al. (Eds.), *Pediatric surgery* (7th ed., pp. 1487–1496). St. Louis, MO: Elsevier, Mosby.

Sonia, C. (2013). Care of surgical patients. In P. A. Potter, A. G. Perry, P. A. Stockert, et al. (Eds.), *Fundamentals of nursing* (8th ed., pp. 1254–1295). St. Louis, MO: Elsevier, Mosby.

QUESTIONS

1. A nurse is performing an assessment of a postoperative patient following the creation of a urinary diversion. Which assessment technique has the nurse performed correctly?

A. Wearing gloves, the nurse gently palpates either side of an approximated and closed incision.
B. The nurse empties the drainage tube container when it is one half full and records the drainage on the I&O record.
C. The nurse uses deep palpation to assess the firmness and tenderness of the patient's abdomen.
D. The nurse checks that the patient has been ambulating at least once in 24 hours and spends time out of bed to increase endurance.

2. The WOC nurse is assessing the stoma of a patient with a new fecal diversion. Which assessment data indicate a finding of edema?

A. The stoma is a deep red color.
B. The stoma is taut and firm to the touch.
C. The lumen location is off center.
D. The skin at the junction of the stoma is not intact.

3. The WOC nurse is assessing the stoma of a patient with a new urinary diversion. Which data represent a normal postoperative finding?

A. The stoma is retracted.
B. Mucus is present in the urine.
C. There is partial skin loss.
D. The stoma is a dark purple color.

4. The WOC nurse is reviewing the operative report of a patient with a new fecal diversion. Which type of stoma function would the nurse expect to find based on this report?

A. The fecal stoma will generally start to function within 3 to 5 days after surgery.
B. When a patient undergoes a laparaoscopic surgical procedure, the patient's stoma will generally function later than when the patient undergoes a laparotomy.
C. Initial stomal output resembles pudding or oatmeal consistency.
D. A low-output fecal stoma, usually a jejunostomy or ileostomy, can cause dehydration.

5. Based on the location of the fecal stoma in the GI tract, the nurse would expect which finding regarding the stoma output in a patient with an established fecal diversion?

A. The output from an ileostomy will vary but is generally about 500 mL in 24 hours.
B. A jejunostomy will have liquid stoma output, and the volume can be as high as 3,400 mL in 24 hours.
C. Colostomy volume will vary from 300 to 500 mL in 24 hours depending on the anatomic location.
D. With a colostomy that is close to the rectum, the output will be pasty to almost formed because the stool has had time to sit in the colon.

6. The nurse is planning care for a patient who has ileostomy output that far exceeds what is considered to be the normal amount. What intervention is expected in this situation?
   A. The use of hypo- and hypertonic fluids
   B. Dietary inclusions of high sugar foods and fluids
   C. The use of isotonic fluids
   D. The restriction of starch-based foods

7. The WOC nurse is assessing a patient with a new urostomy. Which normal finding would the nurse expect?
   A. Minimal output of the stoma should be 800 mL/24 hours.
   B. Mucus should not be found in the output.
   C. Stents are not normally placed at the time of the ureter/conduit anastomosis.
   D. The location of the stoma determines the type of stoma created.

8. Which type of stoma construction would be most commonly found in an obese patient with a short mesentery who requires the creation of an ileostomy?
   A. End stoma
   B. Loop stoma
   C. End loop ileostomy
   D. Mucous fistula

9. Which surgical intervention most commonly results in a loop stoma?
   A. Abdominal perineal resection
   B. Diversion of an obstruction below the stoma
   C. Proctocolectomy
   D. Creation of a Hartmann's pouch

10. Which teaching point would the WOC nurse consider a priority for a postoperative patient who has undergone a fecal and/or urinary diversion?
    A. Teaching a significant other how to empty the ostomy pouch for the patient
    B. Making referrals for follow-up care and psychiatric counseling
    C. Determining if the patient needs a second person involved in stoma care
    D. Teaching the patient to reduce the number of meals consumed per day

ANSWERS: 1.**A**, 2.**B**, 3.**B**, 4.**A**, 5.**D**, 6.**C**, 7.**A**, 8.**C**, 9.**B**, 10.**C**

CHAPTER 10

Selection of Pouching System

Janice C. Colwell

OBJECTIVES

1. Describe factors to consider when selecting pouching systems.
2. Differentiate among product options when selecting pouching systems based on the patient assessment.

Topic Outline

- Skin Barriers
  - Solid Skin Barrier
  - Wear Time
  - Solid Skin Barrier Shapes
  - Fit of the Solid Skin Barrier
  - Skin Barrier Paste
  - Skin Barrier Powder
  - Skin Barrier Ring
  - Skin Barrier Strip Paste
  - Elastic Skin Barrier Strip
  - Liquid Skin Barrier
- Ostomy Pouches
  - One-Piece Pouching system
  - Two-Piece Pouching System
  - Pouch Features
    - Drainable Pouch for Fecal Stoma Management
    - Drainable Pouch for Urinary Stoma Management
    - Nondrainable Pouches
    - Pouch Length
    - Pouch Films
    - Gas Management
- Pouching Accessory Products
  - Belt
  - Adhesive Products
  - Pouch Covers
  - Pouch Liners
  - In-Pouch Deodorant Liquids
  - Oral Odor Eliminators
  - Absorbent Products
- Conclusions

The principles that guide the selection of a pouching system are (1) consistent wear time: the ability to maintain the pouch seal for a predictable amount of time (no leakage between the application and removal of the pouching system); and (2) intact peristomal skin: when the pouching system is removed, the peristomal skin is undamaged.

The pouching system is defined as the products used to collect the stoma effluent, which will provide a secure predictable seal and protect the peristomal skin (Wound Ostomy and Continence Nurses Society [WOCN], 2013). Pouching systems vary among people with an ostomy, and the choices for the products will depend upon a thorough assessment of the patient, his or her stoma, peristomal skin, and his or her self-care abilities coupled with a good understanding of the ostomy products. When the patient has a new stoma, he or she has many reservations and a leading fear is that of leakage and a negative impact on quality of life (Pittman et al., 2008). It is imperative that the most appropriate pouching is chosen for the person with an ostomy and education on how to utilize the pouching system is provided. Periodic review of the fit of the pouching system, wear time, and utilization should be done, keeping in mind that as a person's abdomen changes (loss or gain of weight, abdominal surgery, changing contours due to aging) the stoma and the surrounding tissue can change and an alteration in the pouching system may need to be considered. The pouching system products will include skin barriers, pouches, and accessory products.

Skin Barriers

Skin barriers are available in several configurations, solid sheet integrated with the pouch (a one-piece pouching system), a solid sheet with a flange/coupling mechanism attached (a two-piece pouching system), paste, powder, ring, strip, and liquid. While each of the aforementioned skin barriers provides skin protection, each is unique in its use and purpose (Table 10-1).

Solid Skin Barrier

The solid skin barrier is the interface between the skin and the pouch; it provides the seal (adhesion) and protects the peristomal skin (Fig. 10-1). Solid skin barriers contain many ingredients including hydrocolloids, adhesives, and polymers. The adhesive provides the seal of the skin barrier to the peristomal skin. The purpose of the hydrocolloid is to absorb moisture and maintain the skin barrier seal. If moisture (e.g., from perspiration) is allowed to collect on the skin, the adhesive seal will be lost; thus, absorbing some moisture helps to maintain the seal.

TABLE 10-1 Skin Barriers

Skin Barrier Type	Indications for Use	Considerations	Tips
Solid skin barrier	Protection of the peristomal skin from stoma effluent, integrated into most pouching systems.		Determine the size (stoma opening) and shape (flat or convex) to match the stoma and peristomal assessment. Apply gentle pressure to enhance the seal of the skin barrier/skin seal.
Paste	Prevent undermining of stoma effluent under pouch seal. Fill in uneven areas.	Contains alcohol, will cause stinging if applied to denuded skin. Can be difficult to squeeze tube for application.	Can use as "caulk" around the edge of the skin barrier next to stoma to enhance the seal. Use a moist finger to adjust paste; touching paste with a dry finger will cause the paste to stick to the finger.
Powder	Absorbs moisture of denuded peristomal skin providing a surface to apply pouching system.	Too much powder left on the peristomal skin can cause pouch seal failure.	Sprinkle the denuded area liberally with powder; brush off excess before pouching system application.
Ring	To enhance the seal with a second layer of solid skin barrier. To provide "soft" convexity to a flat pouching system or enhance the convexity of a convex pouching system. Convex rings can be used to provide soft convexity and improve seal.	When placed around a slightly protruding stoma, can be too high a "rise" and may not allow stoma effluent to drain over the ring into the pouch. Can be used in place of paste on denuded skin, as there is no alcohol to cause stinging.	Stretch the ring to the size of the skin barrier opening; place either around the stoma or on the back of the pouch seal. Use on an oval stoma when the pouching system that is used has a round opening; will cover the exposed skin.
Strip	Use around a stoma to enhance the seal as a second skin barrier. Small pieces can be used to fill in uneven areas of the peristomal skin.	Requires manual dexterity to work the strip into the sizes and shapes needed. Can be used in place of paste if there is irritated skin; will not cause further irritation.	Small pieces can be pulled off and rolled into the exact size of the area that needs to be filled or evened out.
Elastic barrier strips	Used to enhance the seal on the outer edge of the pouching system	May not be needed if the pouching system seal remains intact for the wear time.	Can assist in people who have shifts in the peristomal skin such as the person with a peristomal hernia that causes the peristomal skin to move.
Liquid	Used to protect fragile peristomal skin from stripping. Used to seal skin barrier powder to enhance seal.	Select skin barriers will not adequately adhere when a liquid skin barrier is on the skin. Skin barriers with an alcohol base will cause stinging upon application to denuded skin.	Allow liquid skin barrier to dry before pouching system application. The use of a liquid barrier spray will facilitate application onto denuded skin with no discomfort (using a pledget can cause discomfort when rubbing the irritated skin).

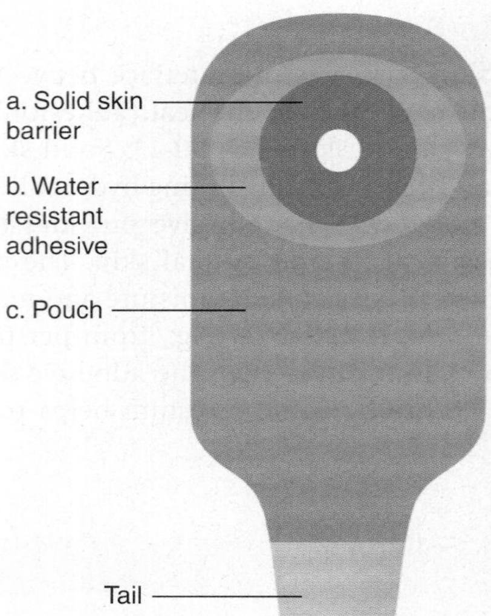

FIGURE 10-1. Pouching system.

Moisture from the stoma (stool or urine) is slowly absorbed by the hydrocolloid, and when an excessive amount of moisture is absorbed the hydrocolloid may lose adhesion and erode. The erosion depends upon several factors, the volume and moisture content of the stoma output, the skin moisture, the use of accessory products (see below), and the type of skin barrier used. Thus, the person with a high-output ileostomy with loose watery stool will note the skin barrier erosion to occur faster than does a person with a pasty infrequent stool. There are two categories of skin barrier materials, regular wear and extended wear. The difference between these two types of skin barriers depends upon the product ingredients: the extended wear barrier has delayed absorption and a higher level of adhesion, generally providing longer wear time (Colwell, 2004). Skin barriers are pressure sensitive, and the bond depends upon the barrier making full contact with the skin surface and is achieved by applying gentle pressure upon application.

CLINICAL PEARL

When teaching a patient to apply a solid skin barrier suggest that they hold their hand over the skin barrier as this will apply even pressure of the skin barrier to the peristomal skin.

A unique solid skin barrier available in a ring or sheet or paste is created from karaya, a vegetable gum produced from tree sap. Karaya has adhesive properties, is acidic in nature, and absorbs moisture rapidly. As karaya absorbs moisture, the adhesive bond is loosened. The use of a karaya skin barrier may be considered when the peristomal skin is damaged from an alkaline environment (such as in crystal buildup on the peristomal skin of a person with a urostomy) or when a patient reports a contact dermatitis from other synthetic skin barriers (karaya is a natural product).

BOX 10-1 Assessment of Pouching System Wear Time

- Ask the patient about the number of normal wear days.
- After pouch removal, examine the skin barrier for signs of erosion.
- Examine the peristomal skin for presence of stool or urine contact.

Wear Time

When considering how a solid skin barrier erodes over time, the challenge becomes how to decide when is the appropriate time to replace the skin barrier (Box 10-1). Changing too soon could lead to medical adhesive–related skin injury (McNichol et al., 2013) (stripping the skin because the adhesive seal was still intact). Changing too late could mean that the stoma effluent can make contact with the skin because the hydrocolloid eroded allowing the output to make contact with the skin or the adhesive seal completely failed and there was leakage under and beyond the pouch adhesive. Average wear time has been reported to be 4 days; however, wear time due to skin barrier erosion is variable and should be determined on a case-by-case basis (Richbourg et al., 2007, 2008).

The back of the skin barrier (the adhesive surface toward the skin) should be examined after removal following several days of wear. The evaluation of the skin barrier integrity starts at the opening that was fitted to the stoma skin junction. The skin barrier material will appear saturated and swollen (Fig. 10-2). If the skin barrier opening is larger

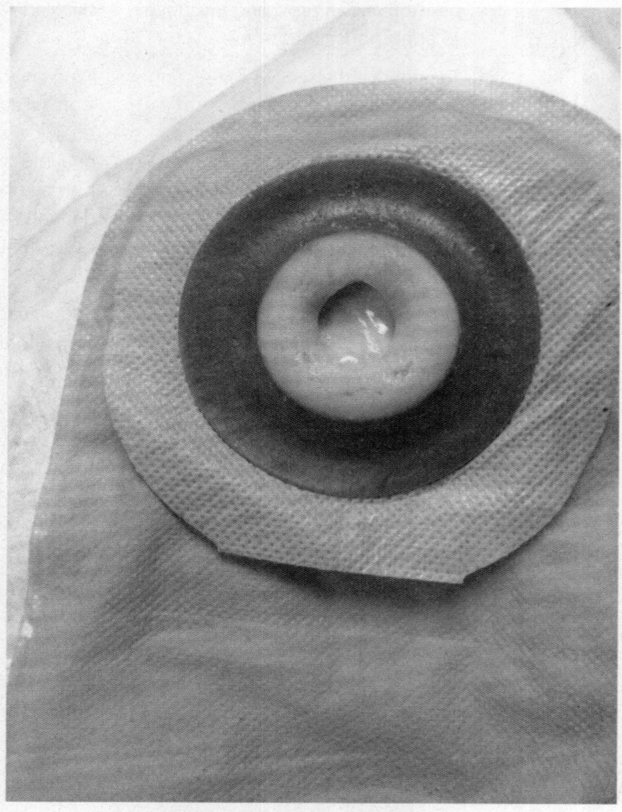

FIGURE 10-2. Saturated skin barrier.

than it was on application, this indicates the ability of the stoma output to make contact with the skin and cause skin injury. If the skin barrier material shows discoloration or undermining of the stoma output, this indicates a break in the seal, with possible skin injury and loss of the seal (leakage). These observations require a decision to be made to decrease wear time, consider a different type of skin barrier, or use an accessory product.

Solid Skin Barrier Shapes

Solid skin barriers are available in several shapes. One distinction is a flat or convex skin barrier; this refers to the skin barrier interface (back of skin barrier, the adhesive surface toward the skin). A flat skin barrier (Fig. 10-3B) has a level or even adhesive surface. A convex skin barrier's adhesive surface is curved or rounded, and the amount of curve varies between products. A convex skin barrier (Fig. 10-3A) can have a minimal amount of curvature (light convexity) to a maximum amount of curve (deep convexity). Convex skin barrier options can also include convexity located next to the skin barrier opening as well as some that extend outward onto more of the skin barrier. Another distinction is flexible versus firm convexity. A flexible convex skin barrier can bend and move with the body; a firm convex skin barrier does not bend, rather it remains rigid. The challenge is deciding which type of convexity will meet the patient's needs.

There are several considerations when deciding when to use a flat or convex skin barrier. The peristomal skin should be examined when the person is lying, standing, and sitting. The area is examined for the presence of creases and/or folds. If the area around the stoma is flat in all positions, a flat barrier should be successful in maintaining the skin barrier seal (WOCN, 2013). If creases and folds are found, these can compromise the seal and a convex barrier can help to flatten the creases. The convex shape can help to keep the peristomal skin flat/even to enhance the seal. The degree of convexity depth (light, moderate, deep) is matched to the depth of the creases and the amount of pressure that may be needed to keep the peristomal skin flat and provide an adequate skin barrier seal.

In some cases, a flexible convex skin barrier is considered when there are deep creases on a soft abdomen and

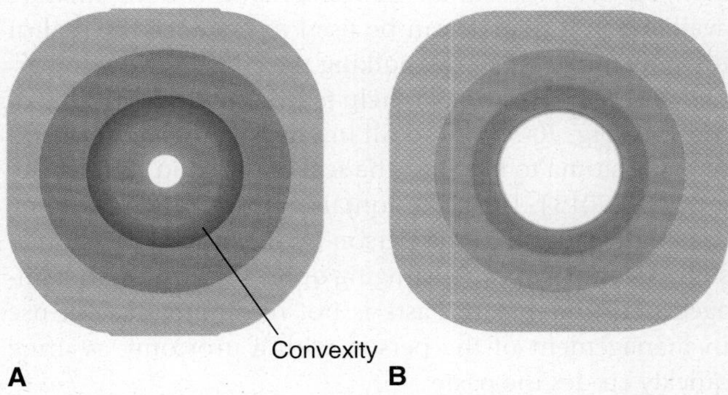

FIGURE 10-3. Convex **(A)** and flat **(B)** skin barrier.

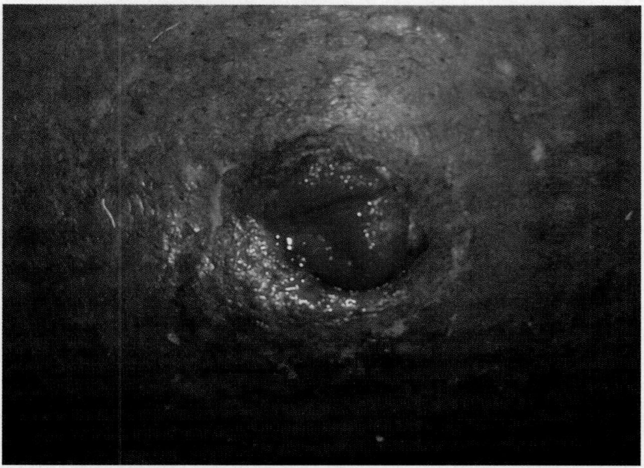

FIGURE 10-4. Stoma with lumen off to side, discharging stoma effluent onto skin.

the rigid convexity appears to pop off the creased area. A second consideration for the use of convexity would be a stoma that does not protrude above the skin barrier causing a seal problem (the stoma effluent discharges under the skin barrier [WOCN, 2013]). A convex adhesive can apply pressure directly around the stoma to help with stoma protrusion (WOCN, 2013). The amount of convexity depth will depend upon the protrusion or lack of protrusion of the stoma. A third consideration for the use of convexity may be when the lumen of the stoma is near or flush to the skin. In some cases, the stoma has adequate protrusion but the lumen is off to the side close to the skin, and the stoma output drains under the skin barrier (Fig. 10-4). The convex skin barrier can help the stoma lumen protrude up over the skin barrier edge.

A second characteristic of a solid skin barrier's shape refers to the outer diameter and the considerations are round, square, or oval. Round skin barriers are circular, a square skin barrier is rectangular, and oval is elliptical (Fig. 10-5). Considerations for use of a round, square, or oval skin barrier are the location of the stoma, if there are skin folds near the stoma that are horizontal (examine the patient sitting, standing, and lying). In some cases, an oval skin barrier can cover more area in the crease than a flat or round skin barrier. In other cases, a round skin barrier may be preferable when there are creases or folds at the edge of the skin barrier, as the use of round skin barrier can avoid creases where a square skin barrier may lie at the edge of the crease causing the outer seal to loosen.

Fit of the Solid Skin Barrier

The opening in the solid skin barrier should be the size of the stoma (WOCN, 2010, 2013) (Fig. 10-6). If the stoma is oval, then the opening should be oval; if the stoma is round the opening should be round. The skin barrier should be blocking access of the stoma effluent to the skin around the stoma. Thus, the opening should fit at the skin–stoma junction. The options to provide this seal include a cut to

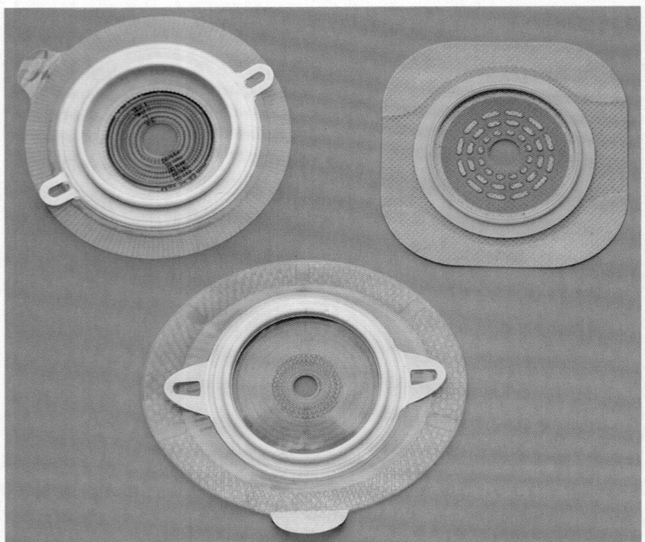

FIGURE 10-5. Skin barrier outer shapes, circular, square, and oval.

fit barrier, a precut round barrier, and a moldable/stretch-to-fit barrier. A cut-to-fit skin barrier has either no opening or a small opening that can be used to start to cut the skin barrier to fit (WOCN, 2010). The opening can be cut to any shape or dimension.

Benefits of the cut-to-fit skin barrier include the ability to change the skin barrier opening as the stoma changes, such as in the immediate postoperative period; the ability to cut the stoma size to match the shape of the stoma, for instance an irregular stoma; and the ability to offset the stoma opening to avoid other structures (incisions, drains). A measuring guide with round shapes or a custom template (for an oval stoma) can be made of the stoma shape and used to cut out additional skin barriers. An

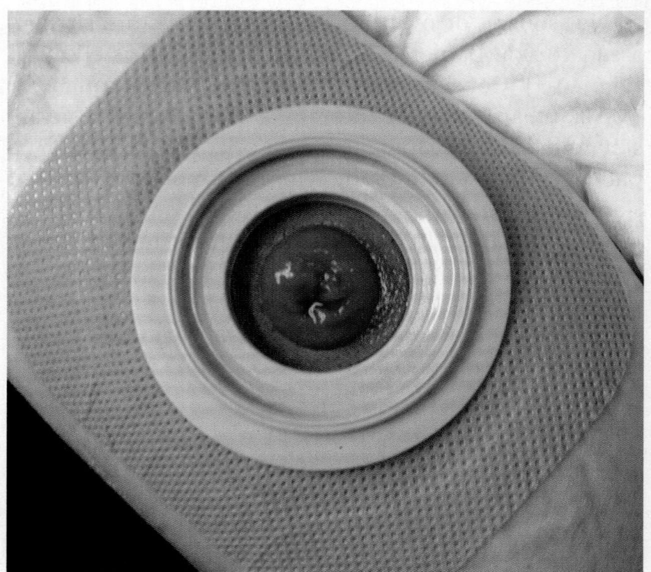

FIGURE 10-6. The skin barrier should fit to the skin–stoma junction.

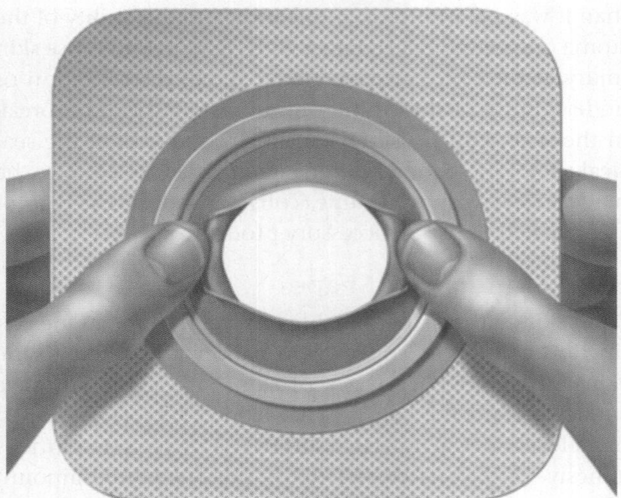

FIGURE 10-7. Moldable skin barrier.

adjustment of the template should be made as the stoma shape changes. A precut opening in the skin barrier can be used for a round stoma, for a stoma in which the size/shape is not thought to change, or for a person who prefers not to cut or may not be able to cut the opening. A measuring guide can be used to determine the size of the stoma, and the skin barrier can be obtained in that size. A newly created stoma should be measured at least every 2 weeks until the size stabilizes. A moldable/shape-to-fit barrier (Fig. 10-7) can be used to stretch the opening to the approximate size of the stoma. The moldable/shape-to-fit skin barrier may be of benefit to someone who does not want to or is unable to cut the skin barrier opening, or if it is anticipated that the stoma size will change over time.

CLINICAL PEARL

Consider the use of a small piece of clear plastic that can be held over the stoma to trace the shape, the shape cut out and traced onto the back of the skin barrier. Save the paper backing from the skin barrier to use for the next pouching system change.

Skin Barrier Paste

Skin barrier paste is an adhesive hydrocolloid mixture available in a tube. It can be used to enhance the seal of the pouching system by caulking the edge of the skin barrier closest to the stoma to help to prevent undermining of the seal (Fig. 10-8) and to fill in uneven areas around and near the stoma to facilitate the seal of the solid skin barrier (WOCN, 2013). The paste contains alcohol and should be used with caution in the person with denuded peristomal skin. Alcohol can cause stinging upon application to damaged peristomal skin. Paste is not recommended for use in management of the person with a urostomy as urine quickly erodes the paste.

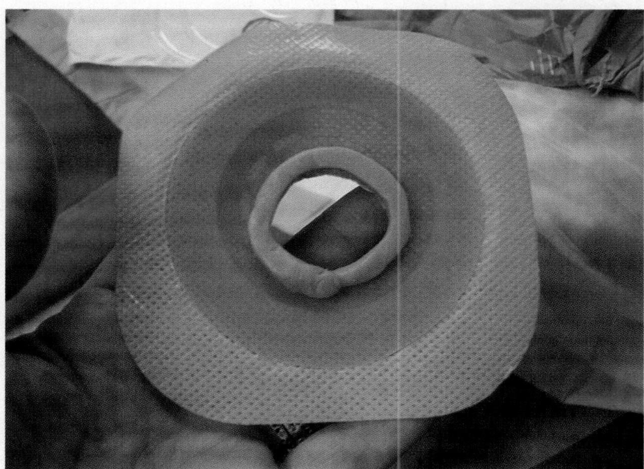

FIGURE 10-8. Skin barrier paste placed at the edge of skin barrier opening to caulk seal.

CLINICAL PEARL

If after application the paste needs to be adjusted or smoothed out, wet a gloved finger or a gauze pad and use to adjust. If paste is touched with a dry pad or gloved finger it will stick to the dry surface and you will not be able to easily make the necessary adjustment.

Skin Barrier Powder

Skin barrier powder is a hydrocolloid that can be used to absorb moisture and can be utilized on denuded peristomal skin. The affected area is sprinkled with skin barrier powder, the powder gently rubbed or patted over the denuded skin and the excess brushed off. The powder will absorb some of the skin moisture helping to secure a seal. Karaya powder, another type of skin barrier powder, is an acidic gum/sap that can be sprinkled on denuded peristomal skin, which may assist in helping to secure the pouching system seal.

CLINICAL PEARL

Do not leave excessive powder on the skin as this will interfere with the skin barrier seal.

Skin Barrier Ring

A skin barrier ring is an adhesive hydrocolloid washer that can be used around the stoma to enhance the seal by providing additional solid skin barrier and/or to level out the area around the stoma (WOCN, 2013). There are several types: a flat hydrocolloid ring (Fig. 10-9) that can be stretched to fit and a convex hydrocolloid ring that is presized either round or oval.

Skin Barrier Strip Paste

A skin barrier strip paste is a band of adhesive hydrocolloid that can be used to fit around a stoma to enhance the seal, or pieces of it can be used to fill in uneven areas such as wrinkles or dips in the peristomal area.

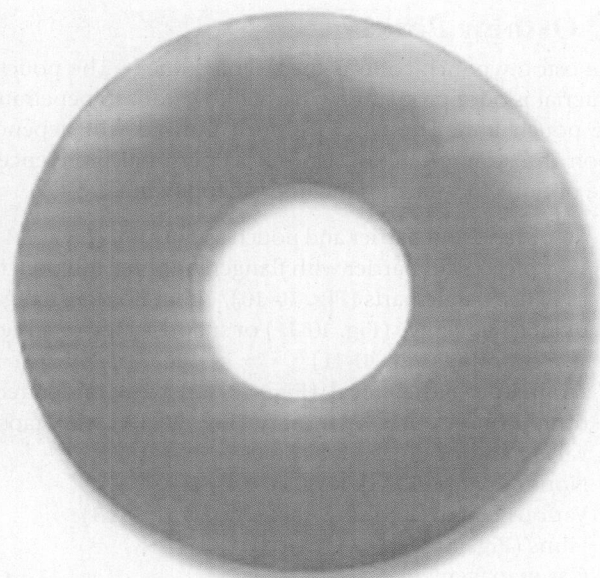

FIGURE 10-9. Skin barrier ring.

Elastic Skin Barrier Strip

An elastic skin barrier strip is a piece of hydrocolloid with elastic that is used to secure the outer seal of the pouching system. Unlike other hydrocolloid products, it is not used directly around the stoma to secure a seal at the interface of the stoma and the pouching system; rather it is used around the outer edge of the barrier for extra security.

CLINICAL PEARL

Since the elastic skin barrier is elastic, it stretches and can be used for people who have a large abdomen and find that the outer seal pulls and detaches with movement.

Liquid Skin Barrier

A liquid skin barrier is an acrylate copolymer or a cyanoacrylate clear film that can be placed on the peristomal skin. The purpose of the liquid skin barrier is to provide skin protection from stoma effluent or adhesive stripping or in some cases to seal skin barrier powder (WOCN, 2013). Cyanoacrylates can be used directly on denuded to skin provide a dry layer to facilitate the pouch seal. Liquid skin barrier films may contain alcohol that could cause a stinging sensation when applied; a no-sting skin barrier film without any alcohol is available. When applied, the liquid skin barrier should be dry before application of the pouching system. Liquid skin barriers are available as a pledget, spray, foam applicator on a stick, or an ampule. Check with the manufacturers of skin barriers, as in some instances, the seal of the solid skin barriers can be decreased with the use of a liquid skin barrier.

Ostomy Pouches

The ostomy pouch collects the stoma effluent. The pouch material is odor proof and will not allow odor to penetrate the pouch film. The type of pouch utilized will depend upon the stoma function as well as personal preference. The options for pouches include the following:

- One piece: skin barrier and pouch as one unit (Fig. 10-1)
- Two piece: skin barrier with flange/coupling and pouch as two separate parts (Fig. 10-10), either floating flange or attached flange (Fig. 10-11) or snap/locking or adhesive coupling (Fig. 10-11)
- Drainable, either fecal (Fig. 10-12) with integrated or add-on closures or urinary (Fig. 10-13) with taps, valves, and/or plugs for closures
- Nondrainable closed; (Fig. 10-14)
- Various lengths and thus capacity; (Fig. 10-15)
- Films (Fig. 10-15)
- Gas management

One-Piece Pouching System

A one-piece pouching system is constructed with the solid skin barrier and the pouch as one unit; the pouch is heat sealed onto the skin barrier (Fig. 10-1). One-piece pouching systems are available with the above-noted skin barrier options: convex/flat, precut/cut to fit, extended/regular wear, outer diameter round, oval, or square. The pouches are available with the following options: drainable/nondrainable, various lengths, clear/opaque film, with or without a gas filter, and with the following closures: integrated, separate and a tap, valve or plug. Most one-piece pouching systems have a water-resistant material framing the solid skin barrier, providing protection of the solid skin barrier when showering or immersing the pouching system in water such as bathing or water sports. Considerations of using a one-piece pouching system are as follows: a flat peristomal profile with the pouch as compared to many of the two-piece pouching systems (WOCN, 2010), only a single seal (no risk of detachment of skin barrier to pouch), and the possible difficulty of placing the pouch over the stoma when using an opaque pouch (can't see through the pouch to center the skin barrier opening over the stoma) and if the stoma is located in a deep crease or skin fold (WOCN, 2010).

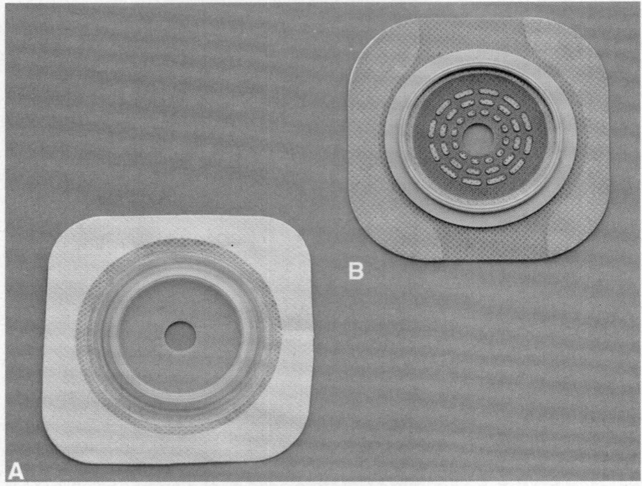

FIGURE 10-11. Two-piece flanges. **A.** Stationary snap coupling. **B.** Floating flange coupling.

Two-Piece Pouching System

A two-piece pouching system consists of a solid skin barrier with a mechanism that accepts the pouch (Fig. 10-10). The solid skin barrier has the characteristics noted above: convex/flat, precut/cut to fit, extended/regular wear, and outer diameter round, oval, or square. The pouch connects to the skin barrier in one of two ways, with a plastic flange that either is fixed to the solid skin barrier or floats above the skin barrier (Fig. 10-11) or with a resealable adhesive coupling. The plastic flange has a rim attached to the skin barrier and a channel or plastic ring on the pouch; the two snap together with pressure to make the connection (Fig. 10-11a). Other two-piece systems use a connection in which the skin barrier flange can be pulled up from the skin barrier (a floating flange) (Fig. 10-11b) and the connection made by pinching the two pieces together. The solid skin barrier in a two-piece system is available both with and without a water-resistant frame on the outer edge of the skin barrier. All two-piece

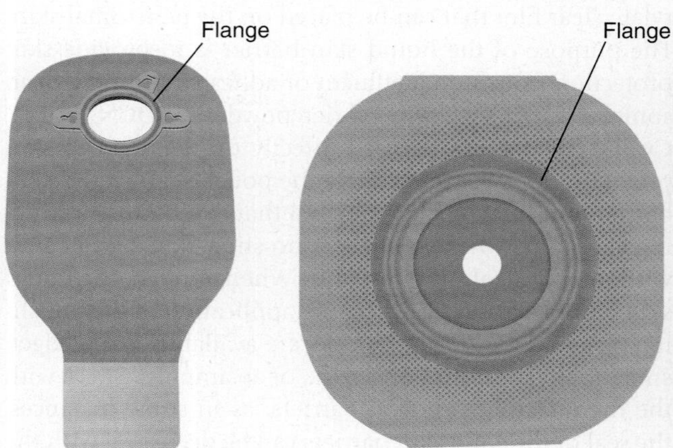

FIGURE 10-10. Two-piece pouching system, flange and pouch.

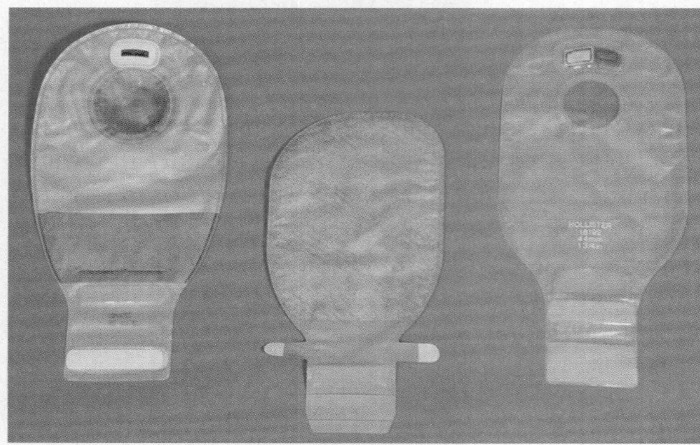

FIGURE 10-12. Drainable pouches.

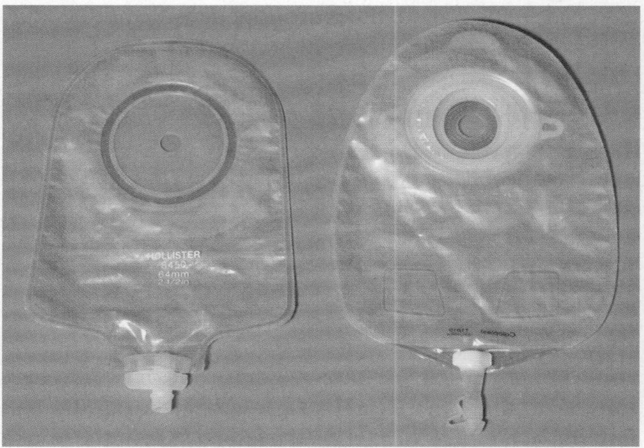

FIGURE 10-13. Urinary pouches with tap.

pouching systems have belt tabs on either the pouch or the skin barrier. Considerations in using a two-piece pouching system are ability to center the skin barrier around the stoma with no pouch in place providing easy visualization, being able to change the pouch without removing the skin barrier, capability to use a pouch liner, profile of the plastic flange under clothing, and security of the pouch and flange connection (see below).

Pouch Features

Drainable Pouch for Fecal Stoma Management

The end of the drainable pouch can be opened to allow the stool or urine to be drained. The end of a pouch for the management of a fecal stoma has a tail that is closed with a closure device when the device is opened, stool is drained, and the end wiped clean and reclosed. The types of closures include the following (Fig. 10-12):

- A rubber or plastic clamp: placed at the end of the pouch, the pouch is folded over the closure and the clamp is snapped closed, a similar clamp uses a rubber band to make the closure.

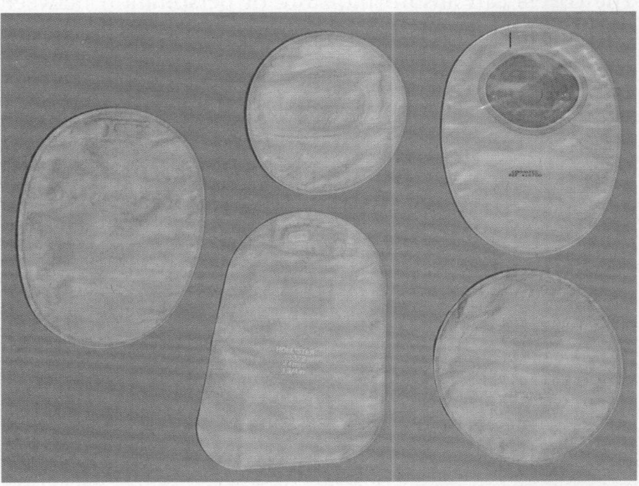

FIGURE 10-14. Nondrainable (closed end) pouch.

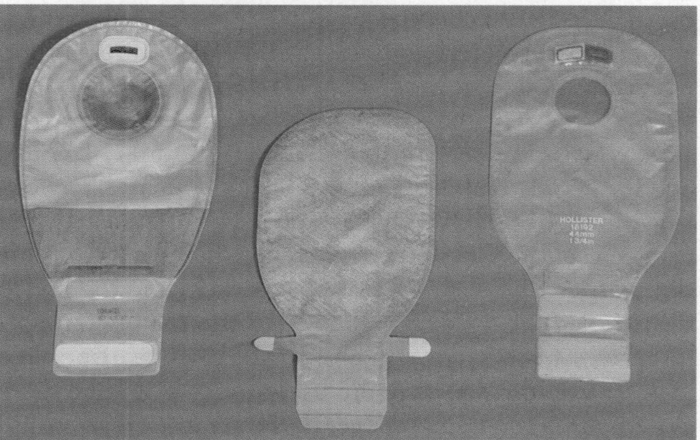

FIGURE 10-15. Various pouch lengths and pouch films.

- Integrated closure/interlocking: the pouch tail is rolled up several times and the plastic interlocking fasteners are pinched closed.
- Velcro closure: the pouch tail is rolled up several times and the tabs of Velcro are smoothed together.
- Some or all of the above closures can be tucked away under the pouch to avoid any discomfort of the pouch closure against the skin.

The type of closure will depend upon the patient's preference as well as abilities to easily open and close the system.

A drainable pouch can be considered for use by a person who has liquid stool that requires the pouch to be emptied more than twice per day (volume of more than 400 mL). The person with a drainable pouch can sit on the toilet far enough back that the water can be seen, the closure opened, and the pouch contents drained. The tail is wiped and the pouch closed.

Drainable Pouch for Urinary Stoma Management

Urostomy pouches have a tap that allows urine to be drained (Fig. 10-13). The types of taps on the bottom of the pouches for a urinary pouch include a cap that is removed, the pouch drained and the cap replaced, and a valve that is twisted or a plug that is pulled out to allow emptying. All urinary systems are drainable, and a feature on a urostomy pouch not found in fecal pouches is an antireflux valve that prevents the urine from refluxing to the top of the pouch and eroding the skin barrier seal, and some urostomy pouches have chambers that distribute the urine throughout the pouch to prevent bulging. A urinary pouching system can be connected to dependent drainage at night with the use of an adapter that attaches the end of the pouch to the dependent drainage collector. Most dependent drainage collectors (or nighttime drainage systems) are closed systems and should be used for 14 days and discarded. If the type of drainage system used can be opened, it is advisable to use either a commercially made solution called a cleanser/decrystallizer or a solution made of one part white vinegar and three parts water for cleansing (United Ostomy Associations of America, Inc., 2014).

Nondrainable Pouches

Nondrainable pouches are closed and will require removal when the pouch is more than half full (WOCN, 2010) (Fig. 10-14). They are used in the management of fecal stomas with low output that is under 400 mL/24 hours, and for people who irrigate and need a pouch in between irrigation. The pouch is either removed from the skin when using a one-piece closed end system or removed from the skin barrier when using a two-piece system and the pouch is discarded. The pouch is then replaced. Many manufacturers of the two-piece systems provide opaque disposable bags to use in discarding the used pouch. The one-piece closed-end pouches have a gentle skin barrier that should not cause peristomal skin trauma when removed.

Pouch Length

Drainable and urostomy pouches are available in several lengths from 9 to 12 inches (Fig. 10-15). Some manufacturers have a high-output pouch that while still 12 inches has a shape that can hold more volume than do the standard drainable pouches. Nondrainable pouch lengths can vary from 3 inches (stoma cap used primarily by people who irrigate) to 12 inches.

Pouch Films

Pouch film is available as clear on both sides (body side and front), clear on the front, material on the body side, opaque on both sides, material or textile on both sides (Fig. 10-15), or material on both sides with a viewing "window," a slit in the material that will allow inspection of the stoma or output. The type of film used will depend on the location of use; for instance right after surgery, the ability to see the stoma and the stoma output is important and a clear pouch may be chosen (WOCN, 2013).

CLINICAL PEARL

Some people who use a pouch with material or textile find that the material is slow to dry after water submersion (bathing or swimming). You can advise your patient to use a towel or a blow dyer on low to dry, or if using a two piece pouching system to use a pouch just for showering and remove the pouch after showering allowing it to dry until the next shower.

Gas Management

Some pouches have an integrated gas filter that can allow gas to pass from the pouch through a gas deodorizing filter and exit the pouch. The filters are generally at the top of the pouch, containing a membrane both in the pouch and on the outside of the pouch with the charcoal between. The challenge for a pouch filter is that the charcoal can become plugged when moist, which happens frequently with stool and humidity in the pouch (WOCN, 2013). Thus, the life of most gas filters is 24 to 36 hours.

A gas vent is an external device that can be placed on the pouch and a hole is made through the pouch film under the vent. The vent has a plug that remains closed until the gas needs to be vented, the plug is opened, the nondeodorized gas is vented, and the vent is closed.

CLINICAL PEARL

Be sure that your patient knows when they use a gas vent the gas is not deodorized and they need to consider where and when they vent the gas.

Pouching Accessory Products

Belt

Some pouching systems have belt tabs (one or two on each side) that allow the wearer to use a belt, fitting the belt into the belt tab(s) located on the lateral side of the pouch adhesive or flange, bringing the belt around the body, and attaching to the belt tab(s) on the other side (Fig. 10-16). The belt is worn snug to the body to apply pressure to the pouching system to enhance the seal. When using a convex pouch, the use of a pouching system belt can help to apply pressure to the convexity and add to the seal.

CLINICAL PEARL

Belts come in several lengths and most are adjustable. The belt should fit snug against the abdomen to apply pressure but not so firm as to damage the skin.

Adhesive Products

There are several ostomy adhesive products that can be used to supplement the seal of the pouching system. They include adhesive sprays applied to the back of the pouching system seal, cement adhesives that are placed both on the pouch seal as well as on the skin, and adhesives that are painted on the pouching system seal. Some of the ostomy adhesive products contain latex and are flammable.

Pouch Covers

Pouch covers can be used to cover or conceal the pouch. The covers can absorb moisture or perspiration between the pouch and skin, decrease rustle (noise of the plastic

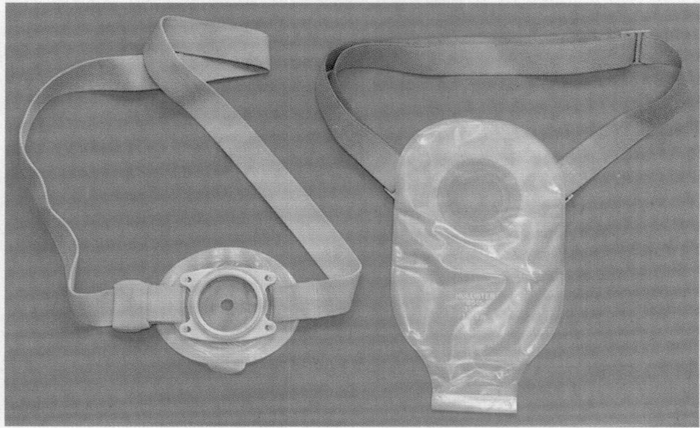

FIGURE 10-16. Pouches with belt tabs.

against the skin) and for some are used during intimacy to conceal the pouch.

Pouch Liners

Pouch liners can be used to line the inside of a two-piece pouching system to collect the stoma output. When the pouch requires emptying (approximately one-third full), the pouch is snapped off of the skin barrier flange, and the liner is removed and deposited into a toilet. A new liner is inserted into the same pouch and reapplied to the flange.

CLINICAL PEARL

When using a pouch liner the patient should poke several holes in the liner (per the manufacturer's instructions) to allow the gas to vent into the pouch.

In-Pouch Deodorant Liquids

In-pouch deodorant liquids and tablets are available to use to decrease or eliminate odor. When a pouch is properly sealed there should be no odor; however, there will be odor when emptying stool, and an in-pouch odor eliminator can be placed in the pouch upon pouch application and after each emptying. The in-pouch deodorants are available as liquid, allowing drops to be placed into the pouch, or as a lubricating solution that can also be placed in the pouch. The lubricating deodorant is squirted into the pouch to lubricate the inside of the pouch to not only eliminate odor but also facilitate stool drainage (WOCN, 2013). The liquid deodorant or odor eliminator will not harm the stoma, but may contain a dye that can change the color of the stool. The majority of the in-pouch deodorizers/eliminators are indicated for use with fecal stoma pouch management.

Oral Odor Eliminators

Oral odor eliminators are over-the-counter pills that are taken to reduce or eliminate odor from stool. The dose is titrated until results are achieved; as many as four pills a day may need to be effective. The two main products contain the following ingredients, bismuth subgallate or chlorophyllin copper complex (known to cause a green discoloration of stool).

Absorbent Products

Absorbent products contained in a packet, sachet, pill, or crystals can be placed into the fecal stoma pouch to turn the effluent into a gel-like substance. The liquid stool is converted into a gel and diverts a high-liquid fecal output away from the pouching system seal and can decrease the noise of the liquid stool in the pouch.

The choice of a pouching system is a decision that is made after a thorough assessment of the following characteristics: the location of the stoma on the abdomen, the amount of stoma protrusion, the location of the lumen of the stoma, the function of the stoma (volume and consistency of the effluent), the peristomal skin integrity, and the peristomal skin geography (flat, creased, soft, or firm tissue). Once pouching options are decided, the patient is educated about the rationale for the suggested pouching system, and an assessment of the patient's abilities to work with the recommended pouching system is done. In some cases, the system chosen may not work out, because the patient does not have the ability to handle the products due to physical or cognition issues. A family member, a significant other, or an assistive worker may need to be educated on the use of the pouching system. Another deciding factor on the choice of a pouching system may be reimbursement. If the desired product is not reimbursed or has poor reimbursement, and the purchase of the items needed cause a hardship for the patient, an alternative product may be needed. It is advisable for the person with a stoma to become familiar with what coverage is available for reimbursement of his or her pouching systems.

Conclusions

Consistent wear time and intact peristomal skin drive the decision of the type of pouching system a person with a stoma should use. However, each of the attributes of a pouching system must be considered as an assessment of the patient's stoma, peristomal skin, abilities, and financial support is done (WOCN, 2010). Reevaluation should be done periodically as the person's body habitus changes such as following an illness and weight gain or loss.

REFERENCES

Colwell, J. C. (2004). Principles of ostomy management. In J. C. Colwell, M. T. Goldberg, & J. E. Carmel (Eds.), *Fecal and urinary diversions: Management principles* (pp. 240–262). St. Louis, MO: Mosby.

McNichol, L., Lund, C., Rosen, T., et al. (2013). Medical adhesives and patient safety: State of the science: Consensus statements for the assessment, prevention, and treatment of adhesive-related skin injuries. *Journal of Wound, Ostomy & Continence Nursing, 40*(4), 365–380.

Pittman, J., Rawl, S. M., Schmidt, C. M., et al. (2008). Demographic and clinical factors related to ostomy complications and quality of life in veterans with an ostomy. *Journal of Wound Ostomy & Continence Nursing, 35*(5), 493–503.

Richbourg, L., Fellows, J., & Arroyave, W. (2008). Ostomy pouch wear time in the United States. *Journal of Wound, Ostomy & Continence Nursing*, 35(5), 504–508.

Richbourg, L., Thorpe, J. M., & Rapp, C. G. (2007). Difficulties experienced by the ostomate after hospital discharge. *Journal of Wound, Ostomy & Continence Nursing, 34*(1), 70–79.

United Ostomy Associations of America, Inc. (2014). *Urostomy fact sheet*. Retrieved October, 2014, from http://www.ostomy.org/ostomy_info/factsheets/facts_urostomy_en.shtml

Wound Ostomy and Continence Nurses Society. (2010). *Management of the patient with a fecal ostomy: Best practice guidelines for clinicians*. Mount Laurel, NJ: Author.

Wound Ostomy and Continence Nurses Society. (2013). *Colostomy and ileostomy products and tips: Best practice for clinicians*. Mount Laurel, NJ: Author.

QUESTIONS

1. A patient with a urostomy reports contact dermatitis under the skin barrier used with a one-piece pouching system. What intervention might the WOC nurse suggest?
   A. Allowing the skin to air dry prior to applying the barrier
   B. Switching to a different manufacturer's one-piece pouching system
   C. Using cortisone cream on the skin under the barrier until it clears up
   D. Switching to a karaya skin barrier

2. The WOC nurse is assessing the seal of a skin barrier for a patient with an ileostomy. The nurse notes that the skin barrier material is undermined with stool. What adverse condition does this finding indicate?
   A. Prolapse of the stoma
   B. Break in the seal with possible skin injury
   C. Peristomal skin infection
   D. Skin barrier that is too large for the stoma

3. The WOC nurse assessing the stoma of a patient in a sitting position notes that there are creases and folds in the peristomal skin. What shape of skin barrier would the nurse recommend for this patient?
   A. Flat.
   B. Convex.
   C. Firm.
   D. Skin barriers are not recommended for skin with creases and folds.

4. What factor determines the size and shape of the opening of a solid skin barrier?
   A. Size and shape of the stoma
   B. Amount of effluent being passed
   C. Desired wear time
   D. Condition of peristomal skin

5. For which patient would the use of skin barrier paste be contraindicated?
   A. A patient with an irregular shape stoma
   B. A patient with a urostomy
   C. A patient with an ileostomy
   D. A patient with folds in the peristomal skin

6. A WOC nurse assesses the area around a patient's stoma and notes that it is not level. What product would be the best option for this patient?
   A. Skin barrier powder
   B. Skin barrier paste
   C. Liquid skin barrier
   D. Karaya powder

7. The WOC nurse is helping a patient with a new urinary diversion choose a pouching system. Upon assessment, the nurse recommends a two-piece pouching system. What is an advantage of this type of system?
   A. It accommodates a flat peristomal profile.
   B. There is no risk of detachment of skin barrier from the pouch.
   C. It allows for application of the skin barrier without the pouch obstructing the view.
   D. It is the best fit when a stoma is located in a deep crease or skin fold.

8. For which patient would a nondrainable pouch be the best option?
   A. A patient with a colostomy
   B. Any patient with a urostomy
   C. A patient who has liquid stool requiring pouch emptying at least two times per day
   D. A patient with an ileostomy

9. A WOC nurse is counseling a patient with a colostomy about gas management for his pouching device. What teaching point accurately describes gas control features?
   A. A gas vent allows deodorized gas to be vented through a plugged opening.
   B. Some pouches have a gas filter at the bottom of the pouch to control gas.
   C. Most pouches with gas filters need to be changed every 24 to 36 hours.
   D. All pouches allow gas to dissipate naturally within the pouch itself.

10. The WOC nurse is teaching a patient with a fecal diversion about accessory products available for use. Which statement accurately describes one of these products?
   A. A once-a-day oral pill is available to reduce or eliminate odor from stool.
   B. Absorbent crystals can be placed in the pouch to turn effluent into a gel.
   C. Liquid pouch deodorant should be discontinued if the stoma becomes irritated.
   D. Pouch liners can be used to cover or conceal the pouch.

ANSWERS: 1.**B**, 2.**B**, 3.**B**, 4.**A**, 5.**B**, 6.**B**, 7.**C**, 8.**A**, 9.**C**, 10.**A**

CHAPTER 11

Patient Education Following Urinary/Fecal Diversion

Margaret T. Goldberg

OBJECTIVE

Distinguish specific ostomy care needs when educating patients and caregivers.

Topic Outline

- Patient Education
- Assessing Readiness
- Pouching Principles
  - How to Empty
  - When to Empty
  - Indications for Pouch Change
  - Preparing Equipment
  - Assessing Peristomal Skin
  - Measuring Stoma
  - Peristomal Skin Cleansing
  - Removal of Pouching System
  - Placement of Pouching System
  - Problem Identification, When to Seek Assistance
- Living with a Stoma
  - Where and when to Obtain Supplies
  - Bathing
  - Clothing
  - Sexual Concerns
  - Dietary Concerns
    - Ileal Conduit
    - Ileostomy
    - Colostomy
  - Medications
  - Follow-up Care
  - Support Groups
- Conclusions

Body image changes and the physical alterations that come with ostomy surgery require major adjustments by the patient. Learning to adapt to these changes as well as acquiring necessary skills for stoma care can present a number of remarkable challenges. The ability to care for the stoma and its output are crucial steps toward the rehabilitation of the person with the new ostomy.

Patient education has become even more challenging in recent years due to changes in health care and the decreasing lengths of hospital stay limiting the time available to present the necessary information. However, it is also thought that preoperative education has an effect on length of hospital stay (WCET, 2014). In addition, comprehensive education delivered by a Wound Ostomy Continence (WOC) nurse can result in a positive adjustment to the ostomy not only in the immediate but also long term (Haugen et al., 2006).

It remains the most important function of the WOC nurse to provide instructions for self-care and encouragement and support to the person having ostomy surgery.

Patient Education

Cheng et al. (2013) found self-care ability strongly associated with psychosocial adjustment, and where possible patients should leave the hospital with optimal self stoma care ability.

The Joint Commission (2012) requires that the patient's learning needs, abilities, preferences, and readiness to learn are assessed. The assessment should consider cultural and religious practices, emotional barriers, desire and motivation to learn, physical and cognitive limitations, language barriers, and financial implications of care choice.

It is important to include any family member that the patient wishes to receive instruction, for in many cases having a "back up" to assist with the technical procedures after discharge will be needed. Altschuler et al. (2009) describe the importance of the support of the patients' partner on the adjustment capabilities of the patient and including them in the instruction process may contribute to their understanding and acceptance of the ostomy.

CLINICAL PEARL

Ostomy education should include a preoperative and postoperative component by a specialized nurse such as a Wound, Ostomy, and Continence (WOC) nurse.

Assessing Readiness

Components of a learning assessment should include the patient's cultural and religious beliefs, emotional barriers, desire and motivation to learn, physical or cognitive limitations, and barriers to communication. A patient's readiness to learn can be affected by physical or psychological comfort such as pain, fatigue, anxiety, anger, or fear. In view of existing time constraints, teaching might begin with encouraging the patient to recognize the need to participate in his or her care. Asking the patient their views of living with the stoma and function, and how we can assist them to assume the necessary tasks that came with the stoma, can be a beginning of their recognition of their need for learning.

While it may seem in these days of shortened lengths of stay that consideration of learner readiness may seem unproductive. O'Shea (2001) states that the patient who does not recognize the need to learn, or is depressed or angry may not be amenable to learning. Recognition of these issues allows the WOC nurse to implement interventions that lead the patient to understand the need for learning and acquiring new skills.

CLINICAL PEARL

Preoperative education may be very limited or not be available in many situations as patients may not arrive at the hospital until just prior to surgery.

The skill set recommended by the WOCN Society Ostomy Consensus Statement (2007) is described as the abilities of the postoperative patient to perform the actions listed in Box 11-1. O'Shea (2001) describes that teaching elder patient may require a longer time to learn, and suggests that relating ostomy teaching to previous learning or experiences helps the aged patient gain the necessary knowledge and skills without any extraneous facts. Teaching illiterate patients should involve verbal explanations, pictures, videos, audio tapes models, and demonstrations. Arrows showing the flow of the procedure in pictures can be helpful. It is also important to recall that illiteracy does not imply a lack of intelligence and these patients self-esteem should be protected.

BOX 11-1 Skill Set for the Postoperative Ostomy Patient

- Manipulate pouch clip or spout
- Empty the pouch
- Remove and apply a pouching system
- Additional skills if possible
  - Bathing
  - Clothing
  - Activity restrictions
  - Influence of medications on ostomy function
  - Dietary considerations
  - Peristomal skin care
  - Monitoring for complications
  - Sexual function (Colwell & Beitz, 2007)
  - Option for colostomy irrigation

Pouching Principles

Regardless of type of ostomy, there are principles that apply when managing a stoma with a pouching system. The pouching system should provide the person with an ostomy consistent wear time and containment of stomal output and protection of the peristomal skin.

There are one- and two-piece types of ostomy systems with both flat and convex skin barriers. The skin barrier is the part of the system that attaches to the skin; it should fit snugly around the stoma so that no peristomal skin will be exposed. Skin barriers are available as precut or cut to size to accommodate the stoma, which is irregularly shaped or is still shrinking. There are also barriers that may be molded to fit around the stoma without cutting. The pouch contains the output from the stoma and can be drainable and emptied several times per day as needed or may have a closed end where the pouch is removed and replaced rather than emptied. Pouch closures may be a separate clip or integrated into the pouch, closing with a spout or a hook and loop closure. There are many accessory products that are usually used to solve problems such as liquid skin barriers used on thin peristomal skin or paste, strips, or rings used to "caulk" around a stoma where the skin surface is uneven. See Chapter 10 for an in-depth discussion on pouching systems and the principles of pouching.

While general instructions for stoma care are described, over time and when back at home in his or her own

CLINICAL PEARL

A convex skin barrier may be useful if the stoma is flush with the skin or retracted below skin level.

environment, the person with the new ostomy is encouraged to find a comfort level with this care and make the techniques and practices his or her own. The WOC nurse might instruct in current practices, but in order to incorporate the ostomy into his or her life, the patient may fine-tune some of these new procedures until they work well for them.

How to Empty

There are many ways of emptying a pouch, and while the WOC nurse will instruct patients on methods of emptying, the person will adjust the practices to suit her or her lifestyle, along with ease of performing the tasks. Once the patient is comfortable enough to rework the instructions into his or her routine, it is a sign of the beginning of adjustment to the stoma.

Emptying the pouch into the toilet after placing toilet tissue in the bowl to prevent splash back is the most common way to empty pouches (Colwell & Fichera, 2005). Sitting on the toilet emptying the pouch between the legs and in the case of a fecal ostomy, cleaning the bottom edge with toilet tissue is a practice used by many people while others turn the end of the pouch back on to itself to form a cuff with a pouch that uses a clamp. Some people find it easier to face the toilet and empty the pouch down into the bowl, while others use a two-piece system, detach the pouch from the skin barrier and empty into the toilet, and then replace the pouch on the flange. This is an area that the patient can adjust to his or her own comfort level, front facing, back facing, or standing, patient preference can be accepted and can help the patient to feel some control over his or her care.

Some people with a fecal ostomy wish to rinse out the pouch, either with each emptying or daily, although this is not necessary, as long as the tail edge of the pouch is kept clean. Pouches are manufactured to be odor proof, which means they will contain the odor in the pouch; however, when the pouch is emptied, there may be some unpleasant odors. Pouches are available with gas filters that are charcoal and allow gas to escape from the pouch while absorbing the odor. These do not perform as well when the output from the stoma is very liquid, as in an ileostomy, as the liquid stool may clog the filter. There are in-pouch deodorants, odor eliminators, and systemic pill deodorants than can assist in the elimination of odor when emptying pouch. (See Chapter 12 and Box 11-2 for simple pouch emptying instructions.)

When to Empty

This is typically the first skill the person with a new ostomy must learn. It is the most frequent task they will have to perform with the ostomy, sometimes four, five, or six times daily with an ileostomy or urostomy, less often with a colostomy. It is very important that this skill be acquired before the patient leaves the hospital, and he or she should be able to demonstrate his or her ability to check the pouch for filling, empty, and close the end spout or use the clip successfully.

Since there is no sensation of urine or stool coming through the stoma, it means the patient must get into the habit of feeling the pouch to see how full it is. The pouch should be emptied when it is half to one third full to avoid strain on the adhesive seal, or sooner if the person finds this uncomfortable. As noted, as soon as they are able, the patient should be responsible for checking the filling of the pouch and alerting to the need for emptying. As recovery continues, the patient should be responsible for pouch emptying before discharge from the hospital, since they will be as soon as they get home.

BOX 11-2 Instructions for Pouch Emptying

1. Sit on the toilet, as far back as possible.
2. Hold up the pouch and remove/open the bottom of the pouch (clamp or plug tip).
3. Turn up the end of the pouch back on itself to form a cuff—plug tip or self-closure mechanisms form a spout when opened.
4. Place a piece of toilet paper into the toilet and drain pouch into the toilet (reduces splash back).
5. Clean cuffed end of the outlet with toilet paper or wipe—rinsing pouch is not necessary.
6. Undo the cuff—close the end of the pouch or fasten plug tip. If needed, in-pouch deodorant may be used at this time.

Based on Doughty, D. (2005). Principles of ostomy management in the oncology patient. *Supportive Oncology, 3*(1), 59–69; Bak, G.P. (2008). Teaching ostomy patients to regain their independence. *American Nurse Today, 3*(3), 30–34.

Indications for Pouch Change

Most pouches are routinely changed twice per week or any time there is evidence of leakage or skin irritation. Usually itching, burning, and feeling of moistness under the skin barrier are indicators that there is moisture in contact with the skin under the barrier. Leakage outside the edges of the barrier should never be "fixed," repaired, or taped over. Doing this merely traps the leakage onto the skin and will result in skin irritation or peristomal irritant dermatitis. Pouching systems should be changed as soon as possible whenever leakage is noted.

Many people with an ostomy will change the pouching system prior to sexual activity to ensure a leak-free experience, others may find that religious observations require a clean pouch; otherwise, most people establish a routine so that the pouching system is changed prior to any signs of leakage.

Preparing Equipment

Before removing the pouch, the patient should assemble all the necessary equipment at hand so that they do not have to look for items once the pouch is removed and while the stoma is functioning. Most people keep their supplies together on a shelf or in a box or bag for all of their ostomy equipment, including the pouching system and any accessory products they are using paste, belt, tape, or scissors. If the stoma has been recently created, a measuring guide may be used to recheck the stoma circumference since it will shrink postoperatively. After a month or so, if stoma size is stable, a presized barrier may be ordered. If not using a presized skin barrier, it is best to trace the size from the measuring guide onto the paper on the back of the skin barrier, and cut out the skin barrier and apply paste (if used) prior to removing pouch. Most pastes contain alcohol, so allowing the alcohol to dry before application of the skin barrier helps to protect the skin from the effects of the alcohol.

Assessing Peristomal Skin

The skin around the stoma should not look very different from the rest of the skin. While the pouch is off, examine the area for any redness, rashes, or open skin areas. Inspect outer edges of where adhesive tape attaches to barrier for any signs of skin irritation.

Examine the adhesive side of the skin barrier to see if there is any erosion especially around the stoma opening. This might indicate that the pouching system has been in place for too long. If there are any changes to the peristomal skin such as breakdown, erosion, or rashes, instructs the patient to contact the WOC nurse for an appointment. It has been noted that many patients accept skin breakdown under the barrier as normal, they should be instructed that this is cause for a follow-up visit with the WOC nurse.

Measuring Stoma

The stoma will shrink for some time after surgery due to decreasing edema. This means the patient will have to resize the stomal opening of the skin barrier until the size stabilizes. Most ostomy equipment comes with measuring guides that allow placing the openings over the stoma to facilitate selection of the correct stoma size. If the stoma size is not round, usually the WOC nurse will send home a pattern for the patient to trace onto to the skin barrier, but the patient must assess that the pattern to see if it remains the correct size while the stoma continues to shrink.

Peristomal Skin Cleansing

There are many products available for cleansing and protecting peristomal skin, if soap is used it should be rinsed off thoroughly and soap with oils should be avoided (Doughty, 2005). Most people use warm water and a paper towel that can be disposed of rather than washcloths that require laundering. The area should be wiped with warm water and patted dry. If the peristomal area has a large amount of hair growth, shaving or clipping should be considered, in case the hair interferes with adhesion of skin barrier or causes discomfort upon pouching system removal.

Removal of Pouching System

Some people remove the pouch in the shower and wash the peristomal skin with mild, non-oily soap and water. Others prefer to remove the pouching system in the bathroom and apply the system they have laid out ready for application. Gentle removal using a push pull technique from the top down helps to protect the peristomal skin from mechanical injury.

Placement of Pouching System

If the person received preoperative stoma site marking, the stoma location should be visible and application of the pouching system easily accomplished. Many people apply the skin barrier while standing, others find sitting or lying down easier, usually this is a matter of patient preference. For most people, it is important that the area around the stoma be as flat as possible to enhance the pouching system seal.

The spout part of the pouch is usually in the 6 o'clock position, which allows the effluent to fall to the bottom of the pouch and ease of emptying into the toilet. If the patient wears a belt this is the position that keeps the belt tabs in the 3 and 9 o'clock locations. This again can vary with patient preference.

Problem Identification, When to Seek Assistance

Many issues with stoma management do not occur until the patient is at home, attempting to integrate the new ostomy into his or her actual existence. Richbourg et al. (2007) in a small survey identified some of the challenges the person with an ostomy commonly faces after discharge from the hospital—these include pouch leakage, skin irritation, odor, depression, or anxiety. Because of this, the authors recommend WOC nurses remaining in contact with their patients and in fact calls for the creation of nurse-run ostomy clinics. These clinics would provide the patient with assistance in incorporating the ostomy into their lives and dealing with these common problems associated with a new ostomy.

The United Ostomy Associations of America (UOAA) has published recommendations for the patient on when to call his or her doctor or nurse (Box 11-3). The person with a urostomy, who develops fever, chills, abdominal or retroperitoneal pain, and bloody, cloudy, or foul smelling urine may have a urinary tract infection, and should seek an appointment for follow up (Bak, 2008).

BOX 11-3 When to Seek Medical Attention

Severe cramps lasting more than 2 or 3 hours.
Deep cut in the stoma.
Excessive bleeding from the stoma opening (or a moderate amount in the pouch at several emptyings).
Continuous bleeding at the junction between the stoma and skin.
Severe skin irritation or deep ulcers.
Unusual change in stoma size and appearance.
Severe watery discharge lasting more than 5 or 6 hours.
Continuous nausea and vomiting.
No stoma output for 4 to 6 hours plus cramping and nausea.
Increase in the frequency the pouch requires emptying.

Adapted from United Ostomy Associations of America. (2014). Frequently asked questions. Retrieved from http://www.ostomy.org/Ostomy_FAQ.html

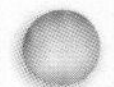

Living with a Stoma

Where and When to Obtain Supplies

The patient may be instructed that many people find it helpful when supplies used in stoma care are kept together on a shelf, in a drawer, or in a box or bag in a dry area away from hot or cold temperatures. They need to order supplies when there is enough equipment to last a month or so, to allow time for delivery.

The WOC nurse should provide the patient written directions and the manufacturer's name and product numbers and a prescription for all materials used in his or her stoma care. Supplies may be ordered from a local pharmacy, from a medical supply store, or a mail order company. The WOC nurse should consider developing a list of area suppliers and mail order companies as well as some online companies that the patient can consider using. Many suppliers will bill Medicare or private insurers directly and the patient should check with his or her health insurance company regarding reimbursement of supply costs, any preferred suppliers and the allowable amounts of supplies.

Bathing

Water is not harmful to the stoma. Patients may take a bath or shower with or without a pouching system in place. Drying the tape or collar of the barrier with a towel or hair dryer can help prevent moisture-associated skin damage. Normal exposure to air or contact with soap and water will not harm the stoma nor will soap irritate it, and water will not flow inwards.

Many patients will swim with the pouching system in place as the pouching system is constructed to enable adhesion in water. The pouching system will remain in place and can be dried or replaced after being in the water.

Before swimming, the pouch should be emptied. When in the water, a support ostomy belt can be left in place if commonly used. Females may wear stretch undergarments made especially for swim suits. Males may want to wear bike shorts or a support garment under their bathing suits.

Many people protect the barrier by taping the edges with waterproof tape. Using a swim suit with a lining for a smoother profile in a dark color or a busy pattern can also help disguise the pouching system. Females may want to choose a suit with a well-placed skirt or ruffle. Men may want to try a suit with a higher waist band or longer leg, or a concealment belt if the stoma is above the belt line. In some instance, a male patient may choose to wear a tank or tee shirt when swimming to conceal the pouching system.

Clothing

For the most part, most patients can wear the same clothing as they wore before surgery. Pouching systems today are predominately unnoticeable even when wearing the most stylish, form fitting clothing for men and women, especially when pouches are emptied routinely and not allowed to overfill. If the stoma is placed above the waistline, over blouses or shirts may be used. In these patients, they may be unable to wear a belt or "tuck in" shirts or blouses, and this does result in a change in clothing style for many people. There are however, some devices available that act as a shield to protect the stoma and allow patients to wear a belt over their pouching system. In a recent report, Gemmill et al. (2010) describe that in a patient population with urinary diversions (n = 307) most did not find the need to change his or her style of clothing after the ostomy. Depending on the activity of the individual, clothing may need to be adjusted, as in swimming or bathing.

Sexual Concerns

It is recognized that ostomy surgery has an effect on intimacy and sexuality (Registered Nurses of Ontario, 2009). Sexual relationships and intimacy can continue after ostomy surgery. There is however, a period of adjustment after surgery and attitude is a key factor in reestablishing sexual expression and intimacy. Sexual function in the female is usually not changed, although dyspareunia (painful intercourse) has been reported. Males may experience damage to nerves that control erection and ejaculation (WCET, 2014). Patients should talk to their doctor and/or WOC nurse about any problems or concerns they or their partner might have. (See Chapters 8 and 14 for discussions of sexual counseling.)

The influence of a partners support on women's psychosocial adjustment to having an ostomy resulting from colorectal cancer is described by Altschuler et al. (2009). The demonstration or withdrawal of support is reported to have a considerable impact on the patient's adjustment both in the long and short term.

Ostomy surgery may present more concerns for single people. When, how, and who to tell about the ostomy is a personal decision, which perhaps could be discussed with an ostomy visitor who has had experience with this issue. However, if a relationship is leading to physical intimacy, it is best the partner is told about the ostomy before discovery is imminent.

CLINICAL PEARL

Patients should be instructed to chew food well, especially fibrous foods to prevent blockage formation.

Dietary Concerns

The UOAA lists foods that affect the person with an ostomy (Table 11-1).

TABLE 11-1 Foods that Affect the Person with an Ostomy

Effect	Foods
Color changes	Asparagus Beets Food coloring Iron pills Licorice Red gelatin Strawberries Tomato sauces
Constipation relief	Coffee, warm/hot Cooked fruits Cooked vegetables Fresh fruits Fruit juices Water Any warm or hot beverage
Diarrhea control	Applesauce Bananas Boiled rice Peanut butter Pectin supplement (fiber) Tapioca Toast
Gas-producing	Alcoholic beverages Beans Soy Cabbage Carbonated beverages Cauliflower Chewing gum Cucumbers Dairy products Milk Nuts Onions Radishes
Increased stools	Alcoholic beverages Whole grains Bran cereals Cooked cabbage Fresh fruits Greens, leafy Milk Prunes Raisins Raw vegetables Spices
Odor control	Buttermilk Cranberry juice Orange juice Parsley Tomato juice Yogurt
Odor-producing	Asparagus Baked beans Broccoli Cabbage Cod liver oil Eggs Fish Garlic Onions Peanut butter Some vitamins Strong cheese
Stoma obstructive	Apple peels Cabbage, raw Celery Chinese vegetables Corn, whole kernel Coconuts Dried fruit Mushrooms Oranges Nuts Pineapple Popcorn Seeds

Adapted from United Ostomy Associations of America Ostomates Food Reference Chart (Pasia, M. (2011). *Diet & Nutrition Guide*. United Ostomy Associations of America. Retrieved from http://www.ostomy.org, info@ostomy.org).

Dietary Concerns

After ostomy surgery, individuals should eat a regular balanced diet that includes the necessary vitamins, minerals, and calories needed for good health (Pasia, 2011). After surgery, when bowel sounds return first foods may be liquid or a low-fiber/low-residue diet until edema subsides, when a regular diet is resumed. New foods should be added gradually to determine their effect on ostomy management.

Some foods cause gas, such as eggs, cabbage, broccoli, onions, fish, beans, milk, cheese, and alcohol. Food should be taken at regular intervals. Skipping meals increase the incidence of watery stools and flatus (gas). Avoid fasting and skipping meals, smoking, chewing gum, and drinking through a straw. Some people benefit from eating six smaller meals, but these should equal three regular meals.

Ileal Conduit

Maintaining adequate fluid intake in the individual with an ileal conduit is important to prevent infection, since the ileal conduit has almost continuous output without any antireflux properties. Patients need to take in 30 cc/kg/d of fluids l at regular intervals throughout the day in order to keep a constant one-way urinary flow (Doughty, 2005).

Ileostomy

Food blockage can occur when insoluble fiber amasses near the fascia-muscle layer. Signs of blockage are constant spurting of liquid or a watery stool, feeling full or bloated, cramping, swollen stoma, nausea and vomiting, and absence of stoma output. Foods known to cause blockage problems include corn, celery, popcorn, nuts, coleslaw, coconut macaroons, grapefruit, and Chinese vegetables such as bamboo shoots, water chestnuts, and raisins.

Insoluble fiber foods should be eaten in small amounts and chewed thoroughly along with fluid intake to prevent the mass from forming. The WOC nurse may perform ileal lavage where 30 to 50 mL of warm saline is instilled though a 14 to 16 French catheter, which is then removed to allow drainage. This is repeated until the blockage is relieved (Doughty, 2005). The UOAA has described interventions for when a blockage is suspected. (See Chapter 12 for listed recommendations.)

Many factors, such as foods, normal bacteria in the intestine, illness, certain medicines, and vitamins can cause odor. Some foods can produce odor: eggs, cabbage, cheese, cucumber, onion, garlic, fish, dairy foods, and coffee. Patient needs to determine which foods cause odor and decide if they need to avoid those foods (Table 11-1). Learning by experience is the only way to discover this, odors may be worse with transverse colostomies. Hints for odor control include:

- Use an odor-resistant pouch.
- Check to see that the skin barrier is properly adhered.
- Empty the pouch often.
- Place special deodorant liquids, odor eliminators, and/or tablets in the pouch.
- Use medicines that control odor; the physician or ostomy nurse can advise about these products and how to use them. Some things may help with odor are chlorophyll tablets, bismuth subgallate, and bismuth subcarbonate.
- Use air deodorizers which can control odor very well when emptying the pouch.

Medications

Absorption may vary with individuals and types of medication. Certain drug problems may arise depending on the type of ostomy the medications used. Patients should be sure to tell their pharmacy or pharmacist about the ostomy to ensure that they are receiving their medications in the appropriate format. Patients with an ileostomy or transverse colostomies should not take laxatives as it could lead to dehydration and extended-release medications (i.e., time-released and enteric-coated medications may pass through the system of people with ileostomies too quickly to be effective). Many patients in the hospice or palliative care setting take long-acting opioids, which are sustained release and dependent on the amount of small bowel still accessible for absorption. In addition, many of these medications can cause constipation and blockage, diarrhea, or altered fluid and electrolyte balances (Tilley, 2012). (See Chapter 12 for a discussion of medications.)

Follow-Up Care

A recent survey of cancer survivors with a urinary diversion (Gemmill et al., 2010) reports the majority of patients reported it took months to feel comfortable with daily care and diet, and problems may continue for years after surgery. Further, it is suggested that long-term access to a WOC nurse is important in improving and maintaining the quality of life of these patients. Sun et al. (2013) describes persistent ostomy concerns and adaptations in long-term (>5 years) colorectal cancer survivors with an ostomy. Most common concerns were identified as stoma location and pouch problems, activity limitations, leakage, odor, pouch adhesive issues, and skin irritation. The authors suggest the need for long-term supportive care strategies. However, being aware of these specific issues, the WOC nurse should intervene early in the preoperative and postoperative course to teach and inform patients in these specific areas, and provide follow up with community resources as well as physician and nursing follow ups.

Listings of ostomy clinics and referral sources for stoma clinics should be given to all ostomy patients at discharge: most ostomy patients will require some measure of lifelong follow up and must receive advice of where to find these services. Appendix B lists ostomy support resources, and Appendix C lists suppliers of ostomy products.

Support Groups

Nurses may refer ostomy patients to support groups and to the online UOAA at http://www.uoaa.org/; the site has active discussion boards for various types of incontinent and continent diversions, along with youth, adult, and parent networks (Dorman, 2009).

CLINICAL PEARL

Some studies relate the presence of an ostomy to a negative impact on the quality of life of these patients. However a consensus of expert opinion is that this is patient specific, many patients after a period of recovery and adjustment manage to overcome many of the negative effects of living with an ostomy.

Conclusions

Adaptation to a new ostomy requires meeting many challenges that the WOC nurse can help the individual with. Education and training in self-stoma care as well as answering the concerns of the patient help the patients to cope with these challenges. The WOC nurse can prepare the patient for living with a stoma and to help to arrange follow-up care when the person goes home from the hospital.

REFERENCES

Altschuler, A., Ramirez, M., Grant M, et al. (2009). The influence of husband's or male partners' support on women's psychosocial adjustment to having an ostomy resulting from colorectal cancer. *Journal of Wound Ostomy and Continence Nursing, 36*(3), 299–305.

Bak, G. P. (2008). Teaching ostomy patients to regain their independence. *American Nurse Today, 3*(3), 30–34.

Cheng, F., Ai-feng, M., Li-Fang, Y., et al. (2013). The correlation between ostomy knowledge and self-care ability with psychosocial adjustment in Chinese patients with a permanent colostomy: A descriptive study. *Ostomy Wound Management, 59*(7), 35–38.

Colwell, J. C., & Beitz, J. (2007). Survey of wound, ostomy and continence (WOC) nurse clinicians on stomal and peristomal complications: A content validation study. *Journal of Wound, Ostomy and Continence Nursing, 34*(1), 57–69.

Colwell, J. C., & Fichera, A. (2005). Care of the obese patient with an ostomy. *Journal of Wound Ostomy and Continence Nursing, 32*(6), 378–383.

Dorman, C. (2009). *Ostomy basics: The nurse's personal feelings toward ostomies play a role in patient outcomes* (pp. 22–27), http://'www.rnweb.com

Doughty, D. (2005). Principles of ostomy management in the oncology patient. *Supportive Oncology, 3*(1), 59–69.

Gemmill, R., Sun, V., Ferrell, B., et al. (2010). *Journal of Wound Ostomy and Continence Nursing, 3*(1), 65–72.

Haugen, B., Bliss, D. Z., & Savik, K. (2006). Perioperative factors that affect long-term adjustment to an incontinent ostomy. *Journal of Wound Ostomy and Continence Nursing, 33*(5), 525–535.

Joint Commission Patient Education Requirements. (2012). Retrieved from http://www.mghpcs.org/eed_portal/Documents/PatientEd/JC_Standards_PatientEd.pdf

O'Shea, H. S. (2001). Teaching the adult ostomy patient. *Journal of Wound Ostomy and Continence Nursing, 28*(1), 47–54.

Pasia, M. (2011). *Diet & Nutrition Guide.* United Ostomy Associations of America. Retrieved from http://www.ostomy.org, info@ostomy.org

Registered Nurses of Ontario. (2009). Toronto, ON. Retrieved from http://www.rnao.org.bestpractices

Richbourg, L., Thorpe, J. M., & Rapp, C. G. (2007). Difficulties experienced by the ostomate after hospital discharge. *Journal of Wound Ostomy and Continence Nursing, 34*(1), 70–79.

Sun, V., Grant, M., McMullen, C. K., et al. (2013). Surviving colorectal cancer. Long-term, persistent ostomy-specific concerns and adaptations. *Journal of Wound Ostomy and Continence Nursing, 40*(1), 61–72.

Tilley, C. (2012). Caring for the patient with a fecal or urinary diversion in palliative and hospice settings: A literature review. *Ostomy Wound Management, 58*(1), 24–34.

United Ostomy Associations of America. (2014). Frequently asked questions. Retrieved from http://www.ostomy.org/Ostomy_FAQ.html

WCET. (2014). WCET International Guideline Recommendations: 3.2 Preoperative education. In K. Zulkowski (Ed.), *WCET international ostomy guideline* (pp. 14–15). Osborne Park, Australia: WCET.

QUESTIONS

1. The WOC nurse is teaching a patient with a new colostomy how to empty the pouch. What is a recommended step in this procedure?
- A. Sit on the front edge of the toilet seat.
- B. Turn up the end of the pouch back on itself to form a cuff.
- C. Clean cuffed end of the outlet with alcohol wipe.
- D. Always rinse pouch prior to reconnecting it.

2. An elderly gentleman with a new ostomy tells the WOC nurse: "I'll never be able to figure out this system, I don't know where anything goes and I'm going home tomorrow!" What patient teaching strategy would best meet this patient's needs?
- A. Provide general written instructions for stoma care and encourage patient describe how they will accomplish this at home.
- B. Encourage the patient to develop a care plan independently and follow it step-by-step in the home environment.
- C. Ensure the patient that there is no recommended procedure for stoma care and that he should figure out a routine that works as soon as possible.
- D. Teach the care plan to the patient's family/caregiver since he is elderly and ask the caregiver to decide if the patient is able to provide self care.

3. What teaching point would the WOC nurse emphasize as a recommended guideline for emptying and changing an ostomy pouch?
- A. Empty pouch after the sensation of urine or stool comes through the stoma.
- B. Empty the pouch when it is three fourth full to avoid strain on the adhesive seal.
- C. If a leak occurs outside the edge of the barrier, the barrier can be taped.
- D. Routinely change the pouch 2 or 3 times per week or if leakage occurs.

4. A patient with a new ostomy is experiencing skin breakdown under the barrier. What would be the priority intervention for this patient?
- A. Schedule a follow-up visit with the WOC nurse.
- B. Change the pouching system more often.
- C. Change the size of the stomal opening of the skin barrier.
- D. Clean the skin around and under the barrier with a petroleum product.

5. The nurse is teaching a patient with a new ostomy tips for successful stoma care. Which tip meets recommended guidelines for care?
A. Always remove the pouch standing up in the shower.
B. Keep pouching system in place until leakage occurs.
C. Remove the pouching system gently using push pull technique.
D. Wash the peristomal skin with mild oil-based soap and water.

6. The WOC nurse is teaching stoma care to a patient with a new ileostomy who is being discharged to home care. Under what condition would the nurse tell the patient to seek medical attention?
A. Pouch is filling twice daily.
B. If there is lots of air in the pouch.
C. If there is severe water discharge lasting more than 5 or 6 hours.
D. If there is no stoma output for 24 hours followed by cramping and nausea.

7. A nutritionist is helping a patient with a new ostomy plan a diet. Which food would the nurse recommend to maintain odor control?
A. Fresh fruits.
B. Tomato juice.
C. Popcorn.
D. Milk.

8. A patient with a new colostomy is complaining of diarrhea. What food would the WOC nurse recommend to help resolve this problem?
A. Cooked vegetables.
B. Fruit juices.
C. Dairy products.
D. Peanut butter.

9. The WOC nurse is advising a patient with a new ileal conduit on how to prevent urinary tract infection. What advice would be appropriate?
A. Drink 30 mL/kg/d of fluids.
B. Avoid insoluble fiber foods.
C. Limit fluids to 10 mL/kg/d.
D. Avoid odor-producing foods.

10. A patient with a new ostomy tells the WOC nurse: "I am a bit nervous about having sex with my partner after this surgery." What should be the nurses response?
A. "Sexuality is not affected by this condition."
B. "You and your partner will need to see if sex is possible."
C. "Most people feel more comfortable if they empty the pouch before engaging in sexual activity."
D. "You need to explore other forms of sexual intimacy besides intercourse."

ANSWERS: 1.**B**, 2.**A**, 3.**D**, 4.**A**, 5.**C**, 6.**C**, 7.**B**, 8.**D**, 9.**A**, 10.**C**

CHAPTER 12

Specific Patient Management Issues

Jane E. Carmel

OBJECTIVE

Analyze specific management issues related to fecal and urinary diversions.

Topic Outline

A fecal and/or urinary diversion presents many concerns for the individual who is adapting and trying to return to their previous life style. The Wound Ostomy Continence (WOC) nurse needs to address many issues related to the type of ostomy the person has as well as whether the diversion is temporary or permanent. This chapter discusses areas related to both fecal and urinary diversions to enable the WOC nurse to provide information to help the person to return to his or her former lifestyle. There are many options and interventions to help to manage his or her concerns, and these are addressed in this chapter.

Temporary Fecal Diversions

Not all fecal diversions are permanent, and this will depend on the patients' diagnosis and prognosis. Types of temporary fecal stomas are end/Hartmann's pouch and loop ileostomy or colostomy. Temporary stomas are created to divert the stool from the distal bowel, allowing the bowel to heal. The surgeon can reverse the stoma within 3 to 6 months with minimal loss of intestinal function (McGrath & Porrett, 2005). There are many conditions that can require a temporary diversion (Box 12-1).

In the Hartmann's procedure, a resection of the diseased bowel is performed, the rectal stump is closed, and an end colostomy is created. This procedure is usually performed for emergency conditions, that is, perforated diverticular disease. The patient will be taught that he or she may experience passing stool or mucus from the anus. This may be a temporary or permanent stoma depending on the indication for the surgery and the patient's condition.

With the loop stoma, a loop of the bowel is brought through the abdominal wall (Figure 7-4 in Chapter 7). An opening is made in the bowel to allow stool to be expelled. A temporary rod or bridge is placed below the loop to prevent retraction of the stoma. Loop ileostomies are more

BOX 12-1 Conditions Requiring Temporary Fecal Stoma

Emergency condition for distal bowel obstruction or distal trauma
To rest distal segment of the bowel that may have a disease process, fistula, or Crohn's disease
To protect an anastomosis

common than are loop colostomies. Reversal surgery for loop ileostomy are easier as a small incision is made around the loop, and the two ends are brought through the incision and reconnected (Cera, 2008).

Although not commonly created, a mucous fistula can be created during emergency surgery at the same time as the ileostomy or colostomy. The proximal end of the remaining colon or rectum is brought out onto the abdomen as a mucous fistula, called a mucous fistula because some mucus will pass from this opening. The purpose of the mucous fistula is to reduce the risk of stump dehiscence, which can occur with active rectal disease and preoperative steroid use (Windsor & Conn, 2008). The patient will be taught to cover the mucous fistula with a stoma cap (**Fig. 12-1**) or a mini drainable pouch or in some cases a gauze pad changed, based on the amount of mucous drainage.

Colostomy

Irrigation

The person with a sigmoid colostomy has the option of managing his or her colostomy with irrigation, and this should be offered as a management method to a person with a left-sided colostomy (**Fig. 12-2**). Managing a colostomy by irrigation is for many people a simple, cost-effective procedure. Carlsson et al. (2010) studied the positive and negative aspects of colostomy irrigation (CI) and found that negative aspects reported were time required for CI, less flexibility to plan CI, and more flatulence. Positive aspects reported were feeling secure, having an empty pouch, sense of freedom, and fewer pouch changes.

CI can be performed daily or every other day with the goal of being "stool free," that is, no stool passing from the stoma between irrigation. Once the colostomy is regulated, the person no longer has to wear a pouching system and can wear a stoma cap. These are available as a one- or two-piece system; some people prefer the two-piece system to use with the irrigation sleeve. Stoma caps are available also as cut-to-fit skin barrier with filter to manage gas and absorb mucous discharge.

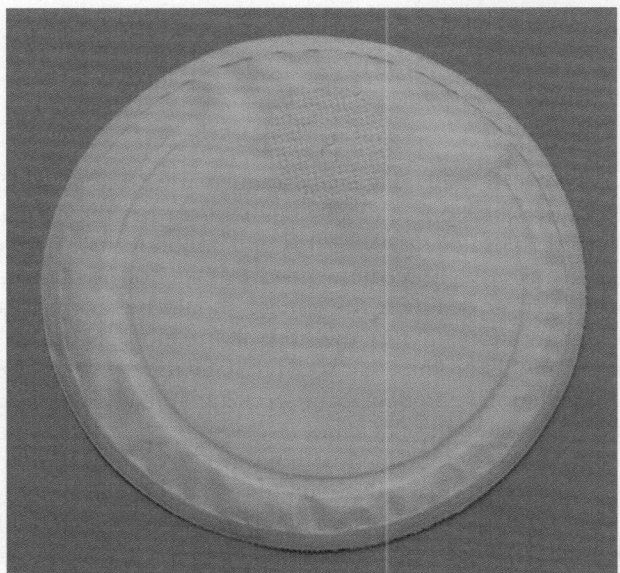

FIGURE 12-1. Stoma cap.

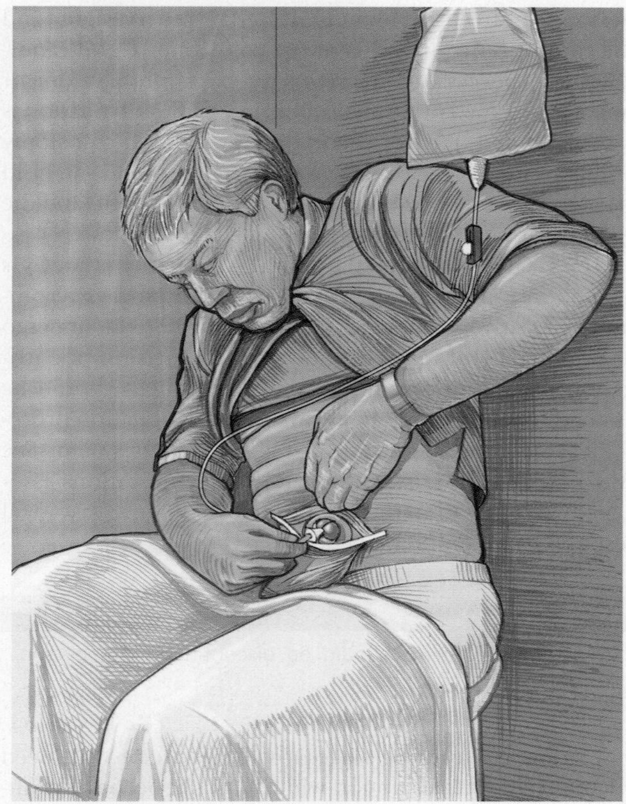

FIGURE 12-2. Colostomy irrigation. From *Nursing 2006*, 36(4), 22.

Patient Selection

Irrigation is not always suitable for all patients with a colostomy. The WOC nurse should evaluate the person's understanding of the irrigation procedure as well as the person's motivation, manual dexterity and eyesight, and the current function of his or her colostomy. Good candidates for a successful outcome with irrigation have one or two semi-formed or formed stools in 24 hours. Irrigation is recommended only for descending or sigmoid colostomy as this section of the colon has less peristalsis and can hold stool for several days; there is less frequent output, and the stool is formed unlike the right-sided colostomies.

The WOC nurse should explain to the patient that CI is an option to manage the ostomy. It is not always recommended early postoperatively. If a patient will undergo chemotherapy or has a healing perineal incision, the irrigation procedure can be delayed. The patient should be assured that he or she can always stop the irrigation procedure at any time and resume using a pouching system. See Box 12-2 for contraindications to CI. Complications associated with irrigation include nonreturn of fluid, vasovagal response, and abdominal cramps.

CLINICAL PEARL

Colostomy irrigations should be discontinued if a person develops a peristomal hernia.

During the learning stage of CI, the person will need encouragement and support while he or she becomes proficient in the procedure. Box 12-3 explains the CI procedure.

Odor and Flatus Management

Odor is a common fear for the person with a diversion; pouching systems are odor proof, but this does not always assure the person there is no odor. Teach the person that odor should only occur when emptying and changing the pouching system, and taking time to clean the inside and outside of the pouch tail prevents odor. If using a pouch clip for open-ended pouch, teach to wash and dry the clip after emptying the pouch to eliminate any risk of odor.

Deodorants/eliminators are available in the form of droplets and liquid that can be added to the inside of the clean pouch to help eliminate the odor of stool. The liquid deodorant/eliminator is placed into the newly applied pouch, and as the stool drains into the pouch, the deodorant/eliminator mixes with the stool to decrease odor. When the pouch is emptied, the deodorant/eliminator is replaced. A lubricating deodorant can be used to both deodorize the stool and lubricate the inside of the pouch for easy emptying.

BOX 12-2 Contraindications to Colostomy Irrigation

Current chemotherapy/radiotherapy
Stoma stenosis
Large parastomal hernia or stoma prolapse
Crohn's disease
Poor prognosis
Diarrhea

BOX 12-3 Colostomy Irrigation Procedure

1. Gather the following equipment*:
   - Irrigation kit: 2-L bag, tubing with flow regulator, soft cone
   - Water-soluble lubricant
   - Irrigation drain sleeve
   - Ostomy belt
   - Warm water
   - Coat hanger or wall hook to hang the irrigation bag from
2. Attach irrigation cone to tubing and fill the bag with 1,000 mL of warm tap water.
3. Hang the irrigation bag from hook at shoulder level when seating on toilet.
4. Open the regulator clamp on the tubing and let the water run through the tube to remove the air. Reclamp the tube.
5. Remove colostomy pouch; if two piece, leave the barrier in place. Place the irrigation sleeve over the stoma or attach to the barrier or secure with an ostomy belt.
6. Lubricate the cone with water-soluble lubricant and gently insert the cone into the stoma until it fits snugly.
7. While holding the cone in place with one hand, open the clamp on the tubing and let 500 to 1,000 mL of water flow slowly into the colon over 5 to 10 minutes. Regulate the flow of water using the clamp. Note start with 500 mL of water.
8. Once the amount of water is instilled, clamp the tube and hold the cone in place for about a minute, and then remove the cone from the stoma.
9. Close the top of the irrigation sleeve, and wait for results to flow into the toilet. Most is expelled in the first 5 to 10 minutes; the rest may take up to 30 to 45 minutes.
10. Once returns are complete, remove the sleeve, clean the skin, and apply the pouching system or stoma cap/mini pouch.
11. Wash the equipment with mild soap and warm water, hang to dry, and store in a clean container.

Adapted from Prinz, A. (2013). Irrigation for the Colostomate-Life without the pouch! Colostomy New Patient Guide. UOAA The Phoenix Magazine; Hayes, D. (2013). Colostomy irrigation: Retraining continence and regaling confidence. *Journal of Stomal Therapy Australia*, *33*(2), 18–20.
*Supplies can be obtained from ostomy companies that have irrigation sets.

There are orally ingested products available to help deodorize the stool internally before it reaches the pouch. Bismuth subgallate (Devrom) is one option for both odor and flatus, usually recommended to take 200 mg before meals and at bedtime. The patient should be taught that this medication will turn the stool dark. Chlorophyllin 100 mg is another product that is taken orally three times a day. This will turn the stool or urine green and initially can cause loose stools, but this is a temporary side effect. Both of these products can be obtained without a prescription, but the patient should discuss this with his or her health care provider and WOC nurse before trying the product; some feel that the green color can mask blood in the stool, which is an important symptom requiring further investigation.

Other recommendations to help control odor from stool include parsley, buttermilk, cranberry juice, and

BOX 12-4
Foods That May Cause Gas and Odor

Asparagus
Beans
Beer
Cabbage family
Carbonated drinks
Eggs (hard boiled)
Fish
Melon
Milk products
Onions
Spiced foods

yogurt. Foods to avoid that can produce odor and gas are listed in Box 12-4.

In the large colon, flatus is formed from bacterial activity related to undigested carbohydrates including cellulose in the colon. About 500 mL of flatus may be expelled daily and can increase based on high-carbohydrate foods eaten (Richards, 2005). Proteins and fats cause little gas. In the small intestine, flatus can occur from swallowing air, chewing gum, eating fast, and using loose-fitting dentures. For flatus management, pouches are available with built-in charcoal filter, vents, and self-sealing filters that can be attached to the outside of the pouch. Integrated pouch filters are usually placed at the top of the pouch and, in many cases, may only last 24 to 36 hours when the filter becomes plugged or wet from stool. Vents, an external device, are designed without a filter and have a plug that needs to be manually opened to release built-up gas in the pouch. These are an alternative to relieving gas and will last as long as the pouch is in place.

Room sprays can be used to eliminate odor rather than mask it and are best used prior to emptying the pouch rather than afterward.

Prevention and Management of Constipation

Constipation can occur in the patient with a sigmoid colostomy; a person with an ileostomy rarely will become constipated as there is little storage capacity in the small bowel. Fiber is recommended for the person with a colostomy to increase bulk to the stool and make it easier to pass. The person being managed with opioid pain medication may also suffer from constipation. Mild constipation can be managed by adjusting the diet in the following ways: increase fluids, high-fiber foods, and exercise. It is recommended that fiber be increased in small increments as it may cause bloating, fullness, and gas. Stool softeners should also be recommended when taking pain medications. There are four types of laxative to consider: bulk forming, stimulant, osmotic, and stool softeners (Table 12-1).

Stimulant laxatives such as senna along with a stool softener may be used in colostomy patient (Tilley, 2012). However, it is not good practice to depend on laxatives. A thorough physical examination and history is important. Digital examination of the stoma needs to be performed by an experienced ostomy nurse, to determine if there is hard stool in the colon. This should be performed by gently inserting a lubricated gloved finger into the stoma lumen to assess for impaction or blockage (Tilley, 2012).

Prevention and Management of Diarrhea

A person with a colostomy who experiences loose stools should first consider if this is related to ingestion of certain foods. The WOC nurse should review the patient's history of foods that caused diarrhea before he or she had a diversion. Causes of diarrhea are osmotic, mechanical, secretory, and pharmacological or a combination of factors (Tilley, 2012). It is also important to review medications and previous history. A person undergoing chemotherapy of following 5-fluorouracil and irinotecan can cause diarrhea (see Chapter 13).

TABLE 12-1 Types of Laxatives

Type	Action	Side Effects
Bulk forming/fiber Example: psyllium (Metamucil, FiberCon)	Absorb water to form soft bulky stool Slow acting 12 h–3 d Adequate fluid intake is necessary for effective fiber therapy	Bloating Cramping Gas
Osmotic Magnesium citrate Magnesium hydroxide (milk of magnesia) Sodium phosphate (Fleet phospho-soda)	Pulls water into the large intestine to soften stool and stimulate peristalsis Rapid onset: 30 min–3 h Should be used short term, no longer than 3 consecutive days	Bloating Gas Cramping Nausea Dehydration
Stimulant Examples: Senna (Senokot) Phenolphthalein (Ex-Lax) Diphenylmethane (Dulcolax)	Stimulates the lining of the bowel causing increased peristaltic activity Considered the most powerful of the laxatives	Cramping Nausea Urine discoloration Diarrhea
Stool softener Example: Colace	Retains water within the stool and promotes the stool to pass easier	Bloating Cramping Gas Bitter taste

Some foods recommended for managing diarrhea are cheese, bananas, applesauce, marshmallows, rice, pasta, and tapioca pudding.

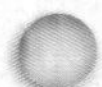 Ileostomy

The person with an ileostomy may have the entire colon, rectum, and anus removed. The WOC nurse needs to explain to the patient that the ileostomy has lost the absorptive function of the colon. Two complications that need to be taught to the patient to recognize are dehydration and obstruction.

Dehydration

The ostomy nurse needs to teach the patient signs of dehydration: increased thirst, lethargy, muscle cramps, dry mouth, abdominal cramps, and decreased urine output. Without the colon, electrolyte deficiency can occur. An important aspect of dietary interventions is to maintain electrolyte levels. The average daily fluid loss for ileostomy can be 500 to 750 mL compared to 100 to 200 mL lost by the average person with an intact colon. Dehydration can occur due to losses of sodium and potassium. The patient may need to increase his or her sodium intake. This can be done by adding high-sodium fluids/foods: broth, canned vegetables, and tomato juice. Potassium is also needed to be added to the diet. Some foods high in potassium are bananas, potatoes, peppers, chicken, beef, and spinach. This should be discussed with the person's physician, and blood work should be monitored. It is important to teach the person to increase fluids especially in hot weather, or when participating in sports.

Food Blockage

Food blockage, or small bowel obstruction, can be partial or complete. A partial blockage can present with abdominal distention, cramping, pain, stoma edema, and watery output. The following instructions can be given: take a warm bath or shower to relax the abdominal muscles, may use a heating pad, and lie on the right side and massage the peristomal area or try the knee–chest position (Box 12-5). Fluids can be taken if there is still some stool output; solid foods should be avoided. The pouch system should be changed and the barrier opening made larger to accommodate the swollen stoma.

If the blockage is complete, there will be little or no stoma activity, nausea and vomiting can occur, and stoma edema. If there is no stoma output, food and fluids should not be taken, and the physician should be called and/or the patient should go to the emergency department (Box 12-6).

Ileal lavage (Box 12-7) is recommended if the obstruction does not resolve. This procedure is performed by a WOC nurse or physician. A soft rubber catheter is lubricated and gently inserted into the stoma up to or if possible beyond the obstruction, and 10 to 20 mL of saline is gently instilled to move the blockage. The fluid is allowed to drain, and the instillation of the fluid is continued several more times to try and break up the blockage. This is not the same as CI. United Ostomy Associations of America (UOAA) has a card for food blockage that the patient can take to the emergency room.

BOX 12-5 Teaching How to Treat an Ileostomy Blockage

Symptoms: Thin, clear liquid output with foul odor; cramping, nausea, vomiting, abdominal pain near the stoma; decrease in amount of output; abdominal and stomal swelling.

Step One: At Home

1. Cut the opening of the skin barrier of your pouching system a little larger than normal because the stoma may swell.
2. If there is some stoma output and you are not nauseated or vomiting, only consume liquids such as soft drinks, sports drinks, or tea.
3. Take a warm bath to relax the abdominal muscles.
4. Try several different body positions, such as a knee–chest position, as it might help move the blockage forward.
5. Massage the abdomen and the area around the stoma as this might increase the pressure behind the blockage and help it to be relieved. Most food blockages occur just inside the stoma.

Step Two: If you are still blocked, are vomiting, or have no stomal output for several hours:

1. Call your doctor or WOC nurse and report what is happening and what you tried at home to alleviate the problem. Your doctor or WOC nurse will give you instructions (e.g., meet at the emergency room, come to the office). If you are told to go to the emergency room, the doctor or WOC nurse can call in orders for your care when you arrive.
2. If you cannot reach your WOC nurse or surgeon and there is **no output** from the stoma, go to the emergency room immediately.

Important: Take all of your pouch supplies with you (e.g., pouch, skin barrier, tail closure, liquid skin barrier).

Adapted from United Ostomy Associations of America (2014).

CLINICAL PEARL

Ileostomy lavage should not be performed until there is a confirmed obstruction.

Diet

After surgery for an ileostomy, the person can gradually go back to his or her usual diet. Patients should be instructed to chew food thoroughly and eat slowly. High-fiber foods should be avoided to prevent the risk of a food blockage. Obstruction can occur when high-fiber foods have difficulty passing through the small intestine and exiting the stoma. Some foods that can contribute to a blockage include Chinese vegetables, corn, celery, and nuts.

Medications

An important consideration when selecting medication for the person with a stoma is the length of the small bowel available for drug absorption. Enteric-coated and sustained-release medications should be avoided by the person with

BOX 12-6
Emergency Staff: Ileostomy Obstruction

Symptoms: No stomal output; cramping abdominal pain; nausea and vomiting; abdominal distention; stomal edema; absent or faint bowel sounds.

1. Contact the patient's surgeon or WOC nurse to obtain history and request orders.
2. Pain medication should be initiated as indicated.
3. Start IV fluids (lactated Ringer solution/normal saline).
4. Obtain flat abdominal x-ray or CT scan to rule out volvulus and determine the site/cause of the obstruction. Check for local blockage (peristomal hernia or stomal stenosis) via digital manipulation of the stoma lumen.
5. Evaluate fluid and electrolyte balance via appropriate laboratory studies.
6. If an ileostomy lavage is ordered, it should be performed by a surgeon or ostomy nurse using the following guidelines:
   - Gently insert a lubricated, gloved finger into the lumen of the stoma. If a blockage is palpated, attempt to gently break it up with your finger.
   - Attach a CI sleeve to the patient's two-piece pouching system. Many brands of pouching systems have Tupperware-like flanges onto which the same size diameter irrigation sleeve can be attached. If the patient is not wearing a two-piece system, remove the one-piece system and attach a CI sleeve to an elastic belt and place it over the stoma.

     Another option: cut a hole over the stoma if they have a one-piece pouching system and do the irrigation and then change the pouch.
   - Working through the top of the CI sleeve, insert a lubricated soft catheter (#14–16 Fr) into the lumen of the stoma until the blockage is reached. Do not force the catheter.

     Note: Slowly instill 30 to 50 mL NS into the catheter using a bulb syringe. Remove the catheter and allow for returns into the irrigation sleeve. Repeat this procedure instilling 30 to 50 mL at a time until the blockage is resolved. This can take 1 to 2 hours.
7. Once the blockage has been resolved, a clean, drainable pouch system should be applied. Because the stoma may be edematous, the opening in the barrier should be slightly larger than the stoma.

Adapted from United Ostomy Associations of America (2014).

high-output ileostomy or short bowel because of slow dissolution properties. People with an ileostomy are at a higher risk for suboptimal drug absorption than is a person with a colostomy. The WOC nurse needs to teach the person with ileostomy to ask his or her pharmacist about medications prescribed, if it will dissolve quickly and be absorbed. Women taking birth control and estrogen replacement medication also need to check with their pharmacist.

Bowel Prep

Any type of bowel prep that may be ordered for different diagnostic procedures or surgeries should not be given to people with ileostomies. The patient and health care clinicians need to know there is a high risk for electrolyte imbalance and dehydration with bowel prep.

BOX 12-7
Colostomy Irrigation Tips

Cramping may occur when instilling water; this may be caused by the flow being too fast or the water being too cold or hot. The irrigation should be stopped until cramps subside, and then the procedure should be resumed.

If water does not go in, the cone tip should be repositioned.

If water leaks around the stoma during instillation, clamp the tube and readjust the cone.

If no return, possible cause may be dehydration; discontinue irrigation, increase oral fluids, and wear a drainable pouch.

Complete return of water and stool may take up to 45 minutes.

Irrigation should be done at the same time of day, every 1 to 2 days.

It may take up to 6 to 8 weeks to achieve a predictable bowel pattern with an irrigation procedure.

Ileal Conduit

Urinary diversions can have a metabolic effect, hyperchloremic metabolic acidosis along with malabsorption syndromes, such as vitamin B_{12} deficiency (Van der Aa et al., 2011). Vitamin B_{12} deficiency may not be clinically apparent until 2 to 5 years after the surgery (Gray & Moore, 2009). Some patients complain of diarrhea; this can be due to diminished bile salt and fat absorption. See Chapter 6 for more information on complications.

Because a continent urinary diversion uses a longer segment of small bowel, there is a greater chance of metabolic changes when compared to the patient with an ileal conduit. Urinary calculi are another possible complication in the patient with an ileal conduit. Long-term follow-up of individuals with urinary diversions is strongly recommended not only from an oncologic but also from metabolic perspective (Khalil, 2010; Stein & Rubenwolf, 2014; Van der Aa et al., 2011).

Urine should be kept acidic. The presence of crystals on stoma and/or peristomal skin is caused by urine alkalosis. See Chapter 15 for management of this condition.

There is no specific diet for a person with a urinary diversion. However, it is important to teach the need for adequate fluid intake. The patient is taught to drink unsweetened cranberry juice, to maintain acidic urine. Vitamin C and cranberry tablets are also another option. People who are on blood thinners (warfarin) should avoid cranberry products. Certain foods and medications can discolor urine and produce strong odor. Foods that cause urine odor are fish and asparagus. Antibiotics may cause odor in urine (Fillingham, 2005).

Stent Management (Urostomy)

Preoperatively, the WOC nurse should teach the patient that stents will be exiting the urostomy. The purpose of the stents is to maintain patency and to allow the ureteral/conduit anastomosis to heal. Sometimes, the surgeon will identify the right from the left stent in some manner; that is, different color stents or cutting on end of the stent straight across and the other obliquely. These are left in place from

7 to 10 days but may be left in longer depending upon the surgeon's preference and the patient's ability to heal.

Stents may fall out, and the patient is instructed not to consider this an emergency. Care must be taken when changing the pouch system not to pull on the stents, as they can migrate and become longer. As the stents lengthen, they may require coiling the stent to place in the pouch due to antireflux valve. The urologist may allow the ostomy nurse to trim the stents as they become too long. It is important that they are cut correctly to distinguish the right from the left ureter. A two-piece ostomy system may help in managing the stents as it is easier to place them in the pouch with a separate barrier/pouch system (two-piece pouch system) due to the length of the stents than trying to place in one-piece pouch system. The WOC nurse should explain that it will be normal to have mucus in the urine and on the stoma postoperatively but it will decrease over time.

CLINICAL PEARL

Stents are not to be irrigated.

Night drainage systems are recommended so that the patient does not have to have his or her sleep disturbed by having to empty the urostomy pouch during the night. An adapter is placed on the nighttime drainage collector to allow attachment of the collector to the pouch. Most pouches have a capacity of 350 mL before they must be emptied, whereas a night drainage system has a capacity of 2,000 mL. However, some people worry about having the tubing become twisted or restricted by the system and prefer not to use the night drainage system. Placing the night drainage system at the bottom of the bed, rather than on the side, may lessen the chances of twisting of the tube. The nighttime bag should be replaced every 30 days.

CLINICAL PEARL

Medicare covers two night drainage systems every 30 days.

A leg bag may also be connected to the end of the pouch; this will provide an extra 500-mL capacity. This is option for people who are traveling and may not have access to a toilet for long period of time. However, some people who use a leg bag find that the leg bag pulls on the pouch adhesive (in various positions) and may not opt to use a leg bag. All of the individuals should be given information about leg bags and encouraged to make their own decisions whether or not to use them.

The WOC nurse should review the medications the patient is taking for any side effects that would cause urine discoloration or odor. Some medications can change the color of urine, including the following:

- Cascara: black color
- Doxorubicin: red color
- Metronidazole: initially red then turns to brown
- Antibiotics: strong odor
- Sulfonamides: greenish-blue color

There may be a need to obtain a urine specimen from the ileal conduit. WOCN has published a procedure for obtaining urine specimen. (Refer to WOCN Best Practice Obtaining Urine Specimen from Ileal Conduit, Appendix D.)

CLINICAL PEARL

Urine specimen from an ileal conduit should be obtained by catheterization of the stoma.

Conclusions

Both fecal and urinary incontinent diversions present with specific management issues that the WOC nurse needs to address when teaching the patient. The patient may have many concerns and fears related to odor, flatus, and returning to former ADLs/social life. The WOC nurse needs to provide positive support along with specific education.

REFERENCES

Carlsson, E., Gylin, M., Nilsson, L., et al. (2010). Positive and negative aspects of colostomy irrigation. A patient and WOC Nurse perspective. *Journal of Wound, Ostomy, and Continence Nursing, 37*(5), 511–516.

Cera, S. (2008, December). Temporary stomas. *The Phoenix*. 48–51.

Fillingham, S. (2005). Care of the patient with urinary stoma. In B. Breckman (Ed.), *Stoma care and rehabilitation* (pp. 93–103). Edinburg, TX: Elsevier.

Gray, M., & Moore, K. (2009). *Urologic disorders adult and pediatric care*. St. Louis: Mosby/Elsevier, Inc.

Hayes, D. (2013). Colostomy irrigation: Retraining continence and regaling confidence. *Journal of Stomal Therapy Australia, 33*(2), 18–20.

Khalil, el-SA. (2010). Long term complications following ileal conduit urinary diversion after radical cystectomy. *Journal of Egyptian National Cancer Institute, 22*(1), 13–18.

McGrath, A., & Porrett, T. (2005). Faecal and urinary stomas and restorative surgical procedures developed to avoid stoma formation. In T. Porrett & A. McGarth (Eds.), *Stoma care* (pp. 18–23). Oxford, UK: Blackwell Publishing.

Prinz, A. (2013). Irrigation for the Colostomate-Life without the pouch! Colostomy New Patient Guide. *UOAA The Phoenix Magazine*.

Richards, A. (2005). Intestinal physiology and its implications for patients with bowel stomas. In B. Breckman (Ed.), *Stoma care and rehabilitation* (pp. 22, 218). Edinburg, TX: Elsevier.

Stein, R., & Rubenwolf, P. (2014). Metabolic consequences after urinary diversion. *Frontiers in Pediatrics, 2*, 15.

Tilley, C. (2012). Caring for the patient with a fecal or urinary diversion in palliative and hospice settings: A literature review. *Ostomy/Wound Management, 58*(1), 24–34.

Van der Aa, F., Joniau, S., Van Den Branden, M., et al. (2011). Metabolic changes after urinary diversion. *Advances in Urology*. Article ID 964325.

Windsor, A., & Conn, G. (2008). Surgery. In J. Burch (Ed.), *Stoma care* (pp. 106–112). West Sussex, UK: Wiley-Blackwell.

Wound, Ostomy, and Continence Nurses Society. (2010). *Management of the patient with a fecal ostomy: Best practice guideline for clinicians*. Mount Laurel, NJ: Author.

Wound Ostomy and Continence Nurses Society. (2012). Obtaining a urine specimen from a urostomy, ileal conduit and colon conduit: Best practice for clinicians. Mount Laurel, NJ: Author.

QUESTIONS

1. Which patient would the WOC nurse recommend as a good candidate for colostomy irrigation (CI)?
   A. A patient who is undergoing radiotherapy
   B. A patient with Crohn's disease
   C. A patient with a sigmoid colostomy
   D. A patient with liquid stools

2. The WOC nurse is teaching a patient with a new colostomy how to perform colostomy irrigation (CI). Which of the following should be included in the teaching plan?
   A. Water should be hung at waist level.
   B. Cramping is normal, and the procedure should be continued if this occurs.
   C. Irrigation should be done daily at the same time each day.
   D. Complete return of water and stool may take up to 2 hours.

3. The WOC nurse is teaching a patient to perform a colostomy irrigation (CI). Which step of the following is correct?
   A. Attach irrigation cone to tubing and fill the bag with 2,000 mL of warm tap water
   B. Hang the irrigation bag from hook at hip level when seated on toilet
   C. Instill the water into the colon over a 15- to 20-minute period
   D. After instillation, close the sleeve and wait up to 45 minutes for complete results

4. A patient calls the WOC nurse with signs and symptoms of an ileostomy blockage. What would the nurse suggest the patient try first to move the blockage forward?
   A. Cut a new skin barrier that is a little smaller than normal to stimulate the stoma.
   B. Take a warm bath to relax the abdominal muscles.
   C. Consume foods high in fiber for a day.
   D. Remain in a knee–chest position for 20 minutes to try to move the blockage.

5. A patient with an ileostomy reports the following symptoms: no stomal output, cramping abdominal pain, nausea, and abdominal distention. The nurse notes no bowel sounds on auscultation and suspects a blockage. After contacting the patient's surgeon or WOC nurse, the ER staff should:
   A. Withhold pain medications until the blockage is confirmed
   B. Start IV antibiotics
   C. Obtain an abdominal x-ray
   D. Force fluids

6. A WOC nurse is performing an ileostomy lavage for a patient with an ileostomy obstruction. Which step in this procedure is performed correctly?
   A. Insert a lubricated, gloved finger into the lumen of the stoma and vigorously break up the blockage.
   B. Attach a colostomy irrigation sleeve to the patient's one-piece pouching system.
   C. Working through the top of the colostomy irrigation sleeve, insert a lubricated soft catheter (#14–16 Fr) into the lumen of the stoma until blockage is reached.
   D. Slowly instill 30 to 50 mL NS into the catheter using a bulb syringe. Remove the catheter and allow for returns into the irrigation sleeve.

7. Which of the following is an osmotic laxative used to soften stool and stimulate peristalsis on a short-term basis?
   A. Magnesium citrate
   B. Dulcolax
   C. Metamucil
   D. Colace

8. The WOC nurse is teaching a patient with an ileostomy how to avoid dehydration due to loss of potassium. Which food would the nurse recommend the patient to include in his or her diet?
   A. Spinach
   B. Dairy products
   C. Apples
   D. Whole grains

9. Which food would the WOC nurse recommend for a patient with a colostomy who is experiencing diarrhea?
   A. Fresh fruits
   B. Potatoes
   C. Leafy vegetables
   D. Cheese

10. A complication of a urinary diversion is:
   A. Hyperchloremic metabolic alkalosis
   B. Vitamin B_{12} deficiency
   C. Kidney failure
   D. Edema

11. A WOC nurse is counseling a patient with a urinary diversion who is taking the medication metronidazole for giardia. What effect of the medication would the nurse describe?
   A. Strong urine odor
   B. Black urine
   C. Red and then brown urine
   D. Greenish-blue urine

ANSWERS: 1.**C**, 2.**C**, 3.**D**, 4.**B**, 5.**C**, 6.**C**, 7.**A**, 8.**A**, 9.**D**, 10.**B**, 11.**C**

CHAPTER 13

Rehabilitation Issues and Special Ostomy Patient Needs

Jane E. Carmel, and Jody Scardillo

OBJECTIVES

1. Identify factors that impact adaptation to an ostomy and implement measures to promote full recovery and adaptation.
2. Assess the needs of special populations and incorporate identified needs into the ostomy plan of care.

Topic Outline

Impact of an Ostomy on Self-Image/Self-Concept

The goals of successful adaptation to an ostomy are to restore or improve the lifestyle the person had before the surgery. This process begins in the period before surgery and continues throughout the postoperative period where the person must learn new self-care techniques and adjust to changes and a lack of control of body functions. Research has shown that some psychological factors related to ostomy adjustment are not disclosed by patients unless asked by the nurse (White, 1998). In the immediate postoperative period, the patient's ability to learn ostomy care is complicated by the need to accept and integrate the fact that the ostomy is present (Sirota, 2006a, 2006b). The WOC nurse can help facilitate transition and adaptation to these changes. Knowledge about self-care is an important factor in adjustment to the ostomy so the WOC nurse can play a pivotal role in patient education. Issues of social isolation, sleep disturbances, sexual dysfunction, and financial concerns have all been identified (Kenderian et al., 2013) in the postoperative period. It is important to discuss the potential for functional problems during preoperative counseling to allow the patient to begin to adjust to the changes and assess for these after surgery to facilitate adaptation.

CLINICAL PEARL

Preoperative appointment with a WOC nurse is very valuable in addressing any fears and anxiety the patient and family may have.

Stages of Adaptation Process

Borwell (2009) defines some milestones of psychological recovery such as beginning to look at and touch the stoma, then allowing others to look at the stoma, expressing interest, asking questions about care, beginning to take responsibility for aspects of stoma care, and finally, socializing with others. Ostomy patients adjust differently, so an individualized plan of care is vital. Gemmill et al. (2010) found that it took from many months to up to 10 years for patients to adjust and accept their urinary diversions.

The ability to adapt and adjust to an ostomy is a significant factor in how well a person can accept these changes in his or her life. Successful adaption is defined by Black (2004) as a return to everyday activities and relationships. Care planning to facilitate adaptation to the ostomy can be guided by the use of a theoretical framework such as the Roy Adaptation Model (Roy, 2009) or Orem's Self-Care Model (Orem et al., 2001). According to Roy, the level of adaptation will affect a person's ability to respond positively or negatively to situations. Roy (2009) described people as adaptive systems with biological and physical processes that are used to adjust effectively to changes in the environment. The two processes for individual coping are the cognator and regulator subsystems, which are integrated life processes that are manifested in a person's behavior. The cognator subsystem include four cognitive–emotive channels of perceptual and information processing, learning, judgment, and emotion (Roy, 2009). According to Roy (2009), the process of adaptation is initiated when input or stimuli from the environment (internal or external) provoke a response in the human system. Three classifications of input or stimuli are identified in this model. The first classification is the focal stimulus or stimuli that are immediately affecting the system. Focal stimuli may be internal or external, and the system is aware of their presence. The contextual stimuli are all other stimuli that contribute to the effect of the focal stimulus, including age, gender, race, education level, insurance coverage, diagnosis, and household living situation. The residual stimuli are unknowns related to the presence of having an ostomy (Roy, 2009). The behaviors that result from the control processes of the regulator–cognator subsystem are observed in four adaptive modes (Roy, 2009) that are the physiologic, self-concept, role function, and interdependence modes. Roy defined the physiologic mode as "the physical and chemical processes involved in the function and activities of living organisms" (p. 89). Elimination is one of five physiologic needs in this mode. According to Roy, physiological integrity or the degree of wholeness attained by adapting to changes in elimination is necessary for individual health and functioning.

Roy (2009) describes the self-concept mode as "the composite of beliefs and feelings held about oneself that is formed from perceptions of others' reactions" (p. 95). It is made up of two subsystems, the physical self and personal self. A person views his or her physical self as a physical being with traits that include bodily appearances, bodily functions, sexuality, healthy states, and illness states. Feelings about the physical self may influence adjustment to having a permanent ostomy, so body image should be assessed.

The ability to engage in self-care activities is reflected in the role function mode (Roy, 2009). How individuals relate with others and the quality of one's support systems constitute the interdependence mode. The level of social engagement was measured to reflect effective or ineffective interdependence mode adjustment.

Orem's theory (2001) consists of three interrelated theories described as self-care theory, self-care deficit theory, and nursing system theory. Self-care theory describes why people act to take care of themselves. This is a learned behavior developed by active participation in self-care. Orem et al. (2001) defines the ability to participate in self-care as self-care agency. The self-care deficit theory defines when nursing is necessary to assist the patient with self-care. This can be determined by a thorough nursing assessment. Nursing systems theory describes the different relationships between the patient and the nurse to meet self-care needs. Orem et al. (2001) describe nursing agency as meeting the self-care needs of the patient while assisting the patient to develop self-care behaviors. Nursing agency occurs in three systems (Orem et al., 2001). The wholly compensatory system occurs when the patient is unable to perform effective self-care activities, so the nurse performs the care. The partly compensatory system occurs when then the patient participates in self-care but cannot meet all self-care demands. In the supportive-education system, the patient is able to perform self-care, so the nurse promotes this.

Orem's theory (2001) uses a three-step nursing process that directs the nurse to use effective interventions to develop effective solutions. Nursing diagnosis and prescription can be determined by assessing the ostomy patient's self-care demands and self-care agency (Martinez, 2005). Design for regulatory operation involves selecting interventions that promote self-care agency and developing a plan to implement these interventions. This includes encouraging the patient to look at the stoma and verbalize concerns about the ostomy (Martinez, 2005). Production and management of nursing systems includes reassessment and modifying interventions as the patient progresses towards self-care.

Factors Affecting Ability to Adapt

There are many factors that impact adaptation to the ostomy. These include the diagnosis that necessitated the ostomy, age, social support, and self-care ability. Bekkers et al. (1996) found that ability to take care of the ostomy using an ostomy pouching system that has a reliable wear time was an important factor in coping and adaptation to the ostomy. Psychosocial needs of ostomy patients can be met by identifying and monitoring those who experience difficulty adjusting to the ostomy and isolating the problem unique to the person (Simmons et al., 2009). The role of religion/spirituality in the ostomy patient's life can be used for support. Li et al. (2012) found that spiritual well-being was associated with psychosocial adjustment to the ostomy.

There are many tools available to measure adjustment to an ostomy. One example is the Ostomy Adjustment Inventory-23 (OAI-23), a 23-item self-report tool that assesses psychosocial adjustment to an ostomy (Simmons et al., 2009). The Ostomy Adjustment Scale (OAS) is a 34-item tool to measure psychological and social adjustment and another example of a way for the WOC nurse to assess adjustment (Olbrisch, 1983).

Self-Esteem/Coping Skills

Persson & Hellstrom (2002) and Williams (2012) found that altered body image was a central theme in adjustment to stoma. Once the initial stress of the surgery and recovery is resolved, body image, physical appearance, and sexuality become greater concerns. Identification of coping skills used for other life stressors may help the patient with a new ostomy apply these skills to adapting to the ostomy. Gemmill et al. (2010) found gender differences in psychological well-being with women having significantly lower scores than did men and found that over 75% of participants had difficulty adjusting to the ostomy. The average participant had undergone surgery 9 years prior to the study concluding that many people have long-term difficulties with ostomy adaptation. They also found that mastering self-care was an important part of adjustment to the ostomy.

Past Experience with Ostomy/Expectations

Identification of previous experiences with ostomy and exploring expectations of the person anticipating ostomy surgery are needed in a baseline assessment. Preoperative counseling should include an assessment of how the disease has affected his or her functional abilities, lifestyle, and sexuality. Negative previous experiences with an ostomy can result in anxiety and fear in the person facing surgery. Exploration of the details of this and education about current management strategies can help allay fears. Anticipation of the change in body function and body image by forward planning allows the ostomy patient to predict the loss and assume a more positive approach that will promote adjustment (Borwell, 2009). The person who has undergone emergency surgery has not had that opportunity prior to surgery, so this should be considered in the postoperative period.

Support Provided by Significant Others

The WOC nurse should discuss the amount of involvement of family or significant others and determine from the patients if this meets their needs. Including significant caregivers in ostomy teaching can ease transition from hospital to home, ease fears, and facilitate adaptation for the patient with a new ostomy.

Assistance Provided by Health Care Team/WOC Nurse

The WOC nurse and the multidisciplinary team including the surgeon, dietician, nursing, and discharge planners collaborate with the patient to provide education, psychosocial support, physical care, management of complications, and long-term follow-up.

Impact of Ostomy Visitor

The support of an ostomy visitor can be invaluable to the patient undergoing a new ostomy procedure. Ostomy visitors are former patients who have an ostomy and have received specialized training, so they can assist the patient's transition to living with an ostomy, and share experiences, although this should not substitute for professional medical advice in any way. Many take advantage of online resources for support and education (see Appendix B).

Ostomy support groups can enhance recovery from surgery and promote adaptation by providing an atmosphere of acceptance and mutual respect and helping to develop coping skills to manage day-to-day life with an ostomy. These groups provide peer support and role modeling for people with ostomies. Many WOC nurses facilitate ostomy support groups. The WOC nurse also can encourage patient participation in these groups as they follow the patient through his or her pre- and postoperative course (Cross & Hottenstein, 2010).

> **CLINICAL PEARL**
>
> The WOC nurse should provide support and be a resource for the Ostomy support group.

Age/Developmental Stage

Knowledge about the lifespan, developmental stage, and basic human characteristics assist the nurse to make an accurate assessment of the individual's psychosocial needs (Sirota, 2006a, 2006b). An adolescent with a new ostomy will have different challenges than an adult in a stable married relationship in terms of sexuality, body image, and socialization (Sirota, 2006a, 2006b). Nursing care must be individualized to the person's situation for best results. The psychosocial phase of adolescence is described by Erickson as identity versus role confusion where altered body image and appearance are the focus. They may also fear loss of sexual function and inability to have a normal relationship (Junkin & Beitz, 2005). The WOC nurse must ensure privacy for the patient, and consider using a low-profile appliance to ensure that the appliance is concealed under clothing. Elastic-type support garments are available to secure the ostomy system. Facilitating an ostomy visitor who is the same age is often beneficial.

For the young adult, intimacy versus isolation is the focus of this phase. The ostomy patient may fear rejection or commitment at the time when long-term relationships may develop. Support of the patient by family and significant others can facilitate adaptation. Educating and including the significant other can allay fears of both partners. Partners sometimes have fears of hurting the patient or the stoma that can be allayed with open communication.

The focus of the middle-aged adult in Erickson's model is generativity versus stagnation. Fears of loss of occupation or spouse and role changes dominate this phase. Assessment of job role and how care of ostomy will impact this are important in the preoperative phase. Does the patient travel? Is heavy lifting required? What are the bathroom facilities like in the work setting? These discussions will help the patient and nurse determine individualized management strategies to ease the transition back to work.

For the older adult, integrity versus despair is the phase. At this stage, loss of spouse and independence, loneliness, and change in living environment are the primary concerns. Physiologic and psychological changes related to the ostomy are compounded by other medical problems. Maintaining a positive attitude, continuing the usual daily routine, and not allowing the ostomy to interfere with normal life are helpful in the elder (Reynaud & Meekder, 2002). Brief frequent teaching sessions with small amounts of information work well for the elder. Assessing and modifying care for the ostomy patient are important for adaptation. Does the patient have arthritis or other conditions affecting mobility? Are vision and memory adequate for self-care? (See Chapter 12).

CLINICAL PEARL

It is important to include another family member during the teaching sessions.

Sexual Function

Potential Impact of Pelvic Dissection on Sexual Function

Pelvic surgery, cancer, and radiation therapy can have a short- or long-term impact on sexual health (Junkin & Beitz, 2005). Men can develop erectile dysfunction, retrograde ejaculation, and loss of libido, while women can experience loss of desire, dyspareunia, and vaginal dryness (Majid & Kingsnorth, 2002) after ostomy surgery. The shape and angle of the vaginal vault change when the rectum is removed. Erectile dysfunction can be temporary or permanent. Men with urinary diversions have a high rate of erectile dysfunction. Pelvic radiation may also cause symptoms of vaginal stenosis and dryness. Vaginal lubricants are helpful for some women as is experimentation with different positions to determine which is most comfortable.

The WOC nurse should reassure the patient that giving and receiving sexual pleasure can continue to be a part of his or her life, even if different because of bodily changes after ostomy surgery (Junkin & Beitz, 2005).

Potential Impact of the Ostomy on Body Image/Sexual Relationships

Persson & Hellstrom (2002) found that altered body image was a central theme in adjustment to stoma.

Concerns about appearance of the stoma and ostomy system, odor, noise, potential for leakage, and fear of abandonment may occur, often after the acute fear of surviving the illness (Lamb, 1990). Careful assessment, guidance, validation of experiences, education about disease and impact on sexual health, and referrals when indicated form the basis of the WOC nurse role in this area of care (Junkin & Beitz, 2005). A baseline preoperative assessment of sexual functioning will assist the WOC nurse to identify postoperative concerns. Basic suggestions for managing sexual relations should be given to the patient and partner including being prepared for sexual activity by having a clean, secure, and empty pouching system and maintaining open and clear communication between partners (Junkin & Beitz, 2005).

The stoma should never be used for sexual purposes. Firm objects may damage the bowel or mucocutaneous junction, cause bleeding, and cause possible scarring and constriction since the bowel does not distend like the rectum. Stimulation of the stoma will not produce the pleasurable response that may be experienced with stimulation of the anal area as the stoma is not an erogenous area.

PLISSIT Counseling Model

Permission, Understanding-Limited Information, Specific Suggestions, Intensive Therapy (PLISSIT) (Anon, 1976) provides four levels of response to issues with sexual health and encourages the nurse to intervene at the level he or she is most comfortable with. WOC nurses should be able to function at permission and limited information stage (Junkin & Beitz, 2005). It is important for the WOC nurse to be aware of his or her own personal attitudes and values toward sexuality in order to identify sexual health needs in their patients (Ayaz, 2009; Junkin & Beitz, 2005). Understanding anatomy and physiology of male and female reproductive system and nervous system function will help to teach patients about bodily changes.

The permission stage is a beginning exploratory phase that helps the person acknowledge that he or she needs assistance to discuss sex. Active listening and sensitivity are needed to assist the patient to express concerns or questions (Borwell, 2009). The use of open-ended questions, such as asking how the ostomy has affected relationship with the partner or what kind of changes the patient has experienced in his or her sexual life will encourage the patient to discuss and ask questions (Ayaz, 2009). It is important to instruct the patient that other ostomy patients may have the same problems they are experiencing.

The understanding-limited information phase allows the nurse to assess if there are any difficulties and if a referral to a WOC nurse is required. A sexual history, identification of problems and goals, and expectations of the patient should be identified so an action plan can be developed (Borwell, 2009). Interventions at this level are geared toward increasing the patient's knowledge level in areas such as treatment side effects, emotional changes, and sexuality (Ayaz, 2009).

The WOC nurse can provide reassurance in the specific suggestion phase. Written information on sexuality can be provided. The United Ostomy Associations of America (UOAA) has many resources including Intimacy after Ostomy Surgery, Sex and the Male Ostomate, Sex and the Female Ostomate, and Sex and the single ostomate available on their Web site www.ostomy.org.

Pouch covers, minipouches, and specialized underwear are available. Internet search or ostomy supply catalogs have many options for undergarments to meet personal preferences. Experimentation with different positions may help if there is discomfort during intercourse.

The intensive therapy stage usually involves WOC nurse involvement to address possible psychological, interpersonal, or physical needs. The WOC nurse should be aware of appropriate resources and refer as needed (Anon, 1976).

CLINICAL PEARL

The WOC nurse should take time to ask and answer any sexual concern the patient may have.

Special Considerations/Needs

Pregnancy

Women with a fecal or urinary diversion can become pregnant and have a normal pregnancy. The female patient who has had an ileostomy may be advised to wait a year after surgery to consider becoming pregnant. Many women with an ileostomy have successful pregnancy delivered by vaginal route.

Management of the ostomy during pregnancy must take into consideration the changing abdominal contour and stoma dimensions. The WOC nurse should be available to assess and recommend changes in ostomy system during the person's pregnancy (Seligman et al., 2011). As the abdomen increases in size, it becomes harder for the person to see the stoma. A partner may need to be taught to assist with ostomy care when the person cannot manage stoma care. Stoma prolapse is another possible complication with the changing body contour.

Medications prescribed during pregnancy, that is, iron can change the color of the stool or urine. The patient should be informed of this potential discoloration and that there is no harm related to this.

Most females who have ulcerative colitis are in the childbearing age and are concerned when having an ileal pouch anal anastomosis (IPAA) whether they can have a safe pregnancy. As the fetus develops, the woman may experience perianal irritation, frequency and urgency, and nocturnal incontinence (Perry-Woodford, 2008). Some of the literature differs on recommendation of vaginal or cesarean delivery. Some surgeons recommend a cesarean section in order to avoid risk of injury to the anal sphincter; however, there is little evidence to support this practice. Studies have found that vaginal delivery appears as safe as cesarean delivery for most females with IPAA. However, there is limited information on long-term function of the pouch in women who have had vaginal deliveries.

Contraception

Women with ileostomy should be advised that most contraceptive pills are absorbed in the duodenum, so a person with an ileostomy or IPAA should have no problems with absorption (Borwell & Breckam, 2005). It is good practice to advise the patient to check with her pharmacist.

Morbid Obesity

The care of the obese patient having ostomy surgery presents a challenge both pre- and postoperatively.

Preoperative stoma siting is a challenge to identify an optimal location for the stoma with the goal of the patient being independent in his or her ostomy care. The ideal site recommended is the upper abdomen above the umbilicus as the patient cannot see his or her lower abdomen. Also the upper abdomen is thinner above the umbilicus making it easier for the surgeon to create a well-vascularized stoma. The surgeon may request that the site be marked at both above and below the umbilicus (Beck, 2011).

Postoperatively, the obese person is at higher risk for complications: mucocutaneous separation, parastomal hernia, stoma retraction, and prolapse (Beck, 2011). Colwell (2014) found that the data were inconsistent on the impact obesity has on surgical risks.

The WOC nurse should be sensitive to the patient's needs when assessing and teaching the obese person. Time must be taken in having the patient find the best position when performing ostomy care. A floor-length mirror on the back of the bathroom door may work well for the patient at home. The WOC nurse in home care has the advantage of assessing the patient's bathroom to make practical suggestions.

End of Life

One of the goals for a person with a fecal and or urinary diversion is to be independent in his or her ostomy care. However, if the patient's conditions changes due to terminal condition or dementia, the WOC nurse will need to help identify a responsible person who can take over the ostomy care when the patient is no longer able to physically manage his or her care. The person with dementia will demonstrate a loss of memory and cognitive and functional skills by not knowing when and how to empty his or her pouch. The role of the WOC nurse is to develop and teach the caregiver the skills for ostomy care that will not overwhelm him or her by providing simple and clear instructions.

Progressive diseases such as Parkinson's, ALS, multiple sclerosis, and dementia will gradually cause functional impairment and lessening cognitive skills. Motor, sensory, and vision can become impaired resulting in the patient needing assistance in his or her ostomy care.

As the patient's condition deteriorates, there may be weight loss that will change the abdominal plane and stoma. The occurrence of tumors and fungating wounds can create a challenge to provide an ostomy pouching system with a good seal. Where needed, the WOC nurse will need to measure the stoma and recommend a new pouching system that will fit better. Catheterization schedules may need to be adjusted in the person with a continent diversion. In the case of abdominal ascites, the ostomy system will also need to be reevaluated for a different system.

The person with end-stage cancer may encounter metastasis to the liver that can result in peristomal varices. With this condition, the caregivers will need to be aware of the risk of bleeding and how to manage it (see Chapter 15). A two-piece system should not be used that would cause pressure on the varices. The patient or caregiver should be instructed to remove the system very gently to avoid trauma. A liquid skin barrier wipe can be used to provide added protection.

Obstruction and constipation may occur related to the disease process, and the caregiver needs to be aware of these conditions and when to call for help.

Many strategies can be implemented to provide a simple procedure for the caregivers to follow: moldable barriers, precut barriers, close end and/or Velcro pouch closure. The person with ileal conduit or high-output ileostomy can be managed with connecting the pouch to a larger capacity drainage system that will not require frequent emptying of the pouch. Indwelling catheters may need to be considered in the person unable to self-catheterize.

Cognitive Deficits

Cognitive changes are usually associated with the older adult. The WOC nurse when teaching the older person needs to allow more time for the patient to process and understand the information. The degree of memory impairment should be assessed and the patient's teaching plan tailored to meet his or her needs. It may be necessary to involve a family member. Written material along with prompts should be given to the patient to review at home (Falvo, 2011).

Psychomotor assessment should be conducted before starting ostomy teaching. This would include motor coordination, muscle strength, energy level, and sensory acuity. There may be cognitive changes associated with aging that may affect the speed at which the person can process the information, working memory, and recall.

The person with learning disabilities will need to have short teaching sessions involving repeating and reinforcing the tasks to learn and demonstrate. It is important to set short-term goals and respect the uniqueness of each individual.

The severely mentally ill person may benefit from using the Makaton signs and symbols as a form of communication. This form of communication uses pictures, signs and symbols, real objectives, photographs, and written word (Black & Hyde, 2004). This teaching option is also used in young children. The pictures and symbols are placed on a large ring for the child to use for communication. With the adult, a scrapbook is more appropriate. Many times, recreational therapy or physical therapy departments are excellent resources for teaching repetitive, physical tasks.

Chemotherapy and Radiation Therapy

Fecal and/or urinary diversion surgery for cancer of colon and/or bladder may not be the only necessary form of treatment. The patient may need to receive chemotherapy and/or radiation therapy, sometimes preoperatively as well as postoperative. It is important that the WOC nurse understands the effects that chemotherapy and/or radiation therapy can have on a patient with a diversion.

Treatment for cancer is classified as:

- Primary—the main treatment
- Neoadjuvant—given before surgery
- Adjuvant—treatment given after surgery aimed at any remaining cancer cells
- Palliative—treatment aimed at limiting effects of disease, where cure cannot be achieved (McGrath & Fulham, 2005)

Chemotherapy

Common side effects associated with chemotherapy are diarrhea, nausea and vomiting, mucositis, anemia, peripheral neuropathy, and palmar–plantar syndrome known as "hand and foot syndrome." The patient with a fecal diversion undergoing chemotherapy will need to be taught to expect changes in his or her bowel output. The WOC nurse will need to advise patients on the possibility of changing their current pouch system to another one to manage diarrhea in order to avoid risk of leakage and peristomal skin problems. A person who has been using a closed-ended pouch will need to change to a drainable pouch, and the pouch will need to be emptied more often. If the colostomy is being managed with irrigation procedure, the patient needs to be advised to wear a pouch system and may have to discontinue irrigation during chemo and radiation therapy. Stoma edema may occur, and the pouch opening will need to accommodate this change.

The person with an ileostomy is at high risk for dehydration from the side effects of nausea, vomiting, and diarrhea. He or she will need to be taught to maintain adequate fluid and food intake. High-calorie, high-protein, low-residue foods should be encouraged, and high-fiber and fatty foods avoided while experiencing diarrhea (McGrath & Fulham, 2005).

Medications may be recommended to manage diarrhea, nausea, and vomiting. The person may find that he or she cannot tolerate his or her normal diet and may have difficulty in maintaining an adequate nutrition and hydration. Antiemetic should be given before the chemotherapy begins.

Oxaliplatin, chemotherapy agent for colorectal cancer, can have a side effect of peripheral neuropathy (numbness in hands and feet). Hand and foot syndrome is a side effect of 5-fluorouracil (chemotherapy agent for colorectal cancer). Manual dexterity can be affected by both these side effects, and the person with a stoma may have difficulty changing and emptying the pouch. The WOC nurse will need to recommend another pouch system the patient can manage better or teach a caregiver to assist the patient in his or her care.

Hamza et al. (2014) studied side effects of oxaliplatin with fluorouracil and leucovorin (FOLFOX) in patients aged 70 years and older compared to patients <70 years of age. The results were no difference in the groups related to tolerance of the toxicity of this regimen.

Mucositis/Stomatitis

Stomatitis can occur with both chemo and radiation therapy. Stomatitis is defined as inflammation of the mucous lining. The patient needs to be taught to practice gentle care of the stoma, as edema and friability of stoma can be common. Patients undergoing chemotherapy and radiation therapy need to also have assessment of their mouth. Oral hygiene is very important. The patient needs to be taught to use a soft toothbrush and antibacterial mouthwash and practice good oral hygiene. Foods that are bland and softer in consistency may be tolerated better with chemotherapy agents commonly used for bowel and bladder cancer (Table 13-1).

Radiation Therapy

Common side effects associated with radiation therapy are fatigue and skin damage. Skin damage is classified as erythema, dry desquamation, moist desquamation, and necrosis (rarely occurs).

The patient needs to be taught not to use any creams or lotions for 2 hours before treatment. Moisturizing creams containing lanolin, alcohol, or petroleum-based creams should be avoided. Radiation treatments may need to be temporarily discontinued if marked stoma friability occurs (Doughty, 2005). Ostomy irrigation should be discontinued during radiation therapy to avoid potential mechanical irritation to intestinal and stoma mucosa (Turnbull, 2007a, 2007b).

Physical and Mental Limitations

Preoperatively, the WOC nurse should assess the patient and his or her level of understanding about his or her surgery and any physical and mental limitations. The WOC nurse needs expertise and patience in understanding of physical, psychosocial, and emotional needs of this population. Assessment of the person who has some challenges may require some innovative techniques to promote optimal ostomy care. The WOC nurse may have to seek other resources to meet their needs.

Visually Impaired

People with limited to total vision loss are still capable of becoming independent in their ostomy care. Legally blind is defined as a person who cannot read one letter on 20/100 line. Most people who are legally blind can see shadows and shapes. However, there is limited literature on ostomy education for the patient visually impaired.

A two-piece system is usually better for managing to apply the barrier to the stoma. Some creative techniques have been developed over the years to assist teaching the person who is visually impaired.

Whiteley (2013) describe a method for ileostomy using a 30-mL syringe barrel (slightly smaller than the stoma), the barrel could be filled with cotton balls if the stoma was active. The syringe barrel is placed over the stoma to maintain a clean, dry peristomal skin, while the barrier is

TABLE 13-1 Chemotherapy Agents for Bladder and Colon Cancer*

Agent	Indication	Adverse Effects
5-Fluorouracil	Colorectal cancer	Diarrhea, photosensitivity, palmar–plantar erythrodysesthesia, alopecia
Irinotecan	Colon cancer	Diarrhea, early onset, neutropenia, alopecia
Oxaliplatin	Colon cancer	Diarrhea, peripheral neuropathy
Mitomycin C	Colon, rectal, and bladder cancer	Fatigue, decreased white blood cells and platelet count, hair loss
Doxorubicin	Bladder cancer	Discolored or red urine, nausea and vomiting, loss of appetite, alopecia
Cisplatin	Bladder cancer	Nausea and vomiting, decrease in WBC and platelet count, bleeding, peripheral neuropathy
Capecitabine	Colon cancer	Stomach pain, loss of appetite, fatigue, dizziness
FOLFOX (fluorouracil, oxaliplatin, leucovorin)	Stage III colon cancer Stronger therapy with more side effects	Fatigue, nausea and vomiting, diarrhea, neurotoxicity especially to cold, neuropathy, low RBC

*Not an all-inclusive list.

placed over the syringe barrel and adhered to the skin. This method can be used for both ileal conduit and colostomy.

Heale (2013) developed a cardboard tube technique for ostomy wafer placement for a stoma with persistent output (ileal conduit, ileostomy). This technique would also be appropriate for a visually impaired person. For a stoma that measured 1 inch, a 5 × 9 cm index card was used to make the tube. The card was wrapped around stoma and secured with tape. Both of these techniques would allow time to treat any peristomal skin conditions. This would also act as a guide to place the barrier for the visually impaired person. However, these techniques can be a challenge for the person with peripheral neuropathy. When developing a teaching plan for the visually impaired, it is important to have all sessions taught by the same WOC nurse and consistently taught exactly the same way.

CLINICAL PEARL

The WOC nurse should consider consulting with an Occupational Therapist in providing techniques to facilitate ostomy management skills.

Hearing Deficit

There are several levels of hearing loss. A person can be born deaf or may start losing his or her hearing after the age of 60. Some people may acquire a hearing aid while others choose not to have an aid. The person who is born deaf may either use sign language or lip reading. The WOC nurse needs to be aware of the persons' preference for communicating.

Some facilities may have a sign language interpreter that can be arranged when the WOC nurse is teaching ostomy care. Another communication method available at some facilities is a live video service with sign language interpreters, called MARTTI, which stands for My Accessible Real-Time Trusted Interpreter (Sattinger, 2007). This on-demand video interpreting service is not only for the deaf or hard of hearing person but also for the person who has English as his or her second language. Over 150 languages are provided.

Cultural Diversity

The ostomy nurse needs to recognize different beliefs, values, and health care practices of different cultures in order to provide appropriate care for people from many multicultural backgrounds. Culture plays an important role in psychosocial adjustment (Sirota, 2006a, 2006b). In Jewish, Muslim, Hindu, and certain other orthodox Christian religions, an intact body and cleanliness are a requirement to perform obligatory religious rituals. It is not unusual for people from these backgrounds to initially refuse stoma surgery even when dispensations have been granted (Blackley, 1998).

Altuntas et al. (2013) conducted a prospective study to analyze the effects of Ramadan fasting on people with a fecal stoma. Ramadan fasting is an Islamic ritual where they fast from sunrise to sunset for 30 days; this occurs in 9th month of the Islamic calendar. Fasting can last up to 18 hours, with no food or drink. Altuntas et al. studied the effects of fasting on nutritional, metabolic status, and quality of life on people with ileostomy and colostomy. Fasting did decrease prealbumin levels, but there was no influence on quality of life. Some noted improvement in flatulence and fecal incontinence during this time period. Results of this study recommend that the decision to fast should be the patient's and the patient should not be prohibited from fasting but close follow-up may be necessary.

Some cultures and religious beliefs may view bodily excretions as polluting them and would not be willing to participate in ostomy care. The Muslim and South Asian cultures view the left hand for cleaning and hygiene and the right hand for eating and touching things (McGrath & Fulham, 2005). Only using the left hand to change the pouching system would be very difficult, and it can be suggested that they wear gloves when changing the pouch (WCET International Ostomy Guideline, 2014). The WOC nurse helps the patient understand ostomy care preoperatively in order to identify any cultural practices that would interfere with adjusting to this change in his or her life.

CLINICAL PEARL

It is important to ask the patient and family about cultural practices and potential impact on ostomy care so that an effective culturally sensitive plan of care is developed.

Effective communication is needed for the non–English speaking patient, or the patient will feel frustrated, angry, and isolated. Selecting a translator is important; family members should not be interpreters. Skilled interpreters are usually available through organizations or arrangements within the health care setting. Some ostomy manufacturers provide education materials in languages other than English on their Web sites and upon request.

The World Council of Enterostomal Therapists (WCET) International Ostomy Guidelines (2014) cites 10 countries with description of cultural and religious belief that can impact ostomy care and adjustment. Vegetarian diets used in the Hindu and Sikh religion can affect stoma output; there may be increase in output and flatus, so the patient should be advised of this effect.

Conclusions

Management of the ostomy patient includes ongoing assessment and teaching with the main goal of the patient becoming independent in his or her ostomy care. Factors such as adjustment, depression, anxiety, sleep difficulties, return to activities of daily living, and sexuality are major issues for the person. The WOC nurse needs to be aware of resources available in order to provide the person with different teaching and communication options to meet individual needs. Care needs to be individualized in those with special needs to promote adaptation and good quality of life. All patients deserve the best quality of life possible.

REFERENCES

Altuntas, Y. E., Gezen, F. C., Sahoniz, T., et al. (2013). Ramadan fasting in patients with a stoma: A prospective study of quality of life and nutritional structure. *Ostomy Wound Management, 29*(5), 26–32.

Anon, J. S. (1976). The PLISSIT model: A proposed conceptual scheme for the behavioral treatment of sexual problems. *Journal of Sex Education Therapy, 2*(2), 1–15.

Ayaz, S. (2009). Approach to sexual problems of patients with stoma by PLISSIT model: An alternative. *Sexual Disability, 27*, 72–81.

Beck, S. (2011). Stoma issues in the obese patient. *Clinics in Colon and Rectal Surgery, 24*(4), 259–262.

Bekkers, M. J., Van Knippenberg, F. C., Van Den Borned, H. W., et al. (1996). Prospective evaluation of psychosocial adaptation to stoma surgery: The role of self-efficacy. *Psychosomatic Medicine, 58*(2), 183–191.

Black, P. (2000). *Holistic stoma care*. Edinburg, TX: Balladeer Tindall.

Black, P. K. (2004). Psychological, sexual and cultural issues for patients with a stoma. *British Journal of Nursing, 13*(12), 692–697.

Black, P., & Hyde, C. (2004). Caring for people with a learning disability, colorectal cancer and stoma. *British Journal of Nursing, 13*(16), 970–975.

Blackley, P. (1998). *Practical stoma wound and continence management*. Australia: Research Publications Pty Ltd.

Borwell, B. (2009). Rehabilitation and stoma care: Addressing the psychological needs. *British Journal of Nursing, 18*(4), S20–S25.

Borwell, B., & Breckam, B. (2005). Specific aspects of care for patients with ileostomies and colostomies. In B. Breckman (Ed.), *Stoma care and rehabilitation* (pp. 69–91). Edinburg, TX: Elsevier.

Colwell, J. (2014). The role of obesity in the patient undergoing colorectal surgery and fecal diversion: A review of the literature. *Ostomy Wound Management, 60*(1), 24–28.

Cross, H., & Hottenstein, P. (2010). Starting and maintaining a hospital-based support group. *Journal of Wound Ostomy Continence Nursing, 37*(4), 393–396.

Doughty, D. (2005). Principles of ostomy management in the oncology patient. *Supportive Oncology, 3*(1), 59–69.

Falvo, D. (2011). *Effective patient education* (4th ed.). Sudbury: Jones and Bartlett.

Gemmill, R., Sun, V., Ferrell, B., et al. (2010). Going with the flow quality of life outcomes of cancer survivors with urinary diversion. *Journal of Wound Ostomy Continence Nursing, 37*(1), 65–72.

Hamza, S., Bouvier, A. M., Rollot, F., et al. (2014). Toxicity of oxaliplatin plus fluorouracil/leucovorin adjuvant chemotherapy in elderly patients with stage III colon cancer: A population-based study. *Annals of Surgical Oncology, 21*(8), 2636–2641.

Heale, M. (2013). Cardboard tube technique for ostomy wafer placement and management of peristomal skin with persistent output. *Journal of Wound Ostomy Continence Nursing, 40*(4), 424–426.

Junkin, J., & Beitz, J. (2005). Sexuality and the person with a stoma implications for comprehensive WOC nursing practice. *Journal of Wound Ostomy Continence Nursing, 32*(2), 121–128.

Kenderian, S., Stephens, E. K., & Jatoi, A. (2013). Ostomies in rectal cancer patients: What is their psychosocial impact? *European Journal of Cancer Care, 23*, 328–332.

Lamb, M. A. (1990). Psychosexual issues: The woman with gynecological cancer. *Seminars in Oncology Nursing, 6*, 237–243.

Li, C., Rew, L., & Hwang, S. (2012). The relationship between spiritual well-being and psychosocial adjustment in Taiwanese patients with colorectal cancer and a colostomy. *Journal of Wound Ostomy Continence Nursing, 39*(2), 161–169.

Majid, A., & Kingsnorth, A. (Eds.) (2002). *Advanced surgical practice*. London, UK: Greenwich Medical Media.

Martinez, L. (2005). Self-care for stoma surgery: Mastering independent stoma self-care skills in an elderly woman. *Nursing Science Quarterly, 18*(1), 66–69.

McGrath, A., & Fulham J. (2005). Understanding chemotherapy and radiotherapy for a person with a stoma. In T. Porrett & A. McGrath (Eds.), *Stoma care*. Oxford, UK: Blackwell.

Olbrisch, M. E. (1983). Development and validation of the ostomy adjustment scale. *Rehabilitation Psychology, 28*(1), 3–12.

Orem, D., Taylor, S., & McLaughlin, K. (2001). *Nursing concepts of practice* (5th ed.). St Louis, MO: Mosby Year Book.

Persson, E., & Hellström, A. L. (2002). Experiences of Swedish men and women 6 to 12 weeks after ostomy surgery. *Journal of Wound Ostomy Continence Nursing, 29*, 103–108.

Perry-Woodford, Z. (2008). Intestinal pouches. In J. Burch (Ed.), *Stoma care* (pp. 149–150). West Suffix: John Wiley & Sons Ltd.

Reynaud, S. N., & Meekder, B. J. (2002). Coping styles of older adults with ostomies. *Journal of Gerontological Nursing, 28*(5), 30–36.

Roy, C. (2009). *The Roy adaptation model* (3rd ed.). Stamford, CT: Appleton & Lange.

Sattinger, A. (2007, November). Video interpreters help hospitals, patient connect. *The Hospitalist*.

Seligman, N. S., Sbar, W., & Berghella, V. (2011). Pouch function and gastrointestinal complications during pregnancy after ileal pouch-anal anastomosis. *Journal of Maternal-Fetal and Neonatal Medicine, 24*(3), 525–530.

Simmons, K. L., Smith, J., & Maekawa, A. (2009). Development and psychometric evaluation of the ostomy adjustment inventory-23. *Journal of Wound Ostomy Continence Nursing, 36*(1), 69–75.

Sirota, T. (2006a). Meeting the psychosocial need of ostomy patients through therapeutic interaction. *World Council of Enterostomal Therapist Journal, 26*(1), 26–31.

Sirota, T. (2006b). Meeting the psychosocial needs of ostomy patients through therapeutic interaction. Part II: Effective uses of nurses' professional competencies. *World Council of Enterostomal Therapist Journal, 26*(2), 5–15.

Turnbull, G. (2007a). Ostomy care and radiation therapy. *Ostomy Wound Management, 53*(11), 24–26.

Turnbull, G. (2007b). Special consideration for patients in a wheelchair. *Ostomy Wound Management, 53*(6), 8 & 10.

White, C. (1998). Psychological management of stoma related concerns. *Nursing Standard, 12*(36), 35–38.

Whiteley, I. (2013). Educating a blind person with ileostomy; enabling self-care and independence. *Journal of Stomal Therapy Australia, 33*(3), 6–10.

Williams, J. (2012). Stoma care: Intimacy and body image issues. *Practice Nursing, 23*(2), 91–93.

World Council of Enterostomal Therapists. (2014). In K. Zulkowski, E. A. Ayello, & D. Stelton (Eds.), *WCET international ostomy guideline*. Perth, Australia: WCET.

QUESTIONS

1. According to Roy's Adaptation Model, an example of focal stimuli is:
A. The stoma itself
B. The person's age
C. The person's gender
D. Insurance coverage

2. A WOC nurse observes a patient's return demonstration of changing the pouching system on a newly created fecal stoma. According to Roy's Adaptation Model, which adaptation mode is this nurse assessing?
A. Physiologic mode
B. Self-concept mode
C. Role function mode
D. Interdependence mode

3. A WOC nurse is needed to assist a patient with ostomy care. This is an example of which of Orem's care theories?
A. Self-care theory
B. Self-care deficit theory
C. Nursing system's theory
D. Self-care agency

4. A patient is able to assist the WOC nurse with ostomy care but cannot perform the procedure independently. Which of Orem's Nursing Agency systems has this patient displayed?
A. Wholly compensatory system
B. Partly compensatory system
C. Supportive-education system
D. Regulatory operation system

5. What psychosocial nursing diagnosis would the WOC nurse find as a common theme in patients' adjustment to stoma?
A. Altered body image
B. Impaired skin integrity
C. Risk for infection
D. Spiritual distress

6. Which strategy for teaching a patient about a new stoma would the WOC nurse find most appropriate for a teenager?
A. Teach the parents or guardian the procedure first.
B. Discuss any limitations in activities or work.
C. Use brief, frequent teaching sessions with small amounts of information.
D. Ensure privacy, and use a low-profile appliance.

7. A WOC nurse is using the PLISSIT model to counsel patients with new ostomies. Which level of response to issues with sexual health would be appropriate for this nurse?
A. Permission and specific suggestions
B. Permission and understanding-limited information
C. Understanding-limited information and specific suggestions
D. Specific suggestion and intensive therapy

8. A patient with colon cancer is receiving chemotherapy as a neoadjuvant treatment. The WOC nurse explains to the patient that this treatment is:
A. The primary treatment for the cancer
B. The treatment given after surgery to eradicate remaining cancer cells
C. The treatment given before surgery
D. The treatment aimed at limiting effects of a cancer than cannot be cured

9. The WOC nurse is caring for a patient who is receiving mitomycin C for rectal cancer. For which common side effects should the nurse alert the patient?
A. Fatigue, decreased white blood cells and platelet count, hair loss
B. Diarrhea, photosensitivity, palmar-plantar erythrodysesthesia, alopecia
C. Stomach pain, loss of appetite, fatigue, dizziness
D. Discolor urine red, nausea & vomiting, loss of appetite, alopecia

10. A WOC nurse is counseling patients with special needs who have new ostomies. Which statement reflects an appropriate teaching point for this population?
A. People with total vision loss are not capable of independent ostomy care.
B. Fasting for Ramadan should be discouraged for people with ostomies.
C. Postoperatively the obese person is at higher risk for complications.
D. Women with ileostomy should not use oral contraceptives for birth control.

ANSWERS: 1.**A**, 2.**C**, 3.**B**, 4.**B**, 5.**A**, 6.**D**, 7.**B**, 8.**C**, 9.**A**, 10.**C**

CHAPTER 14

Assessment and Management of the Pediatric Patient

Kimberly McIltrot

OBJECTIVE

Describe the assessment and management of the pediatric and neonatal patient undergoing fecal and/or urinary diversions.

Topic Outline

Pathology and Management Conditions
- Duodenal Atresia and Stenosis
- Jejunoileal Atresia and Stenosis
- Colonic Atresia
- Malrotation and Volvulus
- Anorectal Malformations
- Necrotizing Enterocolitis
- Hirschsprung's Disease
- Meconium Ileus
- Inflammatory Bowel Disease
- Crohn Disease
- Ulcerative Colitis
- Familial Polyposis Syndromes
- Pediatric Trauma

Management of Fecal Diversions
- Techniques and Indications for Pediatric Pouching
- Refeeding Ostomy Output

Pathology and Management Conditions Leading to Urinary Diversion
- Prune Belly Syndrome
- Myelomeningocele

Construction and Management of Pediatric Urinary Diversions
- Vesicostomy
- Ileovesicostomy

Rehabilitative Issues
- Support and Education for the Child and Family
- Developmental Phase and Implications for Care and Education (Age Specific)
  - Premature Infant/Full-Term Infant
  - Toddler (12 Months to 3 Years) and Preschool (3 to 5 Years)
  - School age (6 to 12 Years)
  - Adolescent (13 to 18 Years)

Conclusions

It is important for the wound, ostomy, and continence nurse (WOC Nurse) to understand the assessment and management of the neonatal and pediatric patient who may undergo surgery for fecal and urinary diversion to assist in decreasing the morbidity and mortality of these often-fragile patients. More than one half of all stomas are placed in the neonatal period and another one fourth in infants younger than 1 year of age (Gauderer, 2012). There has been a decrease in the number of pediatric ostomies created over the past several decades, and the ostomies in childhood are usually not permanent. With "improved surgical approaches and perioperative care, pediatric surgeons were able to safely perform more single-stage procedures, thereby decreasing the need for preliminary decompressing ileostomies and colostomies" (Gauderer, 2012).

Most decompressing intestinal stomas in the pediatric age group are temporary, and after correcting the underlying problem, the diverting stoma is taken down (Gauderer, 2012). Ileostomies are essential in management of neonates with distal intestinal obstruction such as

Hirschsprung's disease (HD), complex meconium ileus (MI), bowel atresias, necrotizing enterocolitis (NEC), and inflammatory bowel disease (IBD) (Gauderer, 2012). Colostomies are stomas of the large bowel and are usually created in congenital hindgut pathologies, such as HD, pelvic malformations, colonic atresia, and severe perineal traumas and burns. Colostomies are common in the adult population where colorectal cancer is the most common indication; however, colostomies are rarely permanent in children (Gauderer, 2012). Urostomies are externalized ileum or colon used as conduits to a urinary system and are less common today with catheterizable stomas. In children, the appendix is often mobilized and used as a catheterizable stoma to the urinary bladder (Gauderer, 2012).

Pathology and Management Conditions

Duodenal Atresia and Stenosis

The most common cause of neonatal intestinal obstruction is duodenal atresia or stenosis, an absence or narrowing of the lumen. This is thought to be caused by a failure of recanalization during the development of the duodenum at 10 weeks of gestation. The duodenal obstructions are classified as atresias (complete obstruction) or stenosis (incomplete obstruction due to web or diaphragm). Atresias are then classified into three types: types I (most common), II, and III (**Fig. 14-1**).

Incidence

The incidence of intestinal atresia is 1 in 6,000 to 10,000 births. No genetic predisposition has been found; however, it is reported among siblings and generations of families. There is an association with trisomy 21 in one third of the patients. Due to early prenatal detection of trisomy 21, and subsequent pregnancy terminations, there has been a decrease in duodenal atresia. Half of the children born with duodenal atresia or stenosis have a congenital anomaly of another organ system (Applebaum & Sydorak, 2012).

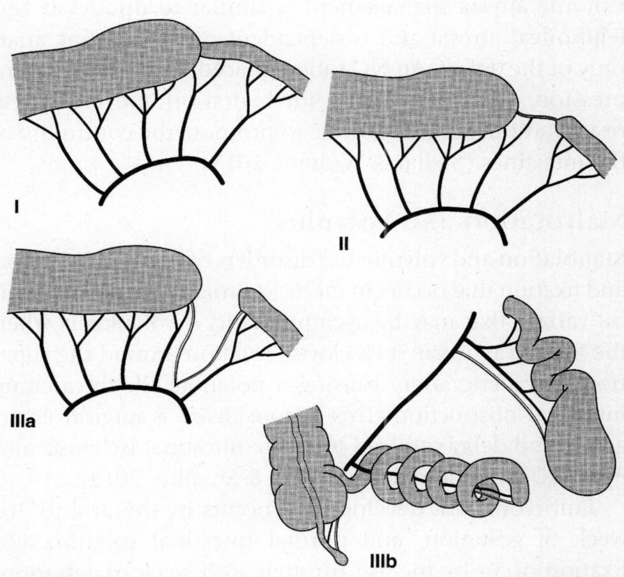

FIGURE 14-1. Duodenal atresia (types I, II, and III): classification of intestinal atresia.

Presentation

Prenatal ultrasound is able to detect most cases of duodenal atresia. It is noted by the classic obstructive sign of the "double bubble" on ultrasound showing the distended stomach and proximal duodenum. The infant may have bilious emesis, the sign of an intestinal obstruction.

Assessment

The ultrasound or abdominal radiograph showing the classic picture of the obstruction is all that is needed to take the infant for an operation once stable. If additional studies are needed, an upper gastrointestinal study may be done to rule out volvulus and is used to rule out partial obstructions or when imaging older children (Applebaum & Sydorak, 2012).

Management

Once volvulus is ruled out, a right upper quadrant incision is made between the liver edge and the umbilicus, or the surgery may be done laparoscopically in some situations. Typically, a duodenoduodenostomy is performed joining the areas of the intestine to bypass the obstruction or stenosed section. If this is unable to be done due to size or anatomy, then a duodenojejunostomy is performed (Aguayo & Ostlie, 2010). Pre- and postoperatively, the patient will have a nasogastric (NG) tube in place for gastric decompression. A peripherally inserted central catheter (PICC) may be placed for nutrition so the anastomoses may heal and to provide nutrition for those children who have a prolonged period of feeding intolerance.

Jejunoileal Atresia and Stenosis

Jejunoileal atresia and stenosis is thought to occur due to a vascular disruption during fetal development. This leads to ischemia, disintegration, and an atretic segment of intestine. The defects are classified into four types (**Fig. 14-2**).

Incidence

Jejunoileal atresia occurs in 1 in 5,000 births, and 1 in 3 infants who are diagnosed are premature.

Presentation

The jejunoileal atresia defect is noted on prenatal ultrasound or by signs and symptoms of obstruction with bilious emesis.

Assessment

Diagnosis is usually made by radiographic study of the abdomen showing proximal loops of bowel with gas and fluid, and the gasless abdomen beyond the defect.

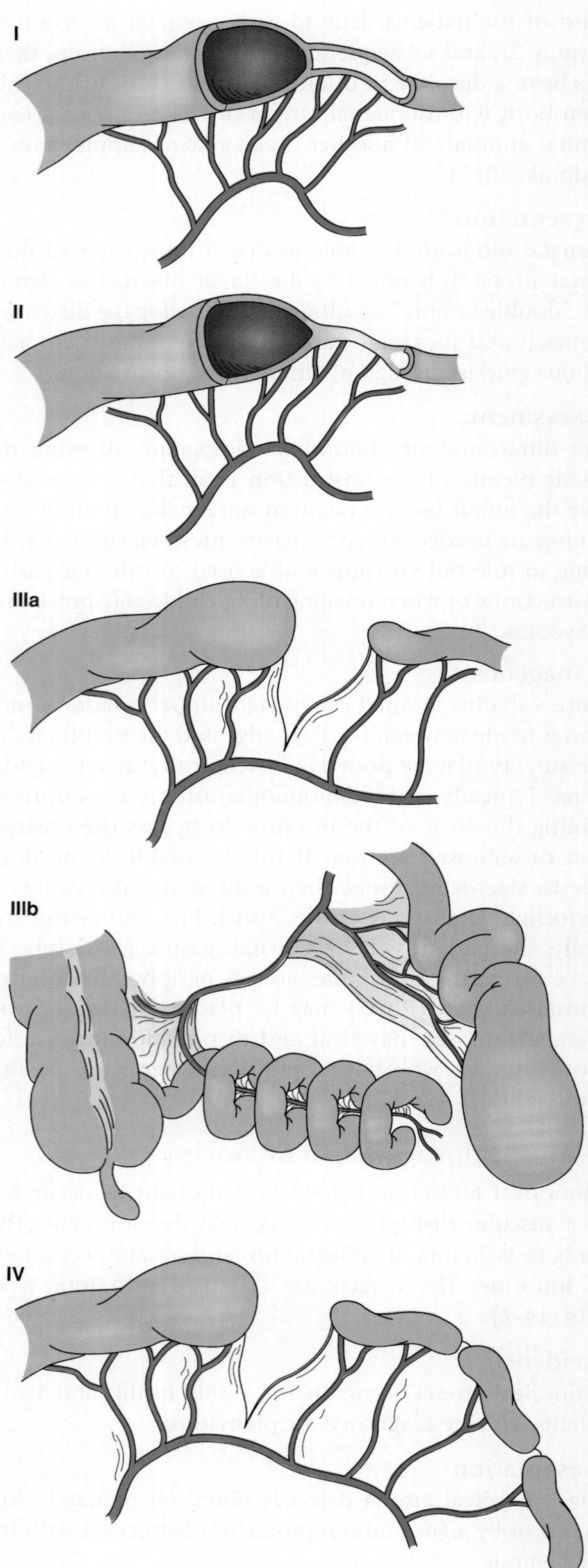

FIGURE 14-2. Classification of intestinal atresia type I, muscular continuity with a complete web. Type II, mesentery intact, fibrous cord. Type IIIa, muscular and mesenteric discontinuous. Type IIIb, apple-peel deformity. Type IV, multiple atresias.

Management

An NG tube is placed for decompression, antibiotics are started if concern exists for perforation or sepsis, and fluids are begun for hydration and electrolyte resuscitation. The most common operation performed is resection of the dilated and hypertrophied proximal bowel with end-to-end anastomosis with or without tapering of the proximal bowel. Normal small bowel length in neonates is 250 cm, in premature infants 160 to 240 cm; approximately 100 cm of intestines is needed for normal intestinal function (Aguayo & Ostlie, 2010). Bowel lengthening procedures can be performed later on in life. Parenteral nutrition will be required until the infant is able to begin oral feeds and longer if feeding intolerance is present.

Colonic Atresia

Colonic atresia is thought to be caused by vascular compromise in utero similar to jejunoileal atresia.

Incidence

Colonic atresia is the least common of the intestinal atresias and occurs 1 in 20,000 births.

Presentation

Colonic atresia presents with signs of a distal intestinal obstruction with feeding intolerance, distention, and bilious vomiting. Minimal or no passing of meconium is noted.

Assessment

Abdominal plain film reading of colonic atresia shows dilated loops of bowel with a cutoff point showing an abrupt end to the intestinal gas pattern. A contrast enema shows a microcolon with a discontinuation of contrast at the atretic point.

Management

Colonic atresia management is similar to duodenal and jejunoileal atresia and is dependent on the specific anatomy of the defect. An NG tube is placed for intestinal compression, and fluids begun for hydration and electrolyte resuscitation. Surgery is done to promote the continuity of the intestines (Stellar & Widmer, 2013).

Malrotation and Volvulus

Malrotation and volvulus are disorders of intestinal rotation and fixation that occurs in utero. Malrotation is an anatomical variant that may be asymptomatic. A volvulus is when the midgut twists in a clockwise rotation around the superior mesenteric artery causing a potential life-threatening intestinal obstruction. This is considered a surgical emergency, and delay can lead to severe intestinal ischemia and necrosis, shock, and death (Zerpa & Shapiro, 2013).

Embryonic gut development occurs by the 2nd to 3rd week of gestation, and normal intestinal rotation and fixation occur by the 4th through 10th week of gestation. Malrotation occurs during the 5th to 8th week when there

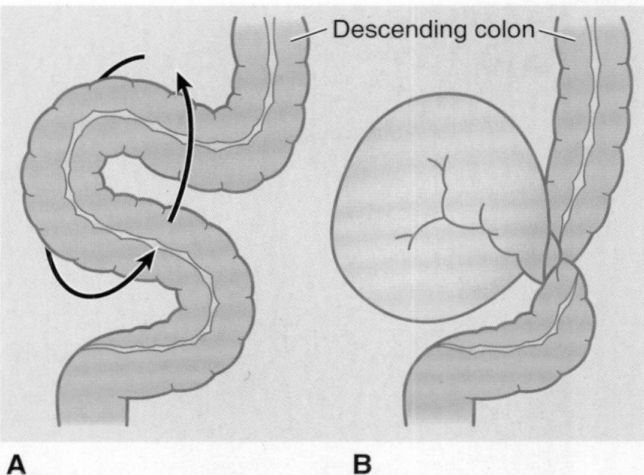

FIGURE 14-3. Volvulus of the sigmoid colon. **A.** Clockwise rotation of colon. **B.** Twistings of colon with obstruction.

is a disruption of the normal process where the intestine projects from the abdominal cavity into the umbilical cord, rotate 270 degrees, and then returns to the abdomen where it fixates between 10th and 12th week of gestation.

In 1932 and 1936, William E. Ladd wrote classic articles explaining the pathophysiology of malrotation with volvulus and its surgical correction for releasing the constricting peritoneal bands called the Ladd procedure. Without the normal 270-degree rotation, the intestines are not stable. Midgut volvulus encompasses the small bowel and is a complication of malrotation since the intestines are not fixed and in proper position. Volvulus occurs when there is at least a 360-degree twisting causing the vascular obstruction (Fig. 14-3).

Incidence

Incidence is difficult to determine as some children have malrotation that is not discovered until years later from an incidental radiograph. Seventy to ninety percent of children with complications present during the neonatal period. Symptomatic malrotation is reported in 1 per 6,000 live births (Zerpa & Shapiro, 2013, p. 333). Patients with omphalocele, gastroschisis, and congenital diaphragmatic hernia (CDH) may have a higher incidence of malrotation. Additional defects seen are intestinal atresias, HD, and Meckel diverticulum (McIltrot & Wilson, 2014).

Presentation

Diagnosis can be difficult because malrotation may range from being asymptomatic to causing episodes of vomiting and abdominal pain. This potentially could take years to diagnose if symptoms are vague, as it may appear to be gastroesophageal reflux disease (GERD) or failure to thrive. Malrotation with midgut volvulus presents with acute worrisome symptoms of a healthy child who suddenly vomits gastric content that becomes bilious vomiting with signs of acute illness (abdominal pain and distention, poor color, and signs of dehydration) (Zerpa & Shapiro, 2013).

Assessment

Malrotation and/or volvulus are diagnosed with radiographic studies. There is much discussion on which studies are most useful, and further research studies need to be done. Plain abdominal radiography may be difficult in small infants; however, the "double bubble" of acute duodenal obstruction or the "gasless" abdomen of the midgut volvulus may give diagnostic clues. Ultrasonography is a good screening tool and can show a vascular "whirlpool" flow and thick-walled bowel loops to the right of the spine. Computed tomography (CT) may show the "whirlpool" flow pattern as well (Dassinger & Smith, 2012). If difficult to diagnose, an upper gastrointestinal contrast study is needed to document the position of ligament of Treitz. The duodenum should be seen traveling across the spine to the left. Abnormal readings are duodenojejunal flexure to the right of the spine, obstruction of the duodenum, and the "beak" or "corkscrew" appearance of the obstructed proximal jejunum (Little & Smith, 2010, p. 419).

Management

The treatment is surgical repair with Ladd procedure for malrotation and detorsion followed by Ladd repair with volvulus. Laparoscopic surgery may be done with malrotation but may be difficult and not as expeditious as an open surgery for volvulus in the emergent situation. Further studies need to be done to assess outcomes of laparoscopic versus open surgical procedures. Postoperative care is determined by the extent of the surgery and damage to the intestines. Management of fluid and electrolytes and pain is crucial. An IV for intravenous fluids and analgesia will be in place postoperatively. An NG tube will be placed to decompress the stomach until bowel function returns. Depending upon the amount of necrotic bowel needing to be removed, there may be a central line and gastrostomy tube (G tube) for feedings and potential ostomy creation.

It is imperative to recognize and surgically treat volvulus right away to help decrease complications. Volvulus is a life-threatening complication of the malrotation where torsion occurs. Bilious vomiting may be the first sign and should be worked up quickly. The prognosis is very good for malrotation and varies depending on the degree of intestinal damage with volvulus. Severe cases may require stoma; however, it is not common.

Anorectal Malformations

Anorectal malformation (ARM) includes a spectrum of congenital defects potentially occurring in the bowel and urinary and reproductive systems. They may range from a low imperforate anus that requires a simple anoplasty within the first few days of life (as seen in Fig. 14-4) to a cloacal exstrophy with involvement of all three systems and a high lesion requiring a three stage repair with (1) diverting colostomy, (2) posterior sagittal anorectoplasty (PSARP), and (3) colostomy closure. The colostomy helps decompress the bowel and prevent infection until surgical site healing is complete. It is important to have an experienced pediatric surgeon who has training in PSARP perineal nerve sparing to have the best outcome for fecal continence (Guardino & Pieper, 2013).

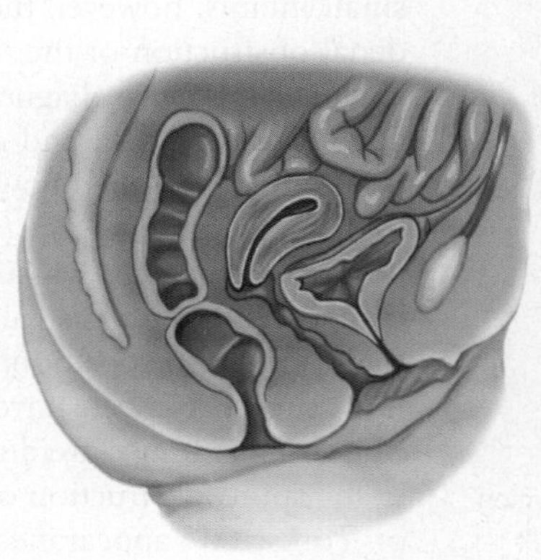

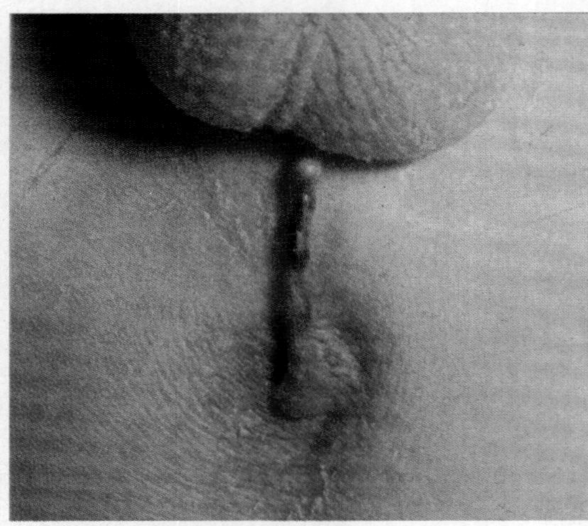

FIGURE 14-4. Anorectal malformation. **A.** Imperforate anus, in which the rectum ends in a blind pouch. **B.** Imperforate anus without fistula. The visible meconium streak along the raphe is consistent with a low imperforate anus.

Incidence

One in 5,000 births worldwide has ARMs with the less severe types being more common. ARMs are more common in boys. Fifty percent of children with ARMs have other associated defects (Guardino & Pieper, 2013). Table 14-1 shows VACTERL association and commonly seen defects with ARMs.

Presentation

The diagnosis of ARMs is often made in the delivery room on examination of the newborn baby or when the nurse attempts to take a rectal temperature and no anus is present. In addition, infants with fistulas are noted to have stool in the wrong location such as in the vaginal vestibule of a female infant. The infant may have absent or displaced anal opening, vomiting, abdominal distention, and meconium in the genitalia of the female or on the perineum of the male away from the anus. Anteriorly displaced anus is common where the anus is not in the correct location, halfway between the coccyx and the base of the scrotum or vagina.

Assessment

A complete physical exam to check anatomy should be done when all infants are born, paying close attention to the genitalia and perianal area. If malformation is found, then the exam should also focus on determining if other commonly associated findings are present.

TABLE 14-1 VACTERL Association

V	**V**ertebral anomalies
A	Imperforate **A**nus
C	**C**ardiac anomalies
T	**T**racheoesophageal fistula
E	**E**sophageal atresia
R	**R**enal anomalies
L	**L**imb anomalies, particularly radical agenesis

Management

Depending upon the malformation, general supportive medical care should be done followed by full workup to rule out other congenital malformations and to determine the severity of the ARM. A team approach is taken including genetics, and multiple radiologic studies may be ordered. Depending upon the exact diagnosis, a surgical plan will be made. For imperforate anus, anoplasty will be done. For complex cloacal exstrophy, urologic, orthopedic, and general surgery will be staged over the next year. An ostomy may be required to decompress the bowel and allow for stool output and will be a priority if there is no outlet for stool. Postoperatively for PSARP, perianal sutures should be gently rinsed clean and antibiotic ointment applied for 1 week. Nothing should be placed in the anus for 2 weeks.

At the 2-week post-op appointment, the family will be taught how to do rectal dilations. If the child was required to have an ostomy, teaching will need to be done with the family immediately postoperatively and follow-up with the clinic appointments. With severe congenital defects such as cloacal defects, pouching may be difficult due to an open, draining bladder on the abdominal wall in close proximity to the stoma. Good skin care and prevention of yeast and denuded skin is a priority to preserve the skin for upcoming surgical repairs. This is a huge adjustment for the family who will be bringing their child to the hospital for many visits and extended hospital stays following surgery in addition to the complex care of the child. Case management, social work, and psychology should be part of the multidisciplinary team.

Necrotizing Enterocolitis

NEC is characterized by necrosis of the mucosal and submucosal layer of the gastrointestinal tract and is the most common surgical emergency in the neonate. It usually affects preterm infants who are in the neonatal intensive care unit

(NICU) and <1,500 g, but 10% of the time does affect the full-term infant. It is unclear exactly what causes NEC; however, it is thought that the immature gastrointestinal tract has altered functions in motility, digestion, intestinal epithelium integrity, circulatory regulation, poor immunologic defense, colonization of bacteria, and feeding intolerance (Rapoport & Nishii, 2013, p. 296). There is hypoxemia of the bowel causing ischemia and then bacteria invade the bowel wall. The schematic is a composite of theories involved in the pathogenesis of NEC (**Fig. 14-5**). Interestingly, few unfed neonates are diagnosed with NEC. The classic study by Lucas and Cole (1990) reported that NEC was 6 to 10 times more common in formula-fed infants than those who were fed breast milk. Mothers are highly encouraged to provide breast milk to their infants especially if they are born prematurely. Careful assessment by the nurse often leads to immediate recognition of the signs and symptoms of NEC, which may improve the outcome for the neonate.

Incidence

In the United States, the NEC incidence is in 0.7 to 1.1 infants per 1,000 births, and the younger the premature infant, the higher the incidence (Rapoport & Nishii, 2013).

Presentation

It is important for early recognition, and initially, the signs may be subtle. The infant may start with temperature instability, apnea and bradycardia, thrombocytopenia, and metabolic acidosis and progress to oliguria, hypotension shock, and deteriorating laboratory and vital signs.

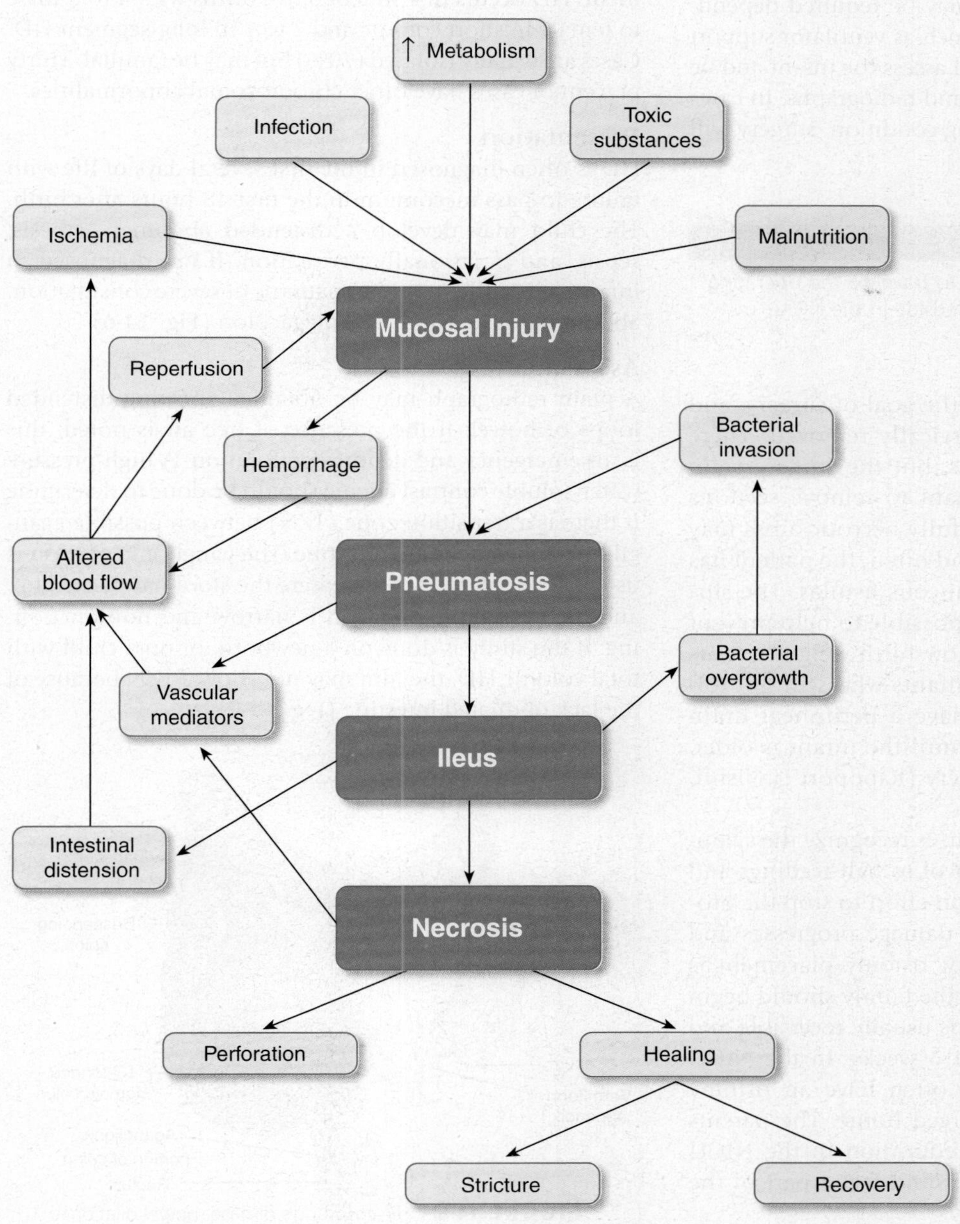

FIGURE 14-5. Necrotizing enterocolitis (NEC). This schematic is a composite of the theories about factors thought to be involved in the pathogenesis of NEC. The progression of this disease is denoted in large type. The factors thought to initiate or propagate the disease process are in smaller type.

Assessment

Radiographic findings may range from normal gas pattern or mild ileus to dilated loops, pneumatosis to pneumoperitoneum. Gastrointestinal findings range from gastric residuals and abdominal distention to bloody stools, absent bowel sounds, abdominal wall edema, and palpable loops of bowel.

Management

The medical and surgical teams are notified, and the infant is placed on NEC watch. Many NICUs have an NEC protocol so if the nurse suspects NEC, he or she can immediately notify the team, halt feedings, make the child NPO (nothing by mouth), start IV antibiotics, and notify the radiology department for serial radiographs. An orogastric (OG) or NG tube is placed to decompress the stomach and intestines. Further support may be required depending upon the infant's condition such as ventilator support and surgery. The surgery team will assess the infant and be on call for worsening symptoms and radiographs. In cases of bowel perforation or worsening condition, surgery will be performed.

CLINICAL PEARL

Occasionally, if the child is too sick to travel to the operating room (OR), surgery is done at the bedside in the NICU.

Bowel length preservation is the goal of surgery, and only fully necrotic bowel is surgically removed. There may be patchy areas of necrosis, but the surgery team may be conservative and reluctant to remove sections that may improve. The severely fully necrotic areas may be resected and anastomosed, and often, the patient has an ileostomy formation with mucous fistulas. The surgeon removes as little bowel as possible to help prevent short bowel syndrome. In very-low-birth weight infants or hemodynamically unstable infants who will not tolerate surgery, the infant may have a peritoneal drain placed to decompress the area until the infant is older, stable, and able to tolerate surgery (Rapoport & Nishii, 2013).

In review, it is vital that the nurses recognize the symptoms and initiate the NEC protocol to halt feedings and begin treatment immediately in an effort to stop the progression of bowel injury. If the damage progresses and surgical intervention is necessary, ostomy placement is common. Ostomy education for the family should begin as soon as possible. The ostomy is usually reversible and will remain in place for at least 6 weeks. In the NICU for the extreme preemies, they often have an ostomy takedown prior to being discharged home. The parents should still be included in the education in the NICU so they may bond with the child and feel a part of the infant's care.

Hirschsprung's Disease

HD is the absence of intraneural ganglion cells and hypertrophic nerves of the bowel, which have created a functional partial or full obstruction. With the lack of ganglion cells, peristalsis does not occur and the stool cannot be pushed through the intestines properly and leads to a blockage. Usually HD occurs in the rectum and sigmoid colon but may be of varying lengths including total intestinal aganglionosis. There are also variant cases such as intestinal neuronal dysplasia (IND) that are characterized by HD symptoms with a rectal biopsy showing ganglion cells. Currently, there is research on these ganglion cells that do not function properly.

Incidence

Intestinal ganglion cells form during early fetal development. HD occurs in 1 in 5,000 live births with 4 to 1 male to female in short colonic and 2 to 1 in long-segment HD. Cases are usually isolated (70%) but may be familial. Thirty percent of cases have other chromosomal abnormalities.

Presentation

HD is often diagnosed in the first several days of life with failure to pass meconium in the first 48 hours after birth. The child may develop a distended abdomen, emesis, sepsis, and occasionally perforation. If not diagnosed in infancy, the child may have patterns of severe constipation, abdominal distension, and megacolon (**Fig. 14-6**).

Assessment

A plain radiograph may be obtained showing distended loops of bowel; if the presence of free air is noted, this is an emergency and denotes perforation. A high-pressure water-soluble contrast enema should be done to determine if there is a transition zone (TZN) between possible aganglionic and ganglionic intestine. The ganglionic portion is usually the enlarged colon where the stool has backed up, and the aganglionic portion is narrow and nonfunctioning. If the study is done on a newborn, or on a child with total colonic HD, the film may not show a TZN because of the lack of dilated intestine (**Fig. 14-7**).

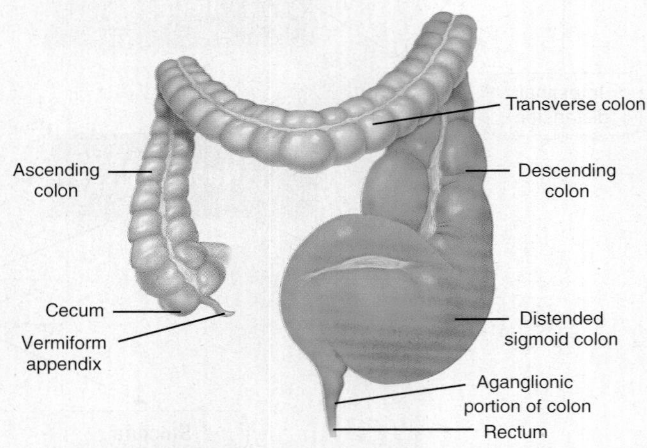

FIGURE 14-6. Hirschsprung's disease: bowel dilation.

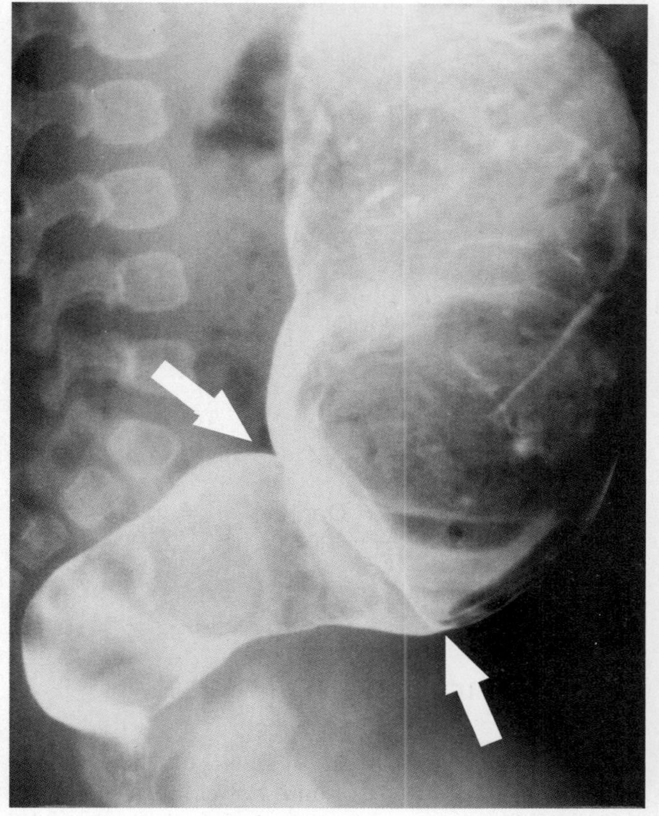

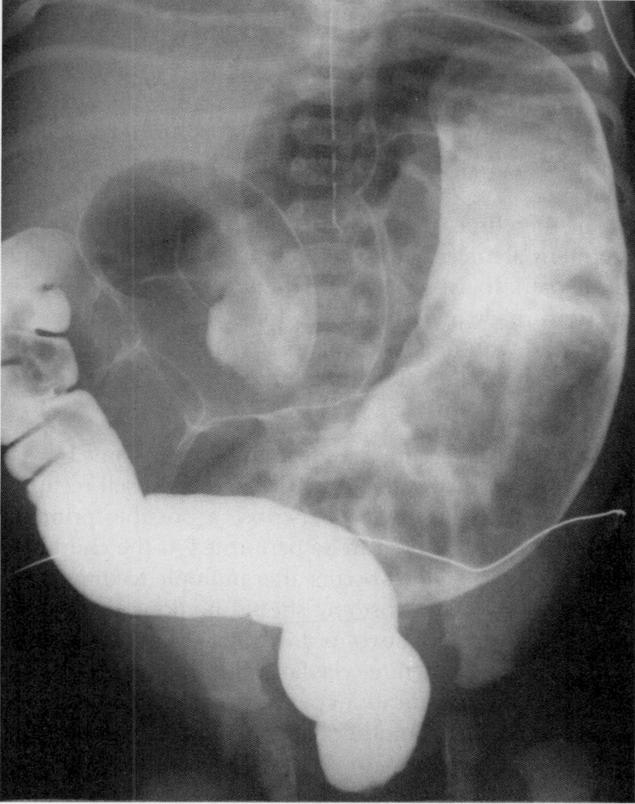

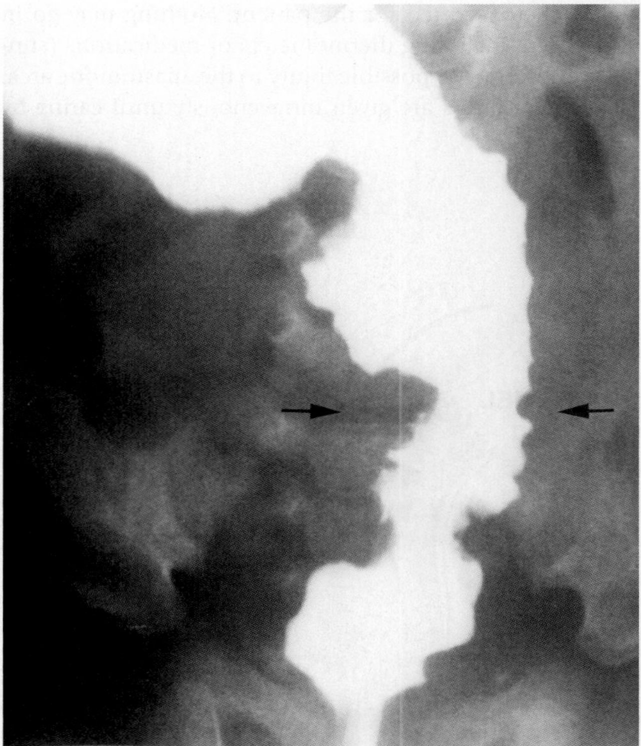

FIGURE 14-7. Hirschsprung's disease. **A.** Characteristic TZN (*arrows*) is seen between the dilated, feces-filled colon above and the relatively narrowed rectum below. **B.** The rectum in this newborn infant is smaller than the sigmoid and descending colon, but a well-defined TZN is not present. **C.** A contrast enema in another infant shows spasm and irregularity of the aganglionic segment (*arrows*).

Anorectal manometry is not widely used in the United States but reportedly done more often in Europe. With this study, pressure-measuring balloon catheters are placed in the anus and rectum to determine the absence of the relaxation reflex of the internal sphincter (Holder & Jackson, 2013). The "gold standard" for diagnosing HD is the suction rectal biopsy. This may be performed in the OR, in the clinic, or at the bedside. Two to three rectal specimens are taken at 2 and 5 cm above the dentate line for the pathologist to determine if ganglion cells are present. If an inadequate biopsy is done or the patient is an older child who requires sedation, a full-thickness biopsy may be done in the OR with anesthesia.

Management

Treatment of HD is surgical resection of aganglionic bowel and anastomosis of ganglionic bowel to the distal rectum. If diagnosed in the neonatal period, a possible primary pull-through procedure can be performed. If the child has distended bowel, which occurs after multiple feedings and buildup of stool, a colostomy should be done to decompress the bowel, and a two- or three-stage surgical repair is performed. There are three classic pull-through procedures, with additional modifications performed per surgeon preference, all of which are modifications based on Dr. Swenson's original surgery in 1964. In addition, there is a single-stage pull-through for HD that is laparoscopic-assisted transanal endorectal pull-through (LATEP) with abdominal exploration and laparoscopic biopsies (Georgeson, 2010).

> **CLINICAL PEARL**
>
> The goal in surgery is to avoid injury to the pelvic nerves to conserve continence and function.

Swenson Technique (1964)

Resection of aganglionic bowel leaving a small portion of aganglionic segment at the dentate line. The ganglionic and aganglionic are anastomosed at an angle to prevent stricture development. The surgery is done with an abdominal incision and the end-to-end anastomosis done by prolapsing the rectum and pulled through ganglionic bowel through the anus to avoid injury to pelvic nerves (**Fig. 14-8**).

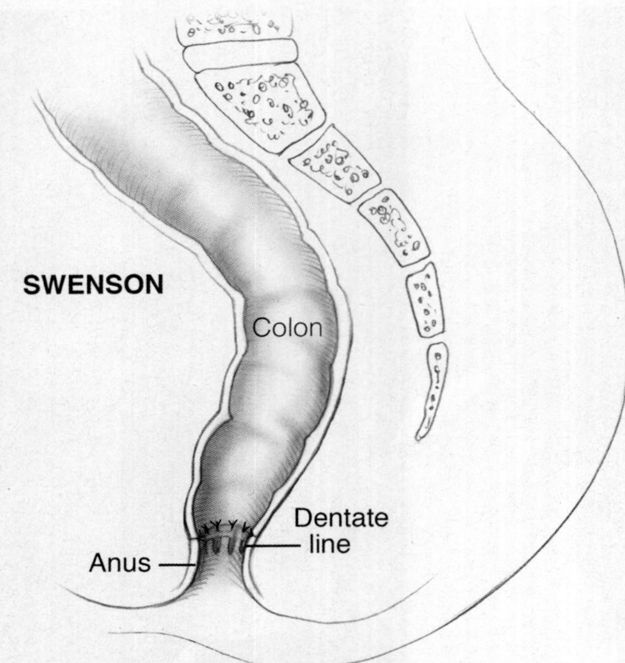

FIGURE 14-8. Swenson procedure.

Duhamel Technique (1960)

Combined abdominoperineal approach of a retrorectal pull-through of ganglionated segment through the aganglionated rectum and sewn to the anus. The septum between the two is then divided using a stapler. This creates a neorectum with an aganglionic anterior wall and ganglionic posterior wall (**Fig. 14-9**).

Soave Endorectal Pull-Through (1964)

Dissection of the mucosal layer from the muscular layer of the aganglionic segment and pulling the ganglionic portion down through the dissected aganglionic muscular cuff (**Fig. 14-10**) (Georgeson, 2010; Holder & Jackson, 2013).

Postoperative care consists of an NG tube placed for 1 to 2 days postoperatively or until bowel function returns. Peripheral intravenous therapy is given for hydration until bowel function begins and a clear liquid advance as tolerated diet is started for the patient. Nothing may go in the rectum including thermometers or medications (suppositories), due to possible injury to the anastomotic area. Pain medications are given intravenously until eating by

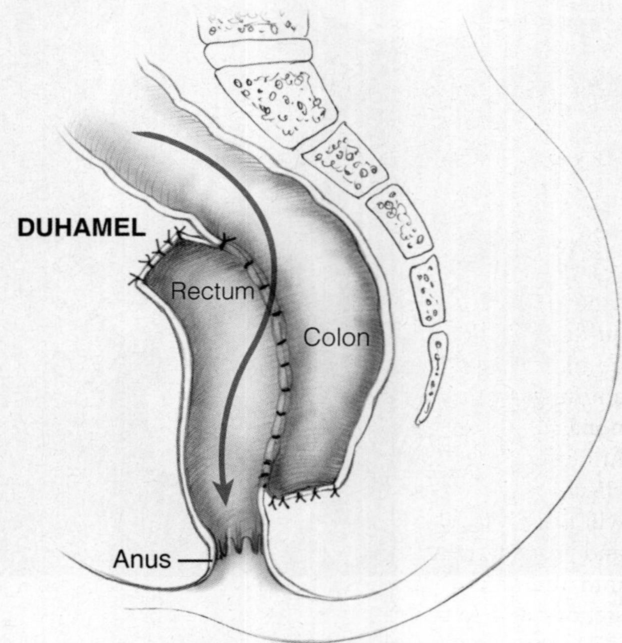

FIGURE 14-9. Duhamel procedure.

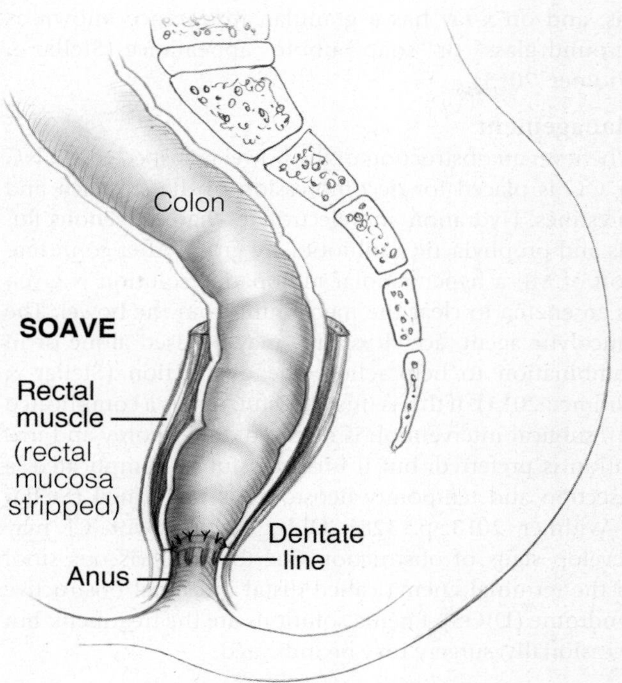

FIGURE 14-10. Soave procedure.

mouth and then a transition to oral pain medications is done prior to discharge home. If the patient has a new ostomy, the stoma is assessed for color, size, shape, and output (see Table 9-2 in Chapter 9). Ostomy care teaching begins immediately with the child and family. If a pull-through procedure was done, care of the perineum is taught. There is frequent stooling after surgery, approximately 6 to 12 stools per day. Contact dermatitis often develops in the diaper area, and the skin can become severely denuded.

CLINICAL PEARL

A nonalcohol skin sealant covered with a thick barrier cream followed by petrolatum is applied to the perineal area.

With diaper changes, gently wipe the stool away and reapply just the cream that was removed. All of the cream can be soaked off with soap and water and the buttocks air-dried daily. If red satellite lesions are noted, this can be indicative of a *Candida* (yeast) skin infection and an antifungal powder can be sprinkled on the skin before the nonalcohol skin sealant and barrier creams are applied. Antifungals should be placed first against the skin to be effective. Two to three weeks after surgery, the surgical team will begin teaching the family how to do rectal dilations and possibly, rectal irrigations. Surgical dilators are passed into the anus to keep the anastomosis from becoming stenotic and to remain open for the passing of stool (see Table 14-2 for appropriate-size dilators for patient age). The patient should pass at least one soft, formed stool daily and adjust diet to prevent constipation or frequent stooling. Toilet training may be delayed; however, bowel management is highly successful, and incontinence rates are low. Reviewing the signs and symptoms of enterocolitis (Box 14-1) is important with each visit to reduce mortality and morbidity.

TABLE 14-2 Rectal Dilator Chart

Age	Dilator Number
1–4 mo	12
4–12 mo	13
8–12 mo	14
1–3 y	15
3–12 y	16
>12 y	17

Meconium Ileus

MI is a blockage in the intestine from abnormal meconium. MI is due to a mutation in the gene for CF transmembrane regulator (CFTR) protein that causes abnormal changes in the chloride, sodium, and water transport that occurs across the apical membrane of epithelial cells. This affects the respiratory, gastrointestinal, biliary, pancreatic, and reproductive systems. MI was considered fatal until 1948, when the first enterotomy was done by Hiatt and Wilson. Then, in 1969, Dr. Helen Noblett discovered a nonoperative treatment with a hyperosmolar enema to remove the abnormal stool (Stellar & Widmer, 2013).

Incidence

Most infants with MI have cystic fibrosis (CF), and 10% to 15% of patients present as neonates. All patients with MI should be tested for CF through sweat chloride testing and genetic testing. CF is the most common life-threatening autosomal recessive disease in the United States (Stellar & Widmer, 2013).

BOX 14-1 Enterocolitis Signs and Symptoms

Enterocolitis: Life-threatening acute inflammation of the mucosa of the small intestinal or colonic epithelium. Enterocolitis may occur preoperatively or postoperatively. If enterocolitis is suspected, instruct the family to report immediately to the closest emergency department for assessment and management of sepsis and shock.

Distended abdomen
Hyperactive bowel sounds
Signs and symptoms of sepsis
Darker green or gray stool
Explosive foul-smelling stool
Lethargy
Fever

Presentation

MI can be simple or complex. Simple MI has intact gastrointestinal tract with obstruction by abnormal meconium in the ileus. Meconium is normally thick, tarry, and green, but with MI, it becomes firm, gray, and pellet-like causing an obstruction due to its failure to pass through the intestines. The child with MI fails to pass meconium, the abdomen becomes distended, and the child develops bilious emesis (Stellar & Widmer, 2013). In complicated MI, the infant will present with additional symptoms of tenderness and abdominal wall erythema. The complicated MI has damage from in utero where a volvulus is isolated, perforated, or developed into atresia. This can occur before the birth of the baby, and this sterile peritonitis may lead to adhesions, calcifications, and meconium cysts.

Assessment

On radiographs, MI is characterized by dilated loops, proximal small bowel, and microcolon with distal ileum and ascending colon filled with pellets of meconium (**Fig. 14-11**). The meconium mixes with swallowed gas, and on x-ray has a granular appearance known as "ground glass" or "soap bubble" appearance (Stellar & Widmer, 2013).

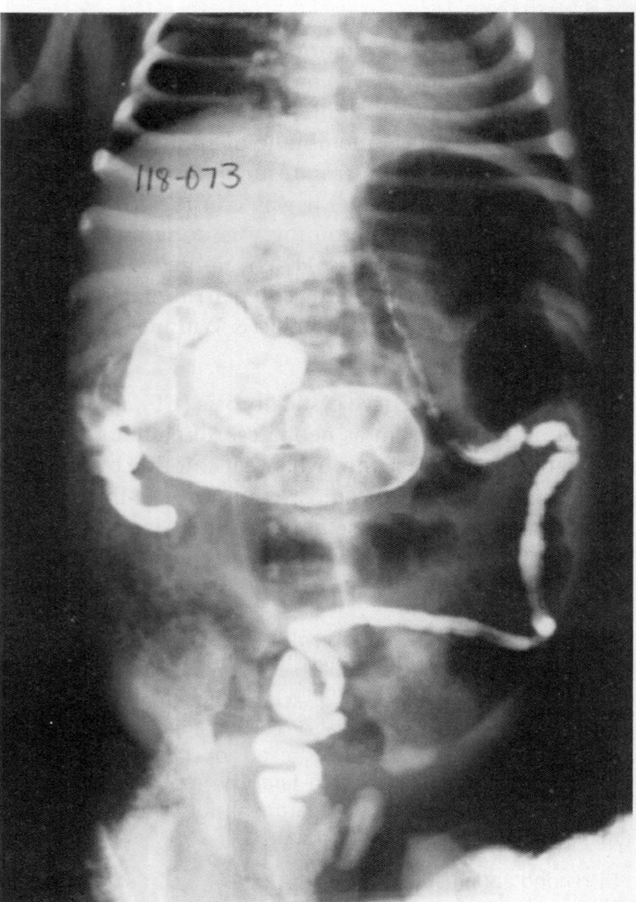

FIGURE 14-11. Meconium ileus. Anteroposterior view from a barium enema performed on an infant with intestinal obstruction in the neonatal period. Microcolon, which may occur in both MI and intestinal atresia, is evident. Unlike in ileal atresia, obstructing plugs of inspissated meconium are present within the lumen of this patient's terminal ileum, a finding suggesting MI.

Management

Whenever an obstruction of the bowel is suspected, an NG or OG is placed for decompression of the stomach and intestines. Hydration and electrolytes via intravenous fluids and prophylactic antibiotics are given. After confirmation of MI, a hyperosmolar radiopaque solution is given as an enema to clear the meconium from the bowel. The mucolytic agent, acetylcysteine, may be used alone or in combination to help relieve the obstruction (Stellar & Widmer, 2013). If this is unsuccessful, or it is a complicated MI, surgical intervention is required. Enterotomy and irrigation is preferred, but if unsuccessful or complicated, a resection and temporary ileostomy is performed (Stellar & Widmer, 2013, p. 328). Older children with CF may develop signs of obstruction due to thick, viscous stool in the terminal enema called distal intestinal obstructive syndrome (DIOS). Enema solutions are the treatment, but occasionally, surgery may be indicated.

Inflammatory Bowel Disease

IBD includes Crohn's disease (CD), ulcerative colitis (UC), and IBD-unclassified or "indeterminate cases." In the pediatric population, 5% to 20% of the cases may be classified as indeterminate due to the difficulties in diagnosing and classifying the disease as either CD or UC. IBD is a chronic, inflammatory disease of the intestinal tract of unknown etiology. There is a relationship of heredity, environmental factors, and immunologic responses. Although there is an in-depth review of IBD in Chapter 4, it is mentioned again in the pediatric chapter due to the fact that 25% to 30% of cases of diagnosed UC and CD occur in childhood. In addition, cases of CD are increasing in childhood, while UC is staying stable. Treatment is medical and surgical management. Good nutrition is imperative as children are rapidly growing, and severe malnutrition and dehydration can permanently stunt the child's growth; corticosteroids can cause osteoporotic effects (Moir, 2010).

Crohn's Disease

CD is a chronic IBD and has no known cure.

Incidence

CD occurs in 0.2 to 8.5 in 100,000 births. It occurs more often in the Northern hemisphere.

Presentation

The child develops ulcers and inflammation with two thirds of the cases occurring in the small bowel and proximal colon (ileocecal). The ulcers can coalesce and also penetrate transmurally creating sinuses, abscesses, and fistulas. The patient develops weight loss, bloody diarrhea, abdominal pain, and perianal disease, and may have a family history of IBD.

Assessment

The patient requires a thorough history and physical and growth evaluation. A rectal exam should be done to observe for perirectal disease. In the anxious child, an exam under anesthesia (EUA) can be scheduled to do a more complete exam, including an anorectal endoscopic exam. Blood work including a complete blood count (CBC), erythrocyte sedimentation rate (ESR), C-reactive protein (CRP), baseline nutritional laboratory tests, stool cultures, and IgA and IgG anti-*Saccharomyces cerevisiae* antibody (ASCA) should be performed (Adibe & Georgeson, 2012).

Management

CD therapy includes medical therapy to achieve remission of the disease and appropriate nutrition to delay surgical procedures as long as possible. Within 10 years of diagnosis, most patients will require surgery and 50% of patients who have had surgery require a second surgery. Surgical procedures are usually due to obstruction from strictures and require a resection or strictureplasty. There is an increased risk of malignancy due to the inflammatory process, and CD patients should follow the recommended guidelines for surveillance (Adibe & Georgeson, 2012).

Ulcerative Colitis

UC is an IBD that affects the lining of the large intestine (colon) and rectum.

Incidence

UC occurs in 2.2 to 4.5 per 100,000 in industrialized countries. Children who are diagnosed are more likely to have pancolitis where the entire colon is involved.

Presentation

Presentation often begins slowly with diarrhea and then blood, mucus, and pus in the stools. Intermittent abdominal cramping, pain, tenesmus (feeling the need to constantly pass stool), tiredness, and anemia due to the blood loss are common. Osteopenia, weight loss, and anorexia with growth retardation are a concern as well, and nutrition becomes crucial with these patients. External hemorrhoids may develop due to the frequent stooling. Fistulas and abscesses are rare and if noted may be suggestive of CD.

Assessment

UC is diagnosed with history and physical, lab work, and colonoscopy. Contrast studies may exacerbate the colitis and so are done less frequently. CT enterography can also provide information but exposes the patients to radiation (Adler et al., 2012).

Management

Management of UC includes medication to promote suppression of the disease and possible surgery that may have side effects but can be curative, avoids a permanent stoma, and helps maintain bowel continence. The surgery of choice (open or laparoscopic) is the ileoanal reservoir or ileal pouch–anal anastomosis (IPAA) with pouch construction to create a reservoir to assist in reducing stool frequency and urgency. A protective loop ileostomy is usually created to help prevent anastomotic leaks and is left in place for several months. UC patients are often undernourished and on high-dose steroids and have rectal inflammation that causes complications with healing (Adler et al., 2012). Many of these UC patients are very sick and hospitalized and receiving medical management prior to surgery and feel significantly better after the ostomy surgery.

The WOC nurse can provide preoperative education and stoma siting followed by postoperative teaching for the ileostomy, pouching, and also pouchitis. Pouchitis is nonspecific mucosal inflammation in the IPAA with increased stooling, nighttime fecal incontinence, pain, and bleeding. It is not life threatening but is life altering with the child feeling ill. There is usually an adequate response with antibiotics or long-term low-dose alternating antibiotics. Patients should be followed long term by the pediatric gastrointestinal service to monitor symptoms, medications, and surveillance of disease.

Familial Polyposis Syndromes

Incidence

Intestinal cancers in children are rare, and surgical procedures are often preventative as in familial adenomatous polyposis (FAP). There is a genetic component to polyps, and children with family members should be followed closely by the pediatric gastrointestinal and surgical team. Large polyps and increased numbers of polyps (often in the thousands) are at a higher risk for becoming malignant. The average age of nonfamilial polyps is noted at age 29.

Presentation

Usually, they are noted by mucus in the stool, blood per rectum, frequency, and bowel habit changes.

Assessment

Obtain a family history of FAP and genetic testing, and perform endoscopic surveillance yearly starting by age 10.

Management

The symptoms are usually not so severe as to require surgery but instead are done prophylactically to prevent cancer. There are varying ages, but the average age of cancer is 39. The risk of cancer and symptoms usually helps determine the timing of surgery, but it is a team approach and often is done during the early teenage years. With FAP, a proctocolectomy and IPAA are performed. Reasons are unclear, but there are fewer complications in FAP patients than in UC patients in regard to pouchitis, nighttime soiling, and incontinence (Moir, 2010). Polyposis syndromes are discussed further in Chapter 5.

Pediatric Trauma

Incidence

Millions of children are injured yearly due to trauma, and hundreds of thousands require hospitalization.

Presentation

Mechanisms of injury vary due to the developmental level of the child. Motor vehicle accidents (MVA) are more common in teenagers, and young children are injured by falls. Boys are more commonly injured in the pediatric age group (McKenna & Pieper, 2013).

Assessment

A full head-to-toe assessment should always be done on the child in addition to obtaining a history from the child and family member or guardian.

Management

Although most children injuring themselves do not require surgery, and even more rarely, an ostomy, it is worth mentioning. Traumas are usually unexpected and if requiring an ostomy, the event is even more stressful and involves comprehensive teaching. Family education and support is necessary. Examples of traumas that may require surgery for an ostomy are blunt abdominal trauma from an MVA with perforation to the intestines, child and sexual abuse such as rectal injury from objects, severe perineal burns requiring diverting ostomy for burn care, and gang violence. Gang violence is being studied around the country, and disturbingly, there is a trend for the gang members to intentionally paralyze and injure the victim with shooting or stabbing so the victim requires a wheelchair and a "bag" (ostomy pouch).

The WOC nurse will provide ostomy education and also help the multidisciplinary team provide psychosocial adjustment. This period of vulnerability of the victim is a time when the team can make a huge difference to change the path of the gang member (Aboutanos, 2014). Safety of the staff, however, is of utmost importance when dealing with potentially violent patients. Refer to WOCN (2011), Surgical indications for fecal diversions (Pediatric ostomy care best practice for clinicians).

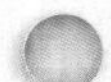

Management of Fecal Diversions

Techniques and Indications for Pediatric Pouching

Stool output should be contained, and the peristomal skin should be kept clear of rashes, denuded skin, and infection. Most often, stool output is contained in a "pouch"; however, stool may be contained in a diaper with good skin care to prevent the output from irritating the peristomal skin. If a stoma has a mucous fistula, they may be pouched together or separately. Fecal stomas and urostomies should not be pouched together due to the risk of infection. Although "baby wipes" are convenient, many brands can be irritating to the skin or leave residual lotions behind on the skin repelling the wafer and preventing it from adhering. The peristomal skin may be washed with water, a basic soap, or stomal wipes.

Younger children are active and frequently dislodge their pouches. They may wear any clothing; however, clothing with snaps between the legs or "onesies" can hold the pouch in place. Pediatric ostomy belts for securing pouches for the toddler age and older may be beneficial; in addition, there are versions of abdominal binders and netting available. Pouches may be secured inside or outside of the diaper per family preference. Children with fragile skin are at risk for developing pressure ulcers and must be monitored to prevent medical device–related pressure ulcers (MDRPU), such as lying on a pouch, spout, or clamp for an extended period of time. Infants may be excessively gassy from crying, sucking, and swallowing air. Pouches with devices such as filters can help easily release the gas.

Older children are embarrassed by smells and sounds. It can be reinforced that if there is a good seal with the pouching system, and no leakage, there should be no odor. Using a deodorizer in the pouch and room atomizers to neutralize the odor when emptying and changing pouches work well. Dropping toilet paper into the toilet bowel will help prevent splashing when emptying pouch contents into the bowl. Before a quiet time in class such as an exam, avoiding foods that cause excessive gas will keep the intestines quieter. The older child will quickly learn what foods affect the stool output. For liquid high-output stomas, crystals placed in the pouch to turn the stool into gel are effective. Typical pouch wear time is anywhere from 24 hours to 5 days. Children may bathe with or without their pouch on depending upon personal preference. Children may play sports and can use ostomy belts or spandex compression garments to help hold their ostomy pouch in place.

Refeeding Ostomy Output

Children with resection of the small bowel causing feeding problems related to bowel length or stomas with high-volume output causing poor growth, long-term total parenteral nutrition, dehydration, and electrolyte imbalance may require refeeding of ostomy output. Refeeding is thought to help intestinal adaptation and improve peristalsis and mucosal growth (Richardson et al., 2006). Refeeding is often done in the premature and full-term infant for short bowel symptoms and occasionally adolescents for rare events such as severe trauma to the intestines (Stellar & Widmer, 2013). To refeed via the stoma, the child must have a patent distal intestinal limb. The patient is on strict intake and output, and the stool output is collected from the ostomy pouch and refed via a pump and catheter. Strict labeling is imperative to avoid accidental administration of stool in intravenous catheters and central lines.

A catheter is placed in to the distal stoma, and the catheter is threaded through an opening created in the ostomy pouch. Initial catheter placement may be done by the surgical team and possibly under radiograph to determine position and length and to closely monitor to prevent intestinal trauma and perforation. Anatomically, if it is possible to pouch the stomas separately, it may be easier to collect stool in one pouch and instill the stool through the second pouch into the mucous fistula. When instilling stool, there may be leakage and frequent catheter displacement.

If leakage occurs, attempt to quantify amount to determine how much needs to be replaced. Refeeding requires a WOC nurse consult, good team communication, and patience and creativity for pouching and tube securement.

Pathology and Management Conditions Leading to Urinary Diversion

Prune Belly Syndrome

Prune belly syndrome (PBS) is a severe congenital malformation with absence of abdominal muscles giving the appearance of a wrinkled prune (Fig. 14-12). The syndrome may also include dilation of the upper urinary tract, clubfeet, and undescended testes (Caldamone & Woodard, 2012). The etiology is unknown with possible distal obstructive disease and mesodermal defect of the abdominal wall and urinary tract.

Incidence

PBS incidence is 1 in 40,000 births with 97% of the cases boys (Caldamone & Woodard, 2012).

Presentation

PBS may be noted on prenatal ultrasound or noted on the birth of the baby with the appearance of the abdomen.

Assessment

Once diagnosed with PBS, further testing may be done to rule out other anomalies. Radiographs are done to assess the internal anatomy of the genitourinary tract. The upper urinary tract with the ureters and kidneys may be severely torturous.

Management

The patient may have surgery for a temporary vesicostomy or ureterostomies to create an outlet for urine so there is no backup of urine to damage the urinary system.

Myelomeningocele

Myelomeningocele or "spina bifida" is a defect in the formation of the neural tube, which causes a spectrum of defects along the brain and spinal cord (Fig. 14-13).

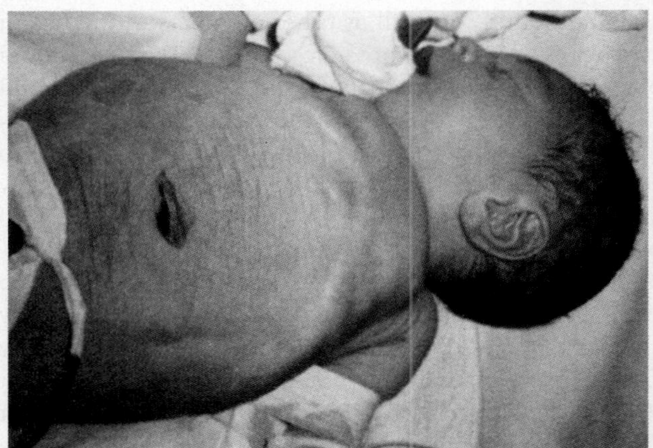

FIGURE 14-12. Prune belly syndrome.

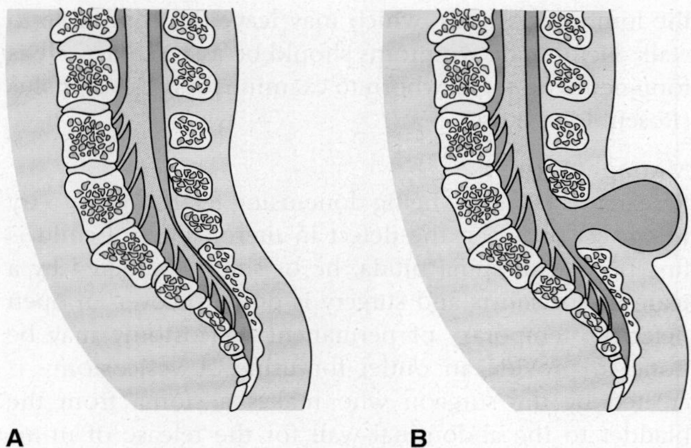

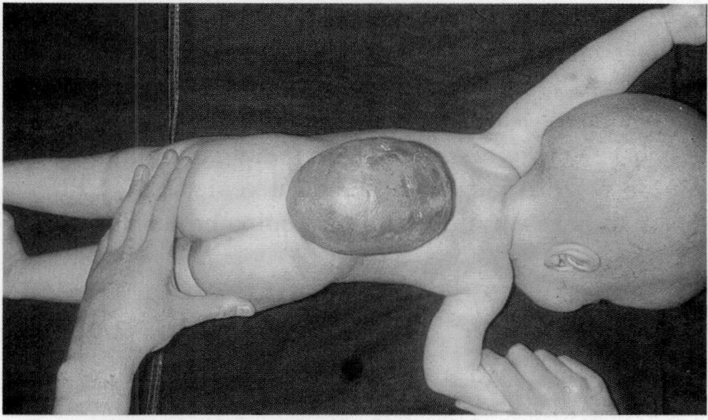

FIGURE 14-13. Myelomeningocele. Spina bifida is incomplete closure of the spinal cord. **A.** Normal spinal cord. **B.** Spina bifida with protrusion of the meninges (meningocele). **C.** Protrusion of the spinal cord and meninges (myelomeningocele).

The etiology is unclear, but genetic factors and environmental factors including folic acid deficiency play a role in neural tube defects (NTD). The malformation of the neural tube involves the laminae and pedicles on the vertebral column. If the neural tube does not close properly on either end or becomes overdistended and ruptures after closure, then an NTD occurs (Rosenblum, 2014).

Incidence

There has been a decrease in incidence in spina bifida with the introduction of folic acid 30 years ago and with antenatal testing procedures that detect NTD, allowing pregnancy termination.

Presentation

Prenatal diagnosis of spina bifida can be made with ultrasonography, fetal amniotic fluid assays, or elevated maternal alpha-fetoprotein. When a child is born with spina bifida, there may be varying degrees of lesions. The dysfunction can be complete paralysis to minimal involvement.

Assessment

A complete physical exam with emphasis on the defect size, level, tissue covering, and if there is any cerebral spine fluid (CSF) leakage. The most common lesion is in the lumbosacral area, which may leave the child able to walk. Neurologic symptoms should be assessed as well as fontanelles on the newborn to examine for hydrocephalus (Rosenblum, 2014).

Management

Research is currently being done using fetal surgery to try to correct or lessen the defect in utero. When a child is first born with spina bifida, he or she is evaluated by a team of specialists and surgery is done to cover an open defect. A temporary or permanent vesicostomy may be done to provide an outlet for urine. A vesicostomy is created by the surgeon who makes a stoma from the bladder to the abdominal wall for the release of urine. Appendicovesicostomy (APV), ileal or colon conduit, may be surgically created when the child is school age for a self-catheterizable urinary stoma. In addition, if the patient has severe constipation and/or to promote independence by not having to wear diapers and/or utilize enemas, a patient may have colostomy surgery. Spina bifida requires a team approach, and many large medical centers or children's hospitals have a multidisciplinary spina bifida clinic.

Construction and Management of Pediatric Urinary Diversions

These are discussed in detail in Chapter 6 and shown in **Figure 14-14**.

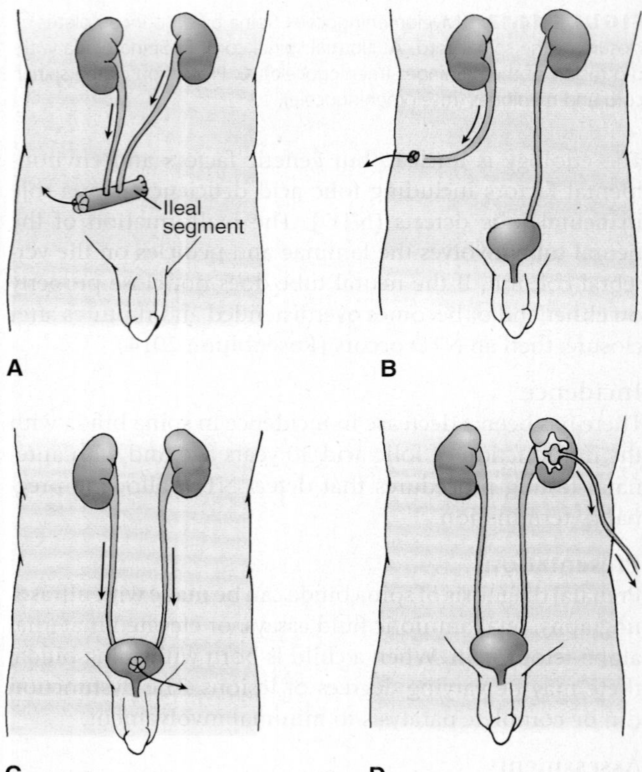

FIGURE 14-14. Pediatric urinary diversions. Types of cutaneous diversions include the conventional ileal conduit (**A**), cutaneous ureterostomy (**B**), vesicostomy (**C**), and nephrostomy (**D**).

Vesicostomy

Vesicostomy is a simple procedure that protects the upper urinary tract, decreases hydronephrosis, and improves kidney function. The bladder is externalized to the abdominal wall so that urine can drain out and not back up in the urinary system (Rouzrokh et al., 2013). This surgery can be performed soon after birth and is often left in place until the child is of school age and can have a catheterizable continent stoma so the patient can be independent. The family will require teaching for peristomal skin care to prevent skin breakdown from constant urine drainage. A diaper that is large enough to cover the vesicostomy can be used to collect the urine. Skin barrier cream is used on the peristomal skin for protection.

Ileovesicostomy

Ileovesicostomy is an effective surgical treatment for patients with neurogenic bladder dysfunction who are unable to perform clean intermittent self-catheterization. Outcomes for ileovesicostomy show improved bladder compliance, reduction of urethral incontinence, and improved quality of life after a successful procedure. Ileovesicostomy surgery is associated with complications in patients with neurogenic bladders with high rates of wound infection (34%), urethral incontinence (28%), and extended hospital length of stay (Vanni et al., 2009). Surgery may be done in open, laparoscopic, or robotic methods. A piece of ileal intestine is removed, and the intestine is sewn back together. The ileal piece is then attached to the bladder and brought to the abdominal wall for the diversion of urine. Refer to WOCN (2011), Surgical indication for fecal diversions (Pediatric ostomy care best practice for clinicians).

Rehabilitative Issues

Support and Education for the Child and Family

It is imperative in pediatrics to provide family-centered care, and the WOC nurse is an invaluable resource for the child and family, as well as other members of the health care team. Whenever possible, the WOC nurse should preoperatively meet the family and then follow the child closely after surgery. From assisting the parents to bonding with their new premature infant with an ostomy, to educating the school nurse of an adolescent with a new and unexpected ostomy, the psychosocial and educational opportunities are limitless. Appendix B lists many support groups. Many busy parents and children enjoy Web sites and chat rooms in order to research in the privacy and convenience of their own home. The Wound Ostomy Continence Nurses Society, Pediatric Ostomy Care: Best Practice for Clinicians (2011) is an invaluable resource for the health care team and may be located on their Web site www.wocn.org.

Developmental Phase and Implications for Care and Education (Age Specific)

Premature Infant/Full-Term Infant

Developmentally, the epidermal barrier is immature and leads to transepidermal water losses and absorption of topical agents through the skin. Premature infants have a weak epidermal and dermal bond, so they are more prone to friction injury and blistering of the skin. There is increased toxicity to chemicals due to immature organs, and nutritional deficiencies should be accounted for due to the immature GI tract. The acid mantle is not developed until day 4 of life, so, younger infants are more prone to invasion of microbes. Fragile skin should be protected, and friction should be minimized. Many of the infant ostomies are temporary and may be closed prior to discharge. For the infant going home with an ostomy, a caregiver should fully demonstrate removing, emptying, and applying an ostomy pouch and explaining the signs and symptoms of complications. The infant will not remember having an ostomy but does experience pain, and the parents need a lot of support bonding and reviewing stoma care and developmentally appropriate care. **Figure 14-15** shows an infant with stoma, and **Figure 14-16** shows an infant with an ostomy pouch.

CLINICAL PEARL

Minimal products should be used on the skin, and manufacturer's guidelines should be followed in regard to age.

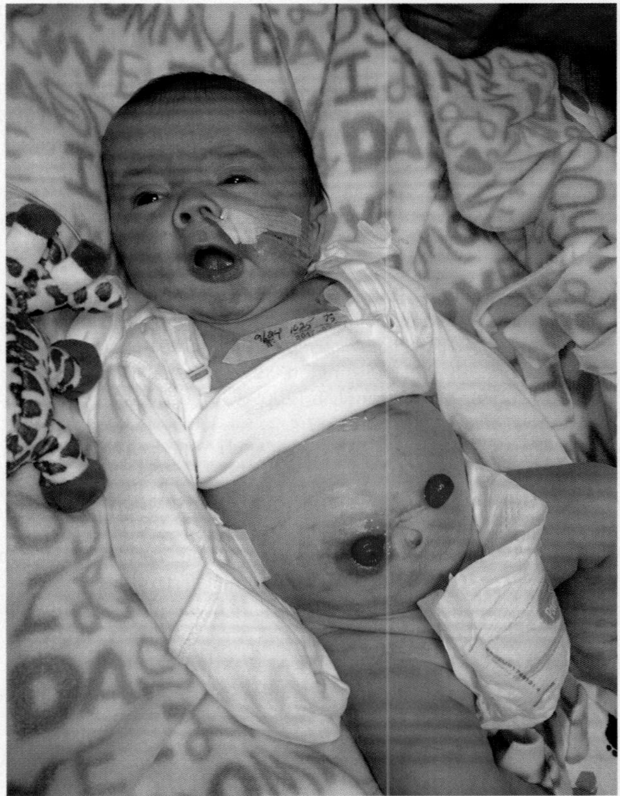

FIGURE 14-15. An infant with stoma.

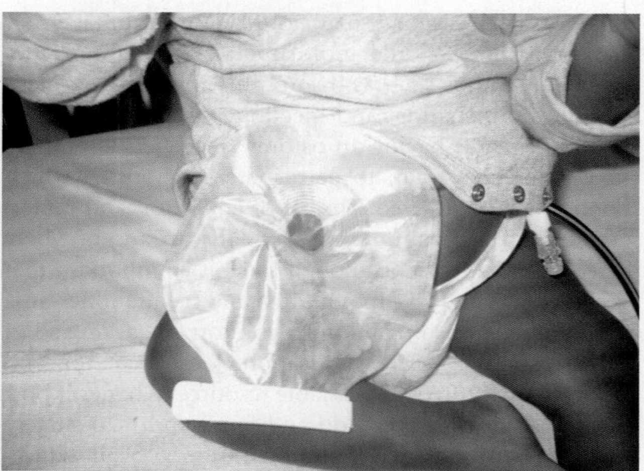

FIGURE 14-16. An infant with ostomy pouch.

Toddler (12 Months to 3 Years) and Preschool (3 to 5 Years)

This age group has a busy and fun time with exploration of the environment and play time is a big part of the child's day. Medical play with dolls and stuffed animals is an effective teaching method with dolls available from some ostomy supply manufacture. Short attention spans should be taken into account when teaching. They are rapidly growing and will have increased improvement with gross motor and fine motor skills, and as their dexterity improves, they can help with more difficult things. Children like to participate and be autonomous. Although the parent or health care provider should change the ostomy pouch, the child can help organize supplies, remove adhesives, and assist per their comfort level. Normal toilet training should take place for urine and stool if not diverted.

School Age (6 to 12 Years)

Advances in cognitive and physical ability should promote independence and support maturity as they grow. They learn readily and enjoy "jobs" as their confidence increases. The older school-aged child can become independent and should participate in overnight sleepovers and camps. Nutrition should be discussed, and the child should participate in meal planning and preparation to help eat nutritious foods for his or her health. They should drink plenty of water and chew food well to prevent blockages.

Adolescent (13 to 18 Years)

Hormonal changes and rapid brain growth during the adolescent years may produce emotional labiality. Extra sensitivity and understanding may be necessary when dealing with this age group. Adolescents can receive full education and should be their own caregivers when dealing with their ostomy with the parents as backup support. Adolescents are very concerned about hygiene, social situations, and sexuality. All of these aspects should be addressed in addition to overall good health, exercise, and nutrition. They may not fully understand their disease process and may rebel or be fearful with this situation. They may participate in risky behaviors at this age and may not plan ahead to take supplies on an outing or order more supplies when running low.

Ostomy camps such as the Youth Rally can be a place for education, sharing, and meeting peers with a similar situation such as having an ostomy. Teenagers appreciate choices and may want to participate in choosing which supplies will be utilized. The art of education and understanding is good communication skills. In an era where there never seems to be enough time, it is important that we slow down and give the children and their families time to form a relationship and to be comfortable asking all of their questions. WOCN publication, Teen Chat: You and Your Ostomy (2013) is a valuable resource. Whenever possible, meeting with the child and family prior to surgery can alleviate some anxiety and be a time to begin education. Stoma siting can be extremely helpful to place the stoma in an appropriate place for anatomical differences and types of clothing the child wears.

Conclusions

There has been a decrease in the number of ostomies performed in childhood with advances in surgical techniques and single-stage procedures. The majority of pediatric stomas are placed during infancy, and they are not usually permanent; a stoma takedown is normally done within 6 weeks to 12 months from the original surgery. However, these patients and especially their families require a large amount of information, education, and emotional support to help them deal with these challenges.

REFERENCES

Aboutanos, M. (2014, June) *Youth gang violence: No lyrics for wounds*. Presented at WOCN 46th Annual Conference, Nashville, TN.

Adibe, O., & Georgeson, K. (2012). Chapter 95: Crohn's disease. In A. G. Coran, N. S. Adzick, T. M. Krummel, et al. (Eds.), *Pediatric surgery* (7th ed., Vol. 1 & 2, pp. 1209–1215). Philadelphia, PA: Elsevier/Saunders.

Adler, J., Coran, A., & Teitelbaum, D. (2012). Chapter 96: Ulcerative colitis. In A. G. Coran, N. S. Adzick, T. M. Krummel, et al. (Eds.), *Pediatric surgery* (7th ed., Vol 1 & 2, pp. 1217–1229). Philadelphia, PA: Elsevier/Saunders.

Applebaum, H., & Sydorak, R. (2012). Chapter 81: Duodenal atresia and stenosis—Annular pancreas. In A. G. Coran, N. S. Adzick, T. M. Krummel, et al. (Eds.), *Pediatric surgery* (7th ed., Vol 1 & 2, pp. 1058–1061). Philadelphia, PA: Elsevier/Saunders.

Aguayo, P., & Ostlie, D. (2010). Chapter 31: Duodenal and intestinal atresia and stenosis. In G. Holcomb & J. Murphy (Eds.), *Ashcraft's pediatric surgery* (5th ed., pp. 400–415). Philadelphia, PA: Saunders/Elsevier.

Caldamone, A., & Woodard, J. (2012). Prune-belly syndrome. In A. Wein (Ed.), *Campbell-Walsh urology* (10th ed., pp. 3310–3324). Philadelphia, PA: Elsevier/Saunders.

Dassinger, M., & Smith, S. (2012). Chapter 86: Disorders of intestinal rotation and fixation. In A. G. Coran, N. S. Adzick, T. M. Krummel, et al. (Eds.), *Pediatric surgery* (7th ed., Vol 1 & 2, pp. 1111–1126). Philadelphia, PA: Elsevier/Saunders.

Gauderer, M. (2012). Chapter 98: Stomas of the small and large intestine. In A. G. Coran, N. S. Adzick, T. M. Krummel, et al. (Eds.), *Pediatric surgery* (7th ed., Vol 1 & 2, pp. 1058–1061). Philadelphia, PA: Elsevier/Saunders.

Georgeson, K. (2010). Chapter 35: Hirschsprung's disease. In G. W. Holcomb & J. P. Murphy (Eds.), *Ashcraft's pediatric surgery* (5th ed., pp. 456–467). Philadelphia, PA: Saunders/Elsevier.

Guardino, K., & Pieper, P. (2013). Chapter 20: Anorectal malformations in children. In N. Browne, L. Flanigan, C. McComiskey, et al. (Eds.), *Nursing care of the pediatric surgical patient* (3rd ed., pp. 359–372). Burlington, MA: Jones & Bartlett Learning.

Holder, M., & Jackson, L. (2013). Chapter 19: Hirschsprung's disease. In N. Browne, L. Flanigan, C. McComiskey, et al. (Eds.), *Nursing care of the pediatric surgical patient* (3rd ed., pp. 347–356). Burlington, MA: Jones & Bartlett Learning.

Little, D., & Smith, S. (2010). Chapter 32: Malrotation. In G. Holcomb & J. Murphy (Eds.), *Ashcraft's pediatric surgery* (5th ed., pp. 416–424). Philadelphia, PA: Saunders/Elsevier.

Lucas, A., & Cole, T. (1990). Breast milk and neonatal necrotizing enterocolitis. *Lancet, 336*, 1519–1523.

McIltrot, K., & Wilson, L. (2014). Chapter 18: The child with altered gastrointestinal status. In V. Bowden & C. Greenberg (Eds.), *Children and their families: The continuum of nursing care* (pp. 783–874). Philadelphia, PA: Lippincott Williams & Wilkins.

McKenna, C., & Pieper, P. (2013). Chapter 31: Pediatric trauma. In N. Browne, L. Flanigan, C. McComiskey, et al. (Eds.), *Nursing care of the pediatric surgical patient* (3rd ed., pp. 513–538). Burlington, MA: Jones & Bartlett Learning.

Moir, C. (2010). Chapter 42: Inflammatory bowel disease and intestinal cancer. In G. Holcomb & J. Murphy (Eds.), *Ashcraft's pediatric surgery* (5th ed., pp. 532–548). Philadelphia, PA: Saunders/Elsevier.

Rapoport, K., & Nishii, E. K. (2013). Chapter 16: Necrotizing enterocolitis. In N. Browne, L. Flanigan, C. McComiskey, et al. (Eds.), *Nursing care of the pediatric surgical patient* (3rd ed., pp. 295–311). Burlington, MA: Jones & Bartlett Learning.

Richardson, L., Banerjee, S., & Heike, R. (2006). What is the evidence in the practice of mucous fistula re-feeding in neonates with short bowel syndrome. *Journal of Pediatric Gastroenterology & Nutrition*, 43 (2): 267–270.

Rosenblum, R. (2014). The child with altered neurologic status. In V. Bowden & C. Greenberg (Eds.), *Children and their families: The continuum of nursing care* (pp. 1021–1103). Philadelphia, PA: Lippincott Williams & Wilkins.

Rouzrokh, M., Mirshemirani, A., Khaleghnejah-Tabaii, A., et al. (2013). Protective temporary vesicostomy for upper urinary tract problems in children. *Iranian Journal of Pediatrics, 23*(6), 648–652.

Stellar, J., & Widmer, T. (2013). Chapter 17: Intestinal atresia, duplications and meconium ileus. In N. Browne, L. Flanigan, C. McComiskey, et al. (Eds.), *Nursing care of the pediatric surgical patient* (3rd ed., pp. 313–329). Burlington, MA: Jones & Bartlett Learning.

Vanni, A., Cohen, M., & Stoffel, J. (2009). Robotic-assisted ileovesicostomy. *Urology, 74*(4), 814–818.

WOCN (2011). Pediatric ostomy care: Best practice for clinicians. Mount Laurel, NJ: Author.

WOCN (2013). Teen chat: You and your ostomy. Mount Laurel, NJ: Author.

Zerpa, J., & Shapiro, T. (2013). Malrotation and volvulus. In N. Browne, L. Flanigan, C. McComiskey, et al. (Eds.), *Nursing care of the pediatric surgical patient* (3rd ed., pp. 333–344). Burlington, MA: Jones & Bartlett Learning.

QUESTIONS

1. What neonatal condition generally necessitates the creation of an ileostomy?
   A. Necrotizing enterocolitis
   B. Colonic atresia
   C. Severe perineal trauma
   D. Pelvic malformation

2. What finding would alert the WOC nurse of a possible intestinal obstruction in an infant?
   A. Gastroesophageal reflux disease
   B. Hypoxemia of the bowel
   C. Thrombocytopenia
   D. Bilious emesis

3. A neonate is diagnosed with malrotation. What life-threatening complication of malrotation may occur where torsion occurs?
   A. Necrotizing enterocolitis
   B. Meconium ileus
   C. Prune belly syndrome
   D. Volvulus

4. A neonate is diagnosed with imperforate anus. For what surgical intervention would the WOC nurse prepare the parents?
   A. Urologic surgery
   B. Anoplasty
   C. General surgery
   D. Creation of an ostomy

5. The nurse is caring for a neonate who failed to pass meconium in the first 48 hours after birth. Upon assessment, the nurse notes a distended abdomen, emesis, and sepsis. What condition would the nurse suspect?
   A. Necrotizing enterocolitis
   B. Hirschsprung's disease
   C. Meconium ileus
   D. Inflammatory bowel disease

6. An 8-year-old female patient is diagnosed with Crohn disease following symptoms of weight loss, bloody diarrhea, abdominal pain, and perianal disease. What should be the priority management goal for this patient?
   A. Surgical resection of the bowel
   B. Medical therapy to achieve remission of the disease
   C. Immediate strictureplasty
   D. Radiation therapy

7. A 10-year-old male patient presents with the following symptoms: intermittent abdominal cramping, pain, tenesmus, fatigue, and anemia. Osteopenia, weight loss, and anorexia with growth retardation are also noted. What condition would the WOC nurse suspect?
   A. Ulcerative colitis
   B. Familial polyposis syndrome
   C. Crohn disease
   D. Inflammatory bowel disease

8. An infant is diagnosed with prune belly syndrome. Which symptom is NOT characteristic of this disorder?
   A. Blood in the stool
   B. Absence of abdominal muscles
   C. Dilation of the upper urinary tract
   D. Clubfeet

9. Which of the following would be the best to recommend for an active toddler to prevent dislodgement of the pouch?
   A. Use one-piece pouch system.
   B. Use a diaper instead of a pouch.
   C. Dress in clothing that has snap crotch.
   D. Restrict active playtime.

10. An infant is diagnosed with myelomeningocele (spina bifida). For what surgery would the wound care nurse prepare the family of this patient?
    A. Colostomy during the first year of life
    B. Appendicovesicostomy at age 2
    C. Vesicostomy
    D. Ileal or colon conduit created when an adolescent/adult

ANSWERS: 1.**A**, 2.**D**, 3.**D**, 4.**B**, 5.**C**, 6.**B**, 7.**A**, 8.**A**, 9.**C**, 10.**C**

CHAPTER 15

Peristomal Skin Conditions

Ginger Salvadalena

OBJECTIVE

Distinguish between peristomal skin conditions and select the associated management strategies.

Topic Outline

The focus of this chapter is peristomal skin conditions. Presented first is information about the scope of the problem, followed by general guidelines for assessment and management of patients who present with peristomal skin conditions. The remainder of the chapter covers specific types of conditions, including their etiology, clinical presentation, assessment, and management.

Scope of the Problem

Peristomal skin problems are common, and they are clinically challenging to prevent and to manage. In prospective studies, the incidence of peristomal skin complications ranged from 29% to 63% (Arumugam et al., 2003; Lindholm et al., 2013; Persson et al., 2010; Salvadalena, 2013). Although individuals with stomas are often unaware that they have a skin problem (Herlufsen et al., 2006; Lyon et al., 2000; Nybaek et al., 2009), peristomal skin issues were shown in a recent study to be the cause of over 30% of the visits to an outpatient stoma clinic (Jemec & Nybaek, 2008). Skin problems cause pain, contribute to higher product usage, adversely affect life satisfaction, and may raise health care costs (Meisner et al., 2012; Nichols & Riemer, 2011; Pittman et al., 2008). Clearly, maintaining and restoring the integrity of the peristomal skin has important implications.

CLINICAL PEARL

Peristomal complications are those that occur in the immediate peristomal area.

The peristomal skin is exposed to mechanical, chemical, and microbial threats on an ongoing basis (Alvey & Beck, 2008). Mechanical threats include abrasion, skin stripping, and pressure injury that can occur due to the use of ostomy skin barriers, tapes, and accessories. The physical forces involved in repeated removal of adhesive products can strip away varying amounts of stratum corneum, pull away hair, and even change the architecture of the skin. Peristomal skin becomes thicker and has higher transepidermal water loss compared to healthy contralateral skin (Nybaek et al., 2010); characteristic changes in the structure of the skin have been identified and vary by the type of skin barrier used for stoma care (Omura et al., 2010).

While there are a number of chemical threats to the peristomal skin, the most noxious is the effluent draining from the stoma; it provides a constant source of moisture, can cause inflammation, and, in the case of an ileostomy, contains enzymes that can damage the skin. Difficulty obtaining the proper fit or size of skin barrier can allow the effluent from the stoma to drain between the skin barrier and the skin, underscoring the importance of carefully selecting of an appropriate stoma site and providing thorough postoperative instruction about ostomy care. Even appropriately selected and applied topical products carry some risk. Products used for stoma care contain a variety of ingredients that may be sensitizing or cause skin irritation, and their selection and application should be done with attention to their intended use and a clear understanding of the patient's individual needs, history, and risk factors.

Peristomal skin is warm and may be moist, increasing its vulnerability to pathogens (Cutting & White, 2002). Pathogens normally present on the skin can proliferate producing infection; the ones that most commonly occur are fungal or bacterial. Moist skin is more susceptible than dry skin to pressure-induced skin damage and reductions in regional blood flow (Mayrovitz & Sims, 2001); thus, the risks for skin problems are likely to be intensified in the presence of leakage. Complicating the mechanical, chemical, and microbial threats are the influences of the host environment: the health conditions of the individual who has the stoma, his or her age, self-care status, and other individual factors impacting his or her risk of illness.

Assessment Guidelines

The general approach to peristomal skin assessment is similar across a variety of skin conditions. Begin the assessment by taking a problem-focused history. Include the following: when and how the problem started, description of the problem, signs and symptoms, what has been done to manage it, and any prior episodes of similar problems. Ask about pouching system wear time (usual and current), presence of any leakage (usual and current), peristomal pain, pruritus, and any other sensations in the area of the skin condition. Review the patient's general health history, allergies, and medications. Ask the patient to describe or list each of the products he or she is using for ostomy care, how it is being applied, and the duration of use.

Begin the physical examination *before* the pouching system has been removed, if possible. Note how the pouching system has been applied, its security, and any areas of leakage, tension, channeling, or pressure. After removing the skin barrier and *before* discarding it, look at the adhesive/skin side of the barrier. Under good lighting, look at the barrier for any signs of erosion, noting its location and any evidence of leakage. The barrier provides important clues about the location of leakage of effluent onto the peristomal skin. When the pouching system has been completely removed (and discarded), examine the peristomal skin in the presence of good lighting. For the purposes of this discussion, the peristomal skin is defined as the area of skin surrounding the stoma that had contact with the skin barrier of the pouching system. For adults, this area is typically 4 inches or less in diameter. Cleanse the skin to allow a thorough evaluation of the peristomal skin. Note the color and condition of the skin. Normal peristomal skin is free of any damage, that is, the skin is unbroken and rash-free. Variations in pigmentation may occur, particularly in individuals with resolving dermatitis and those with darker skin tones (Williams & Lyon, 2010). Lift the stoma to allow visualization of the skin beneath the lower edge of the mucosa, if needed. Palpate any bumps or nodules. Note any areas of localized redness or warmth in the peristomal skin. Note the skin integrity. If wounds are present, measure their size and depth and note their location in relationship to the stoma. If a rash is present, note the type and distribution. A photograph may be useful for documentation and for future comparison purposes.

If the fit of the pouching system is in question, assess the stoma, peristomal skin, and peristomal contours in lying and sitting positions. Look for incisions or scars in the area of the stoma or beneath the skin barrier as these can cause irregular pouching surface and contribute to skin creases and leakage. New incisions may produce drainage that undermines adhesive skin barriers. Measure the size of the stoma. Compare the result to the size the patient has been using to determine whether the skin barrier has been appropriately sized for the stoma. Is the shape of the pouching system or barrier (flat or convex) appropriate for the contour of the peristomal skin? Is the pouching system flexible enough to move with the contours and/or firm enough to keep creases or folds from forming? A careful evaluation and critical appraisal of the patient's situation are important at each encounter.

Guidelines for Management of Peristomal Skin Conditions

The general guideline for managing peristomal skin conditions is to first determine and treat the cause of the peristomal skin condition and identify and address any possible contributing factors. For example, the patient may need to use a different sized barrier opening or change the barrier more or less frequently. The patient may also require a specific type of topical therapy to treat the underlying disorder, manage moisture, or protect healing skin. Generally, products applied for topical therapy of peristomal skin conditions should be used for a limited period of time, only until the condition resolves. Provide patient education about the management plan, including the suspected etiology of the skin condition and how it is managed, how to apply and use any new products, when to discontinue the treatments, and when to return for follow-up care. Finally, consider whether consultations with other health professionals are needed. Multidisciplinary care is important in the management of patients with unusual peristomal skin complications and ones that fail to improve with usual care. Referrals may include surgeons, dermatologists, gastroenterologists, general practitioners, oncologists, and others depending on the type of complications that are encountered.

The overall goal with any peristomal skin condition is to promote healing while maintaining adequate wear time of the pouching system. When the cause of the skin problem is not known, optimize the pouching system, refer the patient for further diagnosis and treatment, and provide patient education about self-care and completing the next steps in the management plan. The following sections will cover additional information about specific peristomal skin conditions, beginning with the most common, those associated with moisture-related skin damage.

Specific Peristomal Skin Conditions

Peristomal Moisture–Associated Skin Damage

Peristomal moisture–associated skin damage (MASD) is a broad category of skin complication that includes several conditions (irritant dermatitis, maceration, and pseudoverrucous lesions). Peristomal MASD is defined as inflammation and erosion of the skin adjacent to the stoma, associated with exposure to effluent such as urine or stool (Colwell et al., 2011; Gray et al., 2013). The affected area typically begins at the stoma–skin junction and can extend outward. Other terms that have previously been used to describe this type of skin problem have included irritant dermatitis, irritant contact dermatitis, and peristomal dermatitis. Peristomal MASD can develop quickly, particularly in patients who have highly corrosive effluent, such as with an ileostomy. While the principal cause is prolonged exposure to stoma effluent, other moisture sources (perspiration, swimming, use of hot tubs, etc.) can also contribute to the development of peristomal MASD.

Peristomal MASD presents as an area of erythema adjacent to the stoma (red hues in light-skinned individuals, or discoloration in darker skin), which may be accompanied by superficial skin loss. The skin loss may be uniform or patchy, and the edges may be well defined or irregular. The affected area mirrors the pattern of exposure of the skin to stoma effluent. If chronic, hyperkeratosis and scarring can contribute to stoma stenosis at the skin level, particularly with urostomy (Farnham & Cookson, 2004). **Figures 15-1** through **15-4** display peristomal MASD associated with leakage. In extreme cases where leaking pouching systems have gone unchanged for a long period of time, the effluent can track into skin folds or dependent areas leaving erythema and skin loss over a large area. The patient with peristomal MASD often reports stinging pain, especially when anything touches the area, including stoma effluent. The patient usually reports difficulty getting the pouching system to adhere.

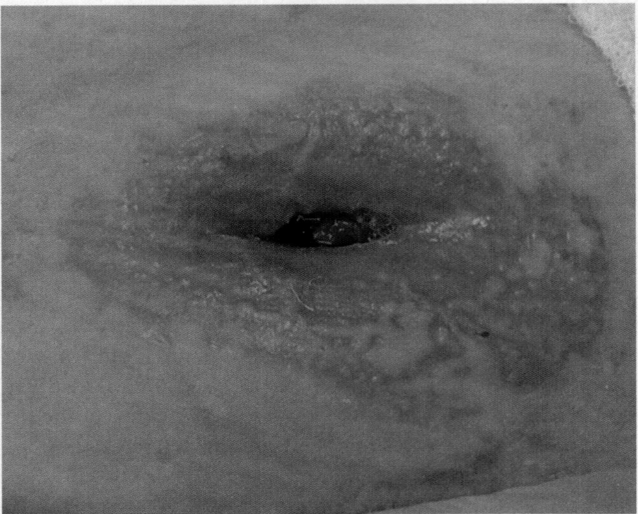

FIGURE 15-1. Irritant dermatitis around a retracted ileostomy stoma where leakage had undermined the skin barrier.

Management of peristomal MASD includes identifying and correcting the cause of the leakage; this may include resizing the skin barrier, modifying the pouching system as appropriate, and selecting accessories that can improve

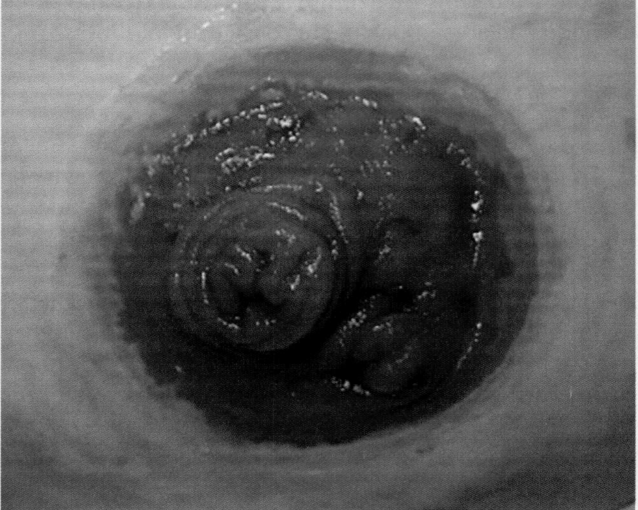

FIGURE 15-2. Irritant dermatitis around a loop stoma where the skin barrier opening was too large.

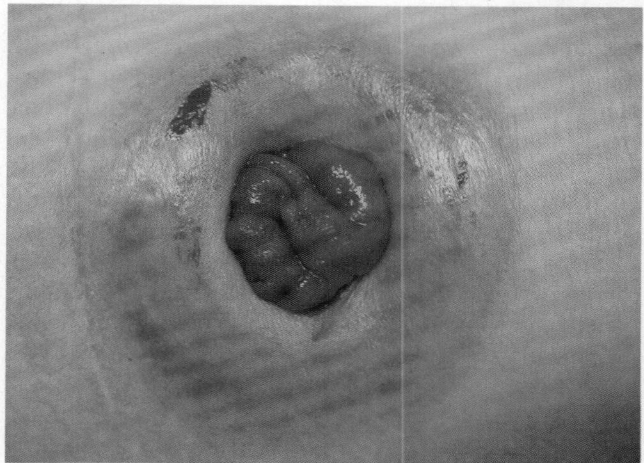

FIGURE 15-3. Irritant dermatitis with patchy areas of skin loss.

the seal of the pouching system to the contours of the patient's abdomen. Manage contributing factors such as excess perspiration and external sources of moisture as appropriate; keep nearby skin folds clean and dry; and dry all aspects of the pouching system after exposure to water from baths, showers, and water sports. Topical care of the affected area usually consists of applying stoma powder to help absorb excess moisture from the areas of damaged skin and provide a dry surface on which the barrier can adhere. A skin barrier film may be applied over the powder and allowed to dry before the pouching system is applied; multiple layers may be added in a process known as "crusting" (Doughty, 2005; Seungmi et al., 2011). If the area of skin damage is large or highly exuding, it may be helpful to apply a thin hydrocolloid sheet dressing before applying the pouching system.

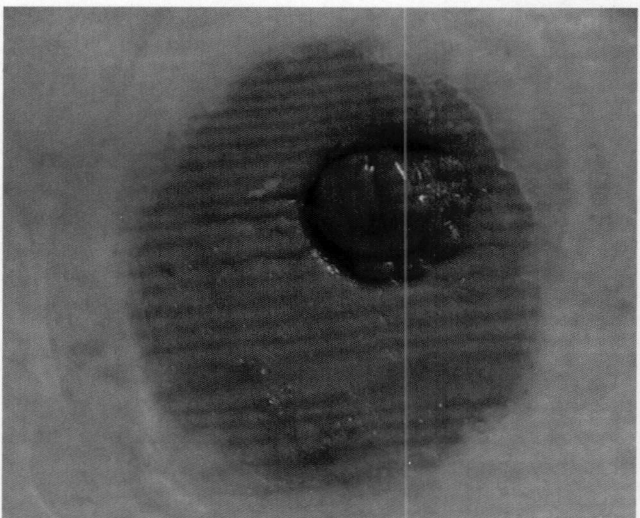

FIGURE 15-4. Irritant dermatitis with even area of partial-thickness skin loss.

Provide the patient with information about the etiology and contributing factors for peristomal MASD, and directions about how to use products. Provide guidance about the frequency of pouch changes, which may need to be done more frequently until the skin has healed. Remind the patient that normal peristomal skin is intact and to seek care if skin problems do not resolve quickly.

Maceration

Maceration presents as soft moist skin that appears waterlogged; it may be whiter or lighter in color than is the skin next to it. The softening of tissue results in increased susceptibility to the damaging effects of friction and irritants (McNichol et al., 2013). **Figure 15-5** illustrates maceration surrounding a leg wound caused by a wet dressing.

Macerated peristomal skin is most common with urostomy stomas, but it can also occur with other stoma types. The patient may present with complaints of pouch leakage or short wear time, or may report that the skin around the stoma appears unusual. This finding is also consistent with patients who are cutting the opening on the skin barrier larger than the stoma size, which allows urine to pool against the peristomal skin.

Management techniques should be directed toward reducing moisture where it is causing the skin to be overhydrated. If urine is pooling around the stoma ensure that the skin barrier opening is sized properly and that the shape of the barrier is preventing urine from getting between the barrier and the skin. Addition of convexity or accessory products (barrier strips, rings, or a stoma belt) may be indicated. Consider whether use of a night drainage bag would help reduce pooling of urine around the stoma during sleep. A barrier film can be applied to the skin to help prevent external moisture from hydrating the skin. If the macerated area is beneath the entire barrier, simply changing the skin barrier more often may suffice. Maceration at the outside edges of the skin barrier or under the tape borders can be reduced by drying the pouching system after swimming and bathing to keep moisture from pooling against the skin and by applying a barrier film to

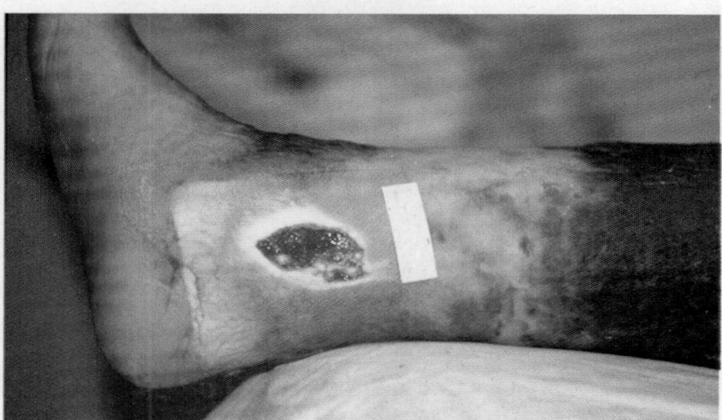

FIGURE 15-5. Periwound maceration related to a wet dressing.

the skin before applying the pouching system. Identify the cause and contributing factors for the maceration; discuss options with the patient, and provide instructions about how to implement the solutions.

CLINICAL PEARL

Use of a hair dryer on a low setting can assist in drying tape borders after swimming or bathing.

Pseudoverrucous Lesions

The term pseudoverrucous lesion refers to an exuberant growth of benign papules that occurs around a stoma when urine or stool irritates the skin. This condition is a type of chronic irritant contact dermatitis that is thought to develop as a result of prolonged exposure to liquid stool and/or urine; it is also sometimes seen in the diaper area during childhood (Fernández et al., 2010). The inflammatory response to the irritant causes thickening and elevation of skin layers next to the stoma. Other terms used to describe this condition are chronic papillomatous dermatitis (CPD), peristomal epitheliomatous hyperplasia (PEH), and pseudoverrucous papules and nodules (PPN). The lesions are often wart-like in appearance, and when biopsied, the lesions have a papillomatous histological appearance with acanthosis, lengthened rete ridges, hyperkeratosis, and dermal inflammation (Williams & Lyon, 2010). One example is shown in **Figure 15-6**. Another condition commonly associated with urostomy and often found in the presence of pseudoverrucous lesions is alkaline encrustation (Szymanski et al., 2010). Crystal deposition occurs when the urine is alkaline and concentrated, and it may be associated with urinary tract infections and renal calculi.

Assessment

The patient presents with a thickened, bumpy, or irregular area that may be higher than the rest of the skin around it, and may appear different in color than the surrounding skin (white, gray, brown, or dark red). The affected area is next to the stoma, where effluent has been in contact with the skin. The patient may report that the lesions itch or that bleeding is seen. Pseudoverrucous lesions often become eroded and tender. Assess the location, distribution, and appearance of the affected area. Gently probe the lesions. Encrustations will feel hard or gritty. Inquire about the product wear time and leakage and confirm appropriate sizing of the skin barrier. Inspect the skin barrier for indications of leakage. If a urostomy, ask the patient about the pattern and volume of fluid intake and determine whether the pouching system has an antireflux valve.

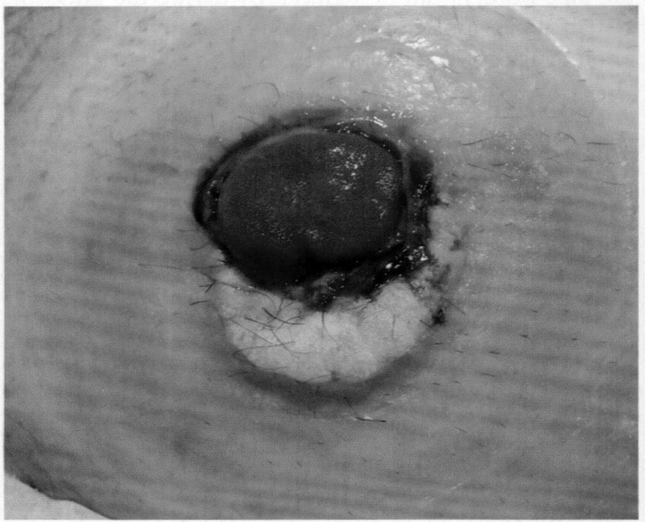

FIGURE 15-6. Pseudoverrucous lesions beneath a urostomy stoma.

Management

The primary aim is to prevent contact of the stoma effluent with the affected area, which will lead to resolution of the condition. Confirm appropriate skin barrier opening size, modify the pouching system to provide a leak-free fit, and change the pouching system frequently enough to prevent leakage or pooling of urine on the skin. Confirm that the urostomy pouch has antireflux, and that the patient is emptying the pouch before the fluid level reaches the level of the stoma (even at night). If urostomy, discuss using a night drainage bag.

If the lesions are elevated and they interfere with getting a good seal between skin barrier and skin, cautery with silver nitrate may be helpful. Several weekly applications may be required. Apply stoma powder to the lesions to absorb excess moisture and to provide a dry adhesion surface. If urostomy, recommend ways to lower the pH of the urine (increase fluid intake; consider adding cranberry juice or cranberry tablets to the diet). If urine encrustations are also present, discuss increasing fluid intake, acidifying the urine, and applying dilute (30% to 50%) vinegar solution to the affected area for 20 minutes when the skin barrier is off for pouching system changes.

Refer the patient if there is no improvement with usual care or in cases where the etiology of the lesions is unclear. Additional diagnostics will include microbiological culture and skin biopsy.

Mechanical Damage

Mechanical damage can result from a variety of causes. When the peristomal skin is injured due to mechanical damage, it often presents as a defined area of skin loss or skin discoloration in a distinct area inconsistent with leakage of stoma effluent. The most common types of mechanical damage seen in the peristomal area are medical adhesive–related skin injuries and pressure ulcers.

Medical adhesive–related skin injuries are common and can occur with any medical product that sticks to the skin, thus, they also occur in the peristomal area. Medical adhesive–related skin injuries are defined as occurrences in which erythema and/or other manifestation such as a blister, tear, or other injury persists more than 30 minutes after the removal of a medical adhesive product (McNichol et al., 2013).

Some of the causes of this condition are preventable, such overuse of tackifiers and bonding agents, improper application of tapes, wrong type of tapes, and repeated application and removal of adhesive products in a short period of time. Other risk factors include extremes in ages, preexisting health conditions (diabetes mellitus, dermatologic conditions, use of immunosuppressive medications and treatments, etc.), malnutrition, and dry or damaged skin. **Figure 15-7** displays peristomal skin with an area of mechanical damage associated with improper removal of a tape bordered skin barrier.

The patient with a peristomal medical adhesive–related skin injury presents with a defined area of skin damage beneath the adhesive portion of the pouching system; it is usually *not* adjacent to the stoma but found further away from the stoma. The patient often reports that the area is painful and moisture from the wound causes the barrier or tape to lift from the skin.

Inquire about the history of the injury and how it occurred. Ask about prior management of the wound and response to date. Gently remove the pouching system and any residual skin barrier. Generally, these types of wounds can be assessed and categorized as partial or full thickness, and measured for length and width. Note the location of the wound relative to the stoma.

Management consists of identifying the cause of the injury and providing patient teaching about how to prevent it from occurring in the future. Modify the pouching system as indicated, and apply a topical product that absorbs exudate and allows the pouching system to adhere while the wound heals. Use products such as adhesive removers, skin barrier sheets, and no-sting skin sealants to ease the application and removal of topical products to the affected area.

Pressure Ulcers

Detection of medical device–related pressure ulcers has increased over the past several years, in part due to increased awareness of the risks of skin injury (Fletcher, 2012). In ostomy care, pressure ulcers are more likely when belts, binders, and firm convex flanges are pressing against the skin for a prolonged period of time. Peristomal pressure ulcers are thought to be more common among patients who have peristomal hernias, perhaps due to the use of convexity and other products that hold products firmly against the body. The clinical presentation of a peristomal pressure ulcer is a partial- or full-thickness wound in an area where there is product-related pressure or friction. A pressure ulcer caused by convexity is shown in **Figure 15-8**. The patient with a peristomal pressure ulcer may complain of pain, and may report that drainage from the wound is interfering with the adherence of the skin barrier and pouching system.

Assessment consists of evaluation of the patient in sitting, standing, and reclining positions in order to determine the forces present between the skin, the pouching products, and any accessories such as belt and closures. The skin is evaluated for changes in color and integrity, and the length, width, and depth of wounds are measured. Management of peristomal pressure ulcers consists of identifying and removing the cause of the pressure, treating the wound while it heals, and providing an alternative pouching system for the patient. Teach the patient how to care for the wound while it is healing, and how to use the new pouching system. Describe the cause of the injury and why it is important to avoid use of the type of product that created the pressure (or how to use it differently so it won't create injury).

Allergic Contact Dermatitis

Expert WOC Nurses define peristomal allergic contact dermatitis as an inflammatory skin response resulting from hypersensitivity to chemical elements (Colwell & Beitz, 2007). When peristomal skin irritation occurs, patients and clinicians often suspect allergy; however, confirmed allergic contact dermatitis is rare (Al-Niaimi et al., 2012;

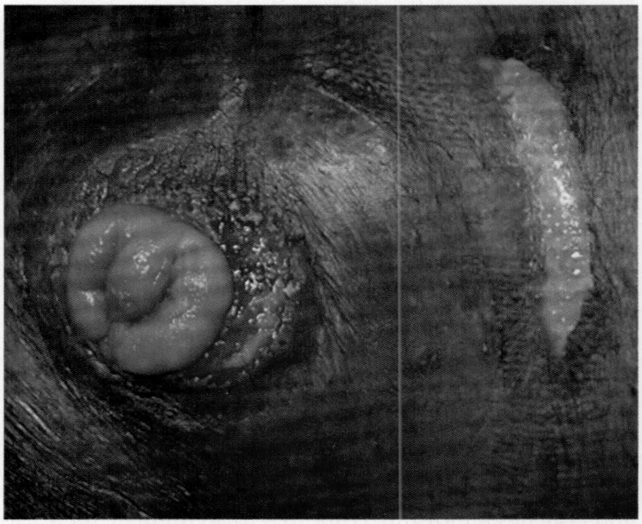

FIGURE 15-7. Peristomal skin tear is shown several inches from the stoma.

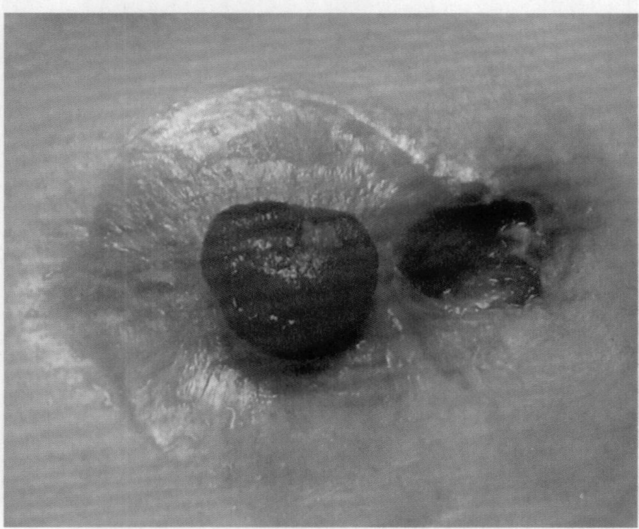

FIGURE 15-8. Peristomal pressure ulcer due to convexity.

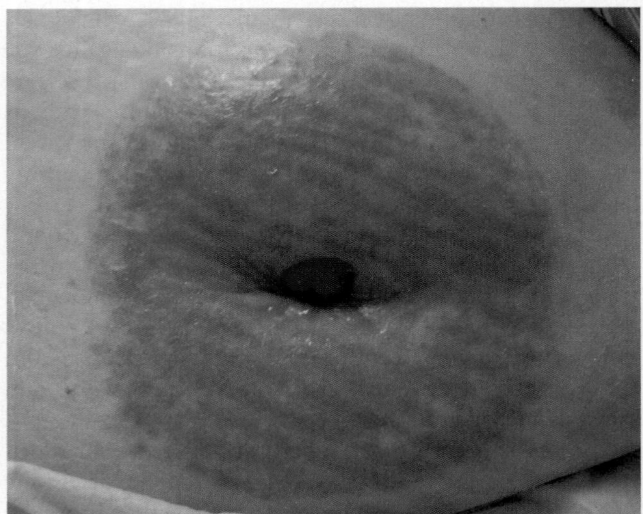

FIGURE 15-9. Allergic contact dermatitis.

Martin et al., 2005). Allergens found to have been involved with peristomal allergic contact dermatitis are components of tapes or skin barriers, dyes, perfumes, preservatives, soaps, and lotions.

Allergic contact dermatitis presents as erythema that may be accompanied by blisters, which are unroofed when the pouching system is removed. Figures 15-9 and 15-10 provide examples of peristomal allergic contact dermatitis. Typically, the affected area at first mirrors the area of contact with the allergen, but as the inflammation progresses the area enlarges, making the original contact area hard to discern. The patient often complains of intense pruritus and may report difficulty with pouch adherence because of the moisture coming from the blistering dermatitis. Ask about all products used on the skin (including soaps, lotions, wipes, and stoma products) and in the pouching system (e.g., lubricants and deodorizers). Ask about prior history of contact allergies, atopic dermatitis, and product sensitivities. Assess the affected area, noting the distribution and characteristics of the condition (rash, peeling, blisters, fissures, etc.). Note any signs of secondary infection. Identify whether the affected area is associated with one or more specific product application areas.

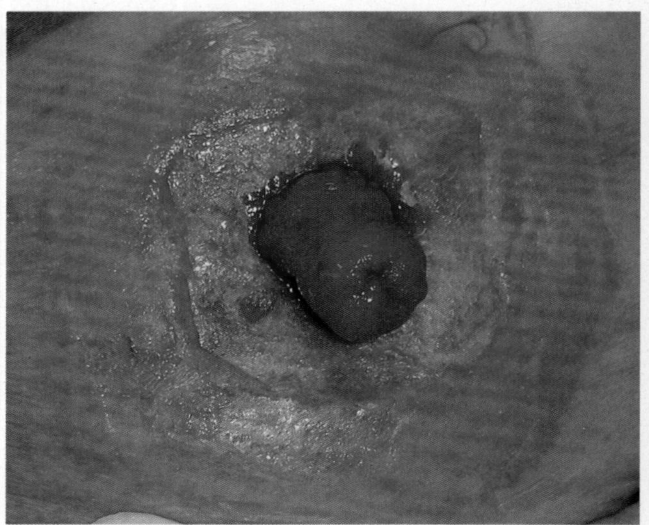

FIGURE 15-10. Allergic contact dermatitis.

Management of allergic contact dermatitis consists primarily of identifying and removing the allergen. In some cases, a simple product change can be made without a full workup, such as using barrier-only products if tape sensitivity is reported. Patch testing using standard dermatologic skin test kits and the patient's products is useful to identify allergens (Landis et al., 2012). Ostomy product manufacturers may provide information about product components upon specific request for assistance in identification of options for patients with specific needs, and a list of chemical ingredients for stoma products was compiled and presented in a recent publication about patch testing in peristomal dermatitis (Al-Niaimi et al., 2012).

Until the dermatitis resolves, a topical corticosteroid spray is often needed to reduce inflammation and provide symptomatic relief. Select products such as sprays that do not impair pouch adhesion, and discontinue use as soon as the condition resolves. Treat secondary infection, if present. If the affected area must be covered by the pouching system, manage excess moisture by applying stoma powder to provide a dry pouching surface. Check skin barrier opening size, modify the pouching system if needed, and alter the frequency of pouching system changes to ensure that the affected area does not become exposed to stoma effluent.

Refer the patient to a dermatologist if standard patch testing is needed, if the source of the skin problem is unclear, or if it persists. Collaborate with consulting providers about appropriate forms of topical medication to ensure that the prescriptive products will be compatible with use of adhesive barrier products changed once or twice a week. Teach the patient about the source of the problem, avoidance of the allergen, how to use any new topical medications, and when to discontinue their use.

Fungal/Candidiasis Infection

Candida albicans is one of the many opportunistic fungal pathogens that are part of the normal microflora in the digestive tract and on the skin; this species accounts for up to 75% of all *Candida* skin infections (Jenkinson & Douglas, 2002). Patients who have had recent treatment with antibiotics are at higher risk to develop cutaneous candidiasis, as are those who are immunosuppressed, who have diabetes mellitus, and who have had corticosteroid therapy or chemotherapy. The infection presents as erythema with a maculopapular rash accompanied by satellite lesions. A typical presentation is shown in Figure 15-11. Fungal rashes start in moist areas; thus, they tend to occur beneath the skin barrier and sometimes beneath tape-bordered products and pouches if moisture is allowed to accumulate there following showers and baths. As the condition worsens, the

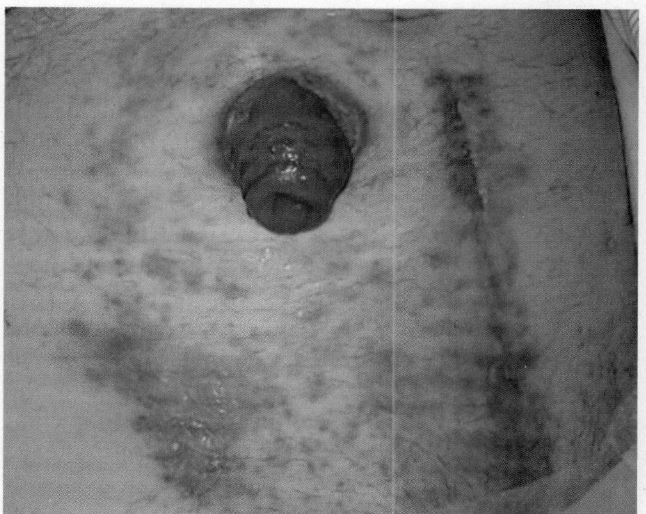

FIGURE 15-11. Peristomal candidiasis.

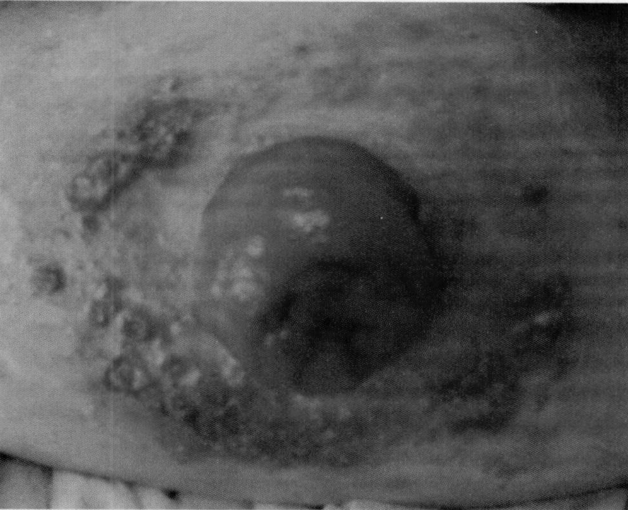

FIGURE 15-12. Complex peristomal skin infection requiring microbial cultures and antibiotics.

inflammation causes extensive redness, the lesions coalesce, and the rash extends to a broader area. The patient usually complains of intense pruritus, a desire to scratch and sometimes to want to remove his or her pouching system. Patients with peristomal candidiasis may have it in other locations, particularly skin folds or creases. Inquire about recent use of antibiotics or immunosuppressive medications that are known to increase risk. Assess the location and extent of the rash, and look at the back of the skin barrier for signs of leakage.

Treatment for peristomal candidiasis includes gentle cleansing of the affected area, drying the skin, and applying a topical antifungal agent. Antifungal powders are dusted onto the affected area; this may be followed by the application of a skin barrier film. After the film dries, the pouching system is applied. Optimize the size of the opening and the fit of the pouching system to prevent leakage of stoma effluent onto the skin (to reduce any sources of moisture that contribute to growth of pathogens).

Teach the patient to thoroughly dry the skin barrier, pouching system, and any tape borders after showers and/or bathing to reduce moisture against the skin. Patients with complicated infections and those with immunosuppression or failure to respond to usual care should be referred for further diagnostics and treatment. An example of a polymicrobial infection of the peristomal skin that required referral is shown in **Figure 15-12**.

Folliculitis

Defined as hair follicle inflammation (Alvey & Beck, 2008); folliculitis typically develops when there is inflammation due to injury or infection (Napierkowski, 2013). **Figure 15-13** displays folliculitis of the torso. In the case of peristomal skin, the mechanism of injury may be multidirectional shaving or pulling of hair when the adhesive skin barrier is removed, followed by secondary infection with gram-positive bacteria such as *Staphylococcus* and *Streptococcus*. The clinical presentation is redness and pustules around the hair follicles under the skin barrier of the pouching system, as shown in **Figure 15-14**. The patient may report that the area is tender to touch, and skin barrier removal is painful. Instruct the patient to clip hair or shave in the direction of hair removal, decrease the frequency of shaving (Lyon, 2010a, 2010b), use an electric shaver, or use a chemical depilatory (Woo et al., 2009). Topical treatment consists of cleansing with antibacterial soap at the time of barrier removal and in some cases, application of a topical antibiotic gel. Cultures may help to differentiate the cause of the infection if it is unclear whether fungal rash or folliculitis is involved. In cases that do not resolve with topical care, an oral antibiotic may be required.

CLINICAL PEARL

Some patients report that use of baby powder on the skin prior to shaving assists with the hair removal.

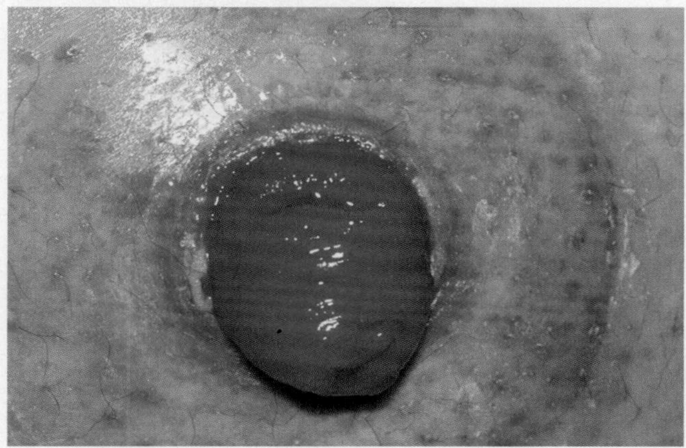

FIGURE 15-13. Folliculitis on the skin of the torso.

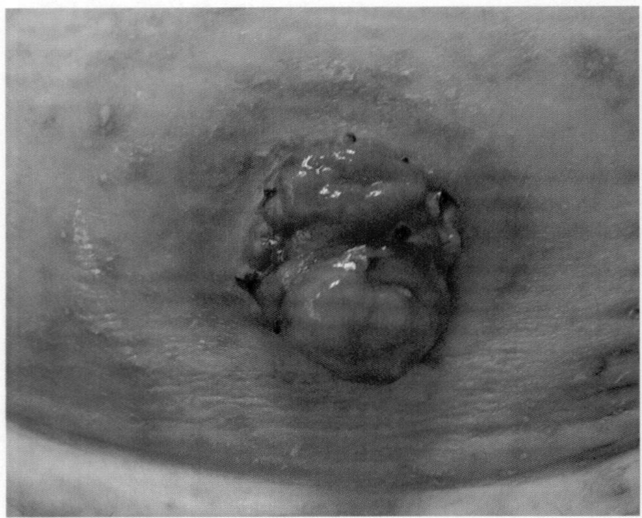

FIGURE 15-14. Peristomal folliculitis.

Varices

Peristomal varices are caused by portal hypertension that leads to enlarged venous channels at locations where the high-pressure portal and low-pressure systemic venous systems meet (Pennick & Artioukh, 2013). The most common causes of portal hypertension are liver cirrhosis and primary sclerosing cholangitis. Peristomal varices occur in up to 5% of individuals with a stoma. These varices may be visible as dilated veins in the submucosal area (referred to as caput medusae), bluish discoloration of the skin in the stoma area (**Fig. 15-15**), and/or a raspberry-like appearing stoma. Varices may also present as spontaneous bleeding from the stoma or mucocutaneous junction without any visible skin changes. The patient may report that the skin bleeds when the pouching system is removed from the skin and/or that there are spontaneous episodes of bleeding from the stoma.

Assessment includes inspection of the skin around the stoma, a problem-focused history, and a review of available laboratory test results. Local pressure should be applied in the event of acute bleeding, and cautery silver nitrate and/or other may be required. To reduce the risk of bleeding when removing the pouching system, it may be helpful to use a barrier film wipe, a one-piece pouch, and standard-wear skin barriers rather than extended-wear skin barriers. Ensure that the opening in the skin barrier does not rub against the mucocutaneous junction, and avoid products that apply pressure to the peristomal skin and mucocutaneous junction, such as convex systems and belts.

Teach the patient how to gently remove the pouching system and gently cleanse the peristomal skin to prevent trauma during self-care. Rebleeding is common; thus, the patient should be referred for further diagnosis and definitive treatment. The transjugular intrahepatic portosystemic shunt (TIPS) procedure has the highest rate of success in preventing recurrent hemorrhage (Pennick & Artioukh, 2013), but other treatments may be discussed such as use of beta-blockers or embolization of vessels.

Granuloma

Another cause of raised reddened lesions is granuloma formation. These tend to be located at the juncture of the stoma and the peristomal skin (**Figs. 15-16** and **15-17**); they occur when there is an immunologic response to foreign material such as retained sutures, in the presence of a moist environment. Granulomas present as raised, red bumps that bleed easily when touched, such as during skin cleansing and pouch changes (Norton et al., 2008). They may be firm or fluid filled if infected. The area may be tender to touch. The patient may report having problems with pouch leakage caused by the moisture from the lesions. The patient may also be concerned by the appearance of the new lesions. Treatment is similar to the management of hypergranulation tissue in wounds (Widgerow & Leak, 2010). Probe each lesion to determine whether loose suture material is present and remove it if possible (Colwell, 2004). Apply topical silver nitrate to the areas of elevated tissue;

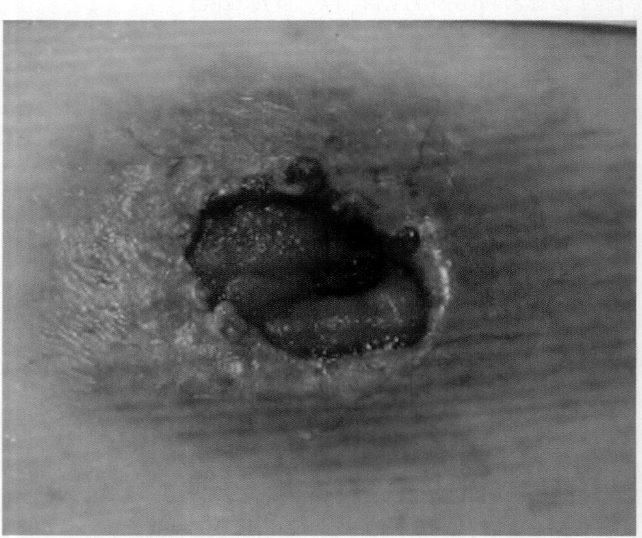

FIGURE 15-15. Peristomal varices.

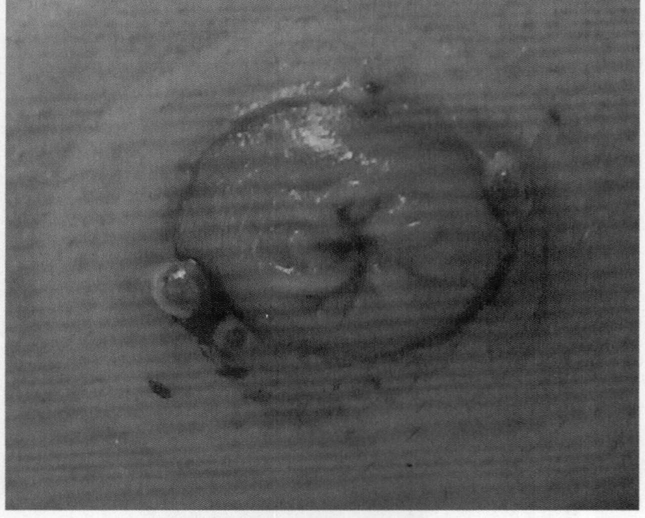

FIGURE 15-16. Granulomas.

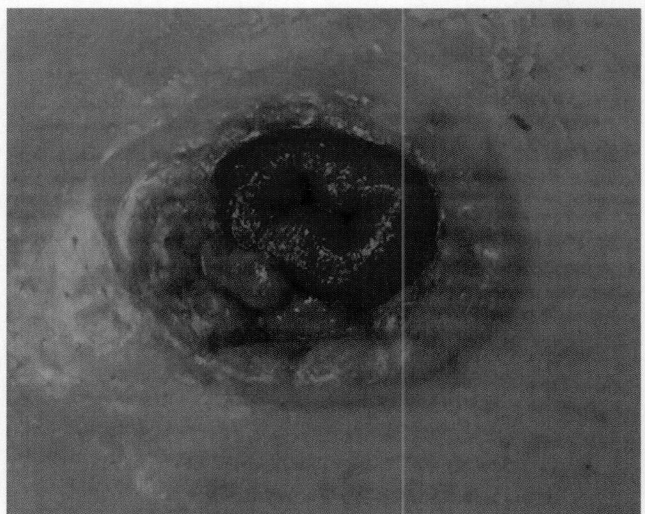

FIGURE 15-17. Granulomas.

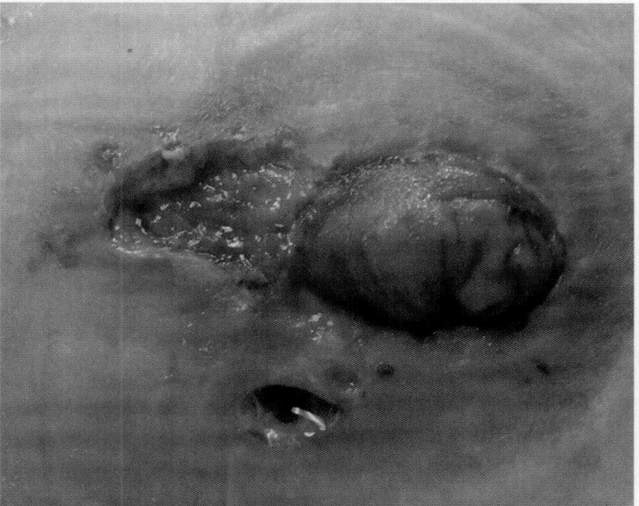

FIGURE 15-18. Peristomal abscess *below* a stoma with a large peristomal wound.

it may be repeated weekly if needed. Apply stoma powder and barrier film to help absorb moisture and protect tender areas during healing. If the affected area is large and moisture is excessive, consider using a foam dressing and convex skin barrier to provide gentle pressure to the area, which may reduce the growth of new lesions. Patients with peristomal granulomas that do not resolve with topical treatment, or who have enlarging granulomas require referral for definitive diagnosis, biopsy, and possible excision.

Peristomal Abscess

Peristomal abscesses can occur at any time; however, acute abscesses are typically seen within 2 weeks after stoma creation. WOC Nurse experts define peristomal abscess as a collection of purulent material beneath the skin; most typically associated with a foreign body (such as a suture) or a disease process (Colwell & Beitz, 2007). Other causes include preoperative colonization of the peristomal skin, infected hematoma, and infected suture granulomas (Kann, 2008). Peristomal abscess occurring near an established stoma may also develop due to underlying disease such as inflammatory bowel disease or pyoderma gangrenosum (PG). Abscesses present as areas of localized redness, swelling, and tenderness in the peristomal area, which may be accompanied by systemic signs of infection. **Figure 15-18** displays an abscess that has opened beneath a stoma, which also has a significant peristomal ulceration.

Patient assessment includes inspection and palpation of the peristomal skin and abdomen, and assessment for signs of systemic infection. If an abscess is suspected, consultation is indicated. Management of a peristomal abscess often requires drainage of the fluid collection, which may include placement of a temporary drain, local wound care with absorbent dressings, and treatment with systemic antibiotics. The affected area needs protection from stoma effluent, but also may require more frequent observation and access for dressing changes; thus, the pouch changes may need to be more frequent.

Provide the patient with information about self-care and completing the next steps in the management plan.

Peristomal Pyoderma Gangrenosum

PG is a neutrophilic dermatosis characterized by recurrent, painful ulcerations. PG classically appears on the lower extremities, most frequently on the tibial areas, but it can also occur in other parts of the body, including the peristomal area. Peristomal pyoderma granulosum (PPG) is often associated with the presence of systemic disease such as inflammatory bowel disease, arthritis, or hematologic disorders; however, the cause is idiopathic up to 50% of the time (Kiran et al., 2005; Moschella & Davis, 2012). The etiology is not fully understood; however, pathergy, causing trivial trauma to initiate and aggravate the lesions, exists up to 30% of individuals with the disorder (Moschella & Davis, 2012).

PPG presents as pustules that enlarge and open into partial- or full-thickness wounds, sometimes with dark-colored, irregular borders and purulent exudate as shown in **Figures 15-19** and **15-20**. These painful undermined

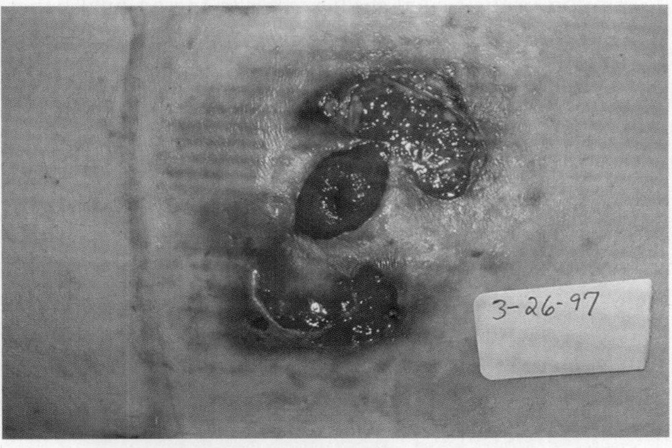

FIGURE 15-19. Pyoderma gangrenosum.

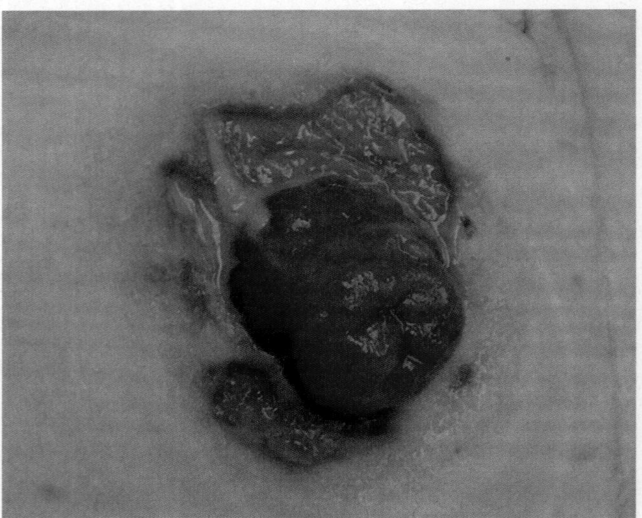

FIGURE 15-20. Pyoderma gangrenosum.

ulcerations progress rapidly and fail to heal with usual treatment. In addition to reports of painful lesions, the patient may complain of difficulty with adherence of the pouching system due to the excessive drainage from the wounds. Assessment includes appearance, size, depth, and location of the wounds and evaluation of possible contributing factors. It can be difficult to determine whether a wound is caused by pressure (such as convexity) or PPG by visual assessment and history; the use of convexity may be a precipitating factor for PPG. Assess the patient for signs and symptoms of local and deep wound infection, and obtain a wound culture if indicated.

Medical management of PPG involves treating infection and reducing the inflammatory process via topical steroids, topical tacrolimus 0.5% preparations, and injection of the periphery of the lesion with triamcinolone hexacetonide or cyclosporine (Altieri et al., 2010; Woo & James, 2005). Topical use of crushed prednisone has recently been reported in a small case series (DeMartyn et al., 2014). In a comprehensive review, Wu and Shen (2013) reported that oral prednisone therapy at a dose of 1 mg/kg/d has usually been effective in controlling PPG, and concomitant use of dapsone and minocycline may provide a steroid-sparing effect. For a complete description of their cited studies, refer to the original paper. When corticosteroids are not effective, options include cyclosporine, 6-mercaptopurine, cyclophosphamide, colchicine, clofazimine, and chlorambucil. Anti-TNF-α medications biologic agents may also be effective in refractory cases.

Local management of PPG lesions includes efforts to remove sources of pressure and friction; thus, a critical evaluation of all pouching products is required. For example, convex products and belts should be avoided or replaced with options that are soft or padded to prevent trauma and pressure to peristomal skin and open wounds. Topical wound management requires absorptive products such as alginates and foam dressings secured by transparent film dressing or thin hydrocolloid sheets to absorb excess wound exudate and provide a dry pouching surface for a predictable period of time between dressing changes. Use standard-wear skin barriers rather than extended-wear skin barriers to prevent damage to peristomal skin due to frequent removal of the pouching system for dressing changes, and consider use of adhesive remover wipes and no-sting skin barrier films to protect the fragile peristomal skin. Nonadhesive pouching systems are also an appropriate option. In cases involving extensive tissue loss and high-volume exudate, PPG wounds have been managed with negative pressure wound therapy. Debridement should be avoided due to the likelihood of pathergy and resultant exacerbation of the wounds.

Referral is indicated for patients presenting with suspected PPG, as medical workup will include evaluation for underlying pathology, culture of lesions, and possible skin biopsy. Biopsies taken from the lesions show neutrophil infiltration and may reveal endothelial edema at the edge of the ulcer, thrombosis of small vessels, necrosis, and extravasation of red blood cells; however, the primary objective of biopsy in PPG is to rule out other causes of ulceration (Wu & Shen, 2013). Instruct the patient about the next steps in the treatment plan and when to return for follow-up care.

Peristomal Psoriasis

Psoriasis is a chronic inflammatory and autoimmune disorder with many clinical variants (Ladizinski et al., 2013). In one cross-sectional study of stoma patients, the incidence of peristomal psoriasis was 7% (Lyon et al., 2000). Peristomal and periwound skin is particularly vulnerable for patients with psoriasis because of the Koebner phenomenon, in which a flare of the disorder occurs in an area of localized skin trauma. This often becomes evident 1 to 2 weeks after a minor skin trauma. Psoriasis most commonly occurs on the extensor surfaces of the extremities, as shown in **Figure 15-21**, but psoriasis can occur for the first time on the peristomal skin (Moriyasu et al., 2006).

The clinical presentation of peristomal psoriasis is a red, inflamed patchy rash with excessive flakiness or scaliness of the skin, which may be shiny or silvery in appearance. Inquire about a history of psoriasis, eczema, or other skin

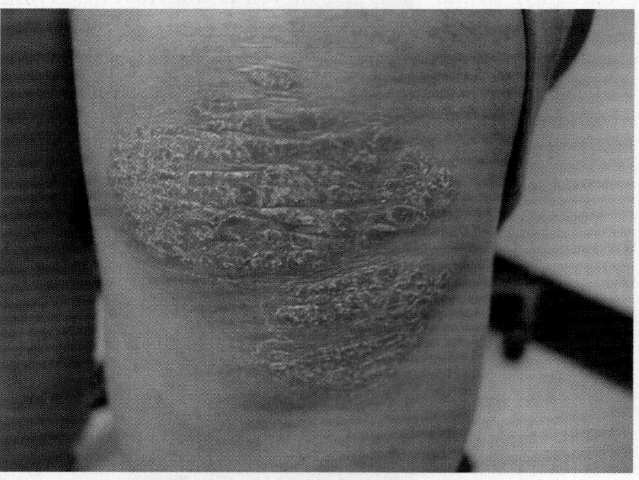

FIGURE 15-21. Plaque psoriasis, mild.

diseases, and obtain a complete history of medications (including topical products). Examine the affected area, noting the color, texture, and integrity of the skin.

Management of peristomal psoriasis is directed at reducing inflammation by use of topical or intralesional corticosteroids. Topical medications used for psoriasis elsewhere on the body may not be appropriate for use under skin barriers due to their occlusive and adhesive properties; thus, collaboration with the prescribing provider is necessary to ensure a successful treatment plan. Use of corticosteroid sprays and lotions and products with low alcohol content are recommended (Ladizinski et al., 2013).

Teach the patient the importance of using a properly sized skin barrier, wearing products that prevent leakage, and changing the pouching system before stoma effluent leaks onto the skin. Prevention of peristomal trauma and irritation may reduce peristomal psoriasis occurrence.

Fistula

An enterocutaneous (EC) fistula is an abnormal connection between the intestine and the skin. EC fistulas can occur on the skin of the abdomen, and they are particularly challenging when the opening is on the peristomal skin undermining the adherence of the pouching system and putting skin integrity at risk. Appearance of a fistula may be indicative of active pathology such as Crohn's disease (Hoentjen, Colwell & Hanauer, 2012) or ulcerative colitis; or occur as a complication of intestinal surgery in patient with malnutrition, infection, and other risk factors.

A patient with a fistula may present with complaints of difficulty maintaining adherence of his or her pouching system, leakage, and peristomal skin irritation accompanied by pain. The patient may notice the fistula is draining fecal effluent or simply describe it as a new open wound. Components of the patient history include onset and duration of symptoms, prior history of fistulas, health history, and medication history. Inquire about any changes in the amount of effluent draining from the stoma since the fistula was first noticed.

Assessment includes examination of the stoma and peristomal skin, including the mucocutaneous juncture where fistulas may be present but easily overlooked. Evaluate draining areas for evidence of warmth, swelling, and fluctuance that may indicate infection or abscess. Evaluate the patient for signs and symptoms of systemic infection. Note the size of the fistula and its location in relationship to the stoma. Note the characteristics and amount of any drainage.

Peristomal fistulas are managed symptomatically while medical evaluation is completed and treatment options are pursued. The initial goal is to protect the peristomal skin from the fistula drainage while also providing a secure pouching system to collect stoma effluent. With a fistula that is close to the stoma, the best option may be to adjust the opening of the skin barrier to simply accommodate the fistula within the same pouching system. Use accessories such as skin barrier rings, strips, paste, or barrier film to customize the opening and protect healthy skin from further damage. Select a two-piece pouching system to allow easy access for subsequent medical evaluations. Fistulas that cannot be pouched with the stoma may be managed by using a wound dressing with adequate skin protection on the surrounding skin or accommodated by a separate pouching system. Appropriate options depend on the location of the peristomal fistula, the volume and type of effluent, the method used to treat the fistula, and the patient's preferences and capabilities.

Refer the patient for evaluation and treatment. Procedures may include radiologic examinations such as fistulogram, CT scan, and insertion of drainage tube. Patients with high-volume drainage or complicated presentations may require hospitalization. Provide the patient with instruction about the next steps in the plan of care, and how to manage stoma care needs until the condition is resolved.

Malignancy

Malignancy of the skin can occur in the peristomal area. The precise incidence is unknown but is thought to be rare (Al-Niaimi & Lyon, 2014; Chang et al., 2014), and it has been reported more often with fecal stomas than urinary stomas. Ileostomy-associated lymphoma, squamous cell carcinoma, and adenocarcinoma have been reported (Chang et al., 2014). The clinical presentation is often a polyp, nodule, lesion, or wound on the peristomal area, stoma, or mucocutaneous junction that does not resolve with usual treatment. For this reason, individuals with peristomal lesions unresponsive to therapy should be referred for biopsy (Chang et al., 2014). Diagnostic tests and treatments depend on the type of malignancy and the stage of the disease. Peristomal metastasis of colorectal cancer may be diagnosed with dermoscopy and subsequent biopsy of suspicious tissue (Ito et al., 2014). Treatment options may include excision of the affected area, stoma relocation, and novel approaches such as electrochemotherapy (Campana et al., 2013).

CLINICAL PEARL

The majority of peristomal complications require local care and attention and management of the underlying cause of the problem.

Conclusions

A variety of conditions can affect the peristomal skin; most of them are related to mechanical, chemical, or infectious causes; some are immunologically mediated or related to systemic disease. Moisture-associated skin damage with irritant dermatitis is the most prevalent, and it is often associated with leakage of stoma effluent under the skin barrier. Because of the high incidence of peristomal skin problems, it is vital that health care providers routinely ask about the condition of the peristomal skin when caring for an individual with a stoma. Ask about the patient's usual skin condition and how the skin appeared at the time of the last pouch change. To evaluate the skin completely, remove the pouching system and examine the skin, the stoma, and the adhesive side of the barrier. Evaluate the appropriateness of the sizing and fit of the pouching products, and determine the etiology of any skin complications. Treatment of the underlying cause of the disorder, identification and management of any contributing factors, and appropriate topical care for open wounds are key steps to restoring normal peristomal skin integrity.

REFERENCES

Al-Niaimi, F., Beck, M., Almaani, N., et al. (2012). The relevance of patch testing in peristomal dermatitis. *British Journal of Dermatology, 167*, 103–109.

Al-Niaimi, F., & Lyon, C. C. (2014). Primary adenocarcinoma in peristomal skin: A case study. *Ostomy Wound Management, 60*(5), 45–47.

Altieri, M., Vaziri, K., & Orkin, B. A. (2010). Topical tacrolimus for parastomal pyoderma gangrenosum: A report of two cases. *Ostomy Wound Management, 56*(9), 32–36.

Alvey, B., & Beck, D. E. (2008). Peristomal dermatology. *Clinics in Colon and Rectal Surgery, 21*(1), 41–44.

Arumugam, P. J., Bevan, L., Macdonald, L., et al. (2003). A prospective audit of stomas—Analysis of risk factors and complications and their management. *Colorectal Disease, 5*(1), 49–52.

Campana, L. G., Scarpa, M., Sommariva, A., et al. (2013). Minimally invasive treatment of peristomal metastases from gastric cancer at an ileostomy site by electrochemotherapy. *Radiology and Oncology, 47*(4), 370–375.

Chang, A., Davis, B., Snyder, J., et al. (2014). Considerations for diagnosis and management of ileostomy-related malignancy: A report of two cases. *Ostomy Wound Management, 60*(5), 38–40, 42–43.

Colwell, J. C. (2004). Stomal and peristomal complications. In J. C. Colwell, M. T. Goldberg, & J. E. Carmel (Eds.), *Fecal and urinary diversions: Management principals* (pp. 308–325). St. Louis, MO: Mosby.

Colwell, J. C., & Beitz, J. (2007). Survey of wound, ostomy and continence (WOC) nurse clinicians on stomal and peristomal complications: A content validation study. *Journal of Wound, Ostomy and Continence Nursing, 34*(1), 57–69.

Colwell, J. C., Ratliff, C. R., Goldberg, M., et al. (2011). MASD part 3: Peristomal moisture-associated dermatitis and periwound moisture-associated dermatitis. A consensus. *Journal of Wound, Ostomy and Continence Nursing, 38*(5), 541–553.

Cutting, K. F., & White, R. J. (2002). Maceration of the skin and wound bed. 1: Its nature and causes. *Journal of Wound Care, 11*(7), 275–278.

DeMartyn, L. E., Faller, N. A., & Miller, L. (2014). Treating peristomal pyoderma gangrenosum with topical crushed prednisone: A report of three cases. *Ostomy Wound Management, 60*(6), 50–54.

Doughty, D. (2005). Principles of ostomy management in the oncology patient. *Journal of Supportive Oncology*, 3, 59–69.

Farnham, S. B., & Cookson, M. S. (2004). Surgical complications of urinary diversion. *World Journal of Urology, 22*(3), 157–167.

Fernández, I. S., Moreno, C., Vano-Galvan, S., et al. (2010). Pseudo-verrucous irritant peristomal dermatitis with an histological pattern of nutritional deficiency dermatitis. *Dermatology Online Journal, 16*(9). Retrieved from http://escholarship.org/uc/item/5sg6m25r

Fletcher, J. (2012). Device related pressure ulcers made easy. *Wounds UK, 8*(2). Retrieved June 25, 2014, from http://www.wounds-uk.com

Gray, M., Colwell, J. C., Doughty, D., et al. (2013). Peristomal moisture-associated skin damage in adults with fecal ostomies: A comprehensive review and consensus. *Journal of Wound, Ostomy and Continence Nursing, 40*(4), 389–399.

Herlufsen, P., Olsen, A. G., Carlsen, B., et al. (2006). Study of peristomal skin disorders in patients with permanent stomas. *British Journal of Nursing, 15*, 854–862.

Hoentjen, F., Colwell, J.C., & Hanauer, S. B. (2012). Complications of peristomal recurrence of Crohn's disease. *Journal of Wound, Ostomy and Continence Nursing, 39*(3), 297–301.

Ito, T., Yoshid, Y., Yamada, N., et al. (2014). Dermoscopy of peristomal polyps and metastasis of colon cancer. *Acta Dermato-Venereologica, 94*, 96–97.

Jemec, G. B., & Nybaek, H. (2008). Peristomal skin problems account for more than one in three visits to ostomy nurses. *British Journal of Dermatology, 159*, 1211–1211.

Jenkinson, H. F., & Douglas, L. J. (2002). Interactions between *Candida* species and bacteria in mixed infections. In K. A. Brogden & J. M. Guthmiller (Eds.), *Polymicrobial diseases*. Washington, DC: ASM Press. Retrieved from http://www.ncbi.nlm.nih.gov/books/NBK2486/

Kann, B. R. (2008). Early stomal complications. *Clinics in Colon and Rectal Surgery, 21*, 23–30.

Kiran, R. P., O'Brien-Ermlich, B., Achkar, J. P., et al. (2005). Management of peristomal pyoderma gangrenosum. *Diseases of the Colon and Rectum, 48*, 1397–1403.

Ladizinski, B., Lee, K. C., Wilmer, E., et al. (2013). A review of the clinical variants and the management of psoriasis. *Advances in Skin & Wound Care, 26*(6), 271–284.

Landis, M. N., Keeling, J. H., Yiannias, J. A., et al. (2012). Results of patch testing in 10 patients with peristomal dermatitis. *Journal of the American Academy of Dermatology, 67*, e91–e104.

Lindholm, E., Persson, E., Carlsson, E., et al. (2013). Ostomy-related complications after emergent abdominal surgery: A 2-year follow-up study. *Journal of Wound, Ostomy and Continence Nursing, 40*(6), 603–610.

Lyon, C. C. (2010a). Infections. In C. C. Lyon & A. Smith (Eds.), *Abdominal stomas and their skin disorders: An atlas of diagnosis and management* (2nd ed., pp. 105–131). London, UK: Informa Healthcare.

Lyon, C. C. (2010b). Skin problems related to the primary abdominal disease. In C. C. Lyon & A. Smith (Eds.), *Abdominal stomas and their skin disorders: An atlas of diagnosis and management* (2nd ed., pp. 177–209). London, UK: Informa Healthcare.

Lyon, C. C., Smith, A. J., Griffiths, C. E. M., et al. (2000). The spectrum of skin disorders in abdominal stoma patients. *British Journal of Dermatology, 143*, 1248–1260.

Martin, J. A., Hughes, T. M., & Stone, N. M. (2005). Peristomal allergic contact dermatitis—Case report and review of the literature. *Contact Dermatitis 52*, 273–275. doi: 10.1111/j.0105-1873.2005.00579.x

Mayrovitz, H. N., & Sims, N. (2001). Biophysical effects of water and synthetic urine on skin. *Advances in Skin & Wound Care, 14*(6), 302–308.

McNichol, L., Lund, C., Rosen, T., et al. (2013). Medical adhesives and patient safety: State of the science. *Journal of Wound, Ostomy and Continence Nursing, 40*(4), 365–380.

Meisner, S., Lehur, P. A., Moran, B., et al. (2012). Peristomal skin complications are common, expensive and difficult to manage: A population based cost modeling study. *PLoS ONE, 7*(5), e37813. doi: 10.1371/journal.pone.0037813

Moriyasu, A., Katoh, N., & Kishimoto, S. (2006). Psoriasis localized exclusively to peristomal skin. *Journal of the American Academy of Dermatology, 54*(2), s55–s56.

Moschella, S. L., & Davis, M. D. P. (2012). Neutrophilic dermatoses. In J. L. Bolognia, J. L. Jorizzo, & J. V. Schaffer (Eds.), *Dermatology* (3rd ed.), 423–438. Elsevier.

Napierkowski, D. (2013). Uncovering common bacterial skin infections. *Nurse Practitioner, 38*(3), 30–37.

Nichols, T., & Riemer, M. (2011). Body image perception, the stoma and peristomal skin condition. *Gastrointestinal Nursing, 9*(1), 22–27.

Norton, C., Williams, J., Taylor, C., et al. (2008). *Oxford handbook of gastrointestinal nursing*. Oxford, UK: Oxford University Press.

Nybaek, H., Knudsen, D. B., Laursen, T. N., et al. (2009). Skin problems in ostomy patients: A case–control study of risk factors. *Acta Dermato-Venereologica 89*, 64–67. doi: 10.2340/00015555-0536

Nybaek, H., Lophagen, S., Karlsmark, T., et al. (2010). Stratum corneum integrity as a predictor for peristomal skin problems in ostomates. *British Journal of Dermatology, 162*(2), 357–361.

Omura, Y., Yamabe, M., & Anazawa, S. (2010). Peristomal skin disorders in patients with intestinal and urinary ostomies: Influence of adhesive forces of various hydrocolloid wafer skin barriers. *Journal of Wound, Ostomy, and Continence Nursing, 37*(3), 289–298.

Pennick, M. O., & Artioukh, D. Y. (2013). Management of parastomal varices: Who re-bleeds and who does not? A systematic review of the literature. *Techniques in Coloproctology, 17*, 163–170.

Persson, E., Berndtsson, I., Carlsson, E., et al. (2010). Stomal related complications and stoma size-a two year follow up. *Colorectal Disease, 12*, 971–976.

Pittman, J., Rawl, S. M., Schmidt, C. M., et al. (2008). Demographic and clinical factors related to ostomy complications and quality of life in veterans with an ostomy. *Journal of Wound, Ostomy, and Continence Nursing, 35*, 493–503.

Salvadalena, G. D. (2013). The incidence of stoma and peristomal complications during the first 3 months after ostomy creation. *Journal of Wound, Ostomy and Continence Nursing, 40*(4), 400–406.

Seungmi, P., Lee, Y. J., Oh, D. N., et al. (2011). Comparison of standardized peristomal skin care and crusting technique in prevention of peristomal skin problems in ostomy patients. *Journal of Korean Academy of Nursing, 41*(6), 814–820.

Szymanski, K. M., St-Cyr, D., Alam, T., et al. (2010). External stoma and peristomal complications following radical cystectomy and ileal conduit diversion: A systematic review. *Ostomy Wound Management, 56*(1), 28–35.

Widgerow, A. D., & Leak, K. (2010). Hypergranulation tissue: Evolution, control and potential elimination. *Wound Healing Southern Africa, 3*(2), 7–9.

Williams, J. D. L., & Lyon, C. C. (2010). Dermatitis: Contact irritation and contact allergy. In C. C. Lyon & A. Smith (Eds.), *Abdominal stomas and their skin disorders: An atlas of diagnosis and management* (2nd ed., pp. 52–104). UK: Informa Healthcare.

Woo, D. K., & James, W. D. (2005). Topical tacrolimus: A review of its uses in dermatology. *Dermatitis, 16*(1), 6–21.

Woo, K., Sibbald, R. G., Ayello, E. A., et al. (2009). Peristomal skin complications and management. *Advances in Skin & Wound Care, 22*(11), 522–532.

Wu, X., & Shen, B. (2013). Diagnosis and management of parastomal pyoderma gangrenosum. *Gastroenterology Report 1*, 1–8. Retrieved from April 19, 2013. doi: 10.1093/gastro/got013

QUESTIONS

1. The WOC nurse is explaining peristomal skin care to patients with new ostomies. Which statement accurately describes a type of mechanical injury that may occur?

A. The physical forces involved in repeated removal of adhesive products can strip away varying amounts of stratum corneum.
B. Effluent draining from the stoma provides a constant source of moisture that may cause inflammation.
C. Products used for stoma care contain a variety of ingredients that may be sensitizing or cause skin irritation.
D. Peristomal skin becomes thinner from adhesive remover use and has higher transepidermal water loss compared to healthy contralateral skin.

2. The WOC nurse is performing an assessment of a patient who presents with peristomal skin irritation. Which action is a recommended step in the assessment process?

A. Erythema in peristomal skin is not a significant finding.
B. Describe the peristomal skin area to be the area surrounding the stoma that had contact with the skin barrier and 6 inches in any direction.
C. Cleanse the skin to allow a thorough evaluation of the peristomal skin noting color and condition of skin.
D. Label any redness or warmth in the peristomal skin as normal conditions.

3. What is the overall goal of peristomal skin care management performed by the WOC nurse?

A. Optimizing the pouching system
B. Promoting intact peristomal skin
C. Making referrals for any skin changes
D. Diagnosing malignancies

4. A patient with an ileostomy presents to the ostomy clinic with peristomal skin irritation. Upon assessment, the WOC nurse notes erythema adjacent to the stoma accompanied by superficial skin loss. What condition would the nurse suspect?

A. Maceration
B. Peristomal moisture–associated skin damage (MASD)
C. Pseudoverrucous lesions
D. Pressure ulcer

5. Which intervention might the WOC nurse recommend to manage peristomal moisture–associated skin damage (MASD)?

A. Cautery with silver nitrate
B. Using an adhesive remover
C. Patch testing to identify allergens
D. Use of skin barrier powder

6. The nurse assessing the peristomal skin of a patient with an ostomy notes erythema and satellite lesions on the skin around the stoma. What condition would the nurse suspect?
   A. Fungal infection
   B. Pressure ulcers
   C. Pseudoverrucous lesions
   D. Maceration

7. A patient is diagnosed with a candidiasis infection of the peristomal skin area. What intervention would the WOC nurse recommend?
   A. Applying a topical antifungal powder to the area
   B. Applying cortisone cream prior to attaching the pouching system
   C. Taking a regimen of an oral antibiotics
   D. Applying a topical antibiotic gel

8. Which patient would the WOC nurse consider at higher risk for development of peristomal varices?
   A. A patient with diabetes mellitus
   B. A patient with latex allergies
   C. A patient with hypertension
   D. A patient with cirrhosis of the liver

9. A patient visiting the ostomy clinic tells the nurse: "I noticed that there are red bumps around my stoma that bleed when I change the pouch." The patient further states that the bumps are painful and that he is having pouch leakage. What condition would the nurse suspect?
   A. Peristomal abscess
   B. Granuloma formation
   C. Peristomal pyoderma gangrenosum
   D. Peristomal psoriasis

10. The nurse is assessing a patient who has a peristomal fistula. What intervention would be appropriate for this patient?
   A. Using topical corticosteroids to reduce infection
   B. Biopsy to check for malignancies
   C. Adjusting the opening of the skin barrier to accommodate the fistula
   D. Drainage of fluid collection

ANSWERS: 1.**A**, 2.**C**, 3.**B**, 4.**B**, 5.**D**, 6.**A**, 7.**A**, 8.**D**, 9.**B**, 10.**C**

CHAPTER 16

Stoma Complications

Joyce Pittman

OBJECTIVE

Distinguish between stoma complications and select the associated management strategies.

Topic Outline

- **Early Complications**
  - Mucocutaneous Separation
  - Stomal Necrosis
  - Stomal Retraction
- **Late Complications**
  - Stomal Stenosis
  - Stomal Prolapse
  - Stomal Trauma
  - Parastomal Hernia
- **Conclusions**

Complications following the surgical creation of an ostomy are a significant problem for many individuals. These complications are often multifaceted involving both physiologic and psychosocial aspects. The physiologic aspect of ostomy complications involves changes of the stoma and peristomal skin (Cottam et al., 2007). In this chapter, we discuss the physiologic aspect of ostomy complications involving the stoma.

Ostomy complications are a significant problem for individuals with an ostomy, yet, definitions and terminology are often not consistent in the literature (Colwell et al., 2001; Salvadalena, 2008). Study design differences, inconsistent definitions and terminology, and timing of measurements make it difficult to accurately measure ostomy complication incidence (Salvadalena, 2008). Due to inconsistent use of terminology, differentiating between stomal and peristomal complications can be difficult.

Overall incidence rates of complications have been reported, although the ranges are very broad. Two comprehensive systematic reviews of the literature on ostomy complications indicated that 18% to 55% of patients with an ostomy experienced peristomal skin irritation, 1% to 37% experienced parastomal herniation, 2% to 25% experienced stomal prolapse, 2% to 10% experienced stenosis, and 1% to 11% experienced retraction of the stoma (Colwell et al., 2001; Salvadalena, 2008). Ratliff et al. (2005) reported that 10% to 70% of all patients with an ostomy develop complications (Ratliff et al., 2005). Putting this into a practical perspective, using the estimates above, stoma complications represent a significant problem with up to 560,000 individuals who receive an ostomy experiencing ostomy-related complications. If we use the annual incidence, up to 84,000 individuals with a new ostomy can be expected to develop ostomy-related complications annually (Pittman, 2011).

Various patient characteristics have been identified as being associated with ostomy complications, but studies with predictive analysis models are limited. Several studies have identified that higher body mass index (BMI), older age, emergent surgery, inflammatory bowel disease, having an ileostomy (vs. colostomy), a diverting "loop" procedure, poor bowel quality, ischemic colitis, stomal retraction, lack of preoperative education, and involvement of a wound, ostomy, and continence (WOC) nurse influence the development of ostomy complications (Bass et al., 1997; Colwell et al., 2001; Duchesne et al., 2002; Park et al., 1999; Pittman et al., 2008). In the landmark retrospective study conducted by Bass at Cook County Hospital in Chicago, complication rates were compared between patients who

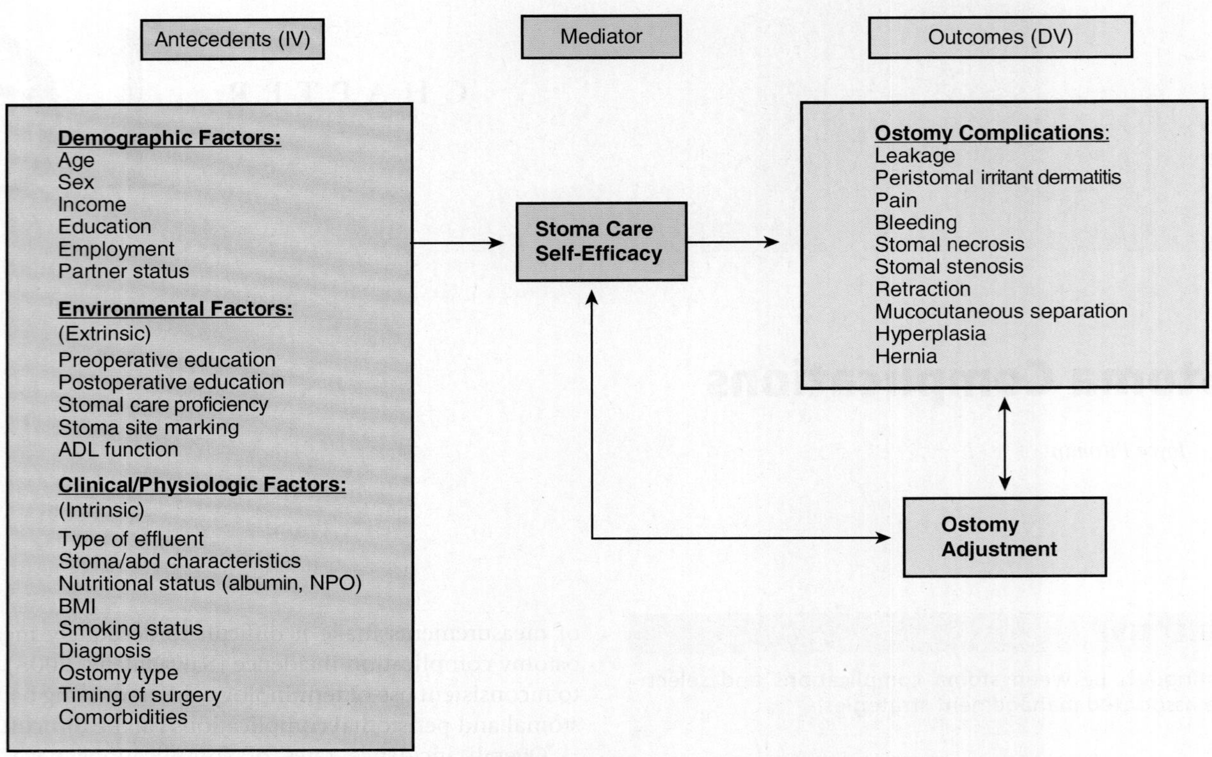

FIGURE 16-1. Pittman Ostomy Complication Conceptual Model.

received preoperative education and stoma site marking by an enterostomal therapist (WOC nurse) and those who did not (Bass et al., 1997). They found that among those who received preoperative education and stoma site marking by an enterostomal therapist, 32.5% developed complications compared to 43.5% of those who did not receive these clinical interventions ($p = 0.05$). The Ostomy Complication Conceptual Model (Fig. 16-1) provides a framework for exploring ostomy complications and the risk factors that contribute to their occurrence (Pittman et al., 2014).

One method of classifying ostomy complications is to separate them into early, within 30 days following surgery, and late complications, >30 days following surgery (Duchesne et al., 2002; Kim & Kumar, 2006; Park et al., 1999; Shabbir & Britton, 2010). In this chapter, we organize our discussion of stomal complications using this classification, recognizing that some complications can occur in both early and late time frames.

Early Complications

Early stomal complications are those that commonly occur within 30 days following surgery and include mucocutaneous separation, stomal necrosis, and stomal retraction.

Mucocutaneous Separation

Etiology/Incidence

Mucocutaneous separation is the detachment of stomal tissue from the surrounding peristomal skin (Colwell & Beitz, 2007) of the stoma, and mucocutaneous junction may be a result of poor healing, tension, or infection. Incidence of mucocutaneous separation has been reported to be from 4% to as high as 24%. Park et al. (1999) reported that 4% of patients had mucocutaneous separation in their review of 1,616 stoma patients (Park et al., 1999). In a prospective study of 3,970 stomas, Cottam et al. (2007) reported that 24% had mucocutaneous separation. In another study of 71 subjects, 13% had mucocutaneous separation (Pittman et al., 2014).

Presentation

Healthy stomas will have a closely approximated and intact mucocutaneous junction (where the stoma is attached to the abdominal wall). As soon as 24 hours after surgery, the stoma and mucocutaneous junction may begin to separate.

Assessment

Assessment of the stoma is done by close visual observation of the stoma and integrity of the mucocutaneous junction. Separation is evident if the stoma detaches from the peristomal skin (Fig. 16-2). Mucocutaneous separation can occur in variable degrees of severity: partial—if it is only a portion of the stomal circumference, or complete—if the entire circumference is involved. The separation can also be superficial, only the skin level, or full thickness, extending to the fascia level (Franchini et al., 1983). Close observation of the area of separation is necessary noting depth, wound base tissue characteristics (necrotic, granular), and type of drainage (serosanguinous, purulent, fecal).

CLINICAL PEARL

Use a cotton tip applicator to assess the depth of the mucocutaneous separation.

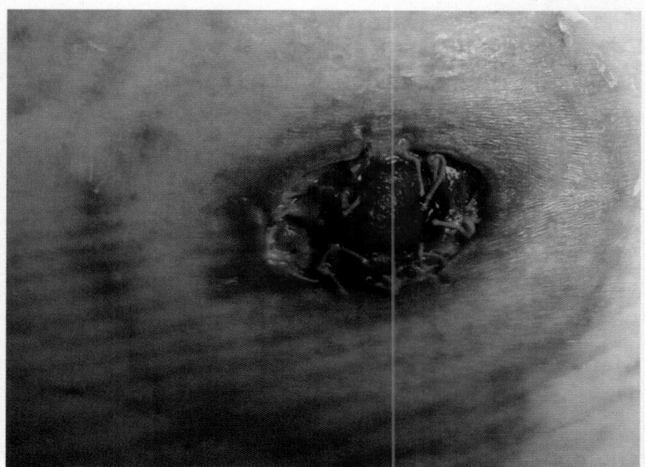

FIGURE 16-2. Mucocutaneous separation.

Management

Management of mucocutaneous separation depends on the degree of the separation. If the separation is partial and superficial, the subcutaneous defect may be small and able to be managed conservatively. The subcutaneous defect may be treated like a wound and filled with an advanced wound product such as skin barrier powder, hydrofiber, or calcium alginate. The skin barrier of the pouching system is fitted over the peristomal skin and defect to provide protection from the stomal effluent. The pouching system is changed as warranted to manage the drainage, assess healing, and reapply the absorbent filler material (Colwell, 2004).

If the defect is large, then fecal contamination of the peristomal subcutaneous defect is likely and infection may occur. The more severe the separation, the more likely retraction of the stoma will occur. With healing, the likelihood of stenosis is high. If the mucocutaneous separation involves the fascial layer (a rarely reported occurrence), the stoma may drop into the abdominal cavity and contamination of the abdomen with fecal effluent and generalized peritonitis may occur. A return to surgery is indicated for repair.

Stomal Necrosis

Etiology/Incidence

Stomal necrosis is defined as death of the stomal tissue resulting from impaired blood flow (Colwell & Beitz, 2007) and has been identified as one of the most common early complications (Duchesne et al., 2002; Kim & Kumar, 2006; Park et al., 1999; Shabbir & Britton, 2010). Ischemia of stomal tissue is usually caused by tension on or inadequacy of the mesenteric vasculature to the intestinal end. It can also be caused by trauma to the stomal tissue during its creation. Stomal necrosis has been associated with obesity and is often a result of the traction that is placed on the mesentery and bowel wall (Colwell & Fichera, 2005).

Presentation

Impending stomal necrosis is evidenced by a progression of discoloration of the stomal tissue from pink to black. The stoma will usually appear dusky and dry within hours to days of surgery progressing to black and flaccid. The degree of necrosis may vary depending on the degree of ischemia. It may encompass the whole stoma, extending below the fascia, or only a portion of the stoma, and above skin level.

Assessment

Assessment of stomal necrosis is done by close visual observation. Within 24 hours of surgery, color changes of the stoma are usually visible. Color of the stoma progresses from dusky red to black (**Fig. 16-3**). To determine the degree or level of stomal necrosis, a clear, glass lubricated tube may be inserted into the stoma. Using a penlight directed into the glass tube, a change in the color of the stoma may be detected thus indicating the level of ischemia.

> **CLINICAL PEARL**
>
> It is advisable to use a clear pouch in the immediate postoperative period to allow for assessment of the stoma color.

A new innovative method of evaluating tissue perfusion is the intraoperative laser angiography using indocyanine green. This vascular imaging technology provides real-time assessment of tissue perfusion that correlates with clinical outcomes and can be used to guide surgical decision making (Gurtner et al., 2013). This method is primarily used intraoperatively to assess perfusion of the stoma and intestine at the time of resection.

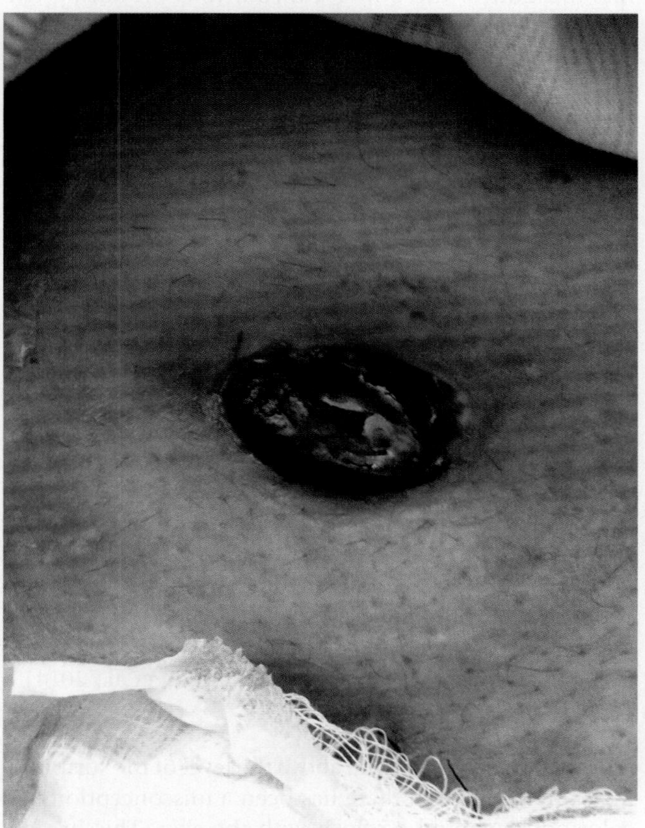

FIGURE 16-3. Stomal necrosis.

Management

Stomal necrosis is often a watch-and-wait situation. If the ischemia and necrosis is above the fascial level, observation may be adequate. Often, if the ischemia and necrosis is superficial, the top layer of the stoma may slough off, leaving a red viable stoma. If the stomal ischemia and necrosis is below skin level but still above the fascial level, the necrotic stomal tissue will become malodorous and flaccid. Debridement is often indicated. After the necrotic tissue is removed or sloughs off, usually there is mucocutaneous separation. As the mucocutaneous separation heals, stenosis may occur. In addition, the level of the stoma above the skin is diminished, and this often leads to pouching challenges. If the ischemia and necrosis extend deeper than the fascial level, urgent surgical intervention may be indicated.

Stomal Retraction

Etiology/Incidence

Retraction is the disappearance of stoma tissue protrusion in line with or below skin level (Colwell & Beitz, 2007). Retraction is usually caused by tension on the stoma from a variety of reasons: short mesentery, thickened abdominal wall, excessive adhesions or scar formation, increased BMI, inadequate initial stoma length, or improper skin excision, stomal necrosis, and mucocutaneous separation (Colwell, 2004). Anecdotal evidence suggests that retraction occurs frequently in overweight patients with larger adipose layers. A shortened and fatty mesentery makes adequate mobilization of the bowel difficult, thus producing tension on the stoma (Cottam, 2005).

Ratliff and Donovan (2001) found that 9 (4%) of 220 ostomy patients had flush or retracted stomas. In a prospective study of 3,970 stomas, Cottam et al. (2007) reported that 40.1% had retraction. In Pittman's prospective study of 71 participants with an ostomy, 24 (39%) had retraction (Pittman et al., 2014). In a 3-year retrospective study of 164 patients who had surgery resulting in an ostomy, retraction occurred in 5% of those patients (Duchesne et al., 2002). Another study of 97 patients with an ostomy found BMI to be associated with retraction ($p = 0.003$) (Arumugam et al., 2003). The incidence of retraction seems to be increasing. Cottam et al. (2007) reported that the incidence of stomal retraction (stoma below the skin level) more than doubled between 1996 and 2004 (22% vs. 51%) (Colwell and Beitz, 2007). In a systematic review of the literature, stoma retraction occurred in 9% to 15% of ileal conduits and 1% to 11% of all stomas (Szymanski et al., 2010). In Pittman's study, patients who did not have their stoma site preoperatively marked by a WOC nurse experienced greater severity of ostomy complications, specifically stomal retraction ($r = 0.32$, $p = 0.01$) (Pittman et al., 2014).

Presentation

A healthy stoma should be above the level of the surrounding skin. In the past, there has been a misconception that colostomies should be flush with the skin. This has not been confirmed in the literature or in practice. In Cottam's study of 1,329 problematic stomas, if the stoma height was <10 mm, the probability of having a problematic stoma was at least 35% ($p < 0.0001$) (Cottam et al., 2007).

Assessment

The stoma needs to be observed without the pouching system in place and in a variety of positions—sitting, supine, and standing. The level of the stoma and the surrounding skin needs to be closely noted. The stoma may disappear in a skin fold or crease when sitting or may become flush or even retracted with position changes and with peristalsis.

Management

The goal of successful pouching of the stoma is to have or create a flat pouching surface. When retraction is present, the goal is to augment the level of the stoma above the skin. This may sometimes be achieved using a convex pouching system and/or belt. If a predictable wear time is not achieved and complications continue, surgical intervention may be necessary to revise the stoma. Local revision may be possible if there is adequate intestine to mobilize above the skin level; if not, a more invasive surgery may be necessary to create a new stoma.

Late Complications

Late stomal complications are those that occur at least 30 days after surgery and often include stomal stenosis, prolapse, and parastomal herniation (Duchesne et al., 2002; Kim & Kumar, 2006; Park et al., 1999; Shabbir & Britton, 2010; Steel & Wu, 2002). With the advance of surgical techniques and laparoscopic surgery, various surgical techniques are being explored to minimize the risk of developing long-term complications (Gurtner et al., 2013; Heiying et al., 2014).

Stomal Stenosis

Etiology/Incidence

Stomal stenosis is the impairment of effluent drainage due to narrowing or contracting of the stomal tissue at the skin or fascial level (Colwell & Beitz, 2007). In the past, stenosis typically occurred early in the postoperative period due to inadequate surgical technique (at fascial level or at skin) or if not matured properly (Hampton, 1992). Due to the improvement in surgical technique, stomal stenosis is rarely seen early but rather late in the recovery process, >30 days following surgery, usually as a result of mucocutaneous separation, stoma necrosis, or retraction of the stoma. As healing occurs, formation of granulation tissue around the stoma constricts the lumen. Other causes of stomal stenosis include chronic disease (Crohn's or tumor), excessive scar formation due to instrumentation (dilatation), or chronic inflammation (peristomal irritant dermatitis or hyperplasia) (Colwell, 2004; Hampton, 1992).

The incidence of stomal stenosis has been reported between 2% and 23%. Of the 316 patients studied, 10.2% were found to have stenosis (Cheung, 1995). In a retrospective study of 150 permanent end ileostomies, Leong and associates (1994) found 23% with stenosis. Pittman et al. (2014) identified 5% in her study of 71 ostomy patients, and Porter et al. (1989) reported a stenosis rate of 11%. In a retrospective study of 1,616 medical records from 1976 to 1995 of patients who had received ostomy surgery, Park et al. (1999) reported that 34% developed ostomy complications with 72% occurring late (more than 30 days postoperatively). The most common late complications were peristomal irritant dermatitis (6%), prolapse (2%), and stenosis (2%) (Park et al., 1999). Finally, in a 3-year retrospective study of 164 patients who had surgery resulting in an ostomy, 17% were reported with stenosis (Duchesne et al., 2002).

Presentation

The appearance of a stenotic stoma opening appears small (Fig. 16-4). Often the patient with a fecal stoma may report pain with stoma evacuation, small ribbon-like stool, or conversely, constipation followed by large explosive evacuations, loud with excessive gas. Patients with urostomies may report frequent urinary tract infections, projectile urine stream, and/or flank pain (Colwell, 2004).

Assessment

Assessment of a stenotic stoma is best performed with a gloved lubricated digit in order to assess the size and mobility of the skin and fascial rings. If a digit cannot be inserted into the stomal opening due to severe stricture, a retrograde contrast study through a small rubber catheter may be performed (Colwell, 2004).

CLINICAL PEARL

When assessing the stoma with a digital exam explain to the patient that the stoma does not contain nerves to cause pain, but if they should feel pressure to let you know so you can stop the exam.

Management

Management of mild stenosis of a fecal ostomy may include low-residue diet, stool softeners, or high liquid intake. Stoma dilation by gradually and incrementally introducing a dilator into the stoma has been a common practice in the past, but there is little evidence in the literature to support this practice. However, chronic dilation has been reported to potentially cause stomal stenosis (Hampton, 1992). Stomal dilation can be used to temporarily aid in evacuation but is not recommended as a long-term practice. For the most severe cases, surgery is warranted. This may involve freeing the stoma from the peristomal skin locally or by performing a laparotomy/laparoscope and resiting the stoma.

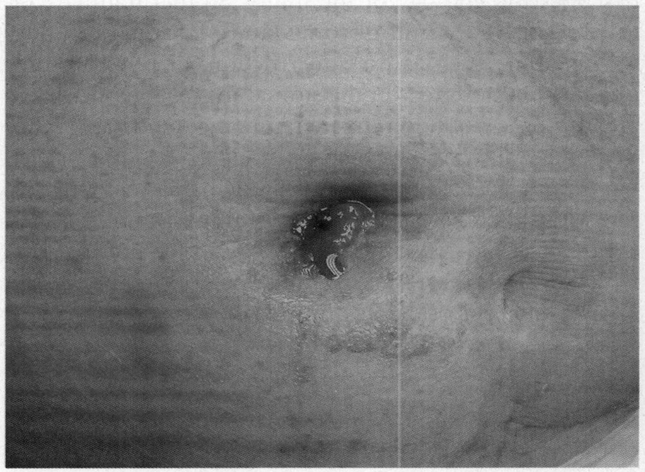

FIGURE 16-4. Stomal stenosis.

Stomal Prolapse

Etiology/Incidence

Stomal prolapse is the telescoping of the intestine through the stoma (Colwell & Beitz, 2007). Prolapse of the stoma can occur for a number of reasons: increased abdominal pressure, obesity, the stomal opening in the abdominal wall is too large, or the stoma was created outside the rectus muscle (Weideman et al., 2012).

All stomas are subject to prolapse, and incidence reports vary. Stoma prolapse is often seen in loop colostomies, and the distal limb is predominantly involved (Shellito, 1998; Gordon et al., 1998). Cheung (1995) reported that 6.8% developed prolapse in 156 end-sigmoid colostomies. In a study of 130 subjects with an end colostomy over a 6-year period, 4% experienced prolapsed stoma (Porter et al., 1989). Stomal prolapse is often seen in children (Franchini et al., 1983; Steinau et al., 2001). In a study of 144 infants with anorectal malformations, the incidence of stomal prolapse was higher in those with loop versus divided colostomies, 17.8% and 2.8%, respectively ($p = 0.005$) (Oda et al., 2014). Chen et al. (2013) performed a meta-analysis including five randomized controlled trials and seven nonrandomized studies with 1,687 patients in total comparing outcomes in temporary ileostomies versus temporary colostomies. They found a lower incidence of stoma prolapse in temporary ileostomy patients compared to temporary colostomy patients in both randomized control trials and nonrandomized trials (RR 0.15, 95% CI: 0.04 to 0.48, $p = 0.001$ and RR 0.26, 95% CI: 0.10 to 0.67, $p = 0.005$, respectively) (Chen et al., 2013). In a systematic review of the literature related to stoma complications following radical cystectomy and ileal conduit diversions, stomal prolapse was identified in 1.5% to 8% at a mean of 2 years following surgery (Szymanski et al., 2010). It has been reported that up to 50% of patients with prolapsed colostomy also had a parastomal hernia (Kim & Kumar, 2006).

Presentation

A prolapsed stoma can present in a variety of degrees of severity and length of stomal protrusion (Fig. 16-5). The length of the prolapsed stoma will guide management. The greater the length of the prolapse, the greater the likelihood of stomal edema, trauma, and ischemia. As the stoma becomes edematous and dependent, it becomes a deep red color (vasodilation). With a very prominent (5 to 13 inches) prolapse, the stoma is susceptible to trauma. Care

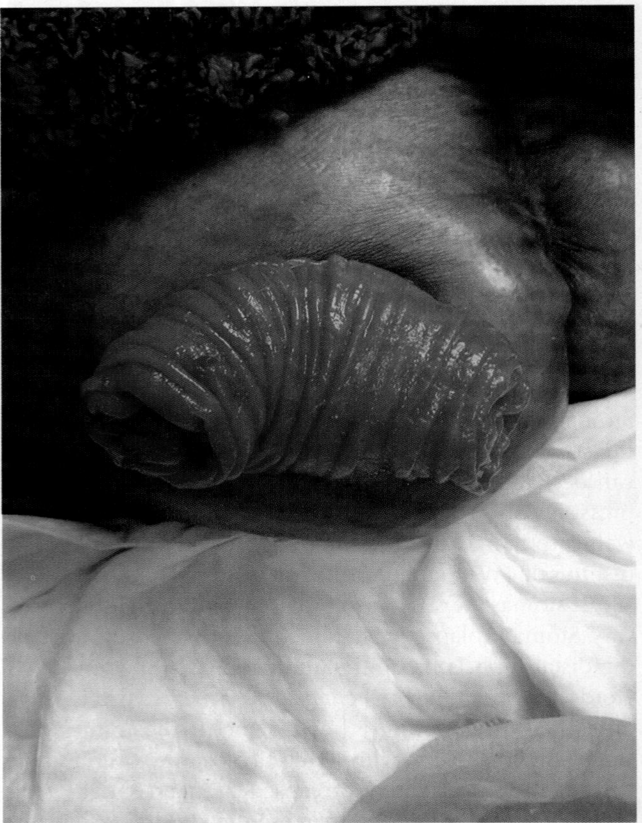

FIGURE 16-5. Stomal prolapse.

needs to include avoiding friction, laceration, or pressure to the stoma. In extreme situations, blood supply to the stoma may become compromised and stomal ischemia may occur.

Assessment

Assessment of the prolapsed stoma is performed by observation and palpation. Close observation must be done to determine the degree of the prolapse, color of the stoma, output characteristics, and pouching management. Palpation is accomplished with the patient in a supine position and attempting to reduce the prolapse with gentle pressure.

Management

Conservative management of the stomal prolapse is usually recommended. It is frequently best to apply the pouching system when the prolapsed is reduced. Have the patient lie flat and apply gentle pressure over the stoma to reduce. Reduction of the prolapse can be augmented by the application of cold (ice packs) to the stoma (over the pouch) for several minutes (Colwell, 2004). The use of sprinkling sugar over the prolapsed stoma has been reported to be effective to reduce prolapse (Fligelstone et al., 1997). Another management technique suggested is to use a hernia support belt with prolapse strap (Table 16-1). However, the strap usually does not provide enough pressure to prevent prolapsing of the stoma but simply provides support.

The pouching system should be adapted to fit the size of the prolapsed stoma. The pouch needs to accommodate the length of the stoma and be flexible to avoid stomal trauma. Education must be provided to the patient to observe the stoma for color changes and to seek immediate attention if the stoma becomes ischemic as surgery may be indicated (Colwell, 2004).

TABLE 16-1 Hernia Support Belt Ordering Information to Determine Appropriate Belt

Belt style	Original panel: for prevention and small bulge flattening Nu-Form style: for support of nonreducible hernia
Belt fabric	Ventilated fabric Solid elastic
Belt size	Measurement of girth standing and lying
Belt width	Varies according to the area needing support (3–9″ or more)
Stoma location	Right or left side of the abdomen
Belt opening	Pouch manufacture product number
Custom options	Auxiliary belt example

Adapted from Nu-Hope Hernia/Ostomy Belt Worksheet (Nu-Hope).

CLINICAL PEARL

If there is significant length to the prolapse it may be advisable to instruct the patient not to use a two piece pouching system as the stoma may be injured by the plastic flange (the stoma can protrude over the flange and be harmed).

Stomal Trauma

Etiology/Incidence

Stomal trauma has been defined as an injury to the stomal mucosa often related to pressure or physical force (Colwell & Beitz, 2007). Trauma as defined by Webster is "an injury (as a wound) to living tissue caused by an extrinsic agent" (Merriam-Webster, 2014). The term stomal trauma describes the etiology of the injury. Stomal trauma typically occurs as a result of some kind of trauma or injury to the stoma such as pressure, friction, or physical force of some kind exerted on the stomal mucosal tissue. There are no studies found in the literature that report incidence of stoma trauma. However, in a study of 71 adult participants with an ostomy, 32% of participants reported stomal bleeding. The cause of the bleeding was not reported (Pittman et al., 2014). In another study of 330 patients with an end colostomy, the investigators reported that 34.5% had mucosal bleeding (Mahjoubi et al., 2005). Again, the cause of the bleeding was not specified.

Presentation

Stomal trauma presents differently depending on the type of trauma, but it is usually localized to the area where the trauma occurred. It could present as a linear injury with

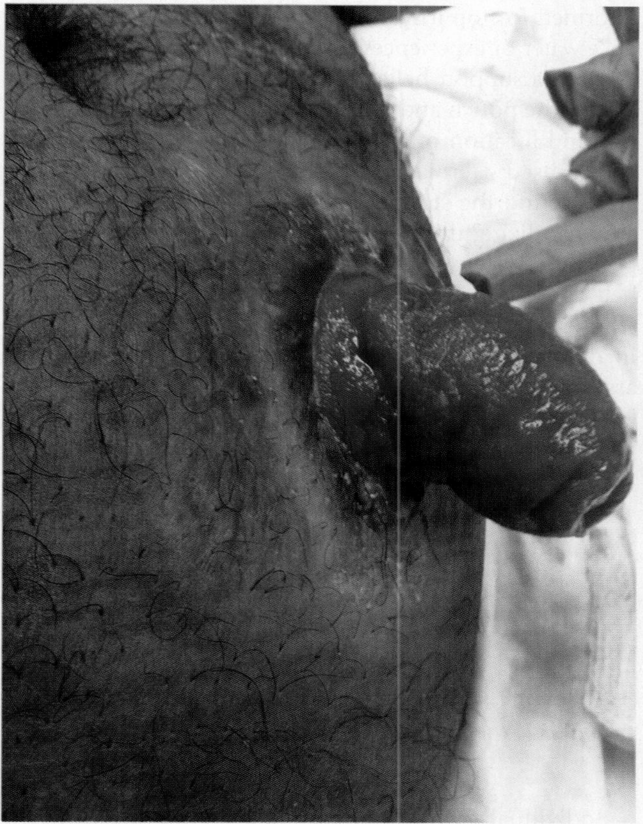

FIGURE 16-6. Stomal trauma.

minimal depth due to a laceration. Or the stomal mucosa could appear denuded with a deep red/dusky friable area that bleeds easily as a result of an abrasive injury (**Fig. 16-6**). The stoma could appear bruised or dusky if there was trauma as a result of pressure such as a seat belt. The appearance of the stomal injury depends on the type of trauma that occurred.

Assessment

A complete history and physical must include information regarding any recent trauma to the stoma. Removal of the pouch and direct visual observation of the stoma must occur in order to assess the stoma for integrity, color, hydration, and bleeding. Any changes in the stoma characteristics warrant further investigation.

Management

In order to treat the stomal trauma injury, the cause of the trauma must be determined and corrected. Stomal trauma injuries usually heal spontaneously once the source of the trauma is eliminated. If the injury was due to a seat belt rubbing across the stoma mucosa, padding the seat belt or shifting seat belt position may be adequate. If the two-piece pouching system flange is too small causing pinching of the stoma, adjusting the size of the pouching system may suffice. Management of stomal trauma includes assessment of the stoma with each pouch change for indications of healing (Colwell, 2004).

Parastomal Hernia

Etiology/Incidence

Parastomal (peristomal) hernia is defined as a defect in abdominal fascia that allows the intestine to bulge into the parastomal area (Colwell & Beitz, 2007). In many patients, the defect enlarges over time and allows the intestines to bulge into the area. The most common abdominal hernias develop at sites where the abdominal wall has natural openings such as the internal inguinal ring, the umbilicus, and the esophageal hiatus. Previous surgical entry sites (incisional hernia and stoma) are also common areas where hernias develop. Factors that increase the pressure in the abdominal cavity, such as obesity, heavy lifting, coughing with chronic lung disease, straining during a bowel movement or urination (prostatism), chronic lung disease, and ascites, have traditionally been considered important in the etiology, especially at these natural openings.

Parastomal hernia is one of the most common ostomy complications with incidence reported from 14% to 50% (Cheung, 1995; De Raet et al., 2008; Israelsson, 2008; Janes et al., 2011; Leong et al., 1994; Porter et al., 1989). DeRaet et al. (2008) reported that 46% of 42 open and lap abdominal–perineal resections developed hernias. These investigators found that when the waist circumference exceeded the calculated threshold of 100 cm, there was a 75% probability to develop a parastomal hernia (De Raet et al., 2008). Janes et al. (2011) reported that the rate of parastomal hernia was 50% after 1 year and 80% after 5 years. In a study comparing complications in 77 patients with laparoscopy surgery versus open surgery, 18% of laparoscopic compared with 2% after open procedures ($p = 0.04$) developed parastomal hernias (Randall et al., 2012).

Poor site selection or technical errors, such as making the fascial opening too large or placing a stoma in an incision, account for some of these hernias. Placing a stoma lateral to the rectus sheath is widely touted as a cause, but this is now being challenged (Israelsson, 2008). Obesity, malnutrition, advanced age, collagen abnormalities, postoperative sepsis, abdominal distention, constipation, obstructive uropathy, steroid use, and chronic lung disease also contribute. Following laparoscopic surgery, removal of the intestinal specimen through the site that was later used to create the stoma may contribute to the development of parastomal hernia (Randall et al., 2012). Novel techniques for stomal reconstruction, such as extraperitoneal tunneling or prophylactic mesh, have had little impact. Fortunately, fewer than 20% of patients with parastomal hernias have a complication that mandates repair.

Presentation

The individual with a parastomal hernia presents with a bulging around or beside the stoma, depending on the size of the defect in the abdominal wall, when abdominal pressure is increased (cough or bears down; **Fig. 16-7**). The individual may not be aware that he or she has a hernia but may report difficulty maintaining the seal of the pouching

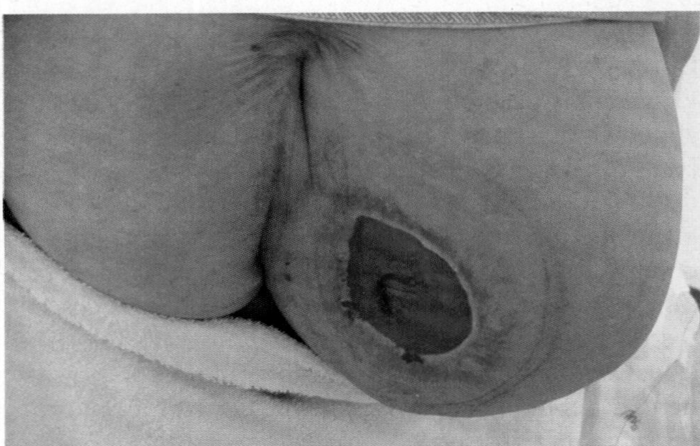

FIGURE 16-7. Peristomal hernia.

system thus experiencing leakage and irritated peristomal skin. This often occurs because of the change in the abdominal skin in contact with the pouching surface causes a shifting of the skin barrier and breakdown of the seal.

Assessment

Assessment of a parastomal hernia includes close visual observation of the patient in a sitting or standing position. An asymmetric bulge is identified next to the stoma and extending outward. Assessment can also be done with the patient in a lying position and asking the patient to cough, bear down, or lift his or her head. Palpate around the stoma as the patient raises his or her head or coughs to feel the extent of the hernia. The size or extent of the hernia varies according to the size of the defect in the abdominal wall. The defect may encompass the entire parastomal area or only a portion. Assessment may also include insertion of a digit into the stoma, feeling for fascial defect around the stoma. An incomplete fascial ring will be felt in the area of the hernia. Radiographic testing can be done to confirm the presence of the parastomal hernia; upper gastrointestinal x-ray with small bowel contrast, retrograde contrast study through the stoma, or computed tomography scan with oral contrast will identify bowel loops around the stoma and above the abdominal wall (Colwell, 2004).

Management

Conservative management and no surgical intervention is the treatment of choice for the asymptomatic patient. Conservative management options include flexible pouching system (avoiding a convex pouching system since the firm ring can cause trauma over the hernia), hernia support belt, spandex garments, regular diet/fluids to ensure soft stool and to prevent constipation, and routine follow-up with a WOC nurse.

A flexible pouching system is recommended in order to accommodate a changing stoma and pouching surface. The pouching system may be either a one-piece or a two-piece system with a floating flange. The stoma should be assessed in both the supine and standing position as the stoma size may enlarge when the hernia is protruding. Individuals who irrigate their colostomy should be informed to stop irrigating if it becomes difficult to introduce water or experience incomplete evacuation.

Hernia support belts are elastic binders with an opening for the pouch and must be custom-fit according to the size and location of the hernia and the type of pouching system used. Hernia support belts provide support to the area around the stoma, decreasing the hernia protrusion and stabilizing the parastomal plane thus improving the pouching system seal. Effectiveness of the hernia support belt varies widely, but it is an option for the individual who is not a surgical candidate. Hernia belts are available in different styles, sizes, and materials, and a thorough assessment should be done prior to ordering the correct belt. The manufacturer of hernia support belts provides a guide/worksheet to use when fitting a person with a belt (Nu-Hope Labs, 2014; Table 16-1).

CLINICAL PEARL

Once a hernia belt is obtained, the patient must be instructed how to apply the belt: the hernia needs to be reduced before belt application. The patient should be supine with the belt under his or her back, the belt pulled up and around the pouch and secured with Velcro. This will support the weakened muscle in a sitting or standing position.

Individuals with a parastomal hernia need to be informed of the importance of a diet and fluids to ensure soft stool and to prevent constipation. Education should also include the necessity of seeking immediate medical attention if the stoma darkens in color or if unremitting pain occurs. In addition, it is important for routine scheduled follow-up with a WOC nurse to monitor the hernia status and condition.

Surgical repair is the option when conservative measures fail. Indications for surgical repair of the stomal hernia depend on degree of severity and include obstruction, incarceration with/without strangulation, stenosis, intractable dermatitis, pouching management failure, large size of hernia, cosmesis, and pain. There are three general types of parastomal hernia repair (Colwell, 2004):

1. Primary fascial repair—an incision is made over the herniated area and the peristomal fascia is reapproximated. There is a high incidence of hernia reoccurrence with this method.
2. Local repair with prosthetic material such as mesh. There is high potential of erosion of the prosthetic material into the intestinal stoma with this method.
3. Stomal relocation to the opposite side of the abdomen. The hernia is repaired and the fascia reapproximated. This is the preferred method.

Conclusions

Research has shown that ostomy complications (stomal and peristomal) negatively affect the quality of life for individuals living with an ostomy and often result in physical and psychosocial limitations for these individuals and their families (Pittman et al., 2008). Not only does the person with an ostomy have to cope with a serious and often life-threatening diagnosis but the placement of an ostomy requires significant changes to one's lifestyle.

As we consider how we can prevent and/or decrease stomal complications, focus needs to be on the modifiable risk factors that contribute to their development and how the WOC nurse can intervene. Nursing interventions that have potential to prevent or decrease the incidence of stomal complications include weight reduction strategies, promoting a healthy lifestyle, and involving of the WOC nurse in preoperative stoma site marking and ostomy management.

REFERENCES

Arumugam, P., Bevan, L., MacDonald, L., et al. (2003). A prospective audit of stomas—Analysis of risk factors and complications and their management. *Colorectal Disease, 5*(1), 49–52.

Bass, E., Del Pino, A., Tan, A., et al. (1997). Does preoperative stomal marking and education by the enterostomal therapist affect outcome? *Diseases of the Colon & Rectum, 40*(4), 440–442.

Chen, J. W., Zhang, D. R., Li, J. R., et al. (2013). Meta-analysis of temporary ileostomy versus colostomy for colorectal anastomoses. *Acta Chirurgica Belgica, 113*(5), 330–339.

Cheung, M. T. (1995). Complications of an abdominal stoma: An analysis of 322 stomas. *Australian and New Zealand Journal of Surgery, 65*(11), 808–811.

Colwell, J. (2004). Stomal and peristomal complications. In J. Colwell, M. Goldberg, & J. Carmel (Eds.), *Fecal and urinary diversions: Management principles*. Philadelphia, PA: Mosby Inc.

Colwell, J., & Beitz, J. (2007). Survey of wound, ostomy and continence (WOC) nurse clinicians on stomal and peristomal complications: A content validation study. *Journal of Wound, Ostomy, and Continence Nursing, 34*(1), 57–69.

Colwell, J. C., & Fichera, A. (2005). Care of the obese patient with an ostomy. *Journal of Wound, Ostomy, and Continence Nursing, 32*(6), 378–385.

Colwell, J., Goldberg, M., & Carmel, J. (2001). The state of the standard diversion. *Journal of Wound, Ostomy, and Continence Nursing, 28*, 6–17.

Cottam, J. (2005). Audit of stoma complications within three weeks of surgery. *Gastrointestinal Nursing, 3*(1), 19–23.

Cottam, J., Richards, K., Hasted, A., et al. (2007). Results of a nationwide prospective audit of stoma complications within 3 weeks of surgery. *Colorectal Disease, 9*, 834–838.

De Raet, J., Delvaux, G., Haentjens, P., et al. (2008). Waist circumference is an independent risk factor for the development of parastomal hernia after permanent colostomy. *Diseases of the Colon & Rectum, 51*, 1806–1809.

Duchesne, J., Wang, Y., Weintraub, S., et al. (2002). Stoma complications: A multivariate analysis. *American Surgeon, 66*(11), 961.

Fligelstone, L. J., Wanendeya, N., & Palmer, B. V. (1997). Osmotic therapy for acure irreducible stomal prolapse. *British Journal of Surgery, 84*(3), 390. DOI: 10.1046/j.1365-2168.1997.02594.x

Franchini, A., Cola, B., Stevens, P. J., et al. (1983). *Atlas of stomal pathology*. New York, NY: Raven Press.

Gurtner, G. J., Neligan, P., Newman, M., et al. (2013). Intraoperative laser angiography using the SPY system: Review of the literature and recommendations for use. *Annals of Surgical Innovation and Research, 7*(1), 1–14.

Hampton, B. (1992). Peristomal and stomal complications. In B. Hampton & R. Bryant (Eds.), *Ostomies and continent diversions: Nursing management*. St. Louis, MO: Mosby Year Book.

Heiying, J., Yonghong, D., Xiaofeng, W., et al. (2014). A study of laparoscopic extraperitoneal sigmoid colostomy after abdomino-perineal resection for rectal cancer. *Gastroenterology Report, 2*(1), 58–62.

Israelsson, L. (2008). Parastomal hernias. *Surgical Clinics of North America, 88*, 113–125.

Janes, A., Weisby, L., & Israelsson, L. A. (2011). Parastomal hernia: Clinical and radiological definitions. *Hernia, 15*, 189–192. DOI: 10.1007/s10029-010-0769-6

Kim, J., & Kumar, R. (2006). Reoperation for stoma-related complications. *Clinics in Colon and Rectal Surgery, 19*(4), 207–212.

Leong, A., Londono-Schimmer, E., & Phillips, R. (1994). Life-table analysis of stomal complications following ileostomy. *British Journal of Surgery, 81*, 727–729.

Mahjoubi, B., Moghimi, A., Mirzaeli, R., et al. (2005). Evaluation of the end colostomy complications and the risk factors influencing them in Iranian patients. *Colorectal Disease, 7*(6), 582–587.

Merriam-Webster. (2014). Trauma from http://www.merriam-webster.com/medical/trauma

Nu-Hope Labs. (2014). http://www.nu-hope.com/beltlit.pdf, accessed 10-9-14.

Oda, O., Davies, D., Colapinto, K., et al. (2014). Loop versus divided colostomy for the management of anorectal malformations. *Journal of Pediatric Surgery, 49*(1), 87–90.

Park, J., Del Pino, A., Orsay, C., et al. (1999). Stoma complications. *Diseases of the Colon & Rectum, 42*(12), 1575–1580.

Pittman, J. (2011). *Ostomy complications and associated risk factors: Development and testing of two instruments*. (Dissertation PhD). Indiana University Purdue University Indianapolis Library.

Pittman, J., Bakas, T., Ellett, M., et al. (2014). Pschometric evaluation of the Ostomy Complication Severity Index. *Journal of Wound, Ostomy, and Continence Nursing, 41*(2), 1–11.

Pittman, J., Rawl, S. M., Schmidt, C. M., et al. (2008). Demographic and clinical factors related to ostomy complications and quality of life in veterans with an ostomy. *Journal of Wound, Ostomy, and Continence Nursing, 35*(5), 493–503.

Porter, J., Salvati, E., Rubin, R., et al. (1989). Complications of colostomies. *Disease of the Colon and Rectum, 32*(4), 299–303.

Randall, J., Lord, B., Fulham, J., et al. (2012). Parastomal hernias as the predominant stoma complication after laparoscopic colorectal surgery. *Surgical Laparoscopy, Endoscopy & Percutaneous Techniques, 22*(5), 420–423.

Ratliff, C., & Donovan, A. (2001). Frequency of peristomal complications. *Ostomy/Wound Management, 47*(8), 26–29.

Ratliff, C., Scarano, K., & Donovan, A. (2005). Descriptive study of peristomal complications. *Journal of Wound, Ostomy, and Continence Nursing, 32*(1), 33–37.

Salvadalena, G. (2008). Incidence of complications of the stoma and peristomal skin among individuals with colostomy, ileostomy, and urostomy: A systematic review. *Journal of Wound, Ostomy, and Continence Nursing, 35*(6), 596–607.

Shabbir, J. B., & Britton, D. C. (2010). Stoma complications: A literature overview. *Colorectal Disease, 12*(10), 958–964.

Steel, M., & Wu, J. (2002). Late stomal complications. *Clinics in Colon and Rectal Surgery, 15*(3), 199–207.

Steinau, G., Ruhi, K. M., Hornchen, H., et al. (2001). Enterostomy complications in infancy and childhood. *Langenbeck's Archives of Surgery, 386*(5), 346–349.

Szymanski, K., St-Cyr, D., Alam, T., et al. (2010). External stoma and peristomal complications following radical cystectomy and ileal conduit diversion: A systematic review. *Ostomy/Wound Management, 56*(1), 28–35.

Weideman, Y., Dunn, D., & Culleiton, A. (2012). *Ostomy management*. Brockton, MA: Western Schools Inc.

QUESTIONS

1. Which patient with an ostomy would be considered at higher risk for developing ostomy complications?
   A. A patient who has a low body mass index (BMI)
   B. A patient whose age is >40 years
   C. A patient who has a colostomy versus an ileostomy
   D. A patient who has a diverting loop procedure performed

2. Which patient would the nurse recognize as having an *early* stomal complication?
   A. A patient experiencing death of the stoma tissue resulting from impaired blood flow
   B. A patient with impairment of effluent drainage due to narrowing or contracting of the stoma tissue at the skin or fascial level
   C. A patient who presents with telescoping of the intestines through the stoma
   D. A patient who has injury to the stomal mucosa related to physical force or pressure

3. Which assessment by the nurse confirms a diagnosis of stomal retraction?
   A. The stoma height is >10 mm.
   B. The stomal tissue turns from pink to black.
   C. The stoma disappears in line with or below skin level.
   D. There is a gap between the stoma and the skin.

4. A patient is diagnosed with stomal retraction. What is *not* a goal of management for this patient?
   A. Use stomal dilation to temporarily aid in evacuation.
   B. Use a convex pouching system to augment level of stoma above skin.
   C. Surgically create a new stoma in a new location.
   D. Revise the stoma with available intestine to mobilize above skin level.

5. The nurse is managing the care of a patient who has a stomal prolapse. Which intervention is appropriate for this patient?
   A. Sprinkle sugar over the prolapsed stoma.
   B. Apply warm compresses to the stoma over the pouch for several minutes.
   C. Apply the pouching system when the prolapse is maximized.
   D. Reduce the prolapse by applying firm pressure to the stoma.

6. A patient with a new stoma complains to the nurse: "I can't always get the pouching system sealed tightly, and then it leaks!" The nurse notes bulging of the peristomal area. What condition would the wound nurse suspect is occurring?
   A. Stomal stenosis
   B. Parastomal hernia
   C. Stomal trauma
   D. Stomal prolapse

7. What is a treatment choice for a patient with parastomal hernia who is asymptomatic?
   A. Loosely fitting garments
   B. Surgical intervention
   C. Convex pouching system
   D. Hernia support belt

8. A patient with a stoma reports pain with stoma evacuation and small, ribbon-like stools. What stomal complication may be present?
   A. Stoma trauma
   B. Stoma prolapse
   C. Stoma stenosis
   D. Parastomal hernia

9. A patient with a new stoma is diagnosed with a large mucocutaneous separation. What condition is likely to occur due to this defect?
   A. Retraction of the stoma
   B. Stomal prolapse
   C. Parastomal hernia
   D. Stomal trauma

10. A patient with a parastomal hernia is scheduled for surgical repair. What type of repair is the preferred method?
   A. Primary fascial repair.
   B. Local repair with prosthetic material such as mesh.
   C. Stomal relocation to the opposite side of the abdomen.
   D. Surgical repair is not an option to correct a parastomal hernia.

ANSWERS: 1.**D**, 2.**A**, 3.**C**, 4.**A**, 5.**A**, 6.**B**, 7.**D**, 8.**C**, 9.**A**, 10.**C**

CHAPTER 17

Fistula Management

Denise Nix and Ruth A. Bryant

OBJECTIVES

1. Describe causative and contributing factors to fistula development.
2. Describe guidelines for medical management of the patient with an enterocutaneous fistula.
3. Outline criteria and guidelines for promotion of spontaneous fistula closure.
4. Explain the significance of pseudostoma formation in the patient with a fistula.
5. Discuss indications for surgical closure of a fistula.
6. Develop and implement individualized management plan for the fistula patient that provides for containment of drainage and odor and protection of perifistular skin.

Topic Outline

Introduction

A fistula (plural fistulas or fistulae) is an abnormal passage between two or more epithelialized surfaces that results in communication between one body cavity or hollow organ and another hollow organ or the skin (Bryant & Best, 2015). An enterocutaneous fistula (ECF) refers to an opening from the intestine to the skin. Although ECFs *can* be located *within* a wound, they should not be confused with a draining wound, surgically placed drain site, or wound dehiscence.

The mortality rates for patients with ECFs range from as low as 5.5% to as high as 30%; death is most often due to sepsis, malnutrition, or fluid and electrolyte imbalance (Kaur & Minocha, 2000; Li et al., 2003; McNaughton et al., 2010). Although the true incidence of ECF development is unknown, Teixeira et al. (2009) reported an incidence of 1.5% in a large study involving 2,373 trauma patients who required laparotomy. They also found that patients with ECFs required significant hospital resources with a statistically significant increase in intensive care unit length of stay (28.5 ± 30.5 vs. 7.6 ± 9.3 days, $p = 0.004$), hospital length of stay (82.1 ± 100.8 vs. 16.2 ± 17.3 days, $p < 0.001$), and mean hospital charges ($539,309 vs. $126,996, $p < 0.001$).

An interdisciplinary team is needed to meet the needs of the patient with a fistula (Canadian Association for Enterostomal Therapy [CAET], 2009). Most authors suggest that essential team members include wound/ostomy nurse, dietitian, pharmacist, nurse, social worker, surgeon, and physician (Haffejee, 2004; Hollington et al., 2004; Lal et al., 2006). Other team members include pain specialists, radiologists, physiotherapists, and occupational therapists (Lal et al., 2006; Oneschuk & Bruera, 1997). ECF management is one of the most difficult clinical challenges for the wound/ostomy nurse. It can also be the most rewarding experience once the patient's quality of life is restored through individualized, unique, and best practice interventions.

TABLE 17-1 Fistula Classification

	Designation	Characteristics
Location	Internal	Tract contained within body
	External	Tract exits through skin
Involved structures (not inclusive)	Colon to vagina	Colovaginal
	Intestine to skin	Enterocutaneous
	Bladder to vagina	Vesicovaginal
	Colon to skin	Colocutaneous
	Rectum to vagina	Rectovaginal
	Colon to vagina	Colovaginal
Volume	High output	>500 mL/24 h
	Moderate output	200–500 mL/24 h
	Low output	<200 mL/24 h
Complexity	Simple	Short direct tract, no abscess, no other organ involvement
	Complex	Type 1—abscess, multiple organ involvement Type 2—opens into the base of a wound

Modified from Bryant, R., & Best, M. (2015). Management of draining wounds and fistulas. In R. Bryant & D. Nix (Eds.), *Acute and chronic wounds: Current management concepts* (5th ed.). St. Louis, MO: Mosby. (In Print.)

Clinical Presentation and Classification

Fever and abdominal pain are the initial indicators of a possible fistula (Nussbaum & Fischer, 2006); however, these are nonspecific indicators. The definitive indicator of a cutaneous fistula is the passage of gastrointestinal (GI) secretions or urine into an open wound bed or through an unintentional opening onto the skin. Manifestations of a fistula tract terminating in the vagina include passage of urine (vesicovaginal fistula) or passage of gas, feces, and/or purulent and extremely malodorous drainage (rectovaginal or enterovaginal fistula). Irradiation-induced rectovaginal fistulas often are preceded by diarrhea, passage of mucus and blood rectally, a sensation of rectal pressure, and a constant urge to defecate (Saclarides, 2002). Fistulas between the intestinal tract and the urinary bladder (e.g., colovesical fistula) present with passage of gas or stool-stained urine through the urethra.

CLINICAL PEARL

The definitive indicator of a cutaneous fistula is the passage of GI secretions or urine into an open wound bed or through an unintentional opening onto the skin.

The pH of the effluent may suggest the origin of the fistula tract. For example, extremely acidic fluid (pH 1.0 to 3.0) suggests a gastric fistula, whereas highly alkaline output (7.8 to 8) is consistent with a pancreatic fistula (Huether, 2002).

Most clinicians describe and classify fistulas according to location, involved structures, and volume of effluent. Although less frequently used, fistulas may also be classified by complexity (see Table 17-1). Mucous fistulas are surgically created openings into the defunctionalized section of bowel; they secrete mucus only, which is relatively easy to contain with dressings or pouches, and they do not increase morbidity or mortality. They are therefore not further discussed in this chapter.

CLINICAL PEARL

Fistulas are typically "named" for the organ of origin and the organ of termination; for example, an ECF is one from the bowel to the skin, and a colovesical fistula is one from the colon to the vagina.

Etiologic Factors

ECFs commonly develop postoperatively, due to anastomotic breakdown, but can also occur spontaneously, as a result of inflammatory bowel disease, cancer, or diverticulitis. The risk of fistula formation is further increased when one of these conditions is complicated by malnutrition, sepsis, hypotension, vasopressors, or corticosteroids (Nussbaum & Fischer, 2006).

Approximately 25% of fistulas develop spontaneously and are associated with an intrinsic intestinal disease (cancer, radiation, diverticulitis, inflammatory bowel disease, appendicitis) or external trauma. Spontaneous fistulas are generally resistant to spontaneous closure. Patients treated for a pelvic cancer are particularly vulnerable to ECFs due to radiation damage; the fistula may develop immediately following radiation or years later (Tran & Thorson, 2008). An analysis of 41 publications reported that 17% of patients receiving pelvic radiation developed ECFs, and the average time frame for fistula development was 3.4 years following completion of radiation therapy (Meissner, 1999). Irradiation-induced ECFs are more likely to occur in patients who receive higher radiation doses (>5,000 cGy), smoke cigarettes, or have atherosclerosis, hypertension, diabetes mellitus, advanced age, pelvic inflammatory disease, or previous pelvic surgery (Hollington et al., 2004; Saclarides, 2002; Tran & Thorson, 2008).

CLINICAL PEARL

Most ECFs occur postoperatively, as a result of anastomotic breakdown; however, fistulas may also develop spontaneously as a result of inflammatory bowel conditions (e.g., diverticulitis, Crohn's disease, radiation enteritis) or trauma.

The majority of ECFs (75% to 85%) are iatrogenic (inadvertently induced from a medical procedure); these fistulas develop postoperatively due to anastomotic breakdown (Nussbaum & Fischer, 2006). A key risk factor for anastomotic breakdown is malnutrition (Mäkelä et al., 2003; Telem et al., 2010). Additional risk factors for postoperative ECF development include existing conditions such as inflammatory bowel disease, cancer, or previous radiation therapy. Surgery-related risk factors include inadequate blood supply, poor suture technique, inadequate bowel prep (e.g., emergency surgery), extensive lysis of adhesions, and trauma surgery (Kassis & Makary, 2008; Nussbaum & Fischer, 2006; Wong et al., 2004). The method of anastomosis (stapled or hand-sewn) has not proven to be a predictor of ECF after surgery for trauma (Demetriades et al., 2002; Kirkpatrick et al., 2003). Patients scheduled for elective surgical procedures should receive adequate nutrition preoperatively in order to minimize the risk of anastomotic breakdown. When emergency surgery is necessary, prevention strategies include adequate intravenous fluids, circulatory support, keeping the patient warm, and broad-spectrum antibiotics (Kassis & Makary, 2008; Maykel & Fischer, 2003). If there are concerns regarding delayed healing of the intestinal anastomosis due to poorly controlled morbidities and extensive intra-abdominal infection, a temporary stoma may be created proximal to the anastomosis to protect the anastomosis during healing; the stoma is closed once healing is complete. In the past, temporary stomas were commonly performed following bowel resection and anastomosis due to traumatic injury; this is no longer standard, as most of these anastomoses have been shown to heal in a timely manner. Interestingly, recent studies indicate that diversion following colonic anastomosis for penetrating colonic injury did not reduce the incidence of septic complications, including abscess and fistula (Demetriades et al., 2001).

Medical Management

Management for this patient population requires a clear understanding of the underlying pathophysiology, astute assessment skills, knowledge about management alternatives and options, competent technical skills, diligent follow-up, and persistence. A comprehensive and effective interdisciplinary approach is required to reduce complications and achieve closure (Bryant & Best, 2015). Spontaneous closure of an ECF is defined as closing with medical management within 6 to 8 weeks (Teixeira et al., 2009). Wong et al. (2004) report 90% of simple type 1 fistulas close spontaneously, whereas <10% of complex type 2 fistulas close spontaneously. Additional factors that correlate with spontaneous closure include postoperative occurrence, low output, absence of sepsis, and adequate nutrition (Campos et al., 1999; Nussbaum & Fischer, 2006). When sepsis is controlled and appropriate nutritional support is provided, approximately 19% to 40% of all fistulas close spontaneously with medical management. The majority of ECFs that close spontaneously do so within 5 weeks (Kassis & Makary, 2008).

CLINICAL PEARL

Only a limited percentage (19% to 40%) of fistulas close spontaneously, even with optimal management; those that do close spontaneously usually do so within 5 to 6 weeks.

Objectives of ECF management are described below and include: (1) maintenance of fluid and electrolyte balance; (2) measures to minimize fistula output; (3) control of infection; (4) nutritional support; (5) definition of the fistula tract; and (6) skin protection and containment of effluent.

Maintenance of Fluid and Electrolyte Balance

Each day 8 to 10 L of fluid flows through the jejunum, depending on oral intake. In the intact functioning intestine, 98% of this fluid is (re)absorbed, leaving only 100 to 200 mL of fluid to be excreted in the stool. Development of a fistula permits abnormal fluid losses, with volume of loss determined in part by size of the fistulous opening and in part by anatomic location within the bowel. For example, fistulas located in the proximal small bowel are generally high output, while fistulas occurring in the colon are typically low output. When providing fluid replacement, the prescribing provider must consider both the volume and the composition of the fistulous drainage, both of which are impacted by fistula location within the GI tract. Severe metabolic disturbances have been noted with ECF output >200 mL/day due to loss of hydrogen, chloride, sodium, and potassium ions (Arebi & Forbes, 2004; Makhdoom et al., 2000). Careful monitoring of tissue perfusion, weight, urine, and fistula output is necessary to evaluate fluid balance. Adequate fluid and electrolyte replacement is critical to prevent hypovolemia and circulatory failure in the patient with a high-output ECF (Makhdoom et al., 2000).

Measures to Minimize Fistula Output

A key intervention for promotion of spontaneous closure is to minimize the amount of fluid flowing through the fistula tract, that is, to reduce oral and enteral intake. This may be done by making the patient NPO (nothing by mouth), or by limiting oral and/or enteral intake to the amount needed to keep the intestinal mucosa healthy. Significantly reduced oral/enteral intake minimizes fistula output by decreasing luminal contents, GI stimulation, and pancreaticobiliary secretion. Administration of H_2 antagonists (e.g., cimetidine), frequently used to prevent stress ulcerations, also decreases gastric, biliary, and pancreatic secretions. Despite this reduction in secretions, H_2 receptors have not been shown to affect either the number of ECFs that close spontaneously or the time to ECF closure (Arebi & Forbes, 2004; Evenson & Fischer, 2006).

Somatostatin and its analog, octreotide, are known to decrease intestinal output in some situations, and have been used as adjunctive therapy in the treatment of ECF. Somatostatin is administered through continuous intravenous infusion due to its short half-life of 1 to 2 minutes. Octreotide's half-life is almost 2 hours, and it is administered three times daily subcutaneously (Makhdoom et al., 2000). In the past, there was lack of consensus as to whether these medications increased closure rates or decreased time to closure (Arebi & Forbes, 2004; Fagniez & Yahchouchy, 1999; Hesse et al., 2001; Sancho et al., 1995; Torres et al., 1992). More recently, a systematic review and meta-analysis conducted by Coughlin et al. (2012) concluded that somatostatin analogs appear to decrease the duration of ECFs (time to closure) and hospital stays, though there was no reduction in number of fistulas that closed and no reduction in fistula-related mortality. Octreotide is not recommended for routine use due to reports of precipitated villous atrophy, interruption of intestinal adaptation, and acute cholecystitis. Some authors recommend a 5- to 8-day trial, with discontinuation of the octreotide if there is no significant reduction in fistula output within that time frame (Draus et al., 2006).

CLINICAL PEARL

Measures to promote spontaneous closure of ECFs include nutritional support, limited oral/enteral intake to reduce the volume of fistula output, and possibly negative pressure wound therapy (NPWT) (to promote wound healing).

Control of Infection

Uncontrolled sepsis and sepsis-associated malnutrition have been shown to be important determinants of mortality in the patient with an ECF (Dubose & Lundy, 2010; Lynch et al., 2004). Symptoms may include localized and then diffuse abdominal pain, ileus, and fever. Presence of abscess can be detected with computed tomographic scanning or ultrasound. CT-guided drainage is the initial management of choice in patients presenting with spontaneous or postoperative intra-abdominal abscess. This can obviate the need for early operative intervention. As seen in **Figure 17-1**, if a fistula develops, a definitive procedure can be deferred with the drain left in place to control further abscess formation (Davis et al., 2000; Lynch et al., 2004). Abscess contents should be cultured after percutaneous or surgical drainage, to assure appropriate antibiotic therapy (Wong et al., 2004).

CLINICAL PEARL

Somatostatin analogs have been shown to reduce the time to fistula closure and the length of hospital stay, but do not increase the number of fistulas that close spontaneously.

Definition of the Fistula Tract

Once the patient is stabilized, definition of the fistula tract should be undertaken. The fistula should be assessed for point of origin, condition of adjacent bowel, presence of abscess, and any distal obstruction or bowel discontinuity.

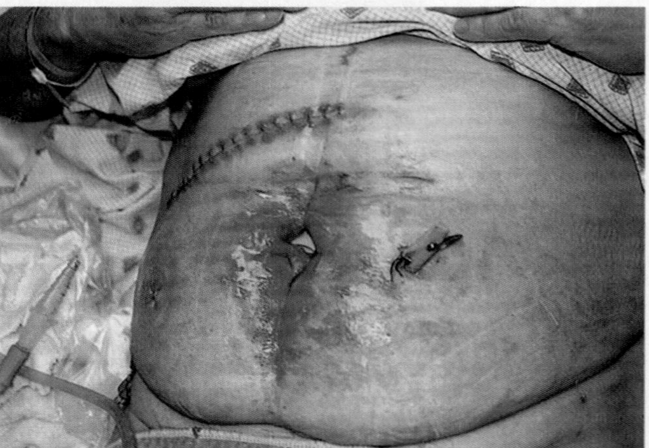

FIGURE 17-1. ECF (small bowel to skin); extensive skin damage due to enzymatic drainage; drain in place for abscess management.

This can be accomplished with a range of radiological examinations: fistulagram, ultrasonography, magnetic resonance imaging (MRI), positive emission tomography (PET) scan, or computerized tomography (Arebi & Forbes, 2004; Schecter et al., 2009).

Nutritional Support

As previously discussed, adequate nutritional support is an essential component of effective management; it is critical to keep the patient in positive nitrogen balance to promote healing of the fistula tract. The route of nutritional support depends on the patient's ability to ingest sufficient quantities, the location of the fistula tract, the absorptive capacity of the bowel mucosa, and the patient's tolerance.

The use of total parenteral nutrition (TPN), accompanied by simultaneous "bowel rest," has revolutionized the care of the fistula patient by allowing for the delivery of nutrition while simultaneously minimizing fistula effluent; this enhances patient management and the potential for spontaneous closure (Dubose & Lundy, 2010). On the negative side, the delivery of TPN through central venous catheters is associated with an appreciable rate of bacteremia and line sepsis. In one study conducted by Wong and colleagues (2004), positive blood cultures were obtained from 24.6% of 88 catheters utilized to deliver TPN to patients undergoing nonoperative management of enteric fistulas.

There is currently increased interest in the use of *enteral* nutrition for prevention and management of patients with ECFs, based on the role of enteral intake on the health and integrity of the intestinal mucosa; low-volume enteral intake can prevent translocation of bacteria; maintain the normal structural, immunologic, and hormonal integrity of the GI tract; and reduce cost relative to TPN (Dubose & Lundy, 2010). During a small retrospective study, Collier et al. (2007) noted that early postoperative initiation of enteral nutrition (≤4 days) resulted in a lower fistula formation rate than did nutritional approaches involving later initiation of enteral feedings (9% vs. 26%, respectively). Researchers also noted that the use of early enteral nutrition resulted in earlier primary abdominal closure and lower hospital charges.

CLINICAL PEARL

Nutritional support is a critical element of effective fistula management; the goals of nutritional management are to maintain positive nitrogen balance (usually through TPN), maintain the integrity of the intestinal mucosa (usually through low-volume enteral intake), and minimize fistula output (usually through reduced oral/enteral intake).

In selected patients, enteral nutrition may be used to maintain nutritional status while promoting fistula closure. It is now known that approximately 4 feet of healthy small intestine (in the adult) are needed to meet nutritional needs via the enteral route (Knechtges & Zimmermann, 2009). Therefore enteral nutrition may be feasible for the patient whose fistula is located in the most proximal or distal portion of a functional GI tract; if the fistula is located in the most proximal segment of the bowel, the enteral feeding must be administered distal to the fistula. Many types of enteral solutions are available, and a dietician should be consulted to recommend the most appropriate solution and administration procedure so that GI intolerance (e.g., diarrhea, abdominal distention) can be avoided.

Skin Protection and Containment

Establishing and maintaining skin protection and containment of the fistula effluent can be a challenging and yet rewarding experience. It is beneficial for WOC nurses managing the patient with an ECF to frequently remind themselves of the four general principles presented by Rolstad and Wong (2004).

1. Assess the pouching system and seal frequently; expect to make changes in the management system.
2. Build flexibility into the care plan.
3. Innovate, using the easiest, most practical approach first.
4. Recognize that care of the patient is frequently provided by inexperienced caregivers.

Skin protection and effluent containment should be initiated as soon as the fistula develops and is not contingent upon medical diagnosis. Goals for topical management of the ECF are listed in Box 17-1 (Bryant & Best, 2015). Methods and techniques for skin protection and containment will be described in the intervention section of the chapter and are presented in Tables 17-2 and 17-3.

CLINICAL PEARL

Skin protection and effluent containment should be initiated as soon as the fistula develops and is not contingent upon medical diagnosis nor the medical plan of care.

BOX 17-1 Goals for Topical Management of the ECF

- Perifistular skin protection
- Containment of effluent
- Odor control
- Patient comfort
- Accurate measurement of effluent
- Patient mobility
- Ease of care
- Cost containment

TABLE 17-2 Fistula Products and their Indications

Product/Accessory	Action	Indications
Skin barrier wipes, wands, or sprays	Provides a protective film to skin	**Low-output fistulae**—provides protective layer to skin. Used in combination with dressings **High-output fistulae**—used in combination with pouches, suction systems, and NPWT to protect against adhesive trauma
Moisture barrier creams, ointments, or pastes	Repels moisture and protects skin	**Low-output fistulae**—provides protection to skin around fistula. May be used in combination with dressings **High-output fistulae**—not indicated. Does not provide enough protection with high-output effluent. Contraindicated with the use of any adhesive products (i.e., pouches), as creams will not allow products to adhere to skin
Pectin barrier rings, strips, and pastes	Provides physical barrier to effluent/stool	**Low-output fistulae**—provides skin protection against effluent **High-output fistulae**—used to fill in uneven surfaces for pouching or as a part of the pouching system
Pouches	Contain effluent/stool and odor from fistula	**Low-output fistulae**—where odor is a problem or the patient prefers to change pouch as opposed to dressings **High-output fistulae**—used to contain stool and odor
Suction systems	Contain effluent in combination with low intermittent suction and dressings or pouches	**Low-output fistulae**—not indicated **High-output fistulae**—where pouching systems to gravity drainage are not effective due to large amounts of liquid effluent. Not a long-term solution
NPWT	Direct pressure closure	**Low-output fistulae**—not indicated **High-output fistulae**—where closure is a possibility. No abscess can be present. The patient must receive bowel rest and nutritional support, e.g., TPN. There should be no evidence of epithelial cells on opening of fistula (no evidence of pseudostoma formation)
Dressings	Absorb drainage	**Low-output fistulae**—used in combination with other skin protectants such as skin barrier wipes, barrier creams and pastes, and pectin wafers **High-output fistulae**—not indicated

NPO, nothing by mouth; NPWT, negative pressure wound therapy; TPN, total parenteral nutrition.

TABLE 17-3 Fistula Containment Options Based on Output and Need for Access

Output volume	<100 mL	<100 mL	>100 mL or dressing change > every 4 h	>100 mL or dressing change > every 4 h
Need for odor control	No	Yes	Yes or no	Yes or no
Need for frequent access	Yes/no	Yes/no	Yes	No
Containment options	Absorptive dressings and perifistular skin protectant (e.g., ointment, paste barrier)	Charcoal cover dressing (placed over absorptive dressings) with environmental deodorants and frequent dressing changes OR Ostomy pouch	Wound management system with window emptied frequently or attached to bedside bag OR Two-piece ostomy pouch emptied frequently Two-piece urostomy pouch emptied frequently or attached to bedside bag (urinary or fecal spout)	Pouching systems OR Closed systems with suction or attached to straight drainage NPWT

Fistula Management for the WOC Nurse

Methods and strategies for fistula management are guided by a thorough assessment; the parameters first described by Boarini and Bryant (1986) remain the standard for fistula assessment today (Bryant & Best, 2015; CAET, 2009).

Assessment

In addition to determining the type of fistula, assessment must include abdominal contours, fistula opening, effluent characteristics, and the condition of the perifistular skin. Each dressing or pouch change represents an opportunity to reevaluate the fistula and to modify the care plan accordingly. All assessments, reassessments, interventions, responses to interventions, and management and follow-up plans should be documented (see Box 17-2).

Progress toward/Impediments to Spontaneous Closure

A critical aspect of assessment is evaluation of progress toward and impediments to spontaneous closure (see Box 17-3). Progress in closure is evidenced by reduced output through the fistula tract along with increased fecal output through the distal bowel (rectum or stoma); thus, fistula output should be monitored, as should the output from any stoma, and the patient with an intact distal bowel should be routinely queried regarding bowel movements. Any indicators of abscess formation (e.g., increasing abdominal tenderness, fever, or purulent drainage mixed with the fecal output) must be promptly reported so that intervention can be initiated. The nurse must also be alert to development of a stomatized fistula, also known as a pseudostoma or an epithelialized stoma; this occurs when the anterior wall of the bowel becomes adherent to the abdominal wall and the fistula tract undergoes mucosal eversion. The end result is a permanent opening into the bowel that must be closed surgically; thus, observation of a "stoma" in the wound bed requires prompt MD notification (see Fig. 17-2).

CLINICAL PEARL

Assessment of the individual with a fistula must include the volume and characteristics of the output, the contours of the abdominal wall and fistula opening, and indicators of progress toward or impediments to spontaneous closure.

Abdominal Contours and Fistula Opening

The fistula opening and abdominal contours should be assessed while the patient is standing, sitting, and lying down if possible. If the pannus is large, more positions may be necessary to observe the changes in perifistular contours that occur with shifts in position of the pannus. Skin contours should be noted, and the abdomen should be inspected for irregular skin surfaces that are created by scars, creases, bony prominences, or other obstacles such as sutures/staples, incisions (dehisced or intact), or stomas. The location of the ECF should be identified, and visible openings should be measured (length and width in cm) and documented. The level at which the fistula empties in relation to the skin (or wound) surface is of critical importance. The fistula opening may be retracted (lower than skin level), level with the skin, above the level of the skin, or in a deep wound (see Fig. 17-2). If the fistula empties directly onto the skin and is level with the skin, a convex pouching system is usually required; in contrast, a

BOX 17-2 Documentation for the WOC Nurse

Focused Assessment
- Fistula source (see **Table 17-1**)
- Pain
- Fistula opening
  - Location
  - Length and width
  - Height (retracted, skin level, protruding)
- Perifistular skin integrity
  - Intact
  - Impaired (erythema, maceration, candidiasis, denudement)
- Abdominal contours and proximity of fistula to: scars, skin folds, bony prominences, drains, or ostomies
- Output/effluent
  - Volume
  - Consistency
  - Color
  - Odor
- Containment system and frequency of changes

Interventions
- Emotional support
- Changes in containment method/procedure with rationale (if any change required)
- Education of patient/family
  - Normal versus impaired skin
  - Signs of infection
  - Containment procedure

Evaluation
- Indicators of progress in closure (or impediments, such as pseudostoma formation)
- Effectiveness of containment system
  - Wear time without leakage
  - Perifistular skin intact or improved
  - Odor control
  - Effects on patient mobility
  - Ease of care
- Patient/family response to interventions
  - Patient satisfaction
  - Comfort
  - Level of activity
  - Learning

Follow-up Plan
- Approximate day of next visit
- Instruction for staff between visits (including what to do if questions/concerns arise)

BOX 17-3 **Factors that Prevent Spontaneous Closure**

- Compromised distal suture line/anastomosis (i.e., tension on suture line, improper suturing technique, inadequate blood supply to anastomosis)
- Distal obstruction
- Foreign body in fistula tract or suture line
- Epithelium-lined tract contiguous with skin (pseudostoma)
- Presence of tumor or disease in site
- Previous irradiation to site
- Crohn's disease
- Abscess
- Hematoma

Adapted from Bryant, R., & Best, M. (2015). Management of draining wounds and fistulas. In R. Bryant & D. Nix (Eds.), *Acute and chronic wounds: Current management concepts* (5th ed.). St. Louis, MO: Mosby. (In Print.)

fistula that has undergone mucosal maturation (pseudostoma formation) and that protrudes above the level of the skin may enable a better pouch seal. The opening might also contain a drain, as seen in **Figure 17-1**, for drainage of an abscess.

CLINICAL PEARL

A "pseudostoma" occurs when the anterior wall of the bowel becomes adherent to the abdominal wall, and the fistula tract undergoes mucosal eversion to create an epithelium-lined tract. Pseudostoma development requires MD notification because it means the fistula will have to be closed surgically.

Assessment of all these parameters will help determine the level of skin protection required, as well as the flexibility, size, and shape of adhesive barrier needed for effective protection of the perifistular skin and avoidance of any areas that could compromise the adhesion of the pouching system or cause discomfort to the patient.

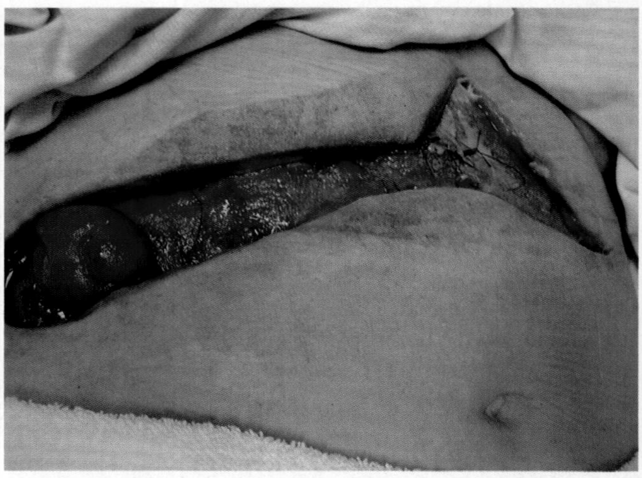

FIGURE 17-2. Pseudostoma in deep wound.

Effluent Characteristics

Assessment of fistula effluent (source, volume, odor, consistency, composition) influences topical management selection by providing insight into the degree of risk for perifistular skin breakdown and odor as well as the type of pouch closure needed. For example, an odorous fistula producing effluent with semi-formed consistency is most likely originating from the left transverse or descending colon. Effluent from the transverse or descending colon will be less damaging to the skin than is output from the small intestine or stomach. (See **Fig. 17-1** for illustration of skin damage related to small bowel drainage.) Thus, the primary goals of topical management for that patient would be containment of effluent and odor control.

ECF output *volumes* >100 mL over 24 hours usually require a pouch or suction or both. In contrast, the ECF with minimal output can often be managed with the application of a perifistular moisture barrier and an absorptive dressing. However, in the presence of odor, even the patient with a low-output fistula may prefer a containment pouch for odor control. It should be noted that odor may originate from numerous sources, including fecal drainage, exudate, necrotic or infected tissue, soiled dressings, and/or chemicals used during treatment.

CLINICAL PEARL

There are multiple options for containment of fistula effluent and perifistular skin protection; the best option for an individual patient is determined by the volume and characteristics of the output and the abdominal contours.

Consistency of effluent is particularly important to selection of a pouching system because it influences the type and number of skin barriers needed as well as the type of drainage outlet required to efficiently empty the pouch. For example, liquid effluent is much more corrosive than is thick effluent and is much more likely to result in premature erosion of the skin barrier; thus, liquid effluent requires the most durable skin barrier/protectant. Liquid effluent is easier to empty from a spout rather than clamp type closure.

Constant exposure of the epidermis to moisture, enzymes, extremes in pH, and mechanical trauma frequently leads to perifistular skin damage. Denudation of perifistular skin is a common complication in fistula patients and often is present when the patient is first seen with the fistula. Perifistular skin is also at risk for fungal infection as a consequence of moisture entrapment against the skin and antibiotic precipitated changes in the normal skin flora. Candidiasis is a common secondary complication and requires treatment with a topical antifungal agent. See Chapter 17 of the wound core curriculum for additional information regarding differential assessment and management of periwound MASD.

In addition to visual inspection, valuable information can be obtained from the patient and nursing staff. For example, patient reports of burning or stinging sensations around the fistula commonly indicate denudation or erosion of the epidermis, and the patient who requires frequent dressing or pouch changes is at risk for skin damage from mechanical injury in addition to damage from exposure to the effluent.

Interventions and Containment Strategies

Fistulas can be managed with skin protection and either dressings or containment devices (pouches, suction, negative pressure). There are a wide number of products available, and the appropriate selection is based on patient assessment. Principles of management warrant repetition: begin with the easiest approach based on assessment and sound rationale, reassess frequently and be flexible, and expect that needs will change. Interventions should be based on established principles and rationale, should include measures for skin protection and containment as well as patient and family support and education, and should be appropriately documented (see Box 17-2). Tables 17-2 and 17-3 present factors to consider when selecting containment methods.

CLINICAL PEARL

The recommended approach to determining the best system for effluent containment and skin protection is to begin with the simplest approach and modify as needed.

Skin Protectants and Barriers

Skin protectant products are available in many types and forms (Table 17-2). Major types include moisture barrier creams, ointments or pastes; solid pectin-based adhesive wafers, rings, or strips; hydrocolloid or karaya-formulated rings; barrier (ostomy) paste formulated with or without alcohol; barrier powder; and liquid barrier film products (skin sealant wipes, wands, and sprays with or without alcohol). As previously stated, product selection must always be based on assessment and a clear understanding of the patient's needs and the properties and indications for use of the various products. For example, moisture barrier products are appropriate only for low-output fistulas managed with dressings. Pectin-based barrier wafers, rings, strips, and paste are widely used to protect the skin and improve adhesion of pouching systems and NPWT systems. Barrier powder is used to treat denuded skin. Liquid barrier film products (also known as skin sealants) are primarily used to protect the skin against adhesive trauma. Table 17-2 provides indications and contraindications for use of each type of barrier product.

CLINICAL PEARL

Moisture barrier ointments are used to protect the skin against moisture and drainage but are appropriate only for low-output fistulas managed with absorptive products; liquid barrier films are used primarily to protect against adhesive trauma; and pectin-based pouches, rings, and pastes are used to promote an effective pouching system and to protect the skin against enzymatic drainage.

Pectin-Based Barrier Products

Most containment pouches have an integrated solid skin barrier attached to the pouch by the manufacturer. Barrier pastes, strips, or rings are frequently needed adjunct products that are used to fill skin defects and create a flatter pouching surface, add convexity, or provide caulking to ensure a effective pouch seal. If the skin is weepy, barrier powder may be lightly applied (as shown in Fig. 17-3) to absorb moisture and improve adhesion of the barrier and pouch to the damaged skin. It is important to realize that application of excessive amounts of powder will impair adhesion. When the skin is extremely denuded, application of the powder can be followed by application of an alcohol-free liquid barrier film; these steps can be repeated up to three times to create a dry surface or crust. When applied and removed appropriately, most of these pectin barrier products are safe to use on damaged as well as intact skin. It should be noted that liquid barrier films (skin sealants) must be allowed to dry so solvents can escape before other products are applied. Some barrier films and barrier pastes contain alcohol and can cause great discomfort when used on damaged skin; the wound/ostomy nurse must provide clear protocols and ongoing staff education to assure that alcohol-free products are the "standard of care" for damaged skin. Great care must be taken to prevent medical adhesive–related skin damage (MARSI) as described in Chapter 17 of the wound core curriculum.

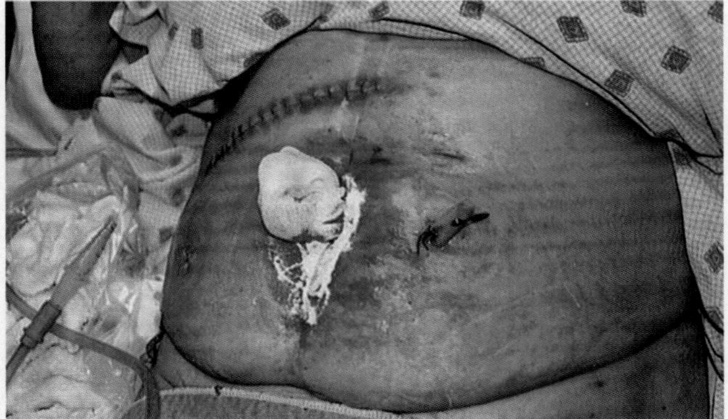

FIGURE 17-3. Pectin powder dusted onto weeping damaged skin; excess powder removed to avoid compromised adhesion of pouch.

CLINICAL PEARL

Pectin powder can be dusted onto areas of denuded skin to create a gummy protective layer; it is important to avoid excessive powder application as this would interfere with adhesion of the pouch.

Absorptive Dressings and Moisture Barriers

Fistulas that are nonodorous with low-volume output (<100 mL/day) and fistulas located in deep creases or anatomical locations that make pouching impossible may require management with dressings and moisture barriers. In these situations, the perifistular skin is protected with a liquid barrier film or a moisture barrier ointment (petrolatum, dimethicone, or zinc oxide–based ointment or paste), and absorptive dressings are then applied. The frequency of changes and reapplication of dressings and barriers is determined by the volume of drainage and the specific products being used. Absorptive dressings include gauze (sponges or strip packing), alginates, hydrofibers, foams, and combinations. When packing is required (e.g., wounds with depth, tunnels, or undermined areas), the wound or ostomy nurse must select a dressing that can be completely retrieved from the wound. If the volume of drainage is such that the dressing must be changed more frequently than every 4 to 8 hours, pouching or closed suction should be considered.

Closed Suction

Closed suction systems can provide skin protection, drainage containment, and odor control, and have been used for years as a reliable and cost-effective method for managing high-output fistulas, or fistulas that are too difficult to pouch (Jeter et al., 1990; Jones & Harbit, 2003; Kordasiewicz, 2004). The wound and surrounding skin are gently cleansed; the periwound skin is then protected with a liquid barrier film and/or hydrocolloid barrier strips. Any major skin defects adjacent to the wound can be filled with barrier strips or paste to improve adhesion of the dressing. The wound base is covered by several layers of moistened gauze to prevent damage to the wound surface by the suction catheter; suction catheters are then placed near the fistula orifice and stabilized with additional layers of moistened gauze. The entire wound is then covered with a transparent adhesive dressing, and paste is applied around the suction catheters, if needed to obtain a secure seal. The suction catheters are then connected to wall suction at a low level of continuous suction (see Fig. 17-4A–C). A Hemovac can provide the suction for short periods to increase the patient's mobility. Effluent must be liquid if suction is to be effective; thick or

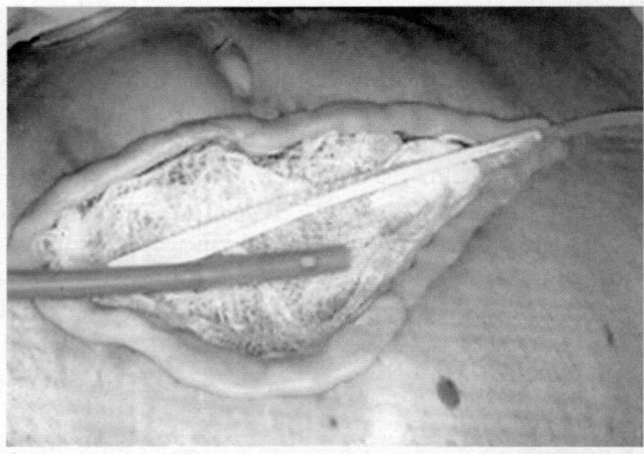

A

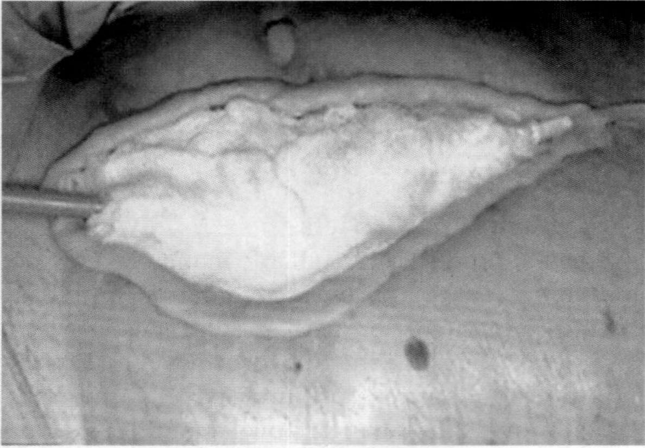

B

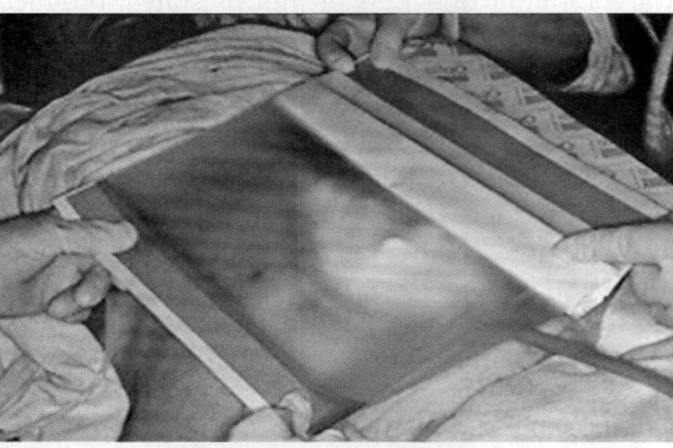

C

FIGURE 17-4. **A–C.** Closed suction procedure.

particulate effluent will occlude the catheter. Typically, these systems are changed every 2 to 3 days to prevent leakage and to permit wound assessment.

CLINICAL PEARL

Closed suction is sometimes a good option for the patient who is not a good candidate for pouching; it provides effective drainage containment and skin protection, but is used only short-term because it severely limits patient mobility.

It must be emphasized that a catheter that is inserted into the fistula tract will act as a foreign body and may interfere with healing and even increase fistula output. On the other hand, a catheter coiled in a defect above the orifice or in the open wound surrounding the fistula opening will not inhibit closure. Because firm tubes can injure fragile tissue, only soft, flexible suction catheters should be used with fistulas. Suction systems should be considered a short-term intervention because of the limitations placed on patient mobility and the time-intensive nature of the care (Dearlove, 1996; Nishide, 1997; Pontieri-Lewis, 2005).

CLINICAL PEARL

A catheter inserted into the fistula tract acts as a foreign body and prevents wound closure.

Negative Pressure Wound Therapy

NPWT incorporates a sponge or gauze and subatmospheric pressure (suction) to promote closure of fistula tracts, the removal and containment of effluent, and/or wound healing. The mechanisms involved in promotion of wound healing include reduction in edema (with associated improvement in perfusion), and mechanical deformation of cells, which has been shown to stimulate the wound repair process. NPWT systems have built-in sensors to alert caregivers to potential and actual breaches in the integrity of the system. NPWT is frequently used for fistulas located in open wounds so long as the following conditions are met: the fistula exhibits the potential for spontaneous closure (i.e., no evidence of pseudostoma formation); there is no evidence of exposed bowel in the wound base; and there is no evidence of abscess or distal obstruction. Caution should be used to prevent any additional fistula formation, that is, a contact layer or the nonporous "white" foam should be used in contact with the wound bed. If the effluent is too thick for suction, or if the fistula has "stomatized" but the wound still needs NPWT for promotion of granulation tissue formation, there are techniques that segregate the fistula for management with pouching while permitting continued use of NPWT for promotion of wound healing (Bruhin et al., 2014; CAET, 2009; Reed et al., 2006) (see Box 17-4). Further information about the application and use of NPWT is presented in Chapter 11 of the wound core curriculum.

BOX 17-4 Procedure for Isolating a Fistula for NPWT

1. Assemble equipment: Ostomy pouch and supplies, NPWT supplies, skin barrier ring, skin barrier paste, transparent dressing.
2. Prepare ostomy/fistula pouch as described in Box 17-5. Apply bead of paste to back of pouch around opening.

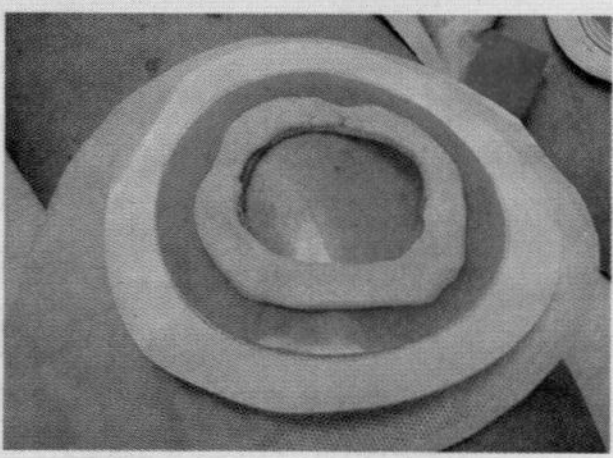

3. Cut a ring out of NPWT sponge dressing material slightly larger than the stomatized fistula; place into wound bed around fistula opening.

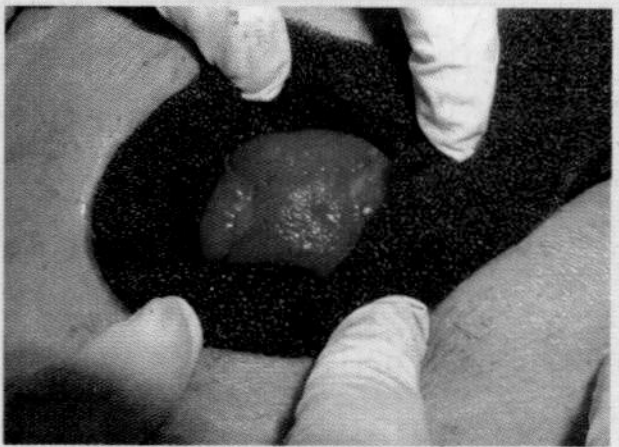

4. Optional: Place skin barrier ring right around fistula and over the NPWT sponge ring; apply bead of paste directly around fistula to caulk area between fistula and barrier ring.
5. Proceed to dress the wound utilizing NPWT procedure/protocol. Initiate suction and assure secure seal.

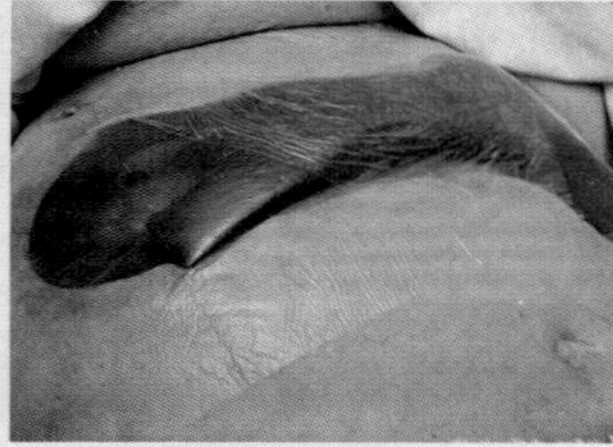

6. Cut an opening in the transparent dressing over fistula.

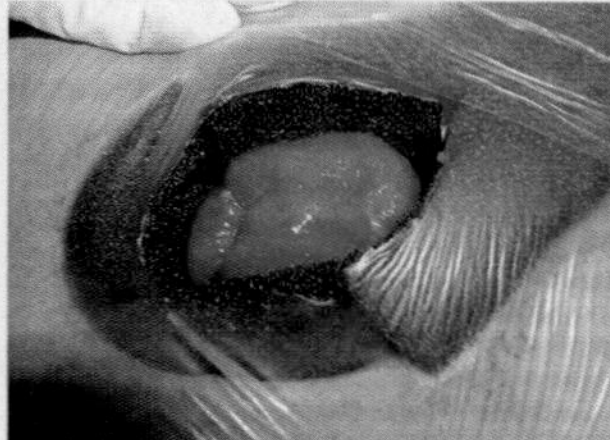

7. Apply the pouch over the fistula on top of the NPWT dressing; close the end of the pouch.

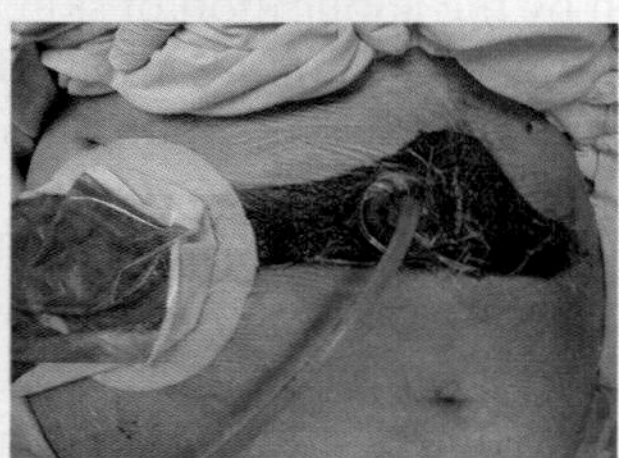

Photos courtesy of: Terri Reed and Diana Economon

CLINICAL PEARL

NPWT can be used to promote wound healing and fistula closure so long as there are no impediments to spontaneous closure; a contact layer or nonporous foam should be used in contact with the wound bed to prevent any additional trauma.

Pouching Systems

Fistula pouches, ostomy pouches (pediatric or adult), retracted penis pouches, and fecal incontinence collectors have all been used for fistula management. Most are preattached to solid-wafer skin barriers. Additional pectin skin barrier products may be required to caulk edges, fill creases, and/or add convexity (see Table 17-2).

When the fistula is located adjacent to an incision, the attached barrier of the pouch sometimes needs to be placed over the incision to prevent leakage onto the incision. When applied and removed appropriately, these products will protect rather than harm an incision. A simple strategy for protection of the incision is to place steristrips or tape strips over the suture line or staple line prior to application of the pouching system.

Strategies to promote adhesion of the pouch to the perifistular skin include assurance of a dry surface; a moist surface will impair pouch adhesion. Pectin barrier powders (NOT talc or corn starch) may be used to absorb moisture from denuded skin and to create a dry surface that supports pouch adherence. The amount of skin barrier powder used should be just enough to absorb the moisture and create a gummy or dry surface; too much powder will impair the adhesion of the pouch. Severely denuded skin may benefit from the "crusting" procedure, as described previously.

CLINICAL PEARL

If a pouching system or NPWT dressing extends over the suture or staple line, steristrips or tape strips should be placed over the incision for protection prior to application of the dressing or pouching system.

Medical adhesive products approved for the skin should be used according to manufacturers' instructions and only when needed. Medical adhesives can be used to enhance the tack of an existing adhesive, extend the adhesive surface on a pouch, or to compensate for the reduced adhesion caused by the application of skin barrier powder onto denuded perifistular skin. Medical adhesives are formulated as liquids/cements, medical adhesive sprays, and adhesive strips, rings, and sheets. Some adhesive products contain potential irritants or allergens, such as latex and/or alcohol; therefore, it is critical for the wound or ostomy nurse to carefully evaluate any adhesive product being considered for use in terms of indications, contraindications,

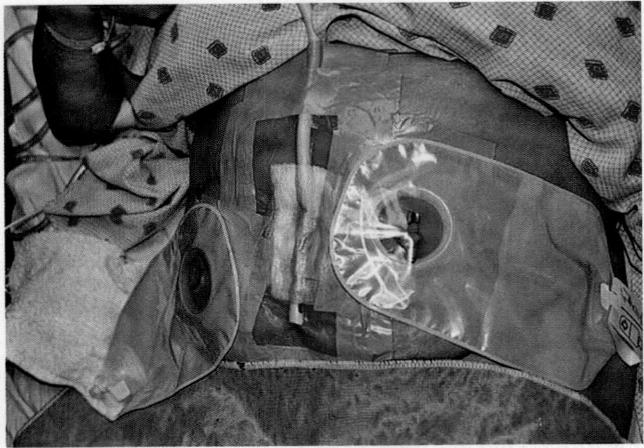

FIGURE 17-5. Two pouches used for separate fistulas.

and guidelines for use. Adhesive liquids and sprays must be allowed to dry completely in order for solvents to evaporate and the adhesive product to become tacky (Bryant, 1994, Bryant & Best, 2015).

If two drainage/fistula sites are too far apart to be included in one pouching system, two pouches may be necessary (see Fig. 17-5) (Davis et al., 2000). When the fistula is located in a deep wound (see Fig. 17-2), it may be helpful to select a pouching system with an integrated window/access cap that facilitates adjunct use of a wound filler dressing such as an alginate or an antimicrobial or saline-moistened gauze. A pattern and procedure for preparation, removal, and application of the pouching system should be created, dated, and kept in the patient's room with instructions and supplies. Figure 17-6 and Box 17-5 present examples of a pattern and pouch change procedure.

Pouching System Adaptations

There are situations in which adaptations of standard pouching techniques are required. Pouching system

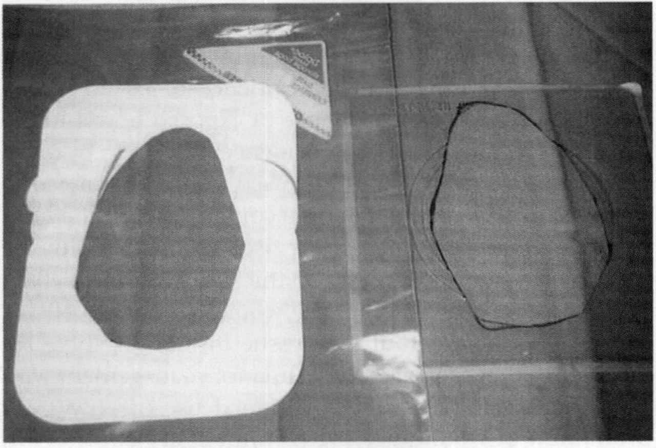

FIGURE 17-6. Pattern for fistula pouch.

BOX 17-5
Fistula Pouch Change Procedure

1. Assemble equipment
   Pouch with integrated skin barrier, pattern, skin barrier paste, scissors, closure device or attachment for bedside bag, water, soft gauze.
2. Prepare pouch.
   A. Trace pattern onto skin barrier surface of pouch. Note: the pattern should provide at least ¼ inch "clearance" of the wound edges (to prevent undermining of drainage under edge of pouch).
   B. Pull the anterior pouch surface away from posterior surface to avoid accidentally cutting hole in pouch surface.
   C. Cut out skin barrier surface according to tracing.
   D. Remove protective backing(s) from the pouch.
3. Remove and apply the pouch.
   A. Remove the pouch, using "push–pull" technique; gently press down on skin with one hand while pulling up on the pouch with the other.
   B. Discard the pouch and save closure clip or attachment device for bedside bag.
   C. Control any discharge with soft gauze.
   D. Clean the skin with water or gentle skin cleanser (without emollients that may impair adhesion of the pouch).
   E. Dry gently and thoroughly.
   F. Position the patient so abdomen has minimal wrinkles and folds (usually supine).
   G. Apply paste around the fistula. Fill in any uneven skin surfaces with paste, barrier rings, or skin barrier strips as needed.
   H. Apply a new pouch, centering fistula/wound site in opening.
   I. Close the bottom of the pouch with clip or attach to bedside bag.

adaptations (e.g., bridging, saddlebagging, and troughing) have been previously described and illustrated by Bryant (1994), and are recognized internationally over two decades later (CAET, 2009; Hoedema & Suryadevara, 2010). These techniques will be briefly described and illustrated (**Figs. 17-7 to 17-9**).

Troughing (**Fig. 17-7**) is a very effective management technique when the fistula is located within an open wound and routine pouching procedures are ineffective. The periwound skin is first protected with overlapping strips of pectin barrier or hydrocolloid wafer and/or barrier paste. The wound is then covered with a transparent adhesive dressing; prior to application of the transparent dressing, an opening is cut into the most dependent portion of the dressing and a pouch is applied over the opening. The opening in the pouch/transparent dressing unit must be placed at the junction between the skin and the inferior aspect of the wound, and must be wider than the diameter of the wound at that point. Since most wounds for which the trough procedure is required are very large, it is helpful to apply the transparent adhesive

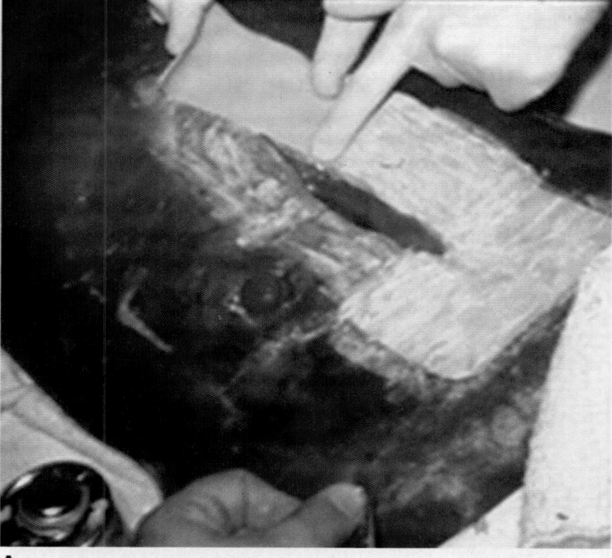
A

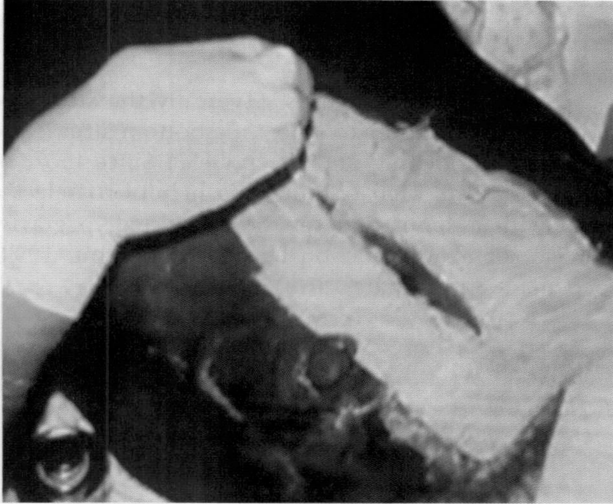
B

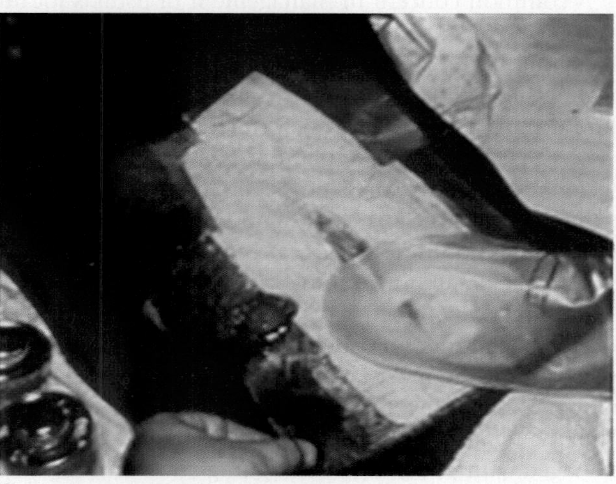
C

FIGURE 17-7. **A–C.** Troughing procedure.

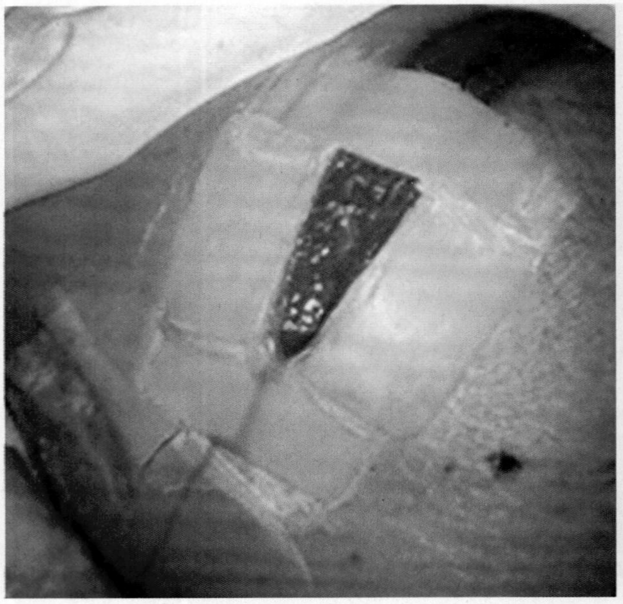

A

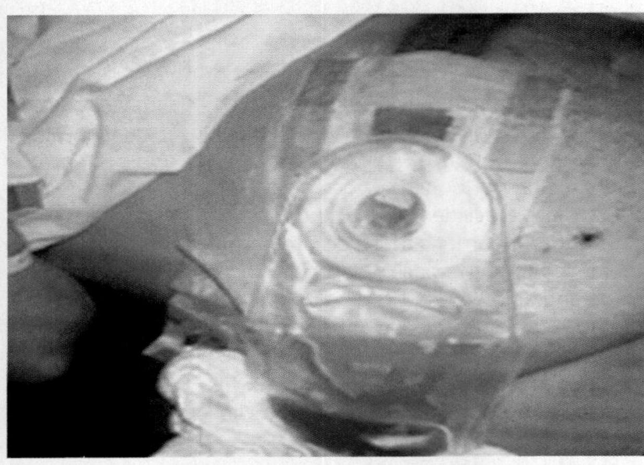

B

FIGURE 17-8. **A** and **B.** Bridging.

dressing in overlapping strips. (Typically the strips are applied from "bottom" to "top"; the bottom strip is the one with the opening and the pouch.) Since most of these fistulas are high output, it is helpful to select a pouch with a spout that can be connected to gravity drainage (or to wall suction if needed) (Bryant, 1994; Hoedema & Suryadevara, 2010).

CLINICAL PEARL

Troughing can frequently be used to provide effective skin protection and containment of effluent for patients in whom a secure pouch seal cannot be maintained.

A common concern in management of fistulas located within open wounds and managed either by pouching or troughing is the impact of small bowel drainage on the healing process. Fortunately, the enzymes in small bowel fluid do not attack the newly formed collagen and blood vessels that comprise granulation tissue, and the very low bacterial counts in small bowel fluid minimize the risk of infection. Clinicians consistently observe that wounds with fistulas continue to heal at the expected rate despite exposure to small bowel effluent.

Bridging (**Fig. 17-8**) may be used when the fistula is located at the inferior aspect of a long vertically oriented wound or at the most lateral aspect of an extensive horizontally oriented wound. The goal is to isolate the fistula from the remainder of the wound so that the fistula can be managed with pouching or troughing and the wound can be managed with moist wound healing or packing. Steps in the bridging procedure are as follows: (1) Identify a point slightly above (or medial to) the fistula at which the bridge will be "built." (2) Apply 1-inch strips of pectin barrier or hydrocolloid wafer in layers to create a structure that fills the wound at that point and extends slightly above skin level. (The white foam used for NPWT therapy can also be used to create a bridge that fills the wound and extends slightly above the skin surface.) (3) Cut a strip of pectin barrier or hydrocolloid wafer that is 1-inch wide (to match the width of the bridge) and long enough to cover the diameter of the wound and 2 inches of skin on either

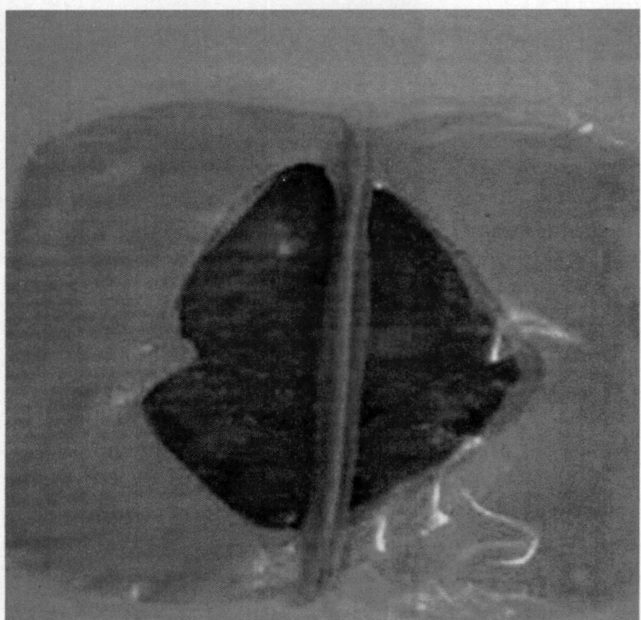

FIGURE 17-9. Saddlebagging: Example of two fistula pouches connected together along the adhesive surface to make one larger adhesive surface.

side of the wound. Place the covering strip over the bridge and onto the surrounding skin. (4) Proceed with pouching or troughing of the fistula and management of the remaining wound according to moist wound healing principles (Bryant, 1994; Hoedema & Suryadevara, 2010).

CLINICAL PEARL

Wounds continue to heal at the expected rate despite exposure to small bowel effluent.

Saddlebagging (Fig. 17-9) is a technique in which two pouches are attached at the skin barrier adhesive edges of each pouch to create one pouch with a larger adhesive surface than standard pouches (Bryant, 1994; CAET, 2009). This technique may be necessary for larger fistulas or fistulas within a large wound that need to be pouched.

Education and Emotional Support

Education and emotional support are critical aspects of the plan of care and its effectiveness. Patients report feelings of loss of control, frustration, embarrassment, hopelessness, isolation, and demoralization due to prolonged hospitalization, financial concerns, alterations in body image, and uncertain outcomes (Haffejee, 2004; Kaushal & Carlson, 2004; Kozell & Martins, 2003; Lloyd et al., 2006; Renton et al., 2006). Unfortunately, these feelings are exacerbated by the inability to eat normally, the possibility/probability of additional surgical procedures, the trial and error process so often required to achieve adequate skin protection and containment of effluent, and the prolonged care trajectory (Kozell & Martins, 2003).

CLINICAL PEARL

Education and emotional support are critical aspects of care for the patient with a fistula and his/her family.

Open communication with the patient and family will decrease anxiety, increase trust, and facilitate independence (Cobb & Knaggs, 2003; Kaushal & Carlson, 2004; Kozell & Martins, 2003). Education should be individualized based on goals of care, specific management approaches, and the patient's needs and learning style. Whenever possible, the patient should learn by participating in his/her care to gain back his/her independence and sense of control. It is important for the wound or ostomy nurse to help the patient and family to establish realistic goals and expectations, and to understand that fistula management and educational needs change over time (Burch & Buchan, 2004; Kozell & Martins, 2003).

Surgical Closure

Surgical intervention to close the fistula is required when impediments to spontaneous closure have been identified, and/or when the fistula fails to close spontaneously. Given the fact that only a minority of fistulas close spontaneously, surgical intervention is required for closure of most fistulas. Surgical procedures may also be indicated for palliation (Nussbaum & Fischer, 2006). Factors known to prevent spontaneous closure are listed in Box 17-3 (Bryant & Best, 2015).

Surgical interventions for ECFs either divert the fecal stream (without resection of the fistula) or provide definitive resection of the fistula tract. Diversion techniques divert the stool away from the fistula site without removal of the fistula by creating a stoma proximal to the fistula or by anastomosing (end-to-end or side-to-side) the two segments of bowel on each side of the fistula. This approach is required when resection of the fistula is not possible or appropriate, such as in the presence of extensive or recurrent malignancy or inadequate perfusion in the vicinity of the fistula due to previous surgery, scar formation, or prior irradiation. The process of resection involves removal of the diseased tissue and fistula tract followed by end-to-end anastomosis of the intestine. To protect the anastomosis, diversion of the fecal stream through a temporary stoma may be indicated. If the fistula involves the colon and the distal colon and rectum are not suitable for anastomosis or the anal sphincters are not competent, a permanent stoma with a Hartmann pouch may be the safest procedure. Enteric fistulas communicating with the urinary tract will always require diversion of the fecal stream proximal to the fistula site to prevent urinary tract infections and pyelonephritis. Timing of surgery depends on the patient's status. Surgery for a type 1 fistula is appropriate when the patient is nutritionally and metabolically stable, the fistula tract has been free of infection for 6 to 8 weeks, and the abdominal wall and peritoneal cavity have returned to a relatively soft, supple, pliable state; the goal is to maximize the potential for successful closure of the fistula, and to minimize the potential for additional complications, including recurrent fistula formation. Judicious timing is warranted for surgical closure of complex type 2 fistulas; surgery is usually delayed for 3 to 6 months, which is extremely frustrating for the patient and family. The wound/ostomy nurse must be able to explain to the patient and family that the extensive intra-abdominal infection associated with the original bowel perforation or anastomotic breakdown resulted in formation of extensive scar tissue within the abdominal cavity (obliterative peritonitis), and that it takes a number of months for the scar tissue to soften enough for the surgeon to separate the loops of bowel and remove the fistula tract without risking additional injury to the bowel and additional fistula formation. Nutritional, metabolic and immunologic status should be restored prior to surgery (Wong et al., 2004); for the patient with an ECF, this usually means that TPN will be required until the fistula is closed. However, the restrictions on oral intake are usually liberalized once it is clear that the fistula will not close spontaneously and that surgical intervention will be required; typically patients are allowed to eat and drink small amounts for pleasure and to keep the bowel mucosa healthy, as discussed earlier.

CLINICAL PEARL

Surgical closure is required for fistulas with known impediments to healing, and for those that "fail" medical management (i.e., fail to close within 5 to 6 weeks of comprehensive management); surgical intervention is usually delayed for several months to permit softening of intra-abdominal adhesions.

Vesicovaginal, Rectovaginal, or Enterovaginal Fistulas

While the vast majority of fistulas involve openings between two loops of bowel or between the bowel and the skin, fistulous openings can also develop between the bladder, rectum, or small bowel and the vagina. Fistulas between the bladder and vagina are typically managed initially by urinary diversion (indwelling urethral or suprapubic catheter or nephrostomy tubes), followed by surgery to close the fistula tract. The urine draining continually from the vagina is usually managed with absorptive pads; alternatively, a balloon-tipped catheter can be placed in the vagina and connected to a leg bag. (If the diameter of the vaginal vault exceeds the diameter of the inflated balloon, causing the catheter to constantly slip out of place, the catheter can be threaded through a baby nipple so that the tip of the catheter rests just above the base of the nipple; the baby nipple/catheter unit is then folded and gently inserted into the vagina so that the base of the nipple rests within the introitus to minimize leakage.) This technique can also be used for management of enterovaginal fistulas; because the drainage is thicker, it is necessary to use a large diameter catheter. Rectovaginal fistulas are typically managed by fecal diversion to permit healing of the fistula tract. For the patient who is not a candidate for surgical intervention, the focus of management should be measures to minimize vaginal contamination, specifically, titration of fiber and fluid intake to maintain soft formed stool that will not pass through the narrow fistulous tract. The patient can also be counseled to use mild antiseptics approved for intravaginal use to reduce or eliminate odor (e.g., TrimoSan).

Conclusions

Caring for a patient with a fistula is one of the most challenging, and rewarding, situations the WOC nurse will encounter (Hoedema & Suryadevara, 2010; McNaughton et al., 2010; Schaffner et al., 1994). Effective management requires a clear understanding of the anatomy of the fistula tract and plan of care, ongoing assessment regarding progress in closure or evidence of failure to close, creativity in developing an effective strategy for containment of effluent and odor, and consistent support and education for the patient and family. The key ingredients to positive outcomes when managing a patient with a fistula are patience; persistence; interdisciplinary collaboration; close surveillance; excellent communication with the patient, family, and colleagues; and a little ingenuity.

REFERENCES

Arebi, N., & Forbes, A. (2004). High output fistula. *Clinics in Colon and Rectal Surgery, 17*(2), 89–98.

Boarini, J., & Bryant, R. A. (1986). Fistula management. *Seminars in Oncology Nursing, 2*, 287.

Bryant, R. (1992). Management of drain sites and fistulas. In R. Bryant (Ed.), *Acute and chronic wounds: Nursing management*. St. Louis, MO: Mosby.

Bryant, R., & Best, M. (2015). Management of draining wounds and fistulas. In R. Bryant & D. Nix (Eds.), *Acute and chronic wounds: Current management concepts* (5th ed.). St. Louis, MO: Mosby. (In Print.)

Bruhin, A., Ferreira, F., Chariker, M., et al. (2014). Systematic review and evidence based recommendations for the use of negative pressure wound therapy in the open abdomen. *International Journal of Surgery, 12*(10), 1105–1114.

Burch, J., & Buchan, D. (2004). Support and guidance for failure and enterocutaneous fistula care. *Gastrointestinal Nursing, 2*(7), 25–32.

Campos, A. C., Andrade, D. F., Campos, G. M., et al. (1999). A multivariate model to determine prognostic factors in gastrointestinal fistulas. *Journal of the American College of Surgery, 188*(5), 483–490.

Canadian Association for Enterostomal Therapy (CAET). (2009). Best practice recommendations for management of enterocutaneous fistulae.

Cobb, A., & Knaggs, E. (2003). The nursing management of enterocutaneous fistulae: A challenge for all. *British Journal of Community Nursing, 8*(9), S32–S38.

Collier, B., Guillamondegui, O., Cotton, B., et al. (2007). Feeding the open abdomen. *Journal of Parenteral and Enteral Nutrition, 31*(5), 410–415.

Coughlin, S., Roth, L., Lurati, G., et al. (2012). Somatostatin analogues for the treatment of enterocutaneous fistulas: A systematic review and meta-analysis. *World Journal of Surgery, 36*(5), 1016–1029.

Davis, M., Dere, K., Hadley, G., et al. (2000). Options for managing an open wound with draining enterocutaneous fistula. *Journal of Wound, Ostomy, and Continence Nursing, 27*(2), 118–123.

Dearlove, J. L. (1996). Skin care management of gastrointestinal fistulas. *Surgical Clinics of North America, 76*(5), 1095–1109.

Demetriades, D., Murray, J. A., Chan, L., et al. (2001). Committee on Multicenter Clinical Trials. American Association for the Surgery of Trauma penetrating colon injuries requiring resection: Diversion or primary anastomosis? An AAST prospective multicenter study. *Journal of Trauma, 50*(5), 765–775.

Demetriades, D., Murray, J. A., Chan, L. S., et al. (2002). Hand sewn versus stapled anastomosis in penetrating colon injuries requiring resection: A multicenter study. *Journal of Trauma, 52*(1), 117–121.

Draus, J. M. Jr., Huss, S. A., Harty, N. J., et al. (2006). Enterocutaneous fistula: Are treatments improving? *Surgery, 140*(4), 570–576; discussion 576–578.

Dubose, J., & Lundy, J. (2010). Enterocutaneous fistulas in the setting of trauma and critical illness. *Clinics in Colon and Rectal Surgery, 23*(3), 182–189.

Evenson, A. R., & Fischer, J. E. (2006). Current management of enterocutaneous fistula. *Journal of Gastrointestinal Surgery, 10*(3), 455–464.

Fagniez, P. L., & Yahchouchy, E. (1999). Use of somatostatin in the treatment of digestive fistulas. *Digestion, 60*(Suppl. 3), 65.

Haffejee, A. A. (2004). Surgical management of high output enterocutaneous fistulae: A 24 year experience. *Current Opinion in Clinical Nutrition and Metabolic Care, 7*, 309–316.

Hesse, U., Ysebaert, B., & de Hemptinne, B. (2001). Role of somatostatin-14 and its analogues in the management of gastrointestinal fistulae: Clinical data. *Gut, 49*(Suppl. IV), iv11.

Hoedema, R., & Suryadevara, S. (2010). Enterostomal therapy and wound care of the enterocutaneous fistula patient. *Clinics in Colon and Rectal Surgery, 23*(3), 161–168.

Hollington, P., Maurdsley, J., Lim, W., et al. (2004). An 11 year experience of enterocutaneous fistulae. *British Journal of Surgery, 91*, 1046–1051.

Huether, S. (2002). The cellular environment: Fluids and electrolytes, acids and bases. In K. McCance & S. Huether (Eds.), *Pathophysiology: The biologic basis for disease in adults and children* (4th ed.). St. Louis, MO: Mosby.

Jeter, K. F., Tintle, T. E., & Chariker M. (1990). Managing draining wounds and fistulae: New and established methods. In D. Krasner (Ed.), *Chronic wound care: A clinical source book for healthcare professionals* (pp. 240–246). King of Prussia, PA: Health Management.

Jones, E. G., & Harbit, M. (2003). Management of an ileostomy and mucous fistula located in a dehisced wound in a patient with morbid obesity. *Journal of Wound, Ostomy, and Continence Nursing, 30*(6), 351.

Kassis, E. S., & Makary, M. A. (2008). Enterocutaneous fistula. In J. S. Cameron (Ed.), *Current surgical therapy* (9th ed.). St. Louis, MO: Mosby.

Kaushal, M., & Carlson, G. L. (2004). Management of enterocutaneous fistulae. *Clinics in Colon and Rectal Surgery, 17*(2), 79–87.

Kaur, N., & Minocha, V. (2000). Review of a hospital experience of enterocutaneous fistula. *Tropical Gastroenterology, 21*(4), 197.

Kirkpatrick, A. W., Baxter, K. A., Simons, R. K., et al. (2003). Intra-abdominal complications after surgical repair of small bowel injuries: An international review. *Journal of Trauma, 55*(3), 399–406.

Knechtges, P., & Zimmermann, E. M. (2009). Intra-abdominal abscesses and fistulae. In T. Yamada et al. (Eds.), *Textbook of Gastroenterology, Vol II* (6th ed.). Philadelphia, PA: Lippincott Williams & Wilkins.

Kordasiewicz, L. M. (2004). Abdominal wound with fistula and large amount of drainage status after incarcerated hernia repair. *Journal of Wound, Ostomy, and Continence Nursing, 31*(3), 150.

Kozell, K., & Martins, L. (2003). Managing the challenges of enterocutaneous fistulae. *Wound Care Canada, 1*(1), 10–14.

Lal, S., Teubner, A., & Shaffer, J. L. (2006). Review article: intestinal failure. *Alimentary Pharmacology and Therapeutics, 24*, 19–31.

Li, J., Ren, J., Zhu, W., et al. (2003). Management of enterocutaneous fistulae: 30-Year clinical experience. *Chinese Medical Journal, 116*(2), 171–175.

Lloyd, D. A. J., Gabe, S. M., & Windsor, A. C. J. (2006). Nutrition and management of enterocutaneous fistula. *British Journal of Surgery, 93*, 1045–1055.

Lynch, A. C., Delaney, C. P., Senagore, A. J., et al. (2004). Clinical outcome and factors predictive of recurrence after enterocutaneous fistula surgery. *Annals of Surgery, 240*(5), 825–831.

Mäkelä, J. T., Kiviniemi, H., & Laitinen, S. (2003). Risk factors for anastomotic leakage after left-sided colorectal resection with rectal anastomosis. *Diseases of the Colon and Rectum, 46*(5), 653–660.

Makhdoom, Z. A., Komar, M. J., & Still, C. D. (2000). Nutrition and enterocutaneous fistulas. *Journal of Clinical Gastroenterology, 31*(3), 195.

Maykel, J. A., & Fischer, J. E. (2003). Current management of intestinal fistulas. In J. L. Cameron (Ed.), *Advances in surgery*. St. Louis, MO: Mosby.

McNaughton, V., Canadian Association for Enterostomal Therapy ECF Best Practice Recommendations Panel, Brown, J., et al. (2010). Summary of best practice recommendations for management of enterocutaneous fistulae from the Canadian Association for Enterostomal Therapy ECF Best Practice Recommendations Panel. *Journal of Wound, Ostomy, and Continence Nursing, 37*(2), 173–184.

Meissner, K. (1999). Late radiogenic small bowel damage: Guidelines for the general surgeon. *Digestive Surgery, 16*, 169.

Nishide, K. (1997). Development of closed-suction pouch drainage for giant fistulae: A report on two cases. *WCET Journal, 17*(1), 16–19.

Nussbaum, M. S., & Fischer, D. R. (2006). Gastric, duodenal and small intestinal fistulas. In C. J. Yeo, et al. (Eds.), *Shackelford's surgery of the alimentary tract* (6th ed.). St. Louis, MO: Saunders.

Oneschuk, D., & Bruera, E. (1997). Successful management of multiple enterocutaneous fistulae in a patient with metastatic colon cancer. *Journal of Pain and Symptom Management, 14*(2), 121–124.

Pontieri-Lewis, V. (2005). Management of gastrointestinal fistulae: A case study. *Medical-Surgical Nursing, 14*(1), 68–72.

Reed, T., Economon, D., & Wiersema-Bryant, L. (2006). Colocutaneous fistula management in a dehisced wound: A case study. *Ostomy Wound Management, 52*(4), 60–64, 66.

Renton, S., Robertson, I., & Speirs, M. (2006). Alternative management of complex wounds and fistulae. *British Journal of Nursing, 15*(16), 851–853.

Rolstad, B., & Wong, W. D. (2004). Nursing considerations in intestinal fistulas. In P. A. Cataldo, & J. M. MacKeigan (Eds.), *Intestinal Stomas: Principles, Techniques, and Management* (2nd ed.). New York, NY: Marcel Dekker.

Saclarides, T. J. (2002). Rectovaginal fistula. *Surgical Clinics of North America, 82*, 1261.

Sancho, J. J., di Costanzo, J., Nubiola, P., et al. (1995). Randomized double-blind placebo-controlled trial of early octreotide in patients with postoperative enterocutaneous fistula. *British Journal of Surgery, 82*(5), 638–641.

Schaffner, A., Hocevar, B. J., & Erwin-Toth, P. (1994). Small-bowel fistulas complicating midline surgical wounds. *Journal of Wound, Ostomy, and Continence Nursing, 21*, 161–165.

Schecter, W. P., Hirshberg, A., Chang, D. S., et al. (2009). "Enteric fistula" principles of management. *Journal of the American College of Surgeons, 209*(4), 484–491.

Teixeira, P. G., Inaba, K., Dubose, J., et al. (2009). Enterocutaneous fistula complicating trauma laparotomy: A major resource burden. *American Surgeon, 75*(1), 30–32.

Telem, D. A., Chin, E. H., Nguyen, S. Q., et al. (2010). Risk factors for anastomotic leak following colorectal surgery: A case–control study. *Archives of Surgery, 145*(4), 371–376.

Torres, A. J., Landa, J. I., Moreno-Azcoita, M., et al. (1992). Somatostatin in the management of gastrointestinal fistulas. A multicenter trial. *Archives of Surgery*, 127(1), 97–99, discussion 100.

Tran, N. A., & Thorson, A. G. (2008). Rectovaginal fistula. In J.L. Cameron (Ed.), *Current surgical therapy* (9th ed.). St. Louis, MO: Mosby.

Wong, W. D., et al. (2004). Management of intestinal fistulas. In P. A. Cataldo & J. M. MacKeigan (Eds.), *Intestinal stomas: Principles, techniques, and management* (2nd ed.). New York, NY: Marcel Dekker.

QUESTIONS

1. The wound care nurse suspects that a patient's surgical wound is developing a fistula. Which of the following is the definitive indicator of a cutaneous fistula?
   A. Fever and infection in the wound bed
   B. Abdominal pain and wound dehiscence
   C. Blood migrating from a wound bed to the gastrointestinal tract
   D. Passage of gastrointestinal secretions or urine into an open wound bed

2. A patient is diagnosed with an enterocutaneous fistula with a high-output volume. Which statement correctly defines this diagnosis?
   A. A passage is created from the intestine to the skin, and the volume is >500 mL/24 h.
   B. A passage is created from the colon to the vagina, and the volume output is >500 mL/24 h.
   C. A passage is created from the bladder to the vagina, and the volume output is 200 to 500 mL/24 h.
   D. A passage is created from the colon to the skin, and the volume output is <200 mL/24 h.

3. The wound care nurse is assessing the wound of a patient diagnosed with a type 1 complex fistula. What data regarding the fistula would the nurse document in the patient record?
   A. Fistula with a short direct tract, no abscess, no other organ involvement
   B. Fistula with an abscess, with multiple organ involvement
   C. Fistula that opens into the base of the wound
   D. Fistula with a tract that is contained within the body

4. What is the etiology of the majority of enterocutaneous fistulas (ECFs)?
   A. Bowel disease
   B. Diverticulitis
   C. Surgical procedures
   D. External trauma

5. The wound care nurse is planning care for a patient with an enterocutaneous fistula (ECF). What is a key initial step in managing a patient with ECF?
   A. Administer H_2 antagonists to decrease ECF closure time.
   B. Use a 2-week trial of octreotide to reduce fistula output.
   C. Limit oral or enteral intake to amount keeping intestinal mucosa healthy.
   D. Force fluids to decrease gastric, biliary, and pancreatic secretions.

6. A patient is diagnosed with an intra-abdominal abscess following a CT scan. What is the initial management of choice for this patient?
   A. CT-guided drainage
   B. Surgical intervention
   C. Pharmacological management
   D. Keeping the patient NPO for 3 days

7. Which of the following assessment findings indicates that the patient will require surgical closure?
   A. Output exceeding 750 mL/24 h.
   B. Evidence of mucosal eversion/pseudostoma formation.
   C. History indicates fistula has been present >14 days.
   D. Hypertrophic granulation tissue in wound bed.

8. The wound care nurse is recommending products for patients with fistulas. Which product is used correctly?
   A. Moisture barrier cream for a high-output fistula
   B. Negative pressure wound therapy (NPWT) for a low-output fistula
   C. Suction system for a low-output fistula
   D. Pouch for a high- or low-output fistula

9. A patient presents with a fistula that has an output volume <50 mL with a need for odor control. What would be a good containment option for this patient?
   A. Wound management system with window emptied frequently
   B. Closed system with suction
   C. Charcoal dressings over dressings with environmental deodorants
   D. Absorptive dressings (e.g., calcium alginate dressings)

10. The wound care nurse is teaching a patient how to change a fistula pouch. Which of the following is a recommended step in this procedure?
    A. Trace the pattern onto the skin barrier surface of the pouch providing at least ¼ inch clearance of wound edges.
    B. Trace the pattern onto the skin barrier of the pouch being careful to size the opening to match the contours of the wound exactly.
    C. Remove the pouch by pulling off the skin quickly while applying gentle pressure on skin with one hand.
    D. Clean the skin with an alcohol wipe or skin cleanser with an emollient and dry gently and thoroughly.

11. The wound care nurse is isolating a fistula for negative pressure wound therapy (NPWT). What step would the nurse take after fitting the sponge around the fistula opening and covering the wound with a transparent drape?

A. Apply the negative pressure suction control device directly over the fistula.
B. Adhere the NPWT ring to the wound bed with the skin barrier ring and paste.
C. Cut an opening in the transparent dressing over the fistula and apply the pouch.
D. Place the suction catheter on the transparent dressing and initiate suction.

12. A patient's fistula is located in an open wound, and routine pouching procedures have been ineffective. What pouching system adaptation would the wound care nurse recommend?

A. Saddlebagging.
B. Bridging.
C. Troughing.
D. The pouching system should be discontinued.

ANSWERS: 1.**D**, 2.**A**, 3.**B**, 4.**C**, 5.**C**, 6.**A**, 7.**B**, 8.**D**, 9.**C**, 10.**A**, 11.**C**, 12.**C**

CHAPTER 18

Nursing Management of the Patient with Percutaneous Tubes

Jane Fellows and Michelle C. Rice

OBJECTIVE

Apply assessment and nursing management techniques to address the complex care needs of a patient with percutaneous tubes.

Topic Outline

Percutaneous tube placement into body organs or spaces is a means for drainage of fluids, maintaining an opening into an organ where obstruction exists, or providing for instillation of fluids, medication, or feeding through the tube. The tubes are usually placed by a physician in surgery, via endoscopy or interventional radiology. The WOC nurse is often consulted for management of these tubes and the complications that may occur with them. Knowledge of the location, purpose, and desired outcome of the tube placement is essential to effectively manage the care of patients with these tubes.

The use of percutaneous tubes is common in the adult and pediatric patient populations across acute care, long-term care, and home care settings. Increasingly they are being used for pain relief and symptom management in palliative care (Requarth, 2011). Common types of these tubes are gastrostomy, jejunostomy, biliary, and nephrostomy.

Gastrostomy and Jejunostomy Tubes

Nasogastric tubes (NGT) are the simplest to insert in the gastrointestinal (GI) tract and the least invasive, but they carry a higher risk for dislodgment and aspiration leading to pneumonia (Hsu et al., 2009). When feeding through the tube or decompression of the GI tract is needed for more than a few weeks, a percutaneous tube is inserted. NGT are indicated for short-term use. Common indications for gastrostomy tube (GT) insertion are obstructing head and neck cancer, benign and malignant esophageal disease, neurologic dysfunction, trauma, and respiratory failure.

GTs have been reported in the literature since the 1800s. Dr. Martin Stamm developed a surgical procedure for placement of a tube directly into the stomach, which is still used today. The standard Stamm gastrostomy involves circumferential purse-string sutures to stabilize the tube within the lumen of the stomach and affix the stomach to the anterior abdominal wall. A later technique developed by Witzel involves creating a serosal tunnel as well as an abdominal wall tunnel through which the tube passes. This is useful when the stomach has been altered so that it cannot be secured to the abdominal wall such as after a gastric bypass surgery or resection of esophageal cancer (Gaurav, 2014). Variations on these open surgical procedures remained the standard of care for feeding or gastric decompression until the 1980s when a procedure for percutaneous endoscopic gastrostomy (PEG) was developed.

PEG is a method of placing a tube into the stomach through the skin, aided by endoscopy (Fig. 18-1). A PEG with a jejunal extension tube can be placed through a preexisting PEG to facilitate more distal feeding while also providing an avenue for gastric decompression when necessary.

PEG tube placement is one of the most common endoscopic procedures performed today, and an estimated 100,000 to 125,000 are performed annually in the United States (Gaurav, 2014).

PEG is now considered the method of choice for enteral access due to the simplicity, effectiveness, and lower cost of the procedure (Miller et al., 2014). However, PEG is not always clinically appropriate, and some of the possible contraindications include the following:

- Uncorrected coagulopathy or thrombocytopenia
- Upper tract obstruction or malformation
- Severe ascites
- Hemodynamic instability
- Sepsis
- Intra-abdominal perforation
- Active peritonitis
- Abdominal wall infection at the selected site of placement
- Gastric outlet obstruction (if PEG tube is being placed for feeding)

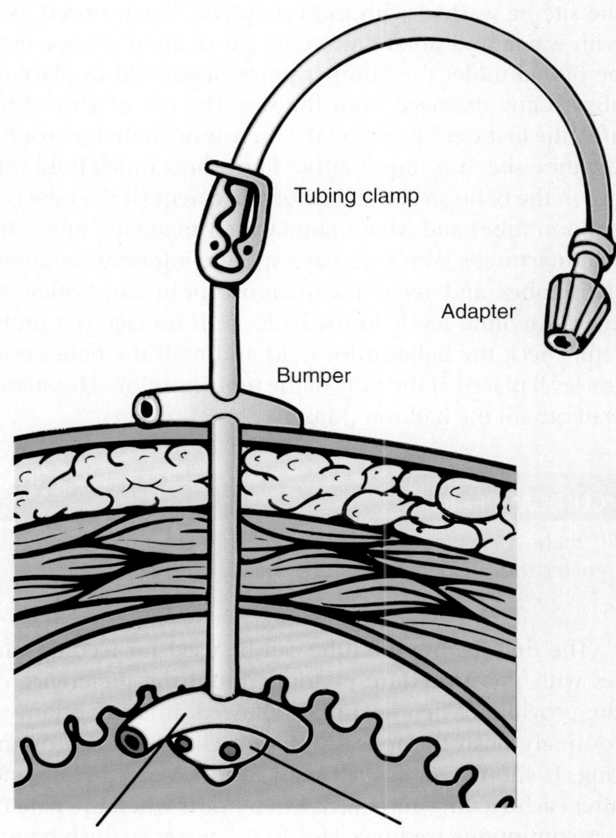

FIGURE 18-1. PEG tube with internal and external bumper.

- Severe gastroparesis (if PEG tube is being placed for feeding)
- History of total gastrectomy

When a PEG is not feasible for the patient, radiologic placement is a possible alternative. This was first described in the literature in the mid-1980s (Duszak, 2014) and avoids the use of an endoscope and is not contraindicated in the presence of upper tract obstruction. It uses fluoroscopy and ultrasound to identify the stomach, and a GT with a balloon is secured against the gastric mucosa with an external bumper on the skin (Fig. 18-2). If gastroesophageal reflux or delaying gastric emptying is a problem, another feeding tube option is a percutaneous gastrojejunal tube (Fig. 18-3). This tube has a balloon and an external skin bumper. There is an extension that is guided through the duodenum and into the jejunum for feeding. These tubes will have a gastric port that can be used for medication or fluid administration or decompression of the stomach and one for the jejunal feeding. A study of 124 patients requiring conversion from a GT to gastrojejunal tube showed a significantly higher success rate using the radiologic placement procedure rather than nonradiologic procedures (Kim et al., 2010). These radiologic procedures require providers with training in interventional radiology, which is not always an option in all facilities.

Both the PEG and radiologic procedures can be done with sedation rather than anesthesia making the procedure safer for the patient, and the time for initial feedings is not delayed. If feeding in the stomach is not possible due to surgical absence of the organ, severe gastroparesis, or gastric outlet obstruction, radiologic intervention is used to place a feeding tube directly into the jejunum. This tube is secured with a stabilizer sutured to the skin.

For those patients who are not candidates for PEG or radiologic procedures, surgical approaches offer the advantage of direct visualization of tube placement into the intended organ (stomach or jejunum). An open laparotomy or laparoscopy is done by a surgeon in the operating room, and the patient receives general anesthesia.

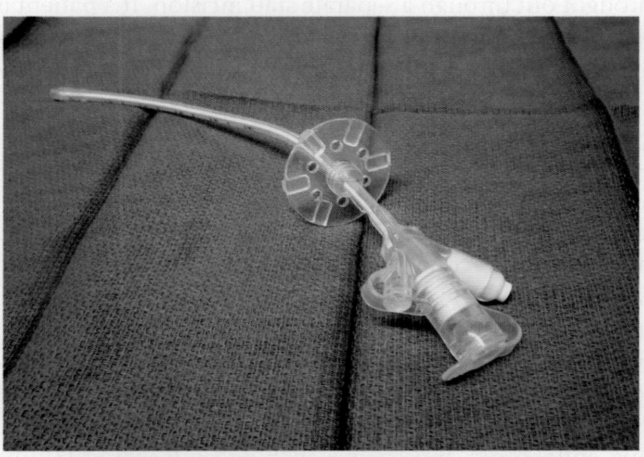

FIGURE 18-2. Balloon-tipped gastrostomy tube.

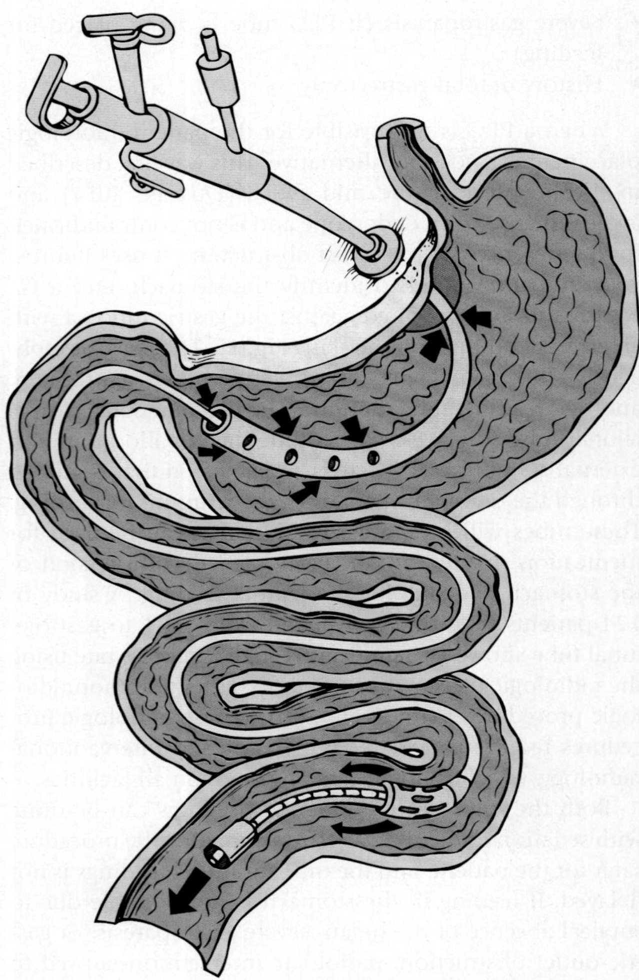

FIGURE 18-3. PEG with jejunal extension.

During the surgical approach, the stomach or jejunum is identified following a laparotomy incision or insertion of the laparoscope. The laparoscopic approach offers smaller incision size, less pain, and decreased risk of incisional hernia (Mizrahi et al., 2014). The appropriate feeding tube is secured within the lumen of the targeted organ and brought out through a separate stab incision. If a patient is scheduled for an open or laparoscopic abdominal surgery and it is expected that a feeding tube may be needed, it should be placed at the time of the surgery.

Comparative Complication Rates

There are many potential complications with these procedures, and most of the patients are malnourished and have significant comorbidities. However, the complication rates are relatively low. The complication rates reported in the literature vary, but it seems generally accepted to be 1% to 3% for PEG placement, 8% to 10% with radiologic procedures, and 7% to 15% with surgical procedures (Miller, 2014). Complications associated with percutaneous endoscopic approaches include endoscopic trauma and perforation of the GI tract, bleeding, skin and soft tissue infection, injury to intra-abdominal viscera such as the liver or colon, tube dislodgment, and fistula creation. Radiologic placement has many of the same risks as do endoscopically placed tubes, but there is no risk of upper tract trauma from the endoscope. Surgically placed tubes are associated most commonly with skin and soft tissue infection, incisional hernia, bleeding, inadvertent removal of the tube, and complications associated with general anesthesia. Issues with inadvertent injury to surrounding intra-abdominal viscera are very rare due to the better visibility during the procedure. In a study comparing laparoscopic versus open laparotomy, the laparoscopic surgery took longer to perform, but the complication rate was higher in the open surgery group (Mizrahi et al., 2014).

Routine Tube Care

Following placement of percutaneous tubes, the external bolster should generally be left in place for at least 4 days. After 4 days, there should be 1/2 to 1 cm of laxity left between the entry point and the bumper of the tube to prevent ulceration of the gastric mucosa or pressure damage to the skin under the bumper. Due to the possibility of edema at the tube site, positioning of the tube should be observed frequently for the first 48 hours after insertion (Miller et al., 2014). Evidence for most effective site care is lacking, but patient education materials recommend that the site be washed with mild soap and water, rinsed well with water, and dried daily. One gauze drain sponge may be placed under the bumper unless it sutured in place to absorb any drainage from the site. The use of a dressing after the first week is optional if there is no drainage around the tube site. It is important to know how much fluid was put in the balloon at the time of placement (if the tube is a balloon tube) and what manufacturer made the tube. The manufacturer's Web sites have specific information about their tubes and recommendations about how often to check the fluid levels in the balloon. If leakage is a problem, check the balloon for fluid and refill the balloon to the level placed at the time of the tube insertion. Use sterile water to fill the balloon (Simons, 2013).

CLINICAL PEARL

If there is crusting around the opening, use a water-moistened cotton-tipped applicator to gently remove.

The time before the tube can be used for feeding varies with the procedure performed and the preference of the provider. When feeding is allowed, it is important to routinely flush the tube to prevent clogging from occurring. It should be flushed with 30 mL water before and after each feeding and every 4 to 6 hours when the patient has continuous feedings. Use 10 mL water to flush before and after giving each medication. If liquid medication is not available, the medication should be finely crushed and mixed with water (Simons & Remington, 2013). If the tube does become clogged, try the following:

- Be sure the tube is not kinked.
- Milk the tube to remove any mechanical obstruction.
- Aspirate any fluid from the tube and then instill 10 mL warm water with a 60-mL catheter tip syringe and pull back and forth on the plunger to try to dislodge the obstruction.
- If it is still clogged, repeat the above step with one pancreatic enzyme tablet and one sodium bicarbonate tablet crushed and mixed in 5 mL of water (WOCN, 2008).
- If the tube cannot be unclogged, contact the physician. Instrumentation or replacement may be necessary.

Managing Skin Complications

There are many types of possible complications with enteral feeding tubes. The most serious adverse effects, such as abscess or necrotizing infection in the skin around the tube; buried bumper syndrome, where the internal tube bumper becomes imbedded in the gastric mucosa; or hemorrhage at the tube site, are uncommon. Complications that may require a consult for the WOC nurse are those that involve skin breakdown (Table 18-1). The most common cause of skin breakdown around the tube site is leakage of gastric contents on the skin. This is caused by movement of the tube that may enlarge the opening in the skin. To stabilize the tube, gently pull up on the tube until the internal anchoring device (bumper) or balloon is against the wall of the stomach and then slide the external stabilizer down

TABLE 18-1 Complications Associated with Enteral Tubes

Type	Contributing Factors	Management
Irritant dermatitis	Leakage of gastric secretions Tube displacement Improper balloon inflation Inadequate tube stabilization Recent weight loss Increased abdominal pressure related to chronic cough, constipation, hypertonicity/spasticity Presence of granulation tissue/hyperplasia Inability to decompress gastric content (i.e., burp) Delayed gastric motility Body structure changes (spinal stenosis, scoliosis) Failure of tract closure related to inadequate wound healing	1. If balloon-tipped tube is in place, check for proper inflation of balloon and add fluid if amount inadequate 2. Check balloon volume weekly 3. Stabilize the tube 4. Apply barrier ointment, such as zinc oxide or nonalcohol skin sealant to irritated skin 5. Use light gauze, or foam dressings to absorb fluid and change whenever wet 6. If unable to stop leakage, consider pouching with nipple device to bring the tube through the front of the pouch (Box 18-1)
Device-related pressure ulcer	Excess tension of the bumper against the skin Failure to rotate bumper after initial insertion Location of tube in a skin fold Weight gain or increased girth Sutured bumpers	1. Ensure the stabilizer rests comfortably against the skin without excess tension 2. Rotate bumper daily if appropriate 3. Consider eliminating the need for the bumper by utilizing a tube anchoring device 4. Depending on characteristics of the ulcer, consider the following: Skin barrier powder, sheet hydrocolloid, or absorptive dressing 5. Ask primary care provider if suture removal is an option
Fungal infection	Chronic moisture in the area of the tube Deep skin fold around the tube On systemic antibiotics Receiving immunosuppression medications	1. Keep the skin dry 2. Use moisture barrier creams or no-sting liquid skin barrier 3. Apply topical antifungal medication twice daily and continue for 2 wk after rash is resolved 4. Recommend systemic treatment if topical is not effective
Cellulitis	Invasive procedure Immunosuppression Diabetes Inappropriate or excessive handling of tube Chronic steroid use	1. Observe the skin for erythema, induration, purulent drainage 2. Assess pain with palpation 3. Recommend a systemic antibiotic if indicated by assessment
Hypertrophic granulation tissue	Moist friable tissue at the site where the tube enters the abdomen. Tissue is composed of connective tissue and tiny blood vessels and bleeds easily	1. Stabilize the tube if the etiology is felt to be a tube that is not secured 2. Consider use of silver nitrate cautery, steroid crème (triamcinolone 0.5% tid) or antimicrobial foam

BOX 18-1 **Procedure for Pouch Application around the Gastrostomy Tube**

Equipment:
Ostomy pouch
Scissors
Skin barrier powder
Wet and dry cloths
No sting skin prep
Cotton-tipped applicators
Gloves
Catheter holder device
Water-resistant tape

Directions:

1. Clamp tube and turn off feeding.
2. Remove the pink tape from around the tube where it exits the pouching system and gently remove the pouch using adhesive remover or warm water. Be careful not to pull or dislodge the tube.
3. Clean the skin with water and pat dry. Cleanse the area under the tube bumper by inserting a cotton-tipped applicator between sutures. Sprinkle skin barrier powder under the bumper to protect the skin.

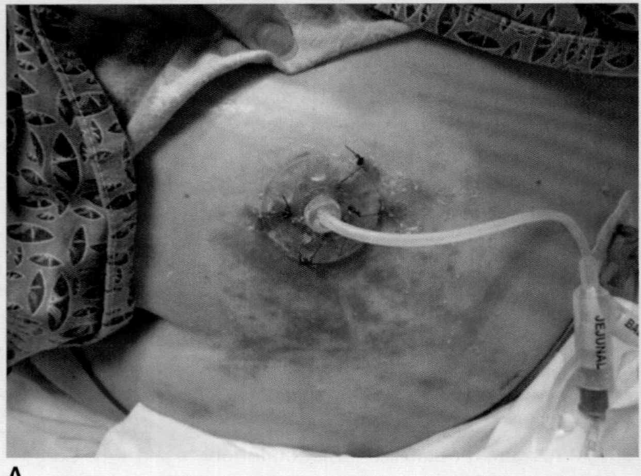

A

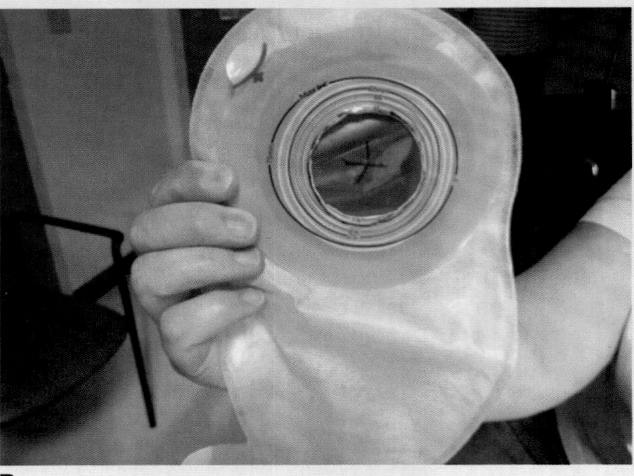

B

4. If there is any skin breakdown **(A)**, sprinkle skin barrier powder on the skin, rub in, and seal with no-sting liquid skin barrier.
5. Cut an opening in skin barrier of the one-piece pouching system to fit around the bumper. Cut an X-shaped opening on the front of the pouch so the gastrostomy tube can be pulled through **(B)**.
6. Place catheter holder device over X cut in front of the pouch to secure the tube and avoid leakage **(C)**. Instructions come with each device. Cut a hole in the nipple large enough to pull the tube through **(D)**.

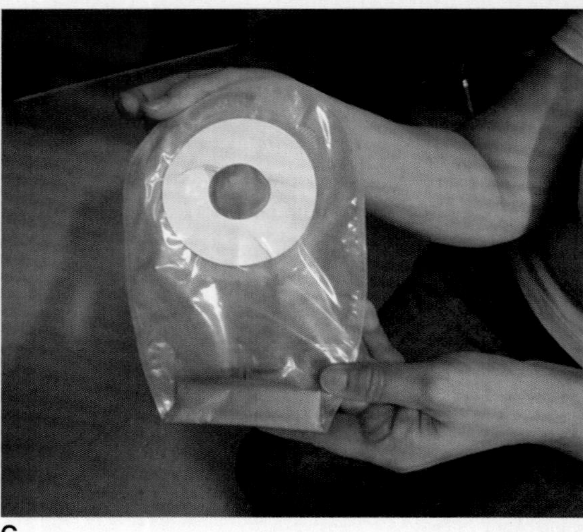

C

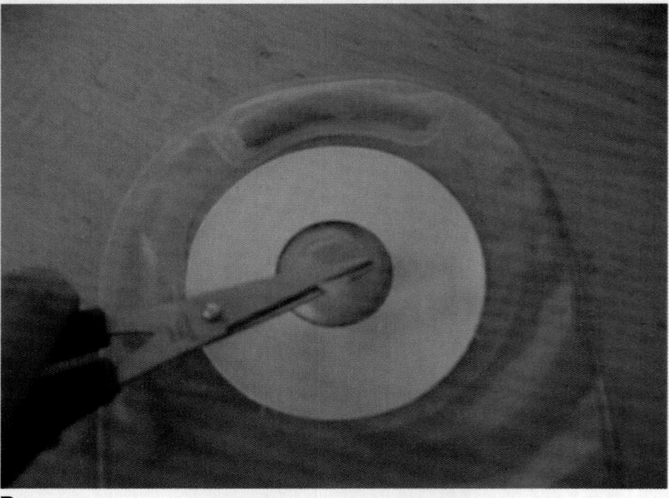

D

BOX 18-1

Procedure for Pouch Application around the Gastrostomy Tube (*Continued*)

7. Pull tube through the opening and place the pouch on the skin. Make sure the skin is dry before placing the pouch **(E)**. Use pink tape around the tube where it exits the pouch to seal the opening in the nipple **(F)**.

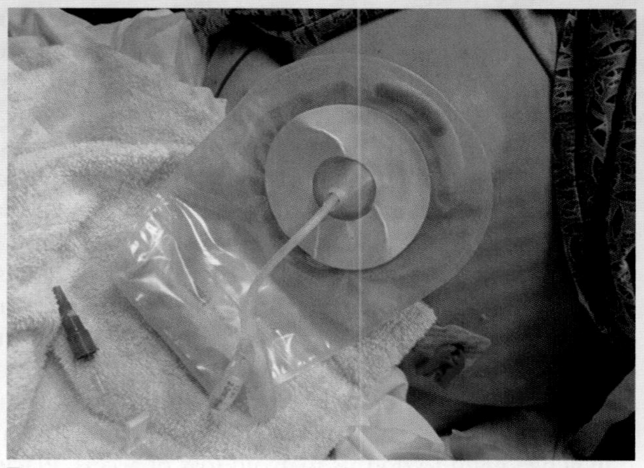

E

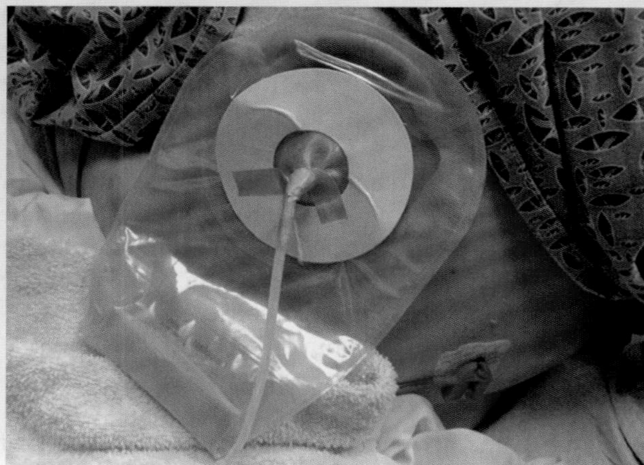

F

to rest comfortably on the skin without excess tension (WOCN, 2008). If there is an external stabilizer sutured to the skin with a jejunostomy and the sutures are no longer intact, it may be necessary to have these replaced. This tube is not secured with an internal bumper or a balloon, so it will migrate if sutures are not present. If there are sutures in the bumper of a PEG tube stabilizer, they may impede the ability to care for the skin and prevent skin complications such as irritant dermatitis and device-related pressure ulcers. It is appropriate to ask if these can be removed after healing has taken place. If there is no external bumper, the use of a commercial stabilizing device to secure the tube (Fig. 18-4) or taping the tube in place may prevent movement. With a balloon-tipped tube, loss of water in the balloon will cause migration of the tube. Replacing a leaking tube with a larger diameter tube in the hopes of obtaining a better seal is not effective and is contraindicated (Stayner et al., 2012). This will further enlarge and distort the leaking tube tract. In rare cases of persistent leakage, the tube must be removed and placed in a different site allowing the original site to close.

FIGURE 18-4. Drain tube attachment device.

CLINICAL PEARL

It is recommended that the amount of water in the balloon is checked weekly and replaced with the correct amount.

Hypertrophic Granulation

It is thought that a poorly secured tube or one that migrates easily in and out of the skin opening may be a causative factor in the development of hypergranulation tissue around an enteral tube. Leakage of fluid, use of hydrogen peroxide, and poor fitting low-profile GT may also contribute to this overgrowth of tissue. The tissue itself is moist and often is friable, which contributes to leakage of formula and enteral fluid round the tube creating a cycle of leakage being both cause and effect. In some cases, it is painful to touch and may bleed easily. The presence of this tissue is not considered a serious complication, but there are reports in the literature linking it to wound infection and cellulitis around the tube (Rahnemai-Azar et al., 2014). A wide variety of treatment options from the application of topical antimicrobial agents and steroid creams to cauterization with silver nitrate and surgical removal have been described in the literature, but the evidence is anecdotal. Nurses in one community health district in the United Kingdom described a care routine for those persons (n = 25) in homes or care facilities with GTs and an overgrowth of granulation tissue around them. They used an antimicrobial cleanser and an antimicrobial foam dressing around the tube for 6 weeks and checked on them at 2-week intervals. At the end of the first 2 weeks, one third ($n = 8$) of the patients no longer had hypergranular tissue present. At the end of 6 weeks, the problem was resolved in six additional patients. The remaining patients received a silver alginate under a foam dressing, and if that did not resolve the hypergranulation, a steroid cream was applied (Warriner & Spruce, 2014). When hypergranulation tissue is present, it is important to stabilize the tube to reduce movement of the tube in the tract. In addition, clinicians use silver nitrate cautery, steroid cream (triamcinolone 0.5% applied tid), or an antimicrobial such as silver in or with a thin foam dressing. Silver nitrate sticks should be used with care to avoid getting the silver nitrate on intact skin as this may cause a burning sensation. More than one application may be needed. In extreme cases, surgical excision of the tissue may be required (WOCN, 2008).

Tube Replacement

GTs may become accidentally dislodged for a variety of reasons. The stabilizer may have loosened, water may have leaked from the balloon, inadvertent traction is placed on the tube, or the patient may have pulled it out. The latter cause is usually secondary to an altered mental state. In these patients, a low-profile tube may be appropriate (Fig. 18-5). The low-profile tube may also be used as a replacement tube when the patient wishes to have one for convenience and ease of concealing the tube under clothing. It is required to measure the stoma tract; there are measuring devices that determine the size tract for low-profile tube needed. This is especially important as a child is growing and may need to order another size tube. GT replacement may be done by a nurse, but verification of workplace policies and regulations of the state board of nursing should guide the decision to do this. In a healthy person, the tract in which the GT is placed would be healed in 2 to 3 weeks. The patients requiring enteral access for feeding are usually malnourished and have chronic conditions that may interfere with healing, so it is advisable to wait 4 to 6 weeks before a nurse should attempt tube replacement (McGinnis, 2013). There is a risk of inserting the tube in the peritoneum if the tract is not healed. When a tube is dislodged unexpectedly after 6 weeks from original placement, it must be replaced as soon as possible before the tract and the opening in the skin begins to close (Box 18-2). For patients at home, a family member may be taught to do this to avoid loss of access. Placing a tube into the opening will solve the immediate problem of maintaining the tract, but the tube should not be used until proper placement has been ascertained by return of gastric fluid through the tube (Juern & Verhaalen, 2014). Replacement GTs are preferred, but a Foley catheter may be used if a GT is not available. The Foley catheter is more readily available and is a less expensive option, but the lumen of the catheter will be smaller and it is less durable, so replacement with a GT should be done when one is available (Ojo, 2013).

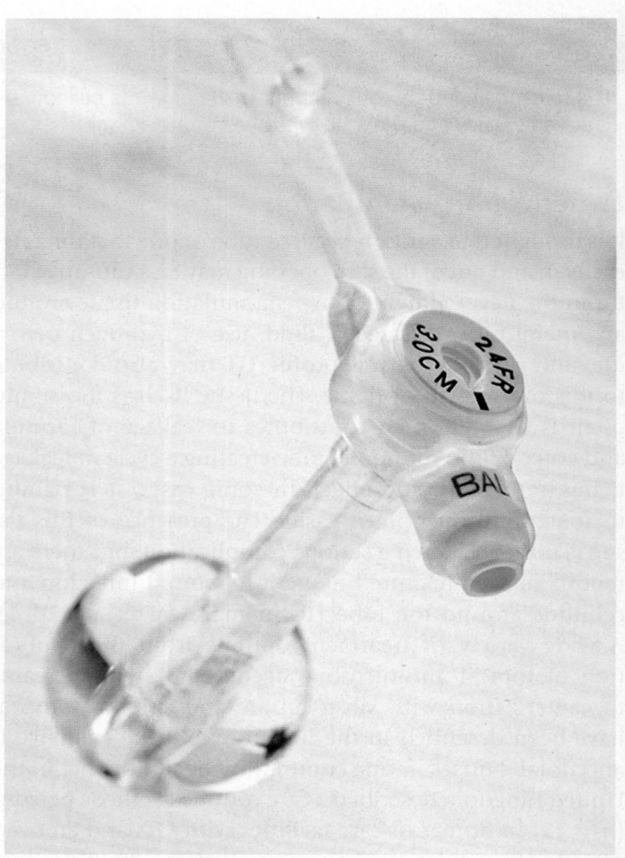

FIGURE 18-5. Low-profile gastrostomy tube.

CLINICAL PEARL

The patient should understand that when the tube falls out they should replace the tube immediately or seek medical attention for replacement.

Pediatric Considerations

The use of enteral feeding tube is a widely used, effective, and standard means of meeting the nutritional needs of child with a dysfunctional GI tract or who is unable to take oral nutrition (Hannah, 2013). The procedure is considered minimally invasive, and patients are discharged a short time after the procedure (Rollins et al., 2013). However, the procedure is not without risks and complications. A review of the literature demonstrates that patients with GTs have significant number of complications and emergency department (ED) visits for nonurgent tube issues. According to Pemberton et al. (2013), anywhere from 11% to 26% of pediatric patients have complications after GT placement. Common complications include leakage, peristomal skin breakdown, dislodgment, and hypergranulation tissue. The management of these complications is the same as for adult patients with a feeding tube. Tube dislodgment may be

BOX 18-2 Procedure for Gastrostomy Tube Exchange with a Balloon-Tipped Tube

Equipment:
Replacement gastrostomy tube of the same size as the one being removed
Water-based lubricant
Empty 10-mL syringe
10-mL syringe filled with water
60-mL catheter-tipped syringe
Gauze pads
Gloves

Directions:
1. Inform the patient of the purpose of the procedure.
2. Place the patient in supine position or elevate the head 30 degrees, as the patient prefers.
3. Test the balloon on the new tube by filling it with water, and ascertain that there is no leak. Remove the water from the balloon.
4. Slide the bumper up the tube to make sure it moves easily.
5. If the old tube is in place (i.e., it has not been inadvertently removed), use an empty syringe to remove the water from the balloon through the aspiration port. Reaspirate to be sure the balloon is empty.
6. Pull the tube gently out. Note the length of the tube from skin level to the tip.
7. Use gauze to wipe away any gastric contents that come out with the tube.
8. Lubricate the replacement tube.
9. Insert the lubricated tube into the stoma opening a couple of centimeters past the length of the tube that was removed.
10. Fill the balloon with water.
11. Pull the tube up until you feel resistance against the stomach wall.
12. Slide the bumper down the tube so that there is only 2 to 3 mm of space between the bumper and the skin. The tube should be able to be turned around freely in the opening.
13. Use the 60-mL syringe to aspirate gastric contents to affirm correct placement.
14. If no gastric contents can be aspirated, connect the tube to a bedside drainage bag and wait 20 minutes to see if the contents drain.
15. If there is no drainage in 20 minutes, tube placement should be confirmed with an abdominal radiograph in the oblique position using contrast.
16. Do not start feeding or flush the tube until there is confirmation of intragastric placement.

decreased with a low-profile tube, and these are used frequently in pediatric patients. A retrospective study by Novotny et al. (2009) of 223 young children who received a standard PEG (n = 110) versus a low-profile PEG (n = 113) showed a significant decrease in tube dislodgment with the low-profile tube and no difference in infection rate. There was also a significantly decreased length of hospital stay in the low-profile tube group. There was not a difference in ED visits for minor complications with the tubes.

According to a 4-year prospective study by Goldberg et al. (2010), infection developed in 37% of patients with the majority taking place during the first 15 days after placement. Hypergranulation tissue was noted in 68% of children with a recurrence in 17% of patients after receiving treatment. A 2009 retrospective cross-sectional descriptive study by Saavedra et al. (2009) showed that over a 23-month period, 77 patients had 181 ED visits for complaints related to the GT. Dislodgment of the GT occurred in 62% of the patients, and 75% of the visits were for GT replacement. In a study of 247 patients treated at a tertiary children's hospital, Correa et al. (2014) found that 20% of patients accounted for 44 ED visits within the first 30 days of discharge for complaints of leaking, mild clogs, and hypergranulation (hyperplasia) tissue. During the time period of 31 to 365 days postdischarge, 40 additional patients returned to the ED a total of 71 times for potentially avoidable visits.

It is clear that care of these children creates substantial stress for family caregivers. Specific education and support needs to be directed to the patients and their families in order to decrease the number of potentially avoidable visits to the ED. This is an area in which a WOC nurse can have tremendous impact on patient and caregiver quality.

Nephrostomy Tubes

Percutaneous nephrostomy tubes are inserted through the skin and into the renal pelvis of the kidney to facilitate drainage of urine after a partial or complete obstruction has occurred. Indications for use include tumors, strictures, dilations, and kidney stone removal. The tube exits through the flank and is connected to extension tubing and drains into a leg or bedside drainage bag (Clinical Center NIH, N.D., p. 3). Important factors in the management of this tube include tube stabilization to prevent pulling, kinking, or dislodgment; possible tube flushing with MD order; prevention of skin irritation; and signs of infection (ACI Urology Network-Nursing, 2012).

Tube stabilization can be accomplished with the use of a commercial catheter holder. Tape may also be used if commercial devices are not available. When securing the tube, consider the tube angle to prevent kinking.

In some instances, flushing of the tube may be needed if there is an absence of urine; persistent flank pain; or presence of clots, debris, or sediment (ACI Urology Network-Nursing, 2012). Consult facility protocols and/or physician guidelines for this practice. Generally, 5 to 10 mL of sterile, normal saline is flushed into the tube. Do not force the saline into the tube. After saline is instilled, reconnect to straight drainage. If unable to instill saline, the physician must be notified.

During the first 2 weeks postprocedure, sterile gauze nephrostomy dressings should be kept dry and be changed daily and as needed for drainage. For sensitive skin, consider the use of adhesive remover to loosen the dressing. If a sterile transparent dressing is in use, it must be changed every 3 days. After the initial 2-week period, the dressing should be changed twice per week and if wet or lifting off (Clinical Center NIH, N.D.). If skin irritation occurs, consider the use of an alcohol-free liquid skin barrier to protect the area. If a fungal rash appears to be present, use an antifungal powder rather than an ointment or cream. If there appears to be sensitivity to the adhesive, consider a dressing with a silicone backing.

Patient and family education includes how to flush the tube if ordered by MD, signs of infection, skin care, how to use and care for a leg or bedside drainage bag, and how often the nephrostomy tube will be changed (usually every 2 to 3 months).

Biliary Tubes

Biliary tubes are necessary when an alternate method of draining bile from the hepatobiliary system is needed. Often, the bile ducts are blocked, resulting in a buildup of bile in the liver that can lead to jaundice, nausea, vomiting, itching, fever, dark urine, and infection (Cote Robson, 2009; Box 18-3). Blockages are caused by tumors, strictures, and gallstones. The thin tube is inserted through the skin into the bile ducts by an interventional radiologist and is connected to a small drainage bag. This procedure is also known as a percutaneous transhepatic cholangiogram (Goodwin & Burnes, 2010).

Management of the biliary tube includes adequate securement of the tube to prevent kinking or dislodgment, flushing of the tube with MD order, dressing changes, and keeping the drain bag below the waist to facilitate proper drainage (Cote Robson, 2009).

Dressing changes should be done weekly and whenever wet or soiled. For sensitive skin, consider the use of adhesive remover to loosen the dressing. If skin irritation develops, an alcohol-free liquid skin barrier may be used to protect the area. Flushing the tube is done twice daily with 10 mL of sterile saline. Never force the saline into the tube. If there is inability to instill, pain occurs, or leakage at the exit site occurs, the physician must be notified (Cote Robson, 2009).

Patient and caregiver education must include routine care of the catheter, assessment of catheter integrity, signs of infection, and signs and symptoms of a blockage.

BOX 18-3 Signs and Symptoms of Biliary Tube Blockage

Leakage at exit site
Decrease in bile drainage output
Inability to flush the tube
Fever, chills, nausea, and increased jaundice
Cote Robson, P. M. (2009). *Caring for your biliary drainage catheter.* Memorial Sloan-Kettering Cancer Center. Retrieved August 30, 2014, from http://www.mskcc.org/cancer-care/patient-education/resources/caring-your-biliary-drainage-catheter

Conclusions

The provision of adequate nutrition support in the hospital setting is the standard of care. The use of the gut for feeding that is provided through enteral access is preferred to the use of parenteral nutrition whenever possible (Miller, 2014). It carries benefits physiologically for the patient as well as decreases the significant risks associated with parenteral nutrition. Patients with higher acuity are candidates for enteral access through endoscopic, radiologic, and surgical techniques available in various care settings. The WOC nurse must know what procedures may be done in his or her practice setting to be prepared for managing the care of these patients and those with other types of percutaneous tubes. Caregiver support and patient education are essential for those patients leaving the hospital with percutaneous tubes, and the WOC nurse can play an important role in preparing both patients and caregivers for discharge (see Care of Feeding Tubes, Appendix I).

REFERENCES

ACI Urology Network-Nursing. (2012). Nursing management of patients with nephrostomy tubes, guidelines and patient information templates. Retrieved from http://www.aci.health.nsw.gov.au/__data/assets/pdf_file/0011/165917/Nephrostomy-Tubes-Toolkit.pdf

Clinical Center NIH. (N.D.). Caring for your percutaneous nephrostomy tube. Retrieved August 30, 2014, from http://www.cc.nih.gov/ccc/patient_education/pepubs/percneph.pdf

Correa, J. A., Fallon, S. C., Murphy, K. M., et al. (2014). Resource utilization after gastrostomy tube placement: Defining areas of improvement for future quality improvement projects. *Journal of Pediatric Surgery*, DOI: http://dx.doi.org/10.1016/j.jpedsurg.2014.06.015

Cote Robson, P. M. (2009). *Caring for your biliary drainage catheter*. Memorial Sloan-Kettering Cancer Center. Retrieved August 30, 2014, from http://www.mskcc.org/cancer-care/patient-education/resources/caring-your-biliary-drainage-catheter

Duszak, R. (2014). Percutaneous gastrostomy and jejunostomy. http://emedicine.medscape.com/article/1821257-overview

Gaurav, A. (2014). Percutaneous endoscopic gastrostomy (PEG) tube placement. http://emedicine.medscape.com/article/149665-overview

Goldberg, E., Barton, S., Xanthopoulos, M. S., et al. (2010). A descriptive study of complications of gastrostomy tubes in children. *Journal of Pediatric Nursing*, 25(2), 72–80. DOI: 10.1016/j.pedn.2008.07.008

Goodwin, M., & Burnes, J. (2010). Biliary drainage. Retrieved August 30, 2014, from http://www.insideradiology.com.au/pages/view.php?T_id=90#.VATKc_ldWSo

Hannah, E. (2013). Everything the nurse practitioner should know about pediatric feeding tubes. *Journal of the America Association of Nurse Practitioners*, 25, 567–577.

Hsu, C. W., Sun, S. E., Lin, S. L., et al. (2009). Duodenal versus gastric feeding in medical intensive care unit patients: A prospective, randomized, clinical study. *Critical Care Medicine*, 37, 1866–1872.

Juern, J., & Verhaalen, A. (2014). Gastrostomy-tube exchange. *New England Journal of Medicine*, *370*, e28. DOI: 10.1056/NEJMvcm1207131

Kim, C. Y., Patel, M. B., Miller, M. J., et al. (2010). Gastrostomy-to-gastrojejunostomy tube conversion: Impact of the method of original gastrostomy tube placement. *Journal of Vascular Interventional Radiology*, *21*(7), 1031–1037.

McGinnis, C. (2013). Replacing gastrostomy tubes. *Critical Care Nurse, 33*(5),75–76.

Miller, K. R., McClave, S. A., Kiraly, L. N., et al. (2014). A tutorial on enteral access in adult patients in the hospitalized setting. *Journal of Parental and Enteral Nutrition, 38*(3), 282–294.

Mizrahi, I., Garg, M., Divino, C. M., et al. (2014). Comparison of laparoscopic vs open approach to gastrostomy tubes. *Journal of the Society of Laparoendoscopic Surgeons, 18*(1), 28–33.

Novotny, N. M., Vegeler, R. C., Breckler, F. D., et al. (2009). Percutaneous endoscopic gastrostomy buttons in children: Superior to tubes. *Journal of Pediatric Surgery, 44*(6), 1193–1196.

Ojo, O. (2013). Balloon gastrostomy tubes for long-term feeding in the community. *British Journal of Nursing, 20*(1), 34–38.

Pemberton, J., Frankfurter, C., Bailey, K., et al. (2013). Gastrostomy matters—The impact of pediatric surgery on caregiver quality of life. *Journal of Pediatric Surgery, 48*(5), 963–970.

Rahnemai-Azar, A., Rahnemai-Azar, A., Naghshizadian, R., et al. (2014). Percutaneous endoscopic gastrostomy: Indications, technique, complications and management. *World Journal of Gastroenterology, 20*(24), 7739–7751.

Requarth, J. (2011). Image-guided palliative care procedures. *Surgical Clinics of North America, 91*(2), 367–402.

Rollins, H., Nathwani, N., & Morridson, D. (2013). Optimising wound care in a child with an infected gastrostomy exit site. *British Journal of Nursing, 22*, 1275–1279.

Saavedra, H., Loske, J. D., Shanley, L., et al. (2009). Gastrostomy tube related complaints in the pediatric emergency department identifying opportunities for improvement. *Pediatric Emergency Care, 25*(11), 728–732.

Simons, S., & Remington, R. (2013). The percutaneous endoscopic gastrostomy tube: A nurse's guide to PEG tubes. *Medsurg Nursing, 22*(2), 77–83.

Stayner, J. L., Bhatnagar, A., McGinn, A. N., et al. (2012). Feeding tube placement: Errors and complications. *Nutrition in Clinical Practice, 27*(6), 738–748.

Warriner, L., & Spruce, P. (2014). Managing overgranulation tissue around gastrostomy sites. *British Journal of Nursing, 21*(5), S20–S25.

WOCN. (2008). *Management of gastrostomy tube complications for adult and pediatric patients*. Mount Laurel, NJ.

QUESTIONS

1. The nurse is assessing a patient who has a nasogastric tube (NGT) in place following gastric surgery. What complication should the patient be monitored for?
A. Fluid and electrolyte imbalance
B. Aspiration pneumonia
C. Constipation
D. Gastroesophageal reflux

2. A percutaneous endoscopic gastrostomy (PEG) tube may be contraindicated in a patient with the following diagnosis?
A. Severe ascites
B. Ulcerative colitis
C. Peptic ulcer
D. Crohn's disease

3. The nurse is assessing a patient who has severe gastroesophageal reflux for placement of a feeding tube. What type of tube would be most appropriate for this patient?
A. Percutaneous endoscopic gastrostomy (PEG) tube
B. Nasogastric tube (NGT)
C. Stamm gastrostomy tube
D. Percutaneous gastrojejunal tube

4. A patient who is undergoing abdominal surgery will need a feeding tube. When would the surgeon place the tube?
A. Prior to surgery
B. During surgery
C. The day after surgery
D. Two to three weeks after surgery

5. Which complication is most commonly associated with surgically placed gastrostomy tubes as opposed to percutaneous endoscopic?
A. Incisional hernia
B. Perforation of the GI tact
C. Injury to intra-abdominal viscera
D. Fistula creation

6. A patient is scheduled for placement of a feeding tube in interventional radiology. What potential complication is avoided by using this method instead of the endoscopic method?
A. Bleeding
B. Soft tissue infection
C. Upper tract trauma
D. Liver trauma

7. The nurse is teaching a patient routine tube care for a newly placed percutaneous endoscopic gastrostomy (PEG) tube. What statement follows recommended guidelines for this care?
A. Following placement of the tube, the external bolster will be left in place for 1 week.
B. A water-resistant dressing should be placed over the tube and insertion site and left in place for 48 hours.
C. The site of the tube should be washed with mild soap and water, rinsed well with water, and dried daily.
D. One gauze drain sponge may be placed under the bumper of a tube that is sutured in place to absorb any drainage from the site.

8. The nurse is providing care for a patient with a gastrostomy tube. What is a recommended intervention when using the tube to administer feedings or medication?
   A. Flush the tube with 60 mL water before and after each feeding.
   B. Use 10 mL water to flush the tube before and after giving medications.
   C. Flush the tube with water every 8 hours with continuous feedings.
   D. Dilute all feedings with water to be sure the tube does not become clogged.

9. What would be the first intervention when a feeding tube becomes clogged?
   A. Milk the tube to remove any mechanical obstruction.
   B. Aspirate fluid from the tube and instill 20 mL warm water into the tube.
   C. If the tube remains clogged after instilling water, use pancreatic enzyme table and sodium bicarbonate table crushed and mixed in 10 mL water.
   D. Use a 60-mL catheter filled with air and pull back and forth on the plunger to dislodge the obstruction.

10. What is the priority intervention when hypergranulation tissue is present around a feeding tube placement site?
   A. Cleaning the area around the tube with hydrogen peroxide
   B. Stabilizing the tube to reduce movement of the tube in the tract
   C. Replacing the tube with another type of tube
   D. Removing the tissue by rubbing briskly with an alcohol-soaked gauze

11. Which of the following would the nurse recognize as indication of biliary tube blockage?
   A. Increase in bile drainage output
   B. A change in the color of the drainage
   C. Cyanosis
   D. Inability to flush the tube

12. What type of tube would be used for a patient who needs kidney stone removal?
   A. Nephrostomy tube
   B. Biliary tube
   C. Gastrostomy tube
   D. Jejunostomy tube

ANSWERS: 1.**B**, 2.**A**, 3.**D**, 4.**B**, 5.**A**, 6.**C**, 7.**C**, 8.**B**, 9.**A**, 10.**B**, 11.**D**, 12.**A**

APPENDIX A

ART CREDITS

Chapter 1

Figure 1-1. McConnell, T. H. (2007). *The nature of disease pathology for the health professions*. Philadelphia, PA: Wolters Kluwer.

Figure 1-2 Archer, P., & Nelson, L. A. (2012). *Applied anatomy & physiology for manual therapists*. Philadelphia, PA: Wolters Kluwer.

Figure 1-3. Moore, K., & Dalley, A. F. (1999). *Clinically oriented anatomy* (4th ed.). Baltimore, MD: Wolters Kluwer.

Figures 1-4 and 1-6. Moore, K. L., Agur, A. M., & Dalley, A. F. (2014). *Essential clinical anatomy*. Philadelphia, PA: Wolters Kluwer.

Figure 1-5. Snell, R. S. (2003). *Clinical anatomy* (7th ed.). Philadelphia, PA: Wolters Kluwer.

Figure 1-7. Snell, R. S. (2011). *Clinical anatomy by regions*. Philadelphia, PA: Wolters Kluwer.

Chapter 2

Figure 2-1. Timby, B. K., & Smith, N. E. (2013). *Introductory medical-surgical nursing*. Philadelphia, PA: Wolters Kluwer.

Figure 2-2. Cohen, B. J. (2012). *Memmler's structure and function of the human body*. Philadelphia, PA: Wolters Kluwer.

Figure 2-3. Cohen, B. J. (2012). *Medical terminology*. Philadelphia, PA: Wolters Kluwer.

Chapter 3

Figures 3-1 and 3-4. Adapted from NCCN guidelines, Colon Cancer. Version 3.2014.

Figure 3-3. Fiser, S. M. (2010). *ABSITE review*. Philadelphia, PA: Wolters Kluwer.

Figures 3-2 and 3-5. Adapted from NCCN guidelines, Rectal Cancer. Version 3.2014.

Figure 3-8. Courtesy of Mary Arnold Long, MSN, RN, CRN, CWOCN-AP, ACNS-BC.

Chapter 4

Figure 4-1. Adapted from Milsom, J. W. (1999). Strictureplasty and mechanical dilation in strictured Crohn's disease. In F. Michelassi & J. W. Milsom (Eds.), *Operative strategies in inflammatory bowel disease* (pp. 259–267). New York, NY: Springer-Verlag.

Figures 4-2 and 4-3. Wexner, S. D., & Fleshman, J. W. (2011). *Colon and rectal surgery: Abdominal operations*. Philadelphia, PA: Wolters Kluwer.

Figure 4-4. McGreer, M. A., & Carter, P. J. (2010). *Workbook for Lippincott's textbook for personal support workers*. Philadelphia, PA: Wolters Kluwer.

Figure 4-6. Dimick, J. B., Upchurch, G. R., & Sonnenday, C. J. (2012). *Clinical scenarios in surgery*. Philadelphia, PA: Wolters Kluwer.

Figure 4-7. Corman, M., Nicholls, R. J., Fazio, V. W., et al. (2012). *Corman's colon and rectal surgery*. Philadelphia, PA: Wolters Kluwer.

Chapter 6

Figure 6-1. Berek, J. S., & Hacker, N. F. (2005). *Practical gynecologic oncology* (4th ed.). Philadelphia, PA: Wolters Kluwer.

Figure 6-2. Scardino, P. T., Linehan, W. M., Zelefsky, M. J., et al. (2011). *Comprehensive textbook of genitourinary oncology*. Philadelphia, PA: Wolters Kluwer.

Figure 6-3. Fischer, J. E., Jones, D. B., Pomposelli, F. B., et al. (2011). *Fischer's mastery of surgery*. Philadelphia, PA: Wolters Kluwer.

Figure 6-4. Reprinted from Hautmann, R. E. (2003). Urinary diversion: Ileal conduit to neobladder. *Journal of Urology, 169*(3), 834–842, with permission.

Chapter 7

Figures 7-1 through 7-11. Reprinted with permission, Cleveland Clinic Center for Medical Art & Photography © 2014. All Rights Reserved.

Chapter 8

Figure 8-1. Courtesy of Jane Carmel, MSN, RN, CWOCN.

Figures 8-2 and 8-4. Fischer, J. E., Jones, D. B., Pomposelli, F. B., et al. (2011). *Fischer's mastery of surgery.* Philadelphia, PA: Wolters Kluwer.

Figure 8-3. From Hurst, R. (1999). Proctocolectomy with ileostomy, abdominal colectomy with ileostomy, and abdominal colectomy with ileoproctostomy. In F. Michelassi & J. W. Milsom (Eds.), *Operative strategies in inflammatory bowel disease* (p. 157). New York, NY: Springer-Verlag.

Chapter 9

Figures 9-1, 9-2 and 9-3. Courtesy of Janice Colwell, MS, RN, CWOCN, FAAN.

Chapter 10

Figures 10-2, 10-4, 10-6, 10-8. Courtesy of Janice Colwell, MS, RN, CWOCN, FAAN.

Figure 10-7. Courtesy of and copyright ConvaTec Incorporated.

Figure 10-9. Courtesy of Hollister Incorporated.

Chapter 14

Figure 14-1. McGahren, E. D., & Wilson, W. G. (2010). *Pediatrics recall.* Philadelphia, PA: Wolters Kluwer.

Figure 14-2. Adapted with permission from Grosfeld, J. L. (1998). Jejunoileal atresia and stenosis. In J. A. O'Neill Jr, M. I. Rowe, J. L. Grosfeld, et al., (Eds.), *Pediatric surgery* (5th ed., pp. 114–118). St. Louis, MO: Mosby.

Figure 14-3. Moore, K. L., Agur, A. M. R., & Dalley, A. F. (2013). *Clinically oriented anatomy.* Philadelphia, PA: Wolters Kluwer.

Figure 14-4. Courtesy of Kevin P. Lally, MD.

Figure 14-5. Adapted with permission from Crouse, D. T. (1993). Necrotizing enterocolitis. In J. J. Pomerance & C. J. Richardson (Eds.), *Neonatology for the clinician* (p. 364). Norwalk, CT: Appleton & Lange.

Figure 14-6. Anatomical Chart Company.

Figure 14-7. Brant, W. E., & Helms, C. A. (2006). *Brant and Helms solution.* Philadelphia, PA: Wolters Kluwer.

Figure 14-11. McMillan, J. A., Feigin, R. D., DeAngelis, C., et al. (2006). *Oski's solution.* Philadelphia, PA: Wolters Kluwer.

Figure 14-12. Courtesy of Karen M. Polise, MSN, RN, Division of Nephrology, The Children's Hospital of Philadelphia.

Figure 14-13. Reprinted with permission from Pillitteri, A. (2008). *Maternal and child health nursing* (5th ed.). Philadelphia, PA: Wolters Kluwer.

Figure 14-14. (2008). *Lippincott's nursing procedures.* Philadelphia, PA: Wolters Kluwer.

Figure 14-15. Bowden, V., & Greenberg, C. S. (2013). *Bowden children and their families.* Philadelphia, PA: Wolters Kluwer.

Figure 14-16. Kyle, T., & Carman, S. (2012). *Essentials of pediatric nursing.* Philadelphia, PA: Wolters Kluwer.

Chapter 15

Figures 15-1, 15-2, 15-4, 15-6 through 15-12, 15-14 through 15-18, and 15-20. Courtesy of Laura Vadman, RN, CWOCN.

Figure 15-3. Courtesy of Janice Colwell, MS, RN, CWOCN, FAAN.

Figure 15-5. Baranoski, S., & Ayello, E. A. (2011). *Wound care essentials.* Philadelphia, PA: Wolters Kluwer.

Figures 15-13 and 15-19. Corman, M., Nicholls, R. J., Fazio, V. W., et al. (2012). *Corman's colon and rectal surgery.* Philadelphia, PA: Wolters Kluwer.

Figure 15-21. Werner, R. (2012). *Massage therapist's guide to pathology.* Philadelphia, PA: Wolters Kluwer.

Chapter 16

Figures 16-2 through 16-6. Courtesy of Janice Colwell, MS, RN, CWOCN, FAAN.

Figure 16-7. Courtesy of Jane Fellows, MSN, RN, CWOCN.

Chapter 17

Figures 17-1, 17-3, 17-5, and 17-6. Reproduced with permission from Davis, M., Dere, K., & Hadley, G. (2000). Options for managing an open wound with draining enterocutaneous fistula. *Journal of Wound, Ostomy & Continence Nursing, 27*(2), 118–123.

Chapter 18

Figures 18-1 and 18-3. Published in (2015). *Essentials for nursing practice* (8th ed., pp. 926–926), copyright Elsevier.

Figure 18-2. Courtesy of Jane Fellows, MSN, RN, CWOCN.

Figure 18-4. Courtesy of Hollister Incorporated.

Figure 18-5. MIC-KEY™ G Feeding Tube is a Registered Trademark or Trademark of Halyard Health, Inc. or its affiliates. Image copyright © 2014 HYH. All rights reserved.

APPENDIX B

SELECTED OSTOMY SUPPORT RESOURCES

American Cancer Society www.cancer.org	Volunteer health organization dedicated to eliminating cancer.
American College of Gastroenterology www.patients.gi.org	Patient resource and education center for GI health.
American College of Surgeons www.facs.org/patienteducation/skills/booklet.html www.facs.org/patienteducation/skills/empty-pouch.pdf	Scientific and educational association of surgeons whose goal is to improve quality of care and set high standards for surgical education and practice. Brochure for patients on emptying and applying ostomy pouch.
American Gastroenterological Association www.gastro.org/patient-center	Patient education information for GI disorders.
American Society of Colorectal Surgeons www.fascrs.org/	Association of surgeons whose goal is to promote high quality patient care by advancing the science through research and education for prevention and management of disorders of the colon, rectum, and anus.
Children's Digestive Health & Nutrition Foundation www.kidsibd.org	Pediatric support group.
Colostomy Association www.colostomyassociation.org.uk/	Provides assistance to those who are new to living with a colostomy as well as those who have been colostomates for many years.
Crohn's & Colitis Foundation of America www.ccfa.org	Mission is finding a cure for Crohn's disease and ulcerative colitis.
Cystic Fibrosis Foundation www.cff.org/	Pediatric support group.
International Foundation for Functional Gastrointestinal Disorders www.iffgd.org	Education and research organization for people affected by GI disorders.
International Ostomy Association www.ostomyinternational.org/	An association of ostomy associations committed to the improvement of the quality of life of ostomates.

SELECTED OSTOMY SUPPORT RESOURCES (CONTINUED)

National Kidney and Urologic Diseases Information Clearinghouse (NKUDIC) http://kidney.niddk.nih.gov/kudiseases/pubs/urostomy/	Informational web page about urostomy.
National Library of Medicine—National Institutes of Health www.nlm.nih.gov/medlineplus/tutorials/	Interactive health tutorial on colostomy and ileostomy.
Pull-Thru Network http://www.pullthrunetwork.org/	Pediatric support group.
Quality Life Association (QLA) www.qla-ostomy.org	Nonprofit nationwide association aimed at meeting the special needs of the continent ostomate.
Short Gut Support www.shortgutsupport.com	Pediatric support group.
Spina Bifida Association www.spinabifidaassociation.org	Education and support for patients with spina bifida and their families.
United Ostomy Associations of America, Inc. www.ostomy.org www.phoenixuoaa.org	Association of affiliated nonprofit support groups dedicated to improving the quality of life of people who have or will have an intestinal or urinary ostomy. *Phoenix* magazine is the leading source for education, information, and inspiration on how to live with a colostomy, ileostomy, or urostomy.
Wound, Ostomy and Continence Nurses Society (WOCN) www.wocn.org	Professional nursing society that supports its members by promoting educational, clinical, and research opportunities to guide the delivery of expert health care to individuals with wounds, ostomies, and incontinence.
https://www.c3life.com/ostomy/	Website supported by Hollister, Inc. that offers education, interactive forums, and information sharing.
www.j-pouch.org	Website offering information and support to those with ileo-anal anastomosis or J-pouch.
Youth Rally www.rally4youth.org	Pediatric support group.

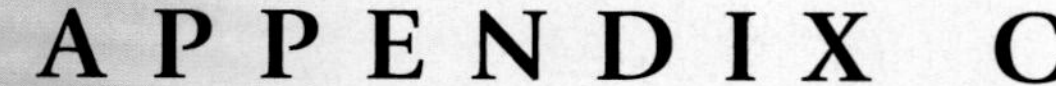

APPENDIX C

SELECTED OSTOMY PRODUCT SUPPLIERS AND MANUFACTURERS

Suppliers stock a large selection; most have toll-free numbers, free shipping, online catalogs with online ordering, and staff who are able to give advice regarding management problems.

Byram Healthcare: www.byramhealthcare.com

Edgepark Medical Suppliers: www.edgepark.com

Liberator Medical Supply Inc: www.liberatormedical.com/ostomy-supplies

Liberty Medical: www.libertymedical.com/ostomy/products

Parthenon Co Inc: www.parthenoninc.com

SGV Medical: http://sgvmedical.com

Shield Healthcare: www.shieldhealthcare.com/products/ostomy

Most major manufacturers of ostomy products will send free samples if requested. Many also have an ostomy nurse on staff.

Cymed: http://cymedostomy.com

Coloplast: www.us.coloplast.com

ConvaTec: www.convatec.com

Genairex: http://genairex.com

Hollister Inc: www.hollister.com/us/ostomy

Marlen International: www.marlen.com

Nu-Hope Laboratories Inc: www.nu-hope.com

Perma-Type Co Inc: www.perma-type.com

Torbot: www.torbot.com

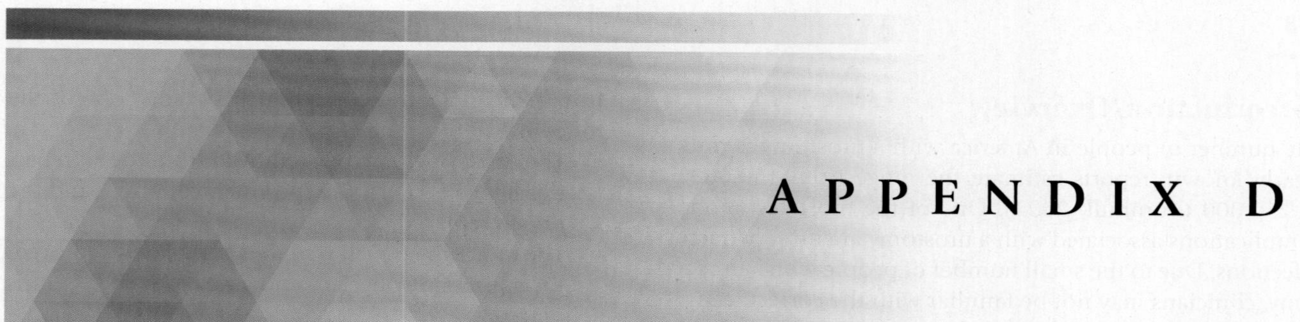

APPENDIX D

PROCEDURE FOR OBTAINING A URINE SAMPLE FROM A UROSTOMY, ILEAL CONDUIT, AND COLON CONDUIT

Best Practice for Clinicians

Acknowledgments

Procedure for Obtaining a Urine Sample from a Urostomy, Ileal Conduit, and Colon Conduit: Best Practice for Clinicians

This document was developed by the WOCN Society's Clinical Practice Ostomy Committee between August 2011 and November 2011.

Mary Mahoney, Chair, BSN, RN, CWON
Wound and Ostomy Nurse
Iowa Health Home Care
Urbandale, IA

Kathryn Baxter, RN, FNP, CWOCN
Nurse Practitioner
St. Luke's Roosevelt Hospital
New York, NY

Joanna Burgess, BSN, RN, CWOCN
Wound, Ostomy, and Continence Nurse
WakeMed Health and Hospitals
Cary, NC

Carole Bauer, MSN, RN, ANP-BC, OCN, CWOCN
Wound, Ostomy, and Continence Nurse Practitioner
Karmanos Cancer Center
Detroit, MI

Cathy Downey, BSN, RN, CWOCN
Program Coordinator
University Medical Center
Las Vegas, NV

Janet Mantel, MA, RN-BC, APN, CWOCN
Advanced Practice Nurse
Englewood Hospital & Medical Center
Englewood, NJ

Jacqueline Perkins, MSN, ARNP, FNP, CWOCN
Wound/Ostomy Nurse Practitioner
VA Central Iowa Health Care System
Des Moines, IA

Michelle Rice, MSN, RN, CWOCN
Ostomy Clinical Nurse Specialist
Duke University Hospital
Durham, NC

Ginger Salvadalena, PhD, RN, CWOCN
Senior Clinical Research Scientist
Hollister Incorporated
Libertyville, IL

Vickie Schafer, MSN, RN, CWON, CCRA
Associate Director, Medical & Scientific Liaison
Medical Affairs North America
Skillman, NJ

Shirley Sheppard, MSN, RN, CWON
Wound Ostomy Skin Care Nurse
University of Illinois Hospital and Health Sciences System
Chicago, IL

Introduction/Overview

The number of people in America with a urostomy is not clearly known; reports estimate the range from 150,000 to 250,000 (Turnbull, 2003). One of the most common complications associated with a urostomy are urinary tract infections. Due to the small number of people with a urostomy, clinicians may not be familiar with the correct technique to obtain a urine sample from a stoma to test for a urinary tract infection. Incorrect sampling techniques may lead to inaccurate culture results, and lead to inappropriate diagnosis and treatment. This document provides a quick and easy resource for correct technique with and without use of a catheter.

Purpose

To obtain an uncontaminated specimen for laboratory analysis (Faller & Lawrence, 1994; Hampton & Bryant, 1992):

- A clean uncontaminated specimen is necessary for accurate laboratory analysis (urine culture).
- Specimens from the urostomy sample often have bacteria; ensure that the specimen obtained is not contaminated.
- The most accurate method of collecting a urine sample for culture, according to limited sources, is the use of a double lumen sterile catheter inserted directly into the stoma.
- Specimens for culture should NEVER be obtained directly from the urostomy pouch or bedside drainage bag (Pagana & Pagana, 2007).
- Antibiotic therapy—it is recommended to use caution when considering antibiotics to treat urinary infection for patients with a urostomy:
  - "Patients should only commence antibiotic therapy if they are symptomatic" (Spraggon, 2008, p. 26).
  - "In the case of ileal conduit or continent urinary diversion, bacteriuria is practically always present, and measurements taken to eradicate the bacterial carriage are fruitless" (Wullt et al., 2004, p. 192).
  - "The detection of urinary infection in these patients is difficult because the ileal loops are almost always colonized. Asymptomatic bacteriuria in the presence of a ureteroileal conduit should not be treated and prophylactic antibiotics are not recommended. Positive urine cultures associated with physical findings of fever, chills, and flank pain should prompt initiation of appropriate bactericidal antibiotics" (Schrier, 2007, p. 884).

Patient Preparation

- Patient with one-piece pouch system: The urostomy pouch system is completely removed, the specimen collected, and a new pouch system is placed.
- In patients with two-piece pouch systems, one of the following options may be chosen:
  - The urostomy pouch is removed from the skin barrier flange (wafer), the specimen collected, and the pouch replaced.
  - The urostomy pouch system is completely removed, the specimen collected, and a new pouch system is placed.

Procedure When Catheter Is Available

Supplies

- Cleansing solution. Check the institution policy. Further research is needed on the use of antiseptic solutions vs. sterile water or saline for cleaning prior to catheter insertion. Some of the solutions recommended are: betadine, chlorhexidine, soap and water (Gould et al., 2009; Unlu et al., 2007).
- Sterile 4 × 4 gauze.
- If a double catheter is not available, a straight catheter may be used. Faller and Lawrence (1994) suggest the use of a 16-French catheter to allow for mucous drainage.
- Sterile specimen container with lid, label, and laboratory bag.
- Sterile and clean gloves.
- New pouch system.
- Soft paper towels and/or wash cloths for cleaning prior to replacing pouch.

Procedure

1. Explain procedure to patient.
2. Wash hands and use standard precautions.
3. Don clean gloves.
4. Open the supplies, maintain sterility.
5. Remove pouch and dispose per institutional policy.
6. Wash hands.
7. Don sterile gloves.
8. Use sterile technique.
9. Cleanse the stoma with cleansing solution, using a circular motion from stoma opening outward (Faller & Lawrence, 1994).
10. Blot the stoma with sterile gauze.
11. Place the open end of catheter into the specimen container.
12. If using a straight catheter, lubricate the catheter with a water soluble lubricant. Gently insert the catheter tip no more than 2 to 3 inches (5.0 to 7.5 cm) into the stoma (never force—if resistance is detected, rotate catheter until it slides; Faller & Lawrence, 1994; Hampton & Bryant, 1992).
    a. If using a double catheter, lubricate the catheter with a water soluble lubricant. Gently insert the catheter tip into the stoma and advance the inner catheter approximately 1 to 2 inches (2.5 to 5.0 cm; Hampton & Bryant, 1992).
13. Hold catheter in position until urine begins to drip. Collect approximately 5 to 10 mL of urine before

removing catheter. Collecting a sufficient amount of urine may take 5 to 15 minutes.

14. Clean and dry the stoma and peristomal skin.
15. Discard supplies according to institution policy.

Procedure to Use if a Catheter Is Not Readily Available

Supplies

- Cleansing solution. Check the institution policy. Further research is needed on the use of antiseptic solutions vs. sterile water or saline for cleaning prior to catheter insertion. Some of the solutions recommended are: betadine, chlorhexidine, soap and water (Gould et al., 2009; Unlu et al., 2007).
- Sterile 4 × 4 gauze.
- Sterile specimen container with lid, label, and laboratory specimen bag.
- Sterile and clean gloves.
- Soft paper towels and/or wash cloths for cleaning prior to replacing pouch.
- New pouching system.

Procedure

1. Explain procedure to patient.
2. Wash hands and use standard precautions.
3. Don clean gloves.
4. Open the supplies, maintain sterility.
5. Remove pouch, and dispose per institutional policy.
6. Wash hands.
7. Don sterile gloves.
8. Use sterile technique.
9. Cleanse the stoma with cleansing solution, using a circular motion from stoma opening outward (Faller & Lawrence, 1994).
10. Blot the stoma with sterile gauze.
11. Discard the first few drops of urine by allowing urine to drip onto sterile gauze.
12. Hold the sterile specimen cup under the stoma. Collect approximately 5 to 10 mL of urine. Collecting a sufficient amount of urine may take 5 to 15 minutes.
13. Clean and dry the stoma and peristomal skin.
14. Discard supplies according to institutional policy.

Aftercare

- Put a lid on the specimen container label: note on label that the specimen is from a urostomy stoma, and put in a laboratory transport bag.
- Apply ostomy pouching system.
- Bring the specimen to lab within 1 hour. In the home care setting, if unable to deliver specimen in 1 hour, refrigerate the specimen and deliver within 24 hours.
- Document in patient's record:
  - Procedure and observations.
  - Instructions given to patient/caregiver.

REFERENCES

Faller, N. A., & Lawrence, K. G. (1994). Obtaining a urine specimen from a conduit urostomy. *The American Journal of Nursing, 94*(1), 37.

Gould, C., Umscheid, C., Agarwal, R., Kuntz, G. & Pegues, D. (2009). *Guideline for prevention of catheter-associated urinary tract infections*. Retrieved November 9, 2011, from http://www.cdc.gov/hicpac/cauti/001_cauti.html

Hampton, B. G., & Bryant, R. A. (1992). *Ostomies and continent diversions: Nursing management* (1st ed.). St. Louis, MO: Mosby.

Pagana, K. D., & Pagana, T. J. (2007). *Mosby's diagnostic and laboratory test reference* (8th ed.). St. Louis, MO: Mosby Elsevier.

Schrier, R. W. (2007). *Diseases of the kidney and urinary tract* (8th ed.). Philadelphia, PA: Lippincott Williams & Wilkins.

Spraggon, E. (2008). The management of ileal conduit urinary diversions. *Continence UK, 2*(1), 17–28.

Turnbull, G. B. (2003). Ostomy statistics: The $64,000 question. *Ostomy/wound Management, 49*(6), 22–23.

Unlu, H., Sardan, Y. C., & Ulker, S. (2007). Comparison of sampling methods for urine cultures. *Journal of Nursing Scholarship: An Official Publication of Sigma Theta Tau International Honor Society of Nursing/Sigma Theta Tau, 39*(4), 325–329. doi: 10.1111/j.1547-5069.2007.00188.x.

Wullt, B., Agace, W., & Mansson, W. (2004). Bladder, bowel and bugs-bacteriuria in patients with intestinal urinary diversion. *World Journal of Urology, 22*(3), 186–195. doi: 10.1007/s00345-004-0432-x.

Acknowledgment about Content Validation

This document was reviewed in the consensus-building process of the Wound, Ostomy and Continence Nurses Society known as Content Validation, which is managed by the Center for Clinical Investigation.

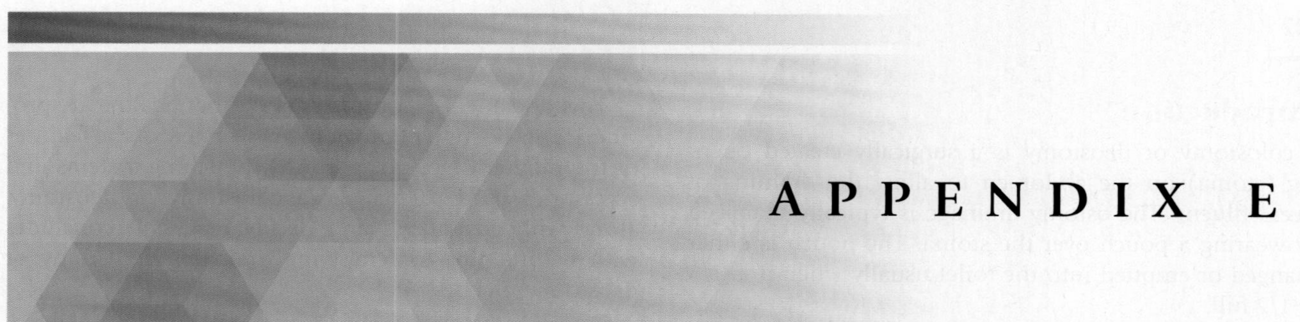

APPENDIX E

COLOSTOMY AND ILEOSTOMY PRODUCTS AND TIPS

Best Practice for Clinicians

Acknowledgments

Colostomy and Ileostomy Products and Tips: Best Practice for Clinicians.

This document was developed by the WOCN Society's Clinical Practice Ostomy Committee between April 2011 and April 2012.

Ginger Salvadalena, Chair, PhD, RN, CWOCN
Senior Clinical Research Scientist
Hollister Incorporated
Libertyville, IL

Carole Bauer, MSN, RN, ANP-BC, OCN, CWOCN
Wound, Ostomy and Continence Nurse Practitioner
The Barbara Ann Karmanos Cancer Center
Detroit, MI

Kathryn Baxter, MS, RN, FNP, CWOCN
Nurse Practitioner, Colon/Rectal Surgery
St. Luke's Roosevelt Hospital
New York, NY

Cathy P. Downey, BSN, RN, CWOCN
Program Coordinator, OP/BCT
University Medical Center
Las Vegas, NV

Kay Durkop-Scott, BSN, RN, CWOCN
Wound Ostomy Continence RN
Porter Adventist Hospital
Denver, CO

Mary F. Mahoney, BSN, RN, CWON
WOC Nurse
Iowa Health Home Care
Des Moines, IA

Barbara Metzger, BSN, RN, CWOCN
WOC Nurse
University of Kentucky Medical Center-Good Samaritan
Lexington, KY

Jacqueline Perkins, MSN, FNP-C, CWOCN
Wound/Ostomy Nurse Practitioner
VA Central Iowa Health Care System
Des Moines, IA

Michelle Rice, MSN, RN, CWOCN
Ostomy Clinical Nurse Specialist
Duke University Hospital
Durham, NC

Victoria Schafer, MSN, RN, CWON, CCRA
Ostomy Care
Associate Director, Medical & Scientific Liaison
Medical Affairs North America
ConvaTec
Skillman, NJ

Shirley Tyler, MS, RN, CWOCN
Wound Care Specialist
Home Care
Mattoon, IL

Introduction

A colostomy or ileostomy is a surgically created opening (stoma) on the abdomen to allow the draining of feces/effluent. The ostomy drainage is typically managed by wearing a pouch over the stoma. The pouch is either changed or emptied into the toilet usually when it is 1/3 to 1/2 full.

This document is for nurses and other health care providers. This document provides an overview of the features of the different types of products, pouching systems and accessories used to manage a colostomy or ileostomy, along with advantages and disadvantages. It concludes with helpful tips for emptying drainable colostomy or ileostomy pouches.

Pouching Systems

Description	Advantages	Disadvantages
Disposable Pouching System		
• System designed to be thrown away after removal. Typically made of lightweight plastic film, which is available in transparent or opaque material. Disposable pouches can be closed-end, or drainable, and part of either one-piece or two-piece pouching systems. May have plastic or fabric backing.	• Odor resistant. • May be worn in bath, shower and swimming pool. • Cleaning usually not necessary. • Drainable pouches are typically changed every 3 to 7 days. Closed pouches are discarded and replaced when 1/3 to 1/2 full of feces/effluent. • Convenient, easy to carry and dispose. • Various sizes/capacity.	• May be more expensive than reusable pouching systems over time. • May require removing stool and then cleaning the end "tail" of pouch for odor control.
Reusable Pouching System		
• Pouch which can be washed and reapplied multiple times. Typically made of vinyl or thick plastic film. Reusable pouches can be closed-end (if used with a liner), or drainable. May be a one-piece or two-piece system comprised of a pouch, also referred to as a skin barrier or wafer.	• Washable. • Able to reuse multiple times. • Some can be used without an adhesive.	• Can retain odors. • Limited number of manufacturers. • Initial cost may be more expensive than disposable pouching system. • May require more time to clean. • Might require a belt and/or adhesive.
One-piece Pouching System		
• The skin barrier and pouch are attached together during manufacturing. Available in drainable and closed styles, with and without filters.	• Many styles are flexible and conform to abdominal contours. • Low profile. • No chance for leakage between skin barrier and pouch as in two-piece systems. • May be less costly than a two-piece system. • May be easier to learn to use. • Often used when abdominal plane contours are uneven, as it can provide greater flexibility than a two-piece system.	• Cannot reposition once applied. • Cannot burp for gas. • Cannot change the pouch without changing the entire system. • Some have less support for loose peristomal skin.
Two-piece Pouching System		
• The skin barrier and pouch are made separately with rigid to semi-rigid rings or with an adhesive coupling system which allows the pouch to be attached to the skin barrier.	• Can provide support to loose peristomal skin. • Can switch between drainable and closed-end pouches without removing the skin barrier. • Can change position of the pouch with patient's position changes (especially for bed-bound patients) to facilitate better drainage.	• Need dexterity and strength to assure attachment of pouch to skin barrier. • Higher profile. • More costly than a one-piece pouch. • Less flexible than a one-piece pouching system and does not mold well to the body contours.

Pouching Systems (*Continued*)

Description	Advantages	Disadvantages
Pouching System with Adhesive Flange		
• The skin barrier and pouch are made separately and designed to stick together without a rigid flange.	• Can change pouch for disposal, emptying or rinsing without removing the skin barrier. • Low profile. • Flexibility similar to a one-piece system. • May be easier to apply than pouching systems with a flange, for those with poor dexterity. • May be used when abdominal plane contours are uneven, such as with a peristomal hernia.	• Less support for flabby peristomal skin. • Limited number of times pouch can be reattached (dependent on manufacturer). • Must have the coordination to apply properly on the skin barrier. • Cannot reuse pouch if adhesive area becomes soiled. • May be more difficult for visually impaired to use.

Types of Pouches

Description	Advantages	Disadvantages
Transparent Pouch		
• Pouch made of clear film.	• Can see stoma for easy application of pouching system. • Able to monitor stoma and effluent appearance, especially in the early postoperative period.	• Appearance of feces/effluent in the pouch may be unpleasant for the patient and/or the significant other.
Opaque Pouch		
• Pouch made of colored film (typically white or beige).	• Cosmetically appealing, unable to see stoma or stool. • More discreet under light-colored clothing.	• May be more difficult to apply when part of a one-piece pouching system.
Drainable Pouch		
• Pouch with an opening at the bottom. A clamp or integrated closure is used to keep the pouch closed until it is time to empty.	• Able to empty frequently. • Cost effective. • Long and shorter lengths are available. • Available with and without filter for gas release.	• Risk of spillage. Can require some skill to drain successfully without spillage of stool. • Need dexterity and strength to manage various closures. • Some versions may be too long for comfort or body size. • Rinsing/cleaning of the pouch may be needed or preferred by some patients.
Closed End Pouch		
• Also called a closed or nondrainable pouch. A pouch without an opening or clamp. It must be removed/discarded when 1/3 to 1/2 full.	• Low profile. • More discreet for intimate situations. • Generally shorter than drainable pouches. • May be easier to use than drainable for some people. • See section on disposable liners. • Available with and without filters for gas release.	• Smaller pouch capacity. • Not practical if having frequent stools or large amounts of fecal/effluent output.
High Output Pouch		
• A drainable pouch which accommodates larger amounts of output. Has a drainage spout at the end of the pouch.	• Used for frequent or high-volume fecal output. • Does not need to be emptied as often. • If stool is liquid, it can be attached to a bedside drainage bag/container.	• More expensive than smaller drainable pouches, but insurance reimbursement is available. • Larger size may make it difficult to conceal. • When connected to bedside drainage bag, tubing and/or pouch can potentially twist and kink, so the tubing should be anchored well and monitored to ensure adequate drainage.

(*Continued*)

Types of Pouches (*Continued*)

Description	Advantages	Disadvantages
Colostomy Irrigation Pouch		
• Long, sleeve–type pouch used during colostomy irrigation. Allows containment of the stool and allows irrigation fluid to flow through the sleeve into the toilet. Some have flanges to use with two-piece system. Some have self adhesive. Pouch size varies by manufacturer.	• Use of colostomy irrigation allows a person with a colostomy to control when they have a bowel movement. May be used to administer an ostomy bowel prep. May eliminate the need for a drainable pouching system between irrigations. • Extra long drain directs effluent into the toilet. • Top opening pouch accommodates a stoma cone. • May be rinsed with cool water for reuse. • May be used as high capacity pouch for short periods of time.	• Irrigation process requires time and appropriate toileting facility. • Pouch is not odor proof.
Stoma Cap		
• A small closed pouch, usually less than 4 inches in diameter, with an absorbent pad inside the pouch. Covers stoma when periods of inactivity can be anticipated, such as after a stoma irrigation. Some are available with a vent or filter for gas release.	• More discreet for intimate situations or under clothes. • Easier to apply than a dressing or bandage–type cover.	• No capacity to contain stool. • Only indicated for use between colostomy irrigations in persons with descending or sigmoid colostomy.
Pouch with Integrated Closure		
• A drainable pouch that has an attached closure at the bottom of the pouch. The closure is part of the drainable pouch, attached during the manufacturing process.	• No clamp/clip to lose. • May be more comfortable. • May be easier to manipulate for those with limited hand dexterity.	• Individuals who have used clips for a long time need instruction and reassurance. • May be harder to remove feces/effluent in order to keep clean and odor free.
Filter		
• A feature available on some pouches which allows gas (but not odor) to escape from the pouch. Filters may be integrated in the pouch during manufacturing or purchased separately and added to a pouch.	• Venting of gas is passive (requires no action on the part of the user). • Low risk of accidental spillage.	• Ineffective if it becomes wet. Newer versions have a barrier film to prevent wetness from entering from either inside or outside the pouch. • May be an added expense. • Add-on filters can become dislodged. • If stool is liquid, may leak through filter and render charcoal ineffective.
Belt Loops		
• A feature on a pouch or skin barrier that allows for use of an elastic belt with a one-piece or two-piece pouching system.	• Belt loops on the skin barrier allow the pouch to be applied and removed without disturbing the belt. • Belt loops on the pouch can add security to the connection between pouch and skin barrier flange.	• Presence of belt loops may make the skin barrier more rigid. • The belt loops may be uncomfortable against the body, and wearing a belt too tightly may lead to a pressure ulcer.

Skin Barriers

The skin barrier is the part of a pouching system that is applied directly to the skin. Adhesive skin barriers are typically made from pectin, karaya gum, and/or synthetic materials. A nonadhesive skin barrier is made from silicone or rubber.

Description	Advantages	Disadvantages
Flat Skin Barrier		
• A skin barrier that has a level or flat appearance. • May be part of a one-piece or two-piece pouching system.	• Used when the peristomal skin surface is flat and the stoma is well budded (protruding at least 1/2 inch above the abdominal wall surface).	• If the peristomal skin surface is not flat and/or the stoma is not well protruded, accessories such as paste or barrier rings may be needed to achieve a better seal around the base of the stoma. • Requires a scissor and dexterity to create a cut-to-fit opening.
Convex Skin Barrier		
• A skin barrier that has a rounded "inverted bowl shape" surface on the side that adheres to the skin used when the stoma is at skin level/flushed or retracted/below skin level. • May be part of a one-piece or two-piece pouching system.	• Used for peristomal skin surface that is concave. • Used for soft peristomal skin surface with a flush or short stoma. • Convexity can be rigid/firm or somewhat flexible and can be useful for stomas that have different depths/degrees of stoma retraction.	• May need to add an ostomy belt to provide added security/support by keeping wafer/barrier in place. • May lift from the skin with body movement and position changes or cause pressure damage if the convexity is too stiff/rigid. • Neither an ostomy belt nor a firm convex barrier should be used in the immediate post-operative period to avoid tension on the suture line of the stoma and to prevent mucocutaneous separation.
Moldable, Shapeable, or Stretchable Skin Barrier		
• A skin barrier that allows the opening for the stoma to be shaped with fingers rather than using scissors.	• Available flat or convex. • Moldable skin barrier has "shape memory" which provides a constant, self-adjusting fit around the base of the stoma. • No scissors needed. • Useful for those with poor hand dexterity or poor eyesight which would make cutting barrier to size difficult.	• May not work consistently with flush, partially flush stomas, or retracted stomas. • May need some dexterity to shape. • Can move over stoma opening over time, leading to leakage. • Option currently only available with a two-piece pouching system.
Skin Barrier with Floating Flange		
• A skin barrier with a flange that is not adhered to the base of the barrier.	• A skin barrier used in a two-piece pouching system. A floating flange allows the pouch to be snapped onto the skin barrier while minimizing the pressure to the patient's abdomen. • Available flat or convex.	• Higher profile than nonfloating flange.
Skin Barrier with Locking Flange		
• A skin barrier with a system to lock the pouch to the flange. • A skin barrier used in a two-piece pouching system.	• Available flat or convex. • May require less dexterity to attach pouch to flange. • Designed for individuals with limited eye-hand coordination. • Allows the pouch to be snapped onto the skin barrier without adding pressure to the abdomen.	• Higher profile than nonlocking flange. • May require more dexterity to attach pouch to flange or coupling mechanism.
Skin Barrier with Smooth Flange		
• A skin barrier with a docking area for the pouch to adhere. • A skin barrier used in a two-piece pouching system.	• The pouch adheres to the skin barrier plate with an adhesive ring. • Available flat or convex. • Can be detached and re-applied. • More flexible than the locking or floating flange.	• Adhesive surface must be dry for good adherence.

(*Continued*)

Skin Barriers (*Continued*)

Description	Advantages	Disadvantages
Tape Border		
• A skin barrier with adhesive tape attached to the edges of the barrier.	• Some skin barriers have a tape border around the outside of the barrier which makes the skin barrier more flexible and lower profile. • Patients may feel more secure with a tape border.	• Patients may have sensitivity to adhesives leading to allergic/contact dermatitis.

Accessories

Description	Advantages	Disadvantages
Pouch Lubricant		
• A lubricant added to the pouch to facilitate the ease of emptying stool from the pouch.	• Pouch sides less likely to stick together. • Stool less likely to stick to sides of pouch. • May also contain an odor eliminator. • Unlike household products, such as mineral oil, nonstick cooking spray, and liquid soap, commercial lubricant will not damage the film of the pouch.	• Extra step and expense.
Gas Vent/Filter		
• Vent added to a pouch to allow wearer to have control over when they release gas.	• Decreases risk of spillage compared to burping or releasing gas from the tail end. • Control when gas is vented. • Accessory filter may also be used.	• Will not deodorize gas without a charcoal filter. • Extra steps are required to apply separate gas vent/filter if it was not integrated into pouch by the manufacturing process. It must be applied 24 hours in advance of using. • Requires dexterity. • Added cost. • May leak liquid effluent from the filter or around connection on pouch. • Gas venting not automatic. Gas vent needs to be manually opened to release gas.
Pouch Liners		
• Placed inside a two-piece pouch and held in place when the pouch is snapped to the flange of the skin barrier. After bowel movement, used liner is removed and flushed and a new liner is placed inside the same pouch.	• Keeps pouch clean—same pouch can be used multiple times. • Weartime of pouch can be extended with use of disposable liners. • May be more discreet for the user because they can be flushed rather than disposed in trash. • Compatible with pouches with or without gas filter.	• Not covered by insurance. • Not compatible with septic systems. • Not compatible with two-piece systems using the Adhesive Coupling Technique. • May adversely affect the security of the pouch adhering to the barrier. • Learning to remove the liner from the pouch without spillage can take time, dexterity, and practice.
Clamp		
• The removable plastic clip used on a drainable pouch.	• Can be cleaned. • Reusable. • Available with curved shape to fit thigh for lower profile. • Several options are available: individuals can often find one that they can handle with their limitations.	• The clamp can break. • Can be dropped or lost when emptying the pouch. • Higher profile (more visible) than integrated pouch closures. • Some styles are difficult for people with limited dexterity. • Added cost if needed to be replaced.

Accessories (*Continued*)

Description	Advantages	Disadvantages
Pouch Cover		
• Cloth envelope-like sleeve to place over ostomy pouch while it is on the body.	• Cosmetically appealing, cannot see stoma or stool. • Can reduce sweating, skin irritation, and provide a more comfortable surface against the skin. • May help reduce noise from vinyl or plastic pouch. • May be integrated within available disposable pouches.	• Added expense with fabric material already covering some pouches.
Skin Sealant		
• Plasticizing agent such as copolymer; some may contain isopropyl alcohol. Available as wipe, spray, gel, liquid, and roll-on.	• Provides a thin protective film to the skin surface. Helps to prevent stripping of the epidermis during adhesive removal and also acts as a moisture barrier. • If applying stoma powder to skin irritation, skin sealant may be added to provide a surface for skin barrier adherence.	• Sealants may not be recommended under some skin barriers because the protective film may reduce the adherence of the barrier. • Skin sealants which contain alcohol can cause pain when applied to irritated skin.
Adhesive Remover		
• Solvent available as gel, wipe, or liquid.	• Aids in the removal of tape, skin adhesives and residue. May be helpful to the patient with sensitive skin to reduce trauma from removal of pouching system.	• Rinsing is typically required to remove residue before pouch application to prevent chemical dermatitis or nonadherence of next pouch.
Skin Adhesive		
• Adhesive made of silicone or latex.	• Used to increase adhesion of an adhesive pouching system or to provide adhesion for a reusable (nonadhesive) system.	• Need to teach patient to allow adhesive to dry to prevent chemical irritation. • May be flammable.
Paste		
• Pectin based product used to help prevent leakage of stoma drainage under the skin barrier.	• Can use to fill in uneven areas and/or as a caulking around the inner edge of the skin barrier to prevent leakage under the skin barrier. • Used to increase the seal of skin barrier to contours of the abdominal surface. • Fills in small creases and depressions and evens out skin contours under a skin barrier. • Used appropriately, will offer a quick seal for the pouching system until the skin barrier adhesive is pressed into place.	• Patients often think this is adhesive paste and use it inappropriately. • Patients often use too much. • Requires dexterity for application to either peristomal skin or skin barrier. May sting when applied to irritated peristomal skin. • May help with improving the fit of barrier. • Is not substantial enough to fill in large creases. Does not hold up well when exposed to urinary or ileal effluent.

(*Continued*)

Accessories (*Continued*)

Description	Advantages	Disadvantages
Skin Barrier Rings		
• Pectin or sodium carboxymethylcellulose based product that is soft and moldable used as a washer around the base of the stoma to help prevent effluent drainage under the skin barrier.	• Used to increase the seal of skin barrier to contours of the abdominal surface. Can be used to enhance the pouching system seal. • Alternative to paste. To help with fitting over contours. • Can be stretched and molded to create custom shapes. • Can be used straight from the package or molded into desired shape to fill in areas that need to be leveled out. • Can be cut, bent, and stacked together to improve the fit of the skin barrier. • For individuals with sensitive skin or limited dexterity. • May prolong skin barrier wear time. • Convex barrier rings can be used to adjust skin barrier thickness for deeper convexity or used to create oval-shaped convexity.	• Requires dexterity for application to either peristomal skin or skin barrier. • Added cost. • Added step.
Stoma Powder		
• Pectin or karaya based powder used to protect peristomal skin and mucocutaneous separation from exposure to stoma discharge.	• Aids healing and protection. • Helps protect open, weeping skin against stoma discharge. Absorbs moisture or exudate from skin prior to placing a skin barrier on peristomal skin for added protection. • May be sealed to the skin by applying a layer of skin sealant before the pouching system is applied.	• If applied improperly, may prevent adhesion of skin barrier.
Strip Paste		
• Pectin based product used to help prevent leakage of stoma drainage under the skin barrier.	• Used to increase the seal of skin barrier to contours of the abdominal surface. Can be used to enhance the pouching system seal. • Can be cut, bent, and stacked together to improve the fit of the skin barrier. • Conforms to irregular skin folds/creases. • Soft and moldable.	• Requires dexterity for application to either peristomal skin or skin barrier. • Added cost. • Added step.
Odor Control Products		
• Air sprays, pouch deodorants, oral deodorants, charcoal filters. • Some sprays have a fragrance which covers up the odor. • Some sprays act by eliminating the odor.	• May decrease odor when emptying pouch.	• Extra step and expense. • May not be effective. • May trigger chemical sensitivities on the stoma or skin. • Oral deodorizers may have side effects. • Diet changes can also be helpful.

Tips For Emptying Drainable Pouches

Description	Advantages	Disadvantages
Prevention of Splashing		
• Place a layer of toilet paper on the water in the toilet before emptying a drainable pouch.	• Can muffle the sound of stool hitting the water. • Can prevent being splashed with toilet water.	• May not work depending on the amount and consistency of stool.
Cuff the End of the Drainable Pouch		
• This technique can be used to empty a drainable pouch without integrated closure. • Hold tail end of pouch up so that stool will not spill out. • Roll tail end of pouch up forming a cuff. • Direct the end of the pouch down and empty. • Clean edge of rolled cuff with toilet paper or moistened paper towel. • Unroll pouch and re-clamp.	• Intended to keep end of pouch and clamp clean, which prevents odor accumulation and soiling of clothing and/or skin. • Enables patient to empty with less risk of soiling hands. • Can reduce time involved in emptying because the inside of the end of the pouch isn't soiled and doesn't need to be cleaned.	• Requires some dexterity. • Difficult when pouch is fairly full or stool is liquid. • Not recommended with pouches that have integrated closure mechanisms.

Acknowledgment about Content Validation

This document was reviewed in the consensus-building process of the Wound, Ostomy and Continence Nurses Society known as Content Validation, which is managed by the Center for Clinical Investigation.

APPENDIX F

WOCN SOCIETY AND AUA POSITION STATEMENT ON PREOPERATIVE STOMA SITE MARKING FOR PATIENTS UNDERGOING UROSTOMY SURGERY

Originated By:

Wound, Ostomy and Continence Nurses Society's (WOCN®) Stoma Site Marking Task Force in collaboration with the American Urological Association (AUA) in 2009 (AUA & WOCN, 2009).

Updated/Revised By:

WOCN Society's Stoma Site Marking Task Force in collaboration with the American Society of Colon and Rectal Surgeons (ASCRS) and the AUA.

Contributing Authors:

Task Force Chair

- **Ginger Salvadalena, PhD, RN, CWOCN**, Principal Scientist, Global Clinical Affairs, Hollister Incorporated, Libertyville, Illinois

Task Force Members

- **Samantha Hendren, MD, MPH**, Associate Professor of Surgery, University of Michigan, Ann Arbor, Michigan
- **Linda McKenna, MSN, RN, CWOCN**, Ostomy & Wound Specialist, Memorial Medical Center, Springfield, Illinois
- **Roberta Muldoon, MD, FACS**, Assistant Professor of Surgery, Vanderbilt University Medical Center, Nashville, Tennessee
- **Debra Netsch, DNP, RN, CNP, FNP-BC, CWOCN**, Mankato Clinic, Ltd, Mankato, Minnesota
- **Ian Paquette, MD**, Assistant Professor of Surgery, University of Cincinnati College of Medicine, Cincinnati, Ohio
- **Joyce Pittman, PhD, ANP-BC, FNP-BC, CWOCN**, Team Lead Wound/Ostomy Adjunct Assistant Professor, Indiana University School of Nursing, Indiana University Health-Methodist, Indianapolis, Indiana
- **Janet Ramundo, MSN, RN, CWOCN**, WOC Nurse, Houston Methodist Hospital, Houston, Texas
- **Gary Steinberg, MD**, The Beth and Bruce White Family Professor and Director of Urologic Oncology; Vice Chairman Section of Urology, The University of Chicago Medicine, Chicago, Illinois

Date Completed:

June 2014

Date Approved by the WOCN Board of Directors:

November 12, 2014

The WOCN Society Suggests the Following Format for Bibliographic Citations:

Wound, Ostomy and Continence Nurses Society. (2014). *WOCN Society and AUA Position Statement on Preoperative Stoma Site Marking for Patients Undergoing Urostomy Surgery*. Mt. Laurel, NJ: Author.

Statement of Position:

Ostomy education and stoma site selection should be performed preoperatively for all patients when an ostomy is a possibility (AUA & WOCN, 2009). Multiple studies indicate that patients who have their stoma site marked preoperatively by a trained clinician have fewer ostomy-related complications (Gulbiniene et al., 2004; Millan et al., 2010; Park et al., 1999; Parmar et al., 2011; Pittman et al., 2008; WOCN, 2010).

An appropriate stoma site may decrease ostomy-related complications such as leakage of the pouching system and peristomal dermatitis. It may also influence the predictability of a pouch's wear time, ability of the patient to adapt to the ostomy and become independent, and may even help control healthcare costs. Preoperatively marking the stoma site allows assessment of the patient's abdomen in multiple positions, which promotes selection of the optimal stoma site. In addition, this preoperative session promotes a patient-centered approach respecting the individuality, values, and information needs of the patient and family. The session may allow time to provide information regarding ostomy management, including pouching options, and provide psychosocial support. While preoperative stoma site marking is strongly supported, it is acknowledged that intra-operative circumstances may not allow for the optimal stoma site to be used in all situations. The final stoma site is chosen by the surgeon after the abdominal cavity is entered and the condition of the bowel is determined.

Urologists and certified ostomy nurses are the optimal clinicians to select and mark stoma sites, as this skill is a part of their education, practice, and training. However, these providers are not always available in emergency situations. All physicians who are called on to choose ostomy sites should familiarize themselves with the principles of proper stoma site selection, including placement of the stoma within the rectus abdominis muscle, use of multiple patient positions to identify appropriate stoma sites, avoidance of folds and scars, and consideration of the clothing/beltline.

Purpose (Rationale for Position):

The WOCN Society in collaboration with the AUA and ASCRS developed the following educational guide to assist clinicians (especially those who are not surgeons or WOC nurses) in selecting an effective stoma site. Marking the optimal location for a stoma preoperatively enhances the likelihood of a patient's independence in stoma care, predictable pouching system wear times, and resumption of normal activities.

Recommendations:

A. Key Points to Consider

1. The stoma site should be located within the rectus abdominis muscle.
2. Positioning issues: Contractures, posture, mobility (e.g., wheelchair confinement, use of a walker, etc.).
3. Physical considerations: Large/protruding/pendulous abdomen, abdominal folds, wrinkles, scars/suture lines, other stomas, rectus abdominis muscle, waist line, iliac crest, braces, pendulous breasts, vision, dexterity, and the presence of a hernia.
4. Patient considerations: Diagnosis, age, occupation, prior experience with a stoma, and preferences about the stoma's location.
5. Surgical considerations: Surgeon's preferences, type of surgery/stoma planned, segment of intestine used, and whether an incontinent versus a continent catheterizable diversion is planned.
6. Multiple stoma sites: If a fecal stoma is also present or planned, consider marking the urinary and fecal stoma sites on different horizontal planes/lines in the event that an ostomy belt is required.

B. Stoma Site Marking Procedure

1. Gather items needed for the procedure: Marking pen, surgical marker, transparent film dressing, and flat skin barrier (i.e., according to the surgeon's preference and/or the facility's policy).
2. Explain the stoma site marking procedure to the patient, and encourage the patient's participation and input.
3. Carefully examine the patient's abdominal surface. If possible, begin with the patient fully clothed in a sitting position with both feet on the floor.
   - Observe the presence of belts, braces, and any other ostomy pouches.
   - Individuals with spinal cord injuries are optimally marked in their usual position, as this will facilitate fitting and care of the pouching system (Cataldo, 2008).
   - If the patient uses a wheelchair, it is best to position them in their own chair and allow time for their body to relax into their usual habitus before marking (Hocevar & Gray, 2008).
4. Have the patient completely remove any clothing that is placed over the abdomen, rather than just moving it out of the way. Waistbands and elastic can create or obscure skin folds that may or may not be present when the clothing is completely removed.
5. Examine the patient's exposed abdomen in various positions (e.g., standing, lying, sitting, and bending forward) to observe for creases, valleys, scars, folds, skin turgor, and contour.
6. Consider an imaginary line where the surgical incision will be located. If possible, choose a point at least 2 inches from the surgical incision where 2 to 3 inches of a flat adhesive skin barrier can be placed.
7. With the patient lying on his or her back, identify the rectus abdominis muscle. This can be done by having the patient do a modified sit up (i.e., raise the head up and off the bed) or by having the patient cough. Palpate the edge of the rectus abdominis muscle. Expert opinion suggests that placement of the stoma within the rectus abdominis muscle may

help prevent a peristomal hernia and/or a prolapse (AUA & WOCN, 2009).

8. Mark a spot on the skin of the abdomen that is located within the rectus abdominis muscle, in the appropriate quadrant for the planned surgery, and within the patient's visual field.
   - Care should be taken to avoid scars or creases; the priority is a flat pouching surface.
   - Individuals who use a wheelchair or have a large, rounded abdominal contour may benefit from having the stoma site marked in an upper quadrant (Hocevar & Gray, 2008).
   - Choose an area that is visible to the patient, and if possible below the belt line to conceal the pouch.
9. If the abdomen is protuberant, choose the apex of the abdominal contour, or if the patient is extremely obese, consider marking the site in an upper abdominal quadrant (Colwell, 2014). In many obese patients the adipose layer is not as thick in the upper abdominal quadrants as compared to the lower quadrants, which may allow better visualization of the stoma (Cataldo, 2008; Colwell, 2014).
10. The mark should initially be made with a sticker or ink pen that can be removed if this is not the optimal spot.
    - It may be desirable to mark sites on the right and left sides of the abdomen to prepare for a change in the surgical outcome, and number the first choice as #1.
    - Have the patient assume sitting, bending, and lying positions to assess and confirm the best choice.
    - It is important to have the patient confirm they can see the site. However, the critical consideration should be a flat pouching surface.
11. After the optimal site is chosen, clean the desired site with alcohol and allow it to dry. Then proceed with marking the selected site with a surgical marker or pen. If desired, cover the site with a transparent film dressing to preserve the final mark. Ensure that any other stray marks have been removed.

C. Examples of Stoma Site Marking

1. See **Figure 1**: Example of marking a stoma site for a female with a protuberant abdomen, creases, and folds.

Step 1
Look at the profile of the patient. Notice where the abdomen curves back under toward the body. The underside of the abdomen is not visisble to the patient. Avoid this area.

AVOID
Line of Sight
Patient cannot see below the line of sight.

Step 2
While patient is seated, look for skin folds and creases. Note and avoid skin folds and creases.

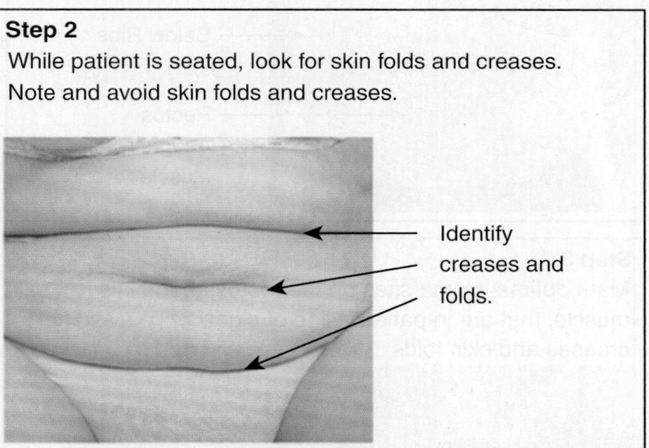

Step 3
Identify and target the rectus abdominis muscle below the ribs.

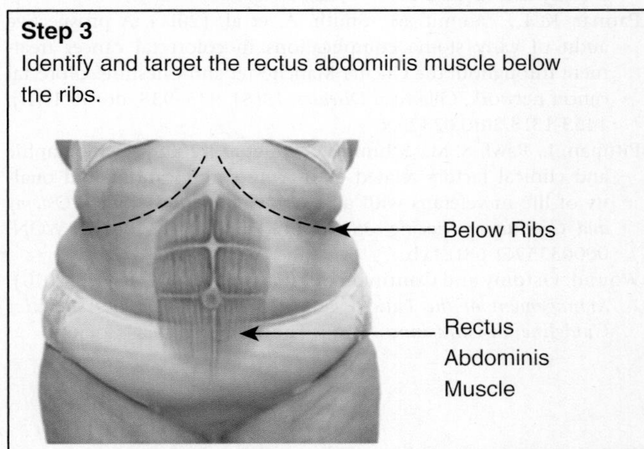

Step 4
Mark optimal stoma sites on the rectus abdominis, that are in patient's line of sight, while avoiding creases and skin folds.

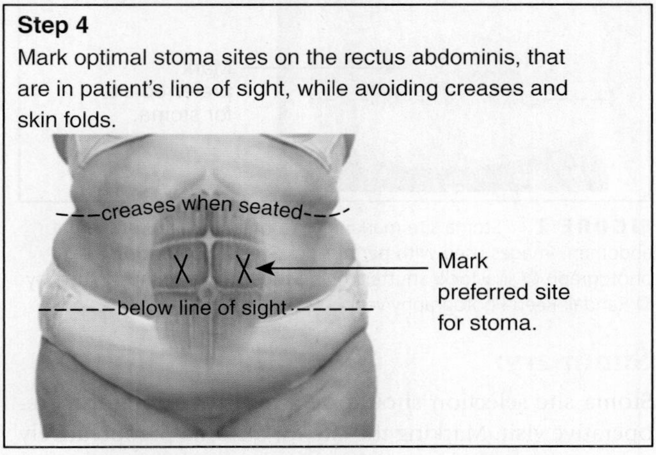

FIGURE 1. Stoma site marking for a female with a protuberant abdomen. Images used with permission: **Step 1**, female photograph © milk122/veer; **Step 2**, female photograph © SeDmi/veer; **Steps 3 and 4**, female photograph © kokhanchikov/shutterstock, and muscle overlay © Randall Reed Photography/veer.

2. See **Figure 2**: Example of marking a stoma site for a male with a protuberant abdomen.

Step 1
Look at the profile of the patient. Notice where the abdomen curves back under toward the body. The underside of the abdomen is not visible to the patient. Avoid this area.

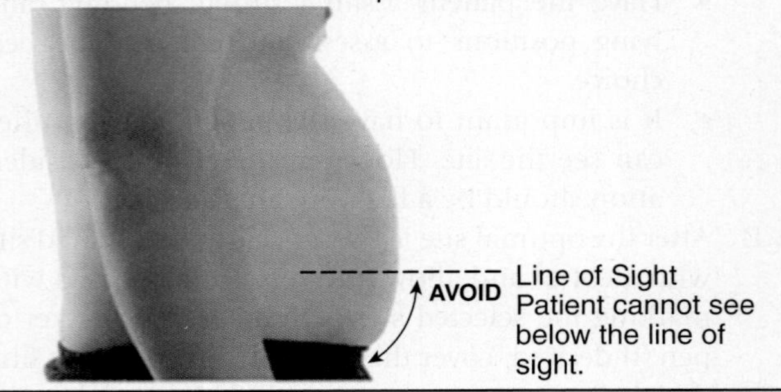

Step 2
Identify and target the rectus abdominis muscle below the ribs.

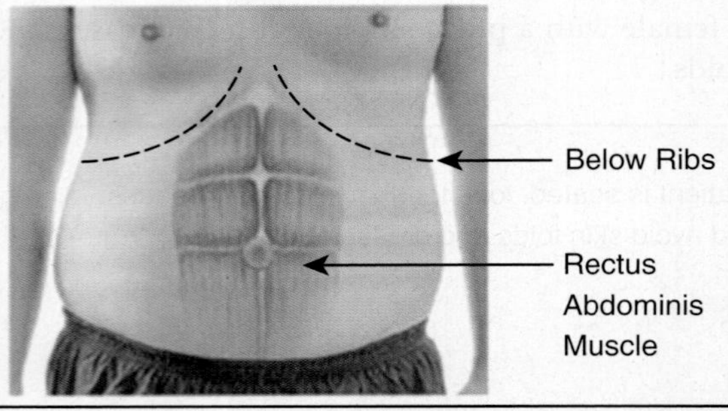

Step 3
Mark optimal stoma sites on the rectus abdominis muscle, that are in patient's line of sight, while avoiding creases and skin folds.

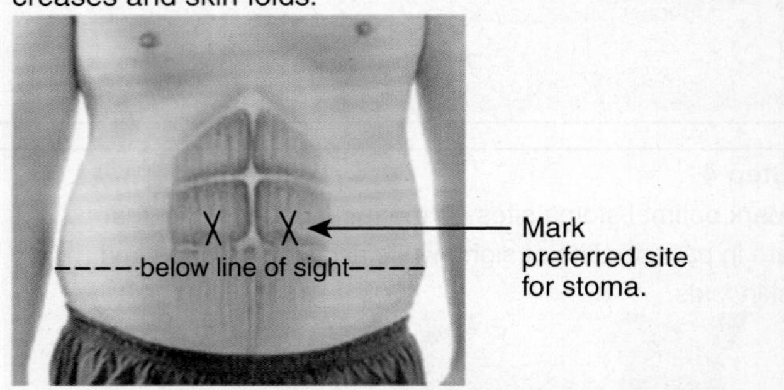

FIGURE 2. Stoma site marking for a male with a protuberant abdomen. Images used with permission: **Steps 1, 2, and 3**, male photograph © sirastock/ shutterstock; **Steps 2 and 3**, muscle overlay © Randall Reed Photography/veer.

Summary:

Stoma site selection should be a priority during the preoperative visit. Marking the site for a stoma preoperatively provides an opportunity to select the optimal site, which can help reduce postoperative problems such as leakage, peristomal dermatitis, and difficulty with self-care of the ostomy. Whenever possible, ostomy education and stoma site selection should be performed preoperatively when an ostomy is a possibility.

Acknowledgment

The task force wishes to acknowledge Christina Augustyn, Industrial Designer, Innovation Management Office, Hollister Incorporated, Libertyville, Illinois, for her contribution in the selection and development of the images.

REFERENCES

AUA & WOCN Society. (2009). AUA and WOCN joint position statement on the value of preoperative stoma marking for patients undergoing creation of an incontinent urostomy. *Journal of Wound, Ostomy and Continence Nursing, 36*(3), 267–268.

Cataldo, P. A. (2008). Technical tips for stoma creation in the challenging patient. *Clinics in Colon and Rectal Surgery, 21*(1), 17–22. doi:10.1055/s-2008-1055317

Colwell, J. C. (2014). The role of obesity in the patient undergoing colorectal surgery and fecal diversion: A review of the literature. *Ostomy Wound Management, 60*(1), 24–28.

Gulbiniene, J., Markelis, R., Tamelis, A. et al. (2004). The impact of preoperative stoma siting and stoma care education on patient's quality of life. *Medicina (Caunas), 40*(11), 1045–1053.

Hocevar, B., & Gray, M. (2008). Intestinal diversion (colostomy or ileostomy) in patients with severe bowel dysfunction following spinal cord injury. *Journal of Wound, Ostomy and Continence Nursing, 35*(2), 159–166. doi:10.1097/01.WON.0000313638.29623.40

Millan, M., Tegido, M., Biondo, S. et al. (2010). Preoperative stoma siting and education by stomatherapists of colorectal cancer patients: A descriptive study in twelve Spanish colorectal surgical units. *Colorectal Diseases, 12*(7 Online), e88–e92. doi:10.1111/j.1463-1318.2009.01942.x

Park, J. J., Del Pino, A., Orsay, C. P. et al. (1999). Stoma complications: The Cook County Hospital experience. *Diseases of the Colon and Rectum, 42*(12), 1575–1580.

Parmar, K. L., Zammit, M., Smith, A. et al. (2011). A prospective audit of early stoma complications in colorectal cancer treatment throughout the Greater Manchester and Cheshire colorectal cancer network. *Colorectal Diseases, 13*(8), 935–938. doi:10.1111/j.1463-1318.2010.02325.x

Pittman, J., Rawl, S. M., Schmidt, C. M. et al. (2008). Demographic and clinical factors related to ostomy complications and quality of life in veterans with an ostomy. *Journal of Wound, Ostomy and Continence Nursing, 35*(5), 493–503. doi:10.1097/01.WON.0000335961.68113.cb

Wound, Ostomy and Continence Nurses Society (WOCN). (2010). *Management of the Patient with a Fecal Ostomy: Best Practice Guideline for Clinicians*. Mount Laurel, NJ: WOCN Society.

APPENDIX G

WOCN SOCIETY AND ASCRS POSITION STATEMENT ON PREOPERATIVE STOMA SITE MARKING FOR PATIENTS UNDERGOING COLOSTOMY OR ILEOSTOMY SURGERY

Originated By:

Wound, Ostomy and Continence Nurses Society's (WOCN®) Stoma Site Marking Task Force in collaboration with the American Society of Colon and Rectal Surgeons (ASCRS) in 2007 (ASCRS & WOCN, 2007).

Updated/Revised By:

WOCN Society's Stoma Site Marking Task Force in collaboration with the ASCRS and the American Urological Association (AUA).

Contributing Authors:

Task Force Chair

- **Ginger Salvadalena, PhD, RN, CWOCN**, Principal Scientist, Global Clinical Affairs, Hollister Incorporated, Libertyville, Illinois

Task Force Members

- **Samantha Hendren, MD, MPH**, Associate Professor of Surgery, University of Michigan, Ann Arbor, Michigan
- **Linda McKenna, MSN, RN, CWOCN**, Ostomy & Wound Specialist, Memorial Medical Center, Springfield, Illinois
- **Roberta Muldoon, MD, FACS**, Assistant Professor of Surgery, Vanderbilt University Medical Center, Nashville, Tennessee
- **Debra Netsch, DNP, RN, CNP, FNP-BC, CWOCN**, Mankato Clinic, Ltd, Mankato, Minnesota
- **Ian Paquette, MD**, Assistant Professor of Surgery, University of Cincinnati College of Medicine, Cincinnati, Ohio
- **Joyce Pittman, PhD, ANP-BC, FNP-BC, CWOCN**, Team Lead Wound/Ostomy Adjunct Assistant Professor, Indiana University School of Nursing, Indiana University Health-Methodist, Indianapolis, Indiana
- **Janet Ramundo, MSN, RN, CWOCN**, WOC Nurse, Houston Methodist Hospital, Houston, Texas
- **Gary Steinberg, MD**, The Beth and Bruce White Family Professor and Director of Urologic Oncology; Vice Chairman Section of Urology, The University of Chicago Medicine, Chicago, Illinois

Date Completed:

June 2014

Date Approved by the WOCN Board of Directors:

November 12, 2014

The WOCN Society suggests the following format for bibliographic citations:

Wound, Ostomy and Continence Nurses Society. (2014). *WOCN Society and ASCRS Position Statement on Preoperative Stoma Site Marking for Patients Undergoing Colostomy or Ileostomy Surgery*. Mt. Laurel, NJ: Author.

Statement of Position:

Ostomy education and stoma site selection should be performed preoperatively for all patients when an ostomy is a possibility (ASCRS & WOCN, 2007). Multiple studies indicate that patients who have their stoma site marked preoperatively by a trained clinician have fewer ostomy-related complications (Gulbiniene et al., 2004; Millan et al., 2010; Park et al., 1999; Parmar et al., 2011; Pittman et al., 2008; WOCN, 2010).

An appropriate stoma site may decrease ostomy-related complications such as leakage of the pouching system and peristomal dermatitis. It may also influence the predictability of a pouch's wear time, ability of the patient to adapt to the ostomy and become independent, and may even help control healthcare costs. Preoperatively marking the stoma site allows assessment of the patient's abdomen in multiple positions, which promotes selection of the optimal stoma site. In addition, this preoperative session promotes a patient-centered approach respecting the individuality, values, and information needs of the patient and family. The session may allow time to provide information regarding ostomy management, including pouching options, and provide psychosocial support. While preoperative stoma site marking is strongly supported, it is acknowledged that intra-operative circumstances may not allow for the optimal stoma site to be used in all situations. The final stoma site is chosen by the surgeon after the abdominal cavity is entered and the condition of the bowel is determined.

Colon and Rectal Surgeons and certified ostomy nurses are the optimal clinicians to select and mark stoma sites, as this skill is a part of their education, practice, and training. However, these providers are not always available in emergency situations. All physicians who are called on to choose ostomy sites should familiarize themselves with the principles of proper stoma site selection, including placement of the stoma within the rectus abdominis muscle, use of multiple patient positions to identify appropriate stoma sites, avoidance of folds and scars, and consideration of the clothing/beltline.

Purpose (Rationale for Position):

The WOCN Society in collaboration with the ASCRS and the AUA developed the following educational guide to assist clinicians (especially those who are not surgeons or WOC nurses) in selecting an effective stoma site. Marking the optimal location for a stoma preoperatively enhances the likelihood of a patient's independence in stoma care, predictable pouching system wear times, and resumption of normal activities.

Recommendations:

A. Key Points to Consider

1. The stoma site should be located within the rectus abdominis muscle.
2. Positioning issues: Contractures, posture, mobility (e.g., wheelchair confinement, use of a walker, etc.).
3. Physical considerations: Large/protruding/pendulous abdomen, abdominal folds, wrinkles, scars/suture lines, other stomas, rectus abdominis muscle, waist line, iliac crest, braces, pendulous breasts, vision, dexterity, and the presence of a hernia.
4. Patient considerations: Diagnosis, age, occupation, prior experience with a stoma, and preferences about the stoma's location.
5. Surgical considerations: Surgeon's preferences, type of surgery/stoma planned, segment of intestine used, and whether an incontinent versus a continent catheterizable diversion is planned.
6. Multiple stoma sites: If a urinary stoma is also present or planned, consider marking the fecal and urinary stoma sites on different horizontal planes/lines in the event that an ostomy belt is required.

B. Stoma Site Marking Procedure

1. Gather items needed for the procedure: Marking pen, surgical marker, transparent film dressing, and flat skin barrier (i.e., according to the surgeon's preference and/or the facility's policy).
2. Explain the stoma site marking procedure to the patient, and encourage the patient's participation and input.
3. Carefully examine the patient's abdominal surface. If possible, begin with the patient fully clothed in a sitting position with both feet on the floor.
   - Observe the presence of belts, braces, and any other ostomy pouches.
   - Individuals with spinal cord injuries are optimally marked in their usual position, as this will facilitate fitting and care of the pouching system (Cataldo, 2008).
   - If the patient uses a wheelchair, it is best to position them in their own chair and allow time for their body to relax into their usual habitus before marking (Hocevar & Gray, 2008).
4. Have the patient completely remove any clothing that is placed over the abdomen, rather than just moving it out of the way. Waistbands and elastic can create or obscure skin folds that may or may not be present when the clothing is completely removed.
5. Examine the patient's exposed abdomen in various positions (e.g., standing, lying, sitting, and bending forward) to observe for creases, valleys, scars, folds, skin turgor, and contour.
6. Consider an imaginary line where the surgical incision will be located. If possible, choose a point at least 2 inches from the surgical incision where 2 to 3 inches of a flat adhesive skin barrier can be placed.
7. With the patient lying on his or her back, identify the rectus abdominis muscle. This can be done by having the patient do a modified sit up (i.e., raise the head up and off the bed) or by having the patient cough. Palpate the edge of the rectus abdominis muscle. Expert opinion suggests that placement of the stoma within the rectus abdominis muscle may help prevent a peristomal hernia and/or a prolapse (ASCRS & WOCN, 2007).
8. Mark a spot on the skin of the abdomen that is located within the rectus abdominis muscle, in the appropriate quadrant for the planned surgery, and within the patient's visual field.

- Care should be taken to avoid scars or creases; the priority is a flat pouching surface.
- Individuals who use a wheelchair or have a large, rounded abdominal contour may benefit from having the stoma site marked in an upper quadrant (Hocevar & Gray, 2008).
- Choose an area that is visible to the patient, and if possible below the belt line to conceal the pouch.

9. If the abdomen is protuberant, choose the apex of the abdominal contour, or if the patient is extremely obese, consider marking the site in an upper abdominal quadrant (Colwell, 2014). In many obese patients the adipose layer is not as thick in the upper abdominal quadrants as compared to the lower quadrants, which may allow better visualization of the stoma (Cataldo, 2008; Colwell, 2014).
10. The mark should initially be made with a sticker or ink pen that can be removed if this is not the optimal spot.
    - It may be desirable to mark sites on the right and left sides of the abdomen to prepare for a change in the surgical outcome, and number the first choice as #1.
    - Have the patient assume sitting, bending, and lying positions to assess and confirm the best choice.
    - It is important to have the patient confirm they can see the site. However, the critical consideration should be a flat pouching surface.
11. After the optimal site is chosen, clean the desired site with alcohol and allow it to dry. Then proceed with marking the selected site with a surgical marker or pen. If desired, cover the site with a transparent film dressing to preserve the final mark. Ensure that any other stray marks have been removed.

C. Examples of Stoma Site Marking

1. See **Figure 1**: Example of marking a stoma site for a female with a protuberant abdomen, creases, and folds.
2. See **Figure 2**: Example of marking a stoma site for a male with a protuberant abdomen.

Step 1

Look at the profile of the patient. Notice where the abdomen curves back under toward the body. The underside of the abdomen is not visisble to the patient. Avoid this area.

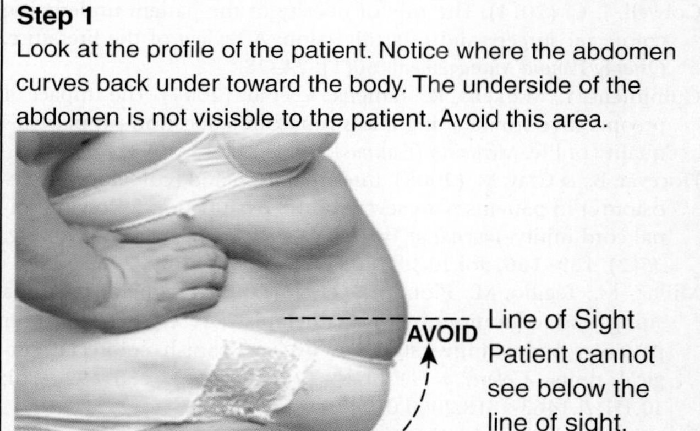

Step 2

While patient is seated, look for skin folds and creases. Note and avoid skin folds and creases.

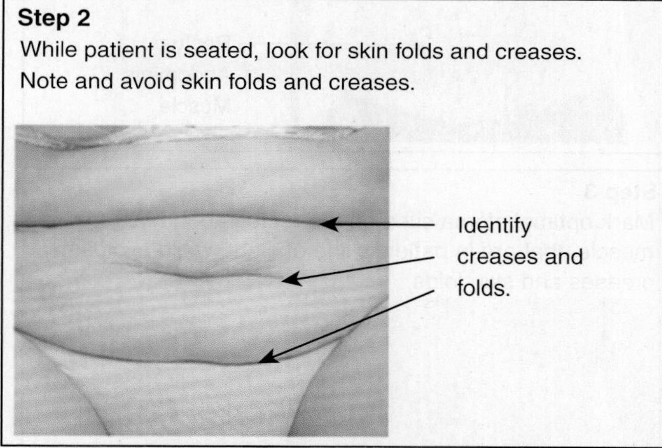

Step 3

Identify and target the rectus abdominis muscle below the ribs.

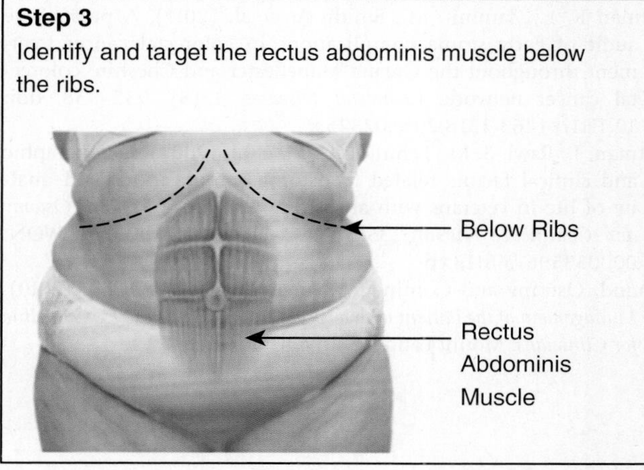

Step 4

Mark optimal stoma sites on the rectus abdominis, that are in patient's line of sight, while avoiding creases and skin folds.

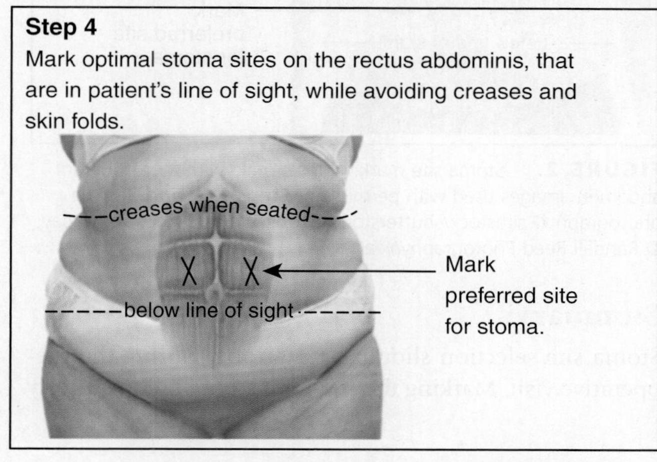

FIGURE 1. Stoma site marking for a female with a protuberant abdomen. Images used with permission: **Step 1**, female photograph © milk122/veer; **Step 2**, female photograph © SeDmi/veer; **Steps 3 and 4**, female photograph © kokhanchikov/shutterstock, and muscle overlay © Randall Reed Photography/veer.

Step 1
Look at the profile of the patient. Notice where the abdomen curves back under toward the body. The underside of the abdomen is not visible to the patient. Avoid this area.

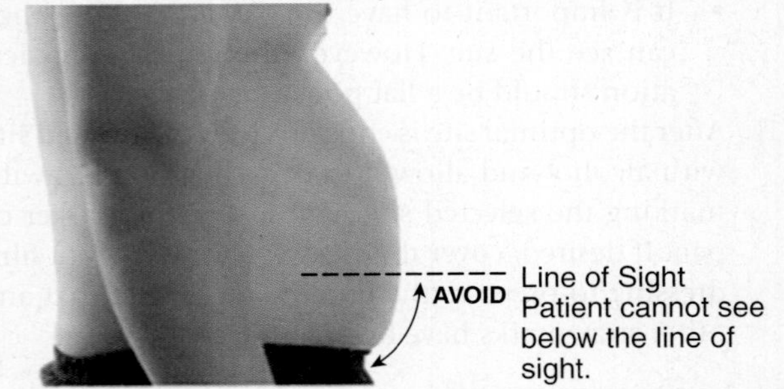

Step 2
Identify and target the rectus abdominis muscle below the ribs.

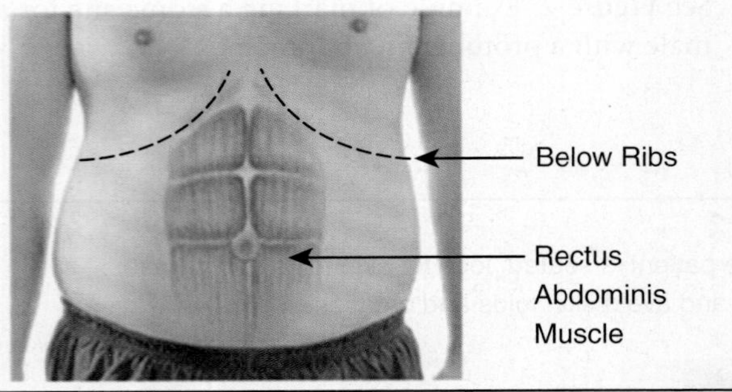

Step 3
Mark optimal stoma sites on the rectus abdominis muscle, that are in patient's line of sight, while avoiding creases and skin folds.

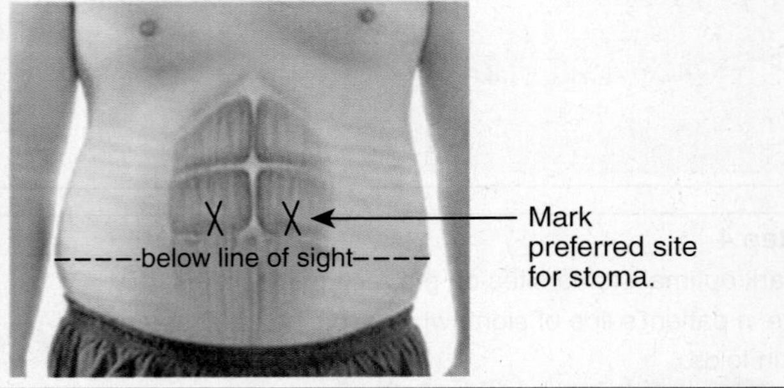

FIGURE 2. Stoma site marking for a male with a protuberant abdomen. Images used with permission: **Steps 1, 2, and 3**, male photograph © sirastock/shutterstock; **Steps 2 and 3**, muscle overlay © Randall Reed Photography/veer.

Summary:

Stoma site selection should be a priority during the preoperative visit. Marking the site for a stoma preoperatively provides an opportunity to select the optimal site, which can help reduce postoperative problems such as leakage, peristomal dermatitis, and difficulty with self-care of the ostomy. Whenever possible, ostomy education and stoma site selection should be performed preoperatively when an ostomy is a possibility.

Acknowledgment

The task force wishes to acknowledge Christina Augustyn, Industrial Designer, Innovation Management Office, Hollister Incorporated, Libertyville, Illinois, for her contribution in the selection and development of the images.

REFERENCES

American Society of Colon and Rectal Surgeons Committee Members & Wound Ostomy Continence Nurse Society Committee Members. (2007). ASCRS and WOCN joint position statement on the value of preoperative stoma marking for patients undergoing fecal ostomy surgery. *Journal of Wound, Ostomy and Continence Nursing, 34*(6), 627–628.

Cataldo, P. A. (2008). Technical tips for stoma creation in the challenging patient. *Clinics in Colon and Rectal Surgery, 21*(1), 17–22. doi:10.1055/s-2008-1055317

Colwell, J. C. (2014). The role of obesity in the patient undergoing colorectal surgery and fecal diversion: A review of the literature. *Ostomy Wound Management, 60*(1), 24–28.

Gulbiniene, J., Markelis, R., Tamelis, A. et al. (2004). The impact of preoperative stoma siting and stoma care education on patient's quality of life. *Medicina (Caunas), 40*(11), 1045–1053.

Hocevar, B., & Gray, M. (2008). Intestinal diversion (colostomy or ileostomy) in patients with severe bowel dysfunction following spinal cord injury. *Journal of Wound, Ostomy and Continence Nursing, 35*(2), 159–166. doi:10.1097/01.WON.0000313638.29623.40

Millan, M., Tegido, M., Biondo, S. et al. (2010). Preoperative stoma siting and education by stomatherapists of colorectal cancer patients: A descriptive study in twelve Spanish colorectal surgical units. *Colorectal Diseases, 12*(7 Online), e88–e92. doi:10.1111/j.1463-1318.2009.01942.x

Park, J. J., Del Pino, A., Orsay, C. P. et al. (1999). Stoma complications: The Cook County Hospital experience. *Diseases of the Colon and Rectum, 42*(12), 1575–1580.

Parmar, K. L., Zammit, M., Smith, A. et al. (2011). A prospective audit of early stoma complications in colorectal cancer treatment throughout the Greater Manchester and Cheshire colorectal cancer network. *Colorectal Diseases, 13*(8), 935–938. doi:10.1111/j.1463-1318.2010.02325.x

Pittman, J., Rawl, S. M., Schmidt, C. M. et al. (2008). Demographic and clinical factors related to ostomy complications and quality of life in veterans with an ostomy. *Journal of Wound, Ostomy and Continence Nursing, 35*(5), 493–503. doi:10.1097/01.WON.0000335961.68113.cb

Wound, Ostomy and Continence Nurses Society (WOCN). (2010). *Management of the Patient with a Fecal Ostomy: Best Practice Guideline for Clinicians*. Mount Laurel, NJ: WOCN Society.

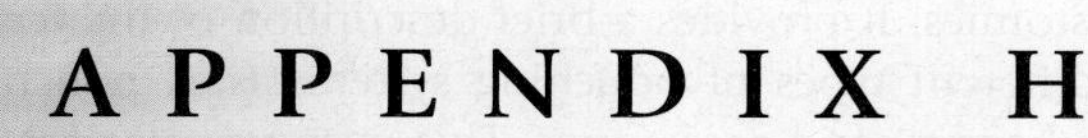

APPENDIX H

UROSTOMY PRODUCTS AND TIPS

Best Practice for Clinicians

Acknowledgments

Urostomy Products and Tips: Best Practice for Clinicians

This document was developed by the WOCN Society's Clinical Practice Ostomy Committee between February 2012 and July 2013.

Mary Mahoney, Chair, MSN, RN, CWON
Wound and Ostomy Nurse
Iowa Health Home Care
Urbandale, IA

Kathryn Baxter, MS, RN, FNP, CWOCN
Nurse Practitioner, Colon & Rectal Surgery
St. Luke's Roosevelt Hospital
New York, NY

Joanna Burgess, BSN, RN, CWOCN
Wound, Ostomy and Continence Nurse
WakeMed Health and Hospitals
Cary, NC

Carole Bauer, MSN, RN, ANP-BC, OCN, CWOCN
Wound, Ostomy and Continence Nurse Practitioner
Karmanos Cancer Center
Detroit, MI

Cathy Downey, BSN, RN, CWOCN
Program Coordinator
University Medical Center
Las Vegas, NV

Janet Mantel, MA, RN-BC, APN, CWOCN
Advanced Practice Nurse
Englewood Hospital & Medical Center
Englewood, NJ

Jacqueline Perkins, MSN, ARNP, FNP, CWOCN
Wound/Ostomy Nurse Practitioner
VA Central Iowa Health Care System
Des Moines, IA

Michelle Rice, MSN, RN, CWOCN
Ostomy Clinical Nurse Specialist
Duke University Hospital
Durham, NC

Ginger Salvadalena, PhD, RN, CWOCN
Senior Clinical Research Scientist
Hollister Incorporated
Libertyville, IL

Vickie Schafer, MSN, RN, CWON, CCRA
Ostomy Care
Associate Director, Medical & Scientific Liaison
Medical Affairs North America
Skillman, NJ

Shirley Sheppard, MSN, RN, CWON
Wound, Ostomy and Skin Care Nurse
University of Illinois Hospital and Health Sciences System
Chicago, IL

Introduction

A urostomy (e.g., ileal conduit or colon conduit) is an opening on the abdomen that is surgically created to drain urine. The urine is typically managed by wearing a pouch on the abdomen. The pouch is drained into the toilet. Additional products are available to accommodate an increased volume of drainage, such as leg bags and bedside drainage collectors.

This document was developed as a resource for nurses and other healthcare providers who care for patients with urostomies. It provides a brief description of the features of different types of pouching systems (i.e., pouch and skin barrier) and accessories. This overview also includes advantages, disadvantages, and special considerations for the use of different types of pouching systems. Additionally, it includes tips for routine pouch care including: emptying the pouch, plus attaching, detaching, and cleaning of drainage collection containers.

Pouching Systems

Product Description	Advantages	Disadvantages	Special Considerations
Disposable Pouching System			
• The pouching system is designed to be discarded upon removal after wearing for a period of time, which varies according to the product or a patient's preference. • Pouches are typically made of lightweight plastic, which is available in transparent or opaque material, and may have a plastic or fabric backing. • Disposable pouches can be part of one-piece or two-piece pouching systems, and are available in various sizes/capacities.	• Odor resistant. • May be worn during a bath, shower, in the swimming pool, and during other water-related activities. • Cleaning is not usually necessary. • Pouches are typically changed every 3 to 7 days.	• Over time, disposables may be more expensive than reusable pouching systems.	
Reusable Pouching System			
• It may be a one-piece or two-piece system, comprised of a pouch with a skin barrier, or a pouch and a silicone ring. The pouch and barrier or rings are made of material that can be cleaned for reuse, and are available in various sizes/capacities. • Pouches are commonly made of vinyl or thick plastic. Rubber products are available. • Barriers are commonly plastic or rubber.	• Can reuse/reapply multiple times with appropriate care and cleansing (length of use dependent on manufacturer). • Some can be used without an adhesive. • Some styles may be removable for daily bathing.	• Can retain odors. • Limited number of manufacturers. • Initial cost may be more expensive than a disposable pouching system. • More time involved with cleaning the system. • Might require use of a belt or adhesive.	
One-piece Pouching System			
• The skin barrier and pouch are fused together during manufacturing.	• Many styles are flexible and conform to abdominal contours. • Low profile. • No chance for leakage between the skin barrier and pouch, which can occur in two-piece systems. • May be less costly than a two-piece system. • May be easier to learn to use than a two-piece system.	• Cannot reposition the pouch once it is applied. • Cannot change the pouch without changing the entire system.	

Pouching Systems (*Continued*)

Product Description	Advantages	Disadvantages	Special Considerations
Two-piece Pouching System with Interlocking Flange			
• The skin barrier and pouch are made separately and have rigid to semi-rigid rings, which allow the user to attach the two parts together.	• Can change the angle of the pouch to accommodate changes in a patient's position. • Can detach the pouch from the barrier to obtain a urine sample from the stoma. • Can detach the pouch from the barrier to change the pouch without removing the barrier.	• Higher profile than a one-piece system. • Less flexible than a one-piece system, and does not mold as well to the body's contours.	• Requires manual dexterity and strength to assure attachment of the pouch to the skin barrier.
Two-piece Pouching System with Flexible Adhesive Flange			
• The skin barrier and pouch are made separately and designed to adhere together without a rigid flange.	• Can change the pouch for disposal or emptying without removing the skin barrier. • Extremely low profile. • Flexibility of a one-piece system. • May be easier to apply for those with poor manual dexterity.	• Limited number of times the pouch can be reattached to the skin barrier (dependent on the manufacturer). • May be difficult to reuse or reattach the pouch if the adhesive area becomes wet. • May be more difficult for visually impaired patients to use.	• Must have good hand-eye coordination to properly attach the pouch's adhesive area to the skin barrier.
Nonadhesive Pouching System			
• The system is reusable and is comprised of a pouch, a nonadherent silicone O-ring seal, and a belt. The silicone O-rings are available in different sizes and thickness. Pouches are available in different sizes and designed with the stoma opening either on the right or left side. • With adequate tension of the belt, the pliable silicone O-ring creates a secure seal between the pouch and abdomen.	• Can reuse/reapply multiple times with appropriate care and cleansing (length of use dependent on manufacturer). • Useful for individuals with allergies to adhesive skin barriers or with other significant skin conditions in the area of the pouch adhesive.	• Nonadhesive systems may not seal well with flush or retracted stomas, or with deep skin folds/creases near the stoma.	• If additional compression is needed to obtain an adequate seal for patients with a softer abdomen or with skin folds, the thicker (taller) O-ring may be needed. • Peristomal skin should be monitored for signs of damage if the belt is worn tightly.

Types of Pouches

Product Description	Advantages	Disadvantages	Special Considerations
• Urostomy pouches have a valve, cap, or plug at the bottom to keep the pouch closed until it is time to empty the pouch or attach to a drainage collection container.	• Urostomy pouches are specifically designed to drain urine. • Most urostomy pouches have an antireflux feature to prevent backflow of urine onto the stoma.		• Requires manual dexterity and strength to manage the various valves or plugs for emptying. • It is not recommended to use fecal pouches for a urostomy.

(*Continued*)

Types of Pouches (*Continued*)

Product Description	Advantages	Disadvantages	Special Considerations
Transparent Pouch			
• Pouch is made of clear lightweight plastic.	• Can see the stoma through the pouch for easy application of the pouching system, if applying as a one-piece. • Can see the stoma while the pouch is in place to monitor the color and appearance of the stoma. • Can see the urine while it is inside the pouch to monitor the color and clarity of the urine.	• May be unpleasant for the patient or their spouse/partner to see the stoma or urine inside the pouch.	
Opaque Pouch			
• Pouch is made of colored lightweight plastic (typically white or beige).	• Cosmetically appealing: cannot see the stoma or urine in the pouch. • More discreet under light-colored clothing.	• May be more difficult to apply when part of a one-piece pouching system because of the inability to visualize the stoma through the pouch for placement.	

Types of Skin Barriers

Product Description	Advantages	Disadvantages	Special Considerations
• Skin Barriers: The part of the pouching system that is attached or placed against the skin. Adhesive skin barriers are made from pectin, karaya gum or synthetic materials. A nonadhesive barrier is made from silicone or rubber. • Skin barriers are available with presized openings (precut) or can be sized to the patient's stoma (cut-to-fit or shapable).			
Flat Skin Barrier			
• A skin barrier that is completely level.	• Useful for flat peristomal skin surfaces.	• May need to add accessories to obtain a better seal if the peristomal skin is not flat.	
Convex Skin Barrier			
• A skin barrier that has a rounded surface on the back (skin contact side) of the barrier. • Convex skin barriers can be rigid or flexible.	• Useful for a peristomal skin surface that is concave or with a flush or retracted stoma.	• May need to add an ostomy belt to enhance the seal. • Barrier may lift from the skin if the convexity is too rigid. • May be more expensive than a flat skin barrier.	
Shapable Skin Barrier			
• The barrier's stomal opening can be molded to fit. • Available flat or convex.	• Allows the opening for the stoma to be stretched and shaped with fingers rather than using scissors to cut the opening.	• May not seal consistently with flush or partially flush stomas. • The barrier can expand over the stomal opening, leading to leakage and decreased wear time.	

Types of Skin Barriers (*Continued*)

Product Description	Advantages	Disadvantages	Special Considerations
Skin Barrier with Stationary Flange			
• A skin barrier used in a two-piece pouching system with a flange that is secured to the barrier. • Available flat or convex.	• Lower profile than a floating flange.	• Snapping the pouch to a barrier that is already attached on the patient's abdomen may cause discomfort.	
Skin Barrier with Floating Flange			
• A skin barrier used in a two-piece pouching system with a flange that raises above the barrier, allowing a person's fingers to fit between the barrier and the flange. • Available flat or convex.	• A floating flange allows the pouch to be snapped onto the skin barrier without adding pressure to the abdomen.	• Higher profile than a nonfloating flange	
Skin Barrier with Locking Flange			
• A skin barrier used in a two-piece pouching system. • Available flat or convex.	• The pouch can be locked into place. • May require less manual dexterity to attach the pouch to the flange. • Allows the pouch to be snapped onto the skin barrier without applying pressure to the abdomen.	• Higher profile than a nonlocking flange.	
Skin Barrier with Plastic Surface			
• A skin barrier used in a two-piece pouching system. The pouch adheres to the skin barrier's plastic surface with an adhesive ring. • Available flat or convex.	• Pouch can be detached and reapplied. • Low profile.	• Pouch does not stick well if the adhesive surface gets wet.	
Skin Barrier with Tape Collar			
• Skin barrier has a wide collar of tape around the outside of the barrier.	• A skin barrier with the tape collar has more flexibility and a lower profile than solid barriers.	• Potential tape sensitivity (rare). • Potential for epidermal skin stripping with tape removal.	

Silicone Ring Barrier

Product Description	Advantages	Disadvantages	Special Considerations
• A nonadhesive ring used instead of a skin barrier. • Rings are available in different sizes to use with disposable or reusable pouches that are available in various shapes/sizes to accommodate individual needs or preferences.	• The nonadhesive quality is helpful for people with allergies, or for people who want to remove the system on a daily basis.	• Need to wear a belt to hold in place. • May not seal well in certain abdominal contours (i.e., deep creases or folds), or with flush or retracted stomas.	

Other Pouch/Skin Barrier Features

Product Description	Advantages	Disadvantages	Special Considerations
Belt Loops			
• A feature on a pouch or skin barrier that allows for use of an elastic belt.	• Belt loops on the skin barrier allow the pouch to be applied and removed without disturbing the belt. • Belt loops on the pouch can add security to the connection between the pouch and skin barrier flange.	• Presence of belt loops may make the skin barrier more rigid. • The belt loops may be uncomfortable against the body and can result in skin damage.	
Adapters (Connectors)			
• Devices specifically designed to allow for attachment of urostomy pouches to other drainage systems.	• Adapters securely connect the pouch outlet to tubing for attachment of a drainage collection container, such as a bedside drainage container or a leg bag. • Adapters are designed to be more secure than pieces of latex or silicone tubing.	• Adapters are not interchangeable between the brands.	• Requires manual dexterity and strength to attach the adapter. • An adapter is replaced when the drainage collection container is replaced.
Drainage Collection Container			
• Consists of a container, which is either a soft plastic container (i.e., leg bag or bedside drainage bag) or a hard plastic jug, and tubing that connects to the regular pouch with an adapter.	• Connecting the pouch to a drainage collection container increases capacity of the pouch and decreases the frequency of emptying. • Extending the frequency of emptying prevents overfilling of the pouch during times when the pouch cannot be emptied, and allows the person the time to rest through the night.	• Patient will need a place to store the collection container when it is not in use. • Tubing may kink.	• To prevent kinking of the tubing, position the tubing down the patient's leg or toward the foot of the bed securing the tubing with leg straps or tape. • Teach the patient to clean the collection container to decrease bacteria and control odor. • There are different methods of cleansing the collection container: follow agency or manufacturer's protocol. • Soft drainage collection containers are replaced twice a month or according to facility or agency policy. • Hard plastic jug containers are replaced every 3 months.

Accessories

Product Description	Advantages	Disadvantages	Special Considerations
Pouch Cover			
• Cloth, envelope-like sleeve to place and wear over the ostomy pouch while it is on the body.	• Cosmetically appealing, cannot see the stoma or urine inside the pouch. • Easily applied by slipping over pouch while it is on the body. • Provides a comfortable surface against the skin to help prevent perspiration, chafing or allergies. • May help reduce noise from a vinyl or plastic pouch. • May be integrated within available disposable pouches.	• Added expense if fabric material is already covering the backing (skin side) of a pouch. • If integrated into the pouch, may take time to dry after bathing, showering or swimming.	
Skin Sealant			
• Plasticizing agent made of ingredients such as silicone or a copolymer. • Contains variable amounts of isopropyl alcohol. • Available as a wipe, spray, gel, liquid, or roll-on.	• Provides a thin protective film to the surface of the skin. • Helps to prevent stripping of the epidermis during adhesive removal, and some also act as a moisture barrier.	• Sealants may not be recommended under some skin barriers because the protective film may reduce the adherence of the skin barrier. • Many sealants contain alcohol that causes pain when applied to irritated skin, and in such situations, an alcohol-free product is needed.	• If applying stoma powder to skin irritation, a skin sealant applied over the powder and dried, provides a dry, smooth surface for adherence of the skin barrier. • May be used to seal antifungal powder when needed to treat peristomal candidiasis.
Skin Adhesive			
• Adhesive products made of silicone or latex.	• Can be used to strengthen the adhesion of an adhesive pouching system, or to provide adhesion for a reusable (nonadhesive) system.	• May cause pain and further irritation to already denuded skin. Recommend "crusting technique" prior to application to denuded skin. • May be flammable.	• Teach the patient to allow the adhesive to dry prior to application of the pouch to prevent chemical irritation.
Adhesive Remover			
• Available as a wipe, spray or liquid.	• Aids in the removal of tape, skin adhesives, and other residue on the skin. • May be helpful to the patient with sensitive skin to reduce trauma from removal of the pouching system.	• Cleaning the skin with mild soap and water is typically required to remove any of the solvent's residue before application of the next pouching system to prevent chemical dermatitis or nonadherence of the pouching system.	• A silicone-based, alcohol free adhesive remover may not require additional cleansing.

(*Continued*)

Accessories (*Continued*)

Product Description	Advantages	Disadvantages	Special Considerations
Paste			
• Pectin-based or karaya products.	• Can be used to fill in uneven areas or as caulking around the inner edge of the skin barrier to prevent stomal drainage getting beneath the skin barrier. • Fills in small creases and depressions and evens out skin/abdominal contours under a skin barrier to increase the fit and adherence of the skin barrier. • Used appropriately, will offer a quick seal for the pouching system until the skin barrier adhesive is pressed into place. • Not commonly used for patients with a urostomy, but some patients find it helpful.	• Most pastes contain some alcohol and may sting when applied to irritated peristomal skin. • Paste is not substantial enough to fill in large creases, as it will wash out. • Patients often think the paste is an "adhesive" and use it inappropriately (i.e., spread the paste like a glue over a large surface area on the skin or skin barrier). • Patients often use excessive amounts of paste, resulting in poor adherence of the pouch and leakage. • Karaya products melt easily when exposed to urine.	• Requires manual dexterity to squeeze paste from the tube and for application of paste to the peristomal skin or skin barrier.
Skin Barrier Rings			
• Pectin or sodium carboxymethylcellulose based product that is soft and moldable formed by the manufacturer into a flat or convex ring. • Available in different sizes and flat or convex.	• Prevent leakage of stomal drainage under the skin barrier. • Increase the seal of skin barriers by molding into contours of the abdominal surface. • May be used as an alternative, or in addition, to paste. • Can be used in their original shape and form, or stretched and molded to create custom shapes to fill in uneven areas. • Can be cut, bent, or stacked together to improve the fit of the skin barrier. • May prolong a skin barrier's wear time. • Leave less residue than paste on the skin after removal. • Conform to irregular skin folds. • Alcohol free and may be used on irritated skin.	• Added cost. • Added step in the application technique.	• Requires manual dexterity for application to the peristomal skin or skin barrier.
Skin Barrier Strip Paste			
• Pectin-based product in soft, moldable, flexible strips.	• Prevents leakage of urine under the skin barrier. • Increases the seal of a skin barrier by molding into contours of the abdominal surface. • May be used as an alternative to paste. • Can be used in the original shape and form, or stretched and molded to create custom shapes to fill in uneven areas.	• Added cost, and may not be covered by insurance. • Added step in the application process.	• Requires manual dexterity for application to the peristomal skin or skin barrier.

Accessories (*Continued*)

Product Description	Advantages	Disadvantages	Special Considerations
Skin Barrier Strip Paste (*Continued*)			
	• Can be cut, bent, or stacked together to improve the fit of the skin barrier. • May extend skin barrier wear time. • Leaves less residue than paste on the skin after removal. • Conforms to irregular skin folds. • Alcohol free and may be used on irritated skin.		
Stoma Powder			
• Pectin or karaya-based powder used to protect peristomal skin and areas of mucocutaneous separation from exposure to stomal discharge.	• Aids in healing of open, irritated peristomal skin. • Absorbs moisture or exudate from the peristomal skin prior to placing a skin barrier for added protection and enhanced adherence of the skin barrier.	• Karaya powder may sting when applied to irritated peristomal skin. • If applied improperly (i.e., excessive amounts), powder may prevent adhesion of the skin barrier.	• Powder may be sealed to the skin by applying a layer of skin sealant over the powder and allowing it to dry, before applying the pouching system, to provide a smooth, dry surface for adherence of the pouching system.
Elastic Barrier Strip			
• Elastic material designed to be placed around the edges of the ostomy skin barrier to hold it securely in place.	• Strips are a skin-friendly alternative to tape. • Use supports longer wear time by decreasing the roll-up on the edges of the barrier. • Due to the elasticity, strips move with the body to hold the skin barrier firmly in place during movement.	• Added cost may not be covered by insurance.	• Store strips in a cool, dry location (away from direct sunlight). • Apply strips while they are at room temperature.
Ostomy Belt			
• Elastic belt with hooks to fasten to the belt loops on the pouch or skin barrier to hold the pouching system firmly in place. • Belts are available in varying sizes and widths, and are adjustable. Most belts are latex free.	• Adds stability and security to the ostomy pouching system. • Often used with convex skin barriers for added security. • Belts are washable and reusable.	• Ostomy belts may be uncomfortable for some patients. • Added cost, and may not be covered by insurance.	• Requires manual dexterity to attach the belt. • Attaching the belt so it lies evenly on the abdomen and is level with the belt loops helps prevent the belt from riding up or down on the abdomen and possibly dislodging the pouching system (American Cancer Society, 2011; American College of Surgeons, n.d.a). • It is important that the tightness of the belt be adjusted so that it does not leave deep grooves or cuts in the skin (American Cancer Society, 2011; American College of Surgeons, n.d.a).

(*Continued*)

Accessories (*Continued*)

Product Description	Advantages	Disadvantages	Special Considerations
Ostomy Belt (*Continued*)			
			• Belt will get wet during showering, bathing, and swimming, which may affect the fit/security of the belt. • It is important for individuals with latex allergies to verify that their chosen belts are latex free.
Ostomy Support Belt			
• Wide, binder-type, belts are designed to support the abdominal muscles, peristomal hernias, or provide pouch support. • Support belts are available in various sizes, widths, and fabrics. Most support belts are latex free. • The belts can be customized for the location and size of the opening for the pouch.	• Support belts can increase the comfort and security of the pouching system to increase wear time. • Can help manage peristomal hernias, or support pendulous, bulging abdomens. • Belts are washable and reusable.	• Support belts may be uncomfortable for some patients. • Added cost, and may not be covered by insurance. • If not fitted correctly, the support belt may dislodge the pouching system.	• Requires manual dexterity to apply the belt. • Manufacturer's directions for measuring and selection of the size and type of support belt must be carefully followed. • For best results with hernias, apply and fasten the support belt in a flat-lying position. • Prolapsed stomas are not common in patients with a urostomy, but prolapse overbelt attachments are available to help manage prolapsed stomas. • It is important for individuals with latex allergies to verify that their chosen support belts are latex free.

Tips for Emptying the Pouch

Product Description	Advantages	Disadvantages	Special Considerations
• Teach the patient to empty the pouch when it is one-third to one-half full. • Teach the following steps for emptying the pouch (American Cancer Society, 2011; American College of Surgeons, n.d.b): 1. Sit on toilet with the pouch between the legs or stand in front of/or alongside the toilet. 2. Place a layer of toilet paper in the toilet to reduce splashing. 3. Point the end of the pouch into the toilet and open the closure on the spout at the end of the pouch to drain the urine. 4. Wipe the end of the pouch/spout with toilet paper. 5. Close the spout on the pouch. 6. Wash hands.	• Regular emptying of the pouch: • Minimizes exposure of the stoma to urine in the pouch. • Prevents excess weight and volume in the pouch to prevent dislodging the skin barrier or pouch. • Prevents bulging of the pouch, to maintain a low profile.		• Requires mobility and manual dexterity. • Requires adaptation of the emptying technique for patients with visual, physical, and other mobility or functional limitations (e.g., bedbound, wheelchair bound, hemiplegia, paraplegia, blindness, severe arthritis in hands).

Tips for Attaching the Pouch to a Drainage Collection Container (Drainage Collector)

Product Description	Advantages	Disadvantages	Special Considerations
• Teach the patient to use the correct adapter for the brand of pouch they are using when connecting to a drainage collector. • Steps in connecting to a drainage collector (American Cancer Society, 2011; American College of Surgeons, n.d.a; United Ostomy Associations of America, Inc., n.d.): 1. Leave a small amount of urine in the pouch prior to attaching the drainage collector to prevent creating a vacuum in the system. 2. Wash hands. 3. Attach the adapter to the tubing or spout on the drainage collector. 4. Connect the end of the pouch to the adapter on the drainage collector. 5. Open the closure on the pouch's drainage spout to allow the urine to flow. 6. Position the drainage collector below the level of the urostomy pouch.	• A drainage collector adds capacity to the ostomy pouch.	• Needs to be rinsed and kept clean/dry. • Takes extra time to care for the drainage collection container. • Additional cost, and may not be covered by insurance.	• Requires manual dexterity to attach.

Tips for Detaching and Cleaning a Drainage Collection Container (Drainage Collector)

Product Description	Advantages	Disadvantages	Special Considerations
• Teach the patient how to detach and clean the drainage collector. • Steps in detaching the drainage collector (American College of Surgeons, n.d.a): 1. Wash hands. 2. Close the spout of the urostomy pouch to prevent leakage. 3. Detach the drainage collector along with the adapter from the urostomy pouch. 4. Empty the urine from the drainage collector and rinse with cool water. 5. Clean the drainage collector (tubing and adapter) daily or every other day with a vinegar and water solution (1 part white vinegar and 3 parts water); or according to agency or manufacturer's protocol (American Cancer Society, 2011; Einstein Healthcare Network, n.d.; United Ostomy Associations of America, Inc., n.d.).	• Regular rinsing and cleansing reduces odor of the drainage collector.		• Requires manual dexterity to detach and clean the drainage collector. • Requires a space to hang the collector to dry when it is not in use.

(Continued)

Tips for Detaching and Cleaning a Drainage Collection Container (Drainage Collector) (*Continued*)

Product Description	Advantages	Disadvantages	Special Considerations
6. Instill the vinegar and water solution through the tubing or spout into the container and let it sit for an hour; then empty and rinse with cool water (Einstein Healthcare Network, n.d.). 7. Allow the drainage collector to air dry with the closure open.			

REFERENCES

American Cancer Society. (2011). *Urostomy: A guide*. Retrieved July 2013, from http://www.cancer.org/acs/groups/cid/documents/webcontent/002931-pdf.pdf

American College of Surgeons. (n.d.a). *Empty the pouch SKILL*. Retrieved July 2013, from http://www.facs.org/patienteducation/skills/empty-pouch.pdf

American College of Surgeons. (n.d.b). *What is a urostomy?* Retrieved July 2013, from http://www.facs.org/patienteducation/skills/your-urostomy.pdf

Einstein Healthcare Network. (n.d.). *Urostomy: Using a night drainage system*. Retrieved July 2013, from http://www.einstein.edu/einsteinhealthtopic/?articleId=89997&articleTypeId=3&healthTopicid=-I&healthTopicName=HealthSheets

United Ostomy Associations of America, Inc. (n.d.). *Urostomy guide*. Retrieved July 2013, from http://www.ostomy.org/ostomy_info/pubs/UrostomyGuide.pdf

Acknowledgment about Content Validation

This document was reviewed in the consensus-building process of the Wound, Ostomy and Continence Nurses Society known as Content Validation, which is managed by the Center for Clinical Investigation.

APPENDIX I

CARE OF FEEDING TUBES

Jane Fellows, MSN, RN, CWOCN

Introduction

There are many reasons why people need feeding tubes. Some need feeding tubes for a short while and others need them for a lifetime. The choice to place a feeding tube can be difficult.

This document is designed to help you make the choice that is best for you and your family. These pages show the proper care of a feeding tube. Please note that while this document was put together as a general guide for those caring for a feeding tube, there may be information in it that does not apply to you or may be slightly different than what your health care provider has told you. Please use this tool as a reference and always consult your primary provider.

My Feeding Tube

Date of procedure: ______________________

Health care provider performing the procedure: ______________________

Procedure: ______________________

Contact information: ______________________

Current feeding tube type:

☐ Gastrostomy tube or G-tube or PEG tube

Type: ______________________

☐ Gastrojejunostomy tube or G-J tube

Type: ______________________

☐ Jejunostomy tube or J tube

Type: ______________________

For balloon-retained feeding tubes:

Amount of water in balloon: _____mL

Some tubes have to be removed by the doctor in the operating room. Some tubes can be removed in a clinic setting.

☐ Your tube: Can be removed in a clinic setting

☐ Must be removed in the operating room

Health care provider managing my tube feeds: ______________________

Contact information: ______________________

My Primary Physician: ______________________

Contact information: ______________________

Home Health Agency: ______________________

Contact information: ______________________

Home Care Supplies: ______________________

Contact information: ______________________

Why do I need a feeding tube?

Your body needs food and drink to heal, have energy, and help you feel better. Since you have trouble swallowing or cannot eat enough calories, giving you food and liquids through the tube in your stomach or intestines helps your body to get the food and water it needs.

What is a feeding tube?

A *feeding tube* is a tube used to provide food and water directly into your stomach or intestines. The tube is placed by a doctor. An opening is made in your skin and the tube is put through this opening into your stomach or intestines.

What are the different types of feeding tubes?

Gastrostomy tube

A gastrostomy tube is a tube which goes through your skin and abdominal wall into your stomach. It is also called "G-tube" or "PEG tube".

PEG stands for:

P = percutaneous (Going through the skin)

E = endoscopic (Looking into your body with a camera and light)

G = gastrostomy (An opening put in your stomach by a doctor)

The tube may be inserted in the endoscopy department or in the operating room.

The gastrostomy tube can be used to put liquid food into the stomach. It can also be used to pull out air and liquid if the stomach isn't working properly and needs to be emptied of extra pressure. Liquid or crushed medications can also be given through the tube.

Gastrojejunostomy tube

This tube is often called a "GJ-tube." The "J" stands for jejunum, which is a part of the small intestine. A GJ tube is actually made of two different tubes that are combined together—one that leads from the outside of your body into the stomach (a G-tube), and an extension that goes into your intestines. A GJ tube has two openings or "ports." One goes into the stomach (G-port) and one goes into the intestine (J-port). The G-port can be used just like a G-tube, as described above. The J-port can only be used for liquid nutrition. If you need to use the J-tube for medications, then the medications or crushed pills should be the same consistency as formula. Typically, medications are not given through the J-tube, however there may be times when this is the only option for you. Prior to using the J-tube for medication, you should talk with your provider. Crushed pills can clog the tube.

Jejunostomy tube

This tube is also called a "J-tube." This tube goes through the skin directly into the intestine (the jejunum). A J-tube is very small and can only be used for liquid nutrition. Crushed pills should NOT be put into the J-tube as they could clog the tube. Suction should never be applied to the J-tube.

What are the parts of a feeding tube?

Here are the parts of your tube you will need to know so you can use and care for your tube:

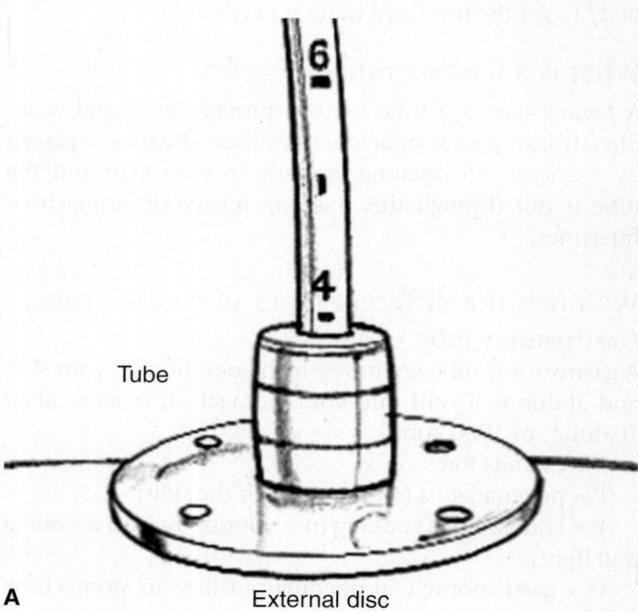

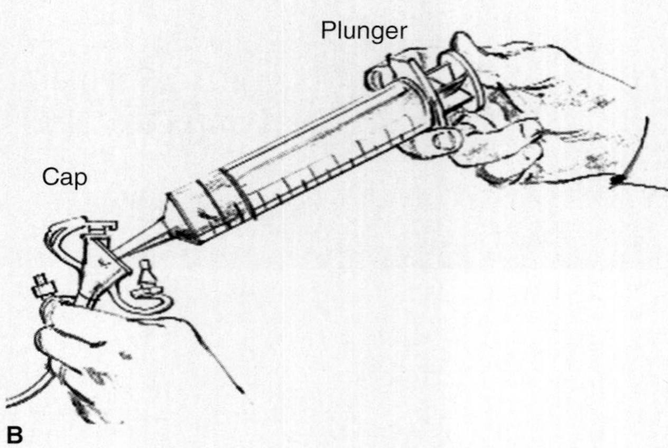

Cap—the cover to the opening of the tube where the feeding goes in

Tube—plastic or silicone tubing that may have numbers on it

External disc—Also called an 'external bumper' or 'bolster.' This is a plastic disc outside of your skin which helps keep the tube secure

G-tubes and GJ-tubes often have an internal 'bumper' or a balloon attached to the tube on the inside of the stomach to help hold it in place.

T-fasteners—In some cases, your doctor will use these to help perform the surgery. You may see one or more little 'buttons' made of hard plastic or cotton, which are stitched to your skin.

Syringe—a 60 mL (2 ounces) tube with a plunger. It is used:

- As a funnel for feedings
- To flush the tube with water
- To give yourself liquid or crushed medicines

Low-profile button—is a feeding tube that sits closer to the skin and attachments are needed for use

Extension sets—are the tubes used with low-profile buttons for feeding and venting

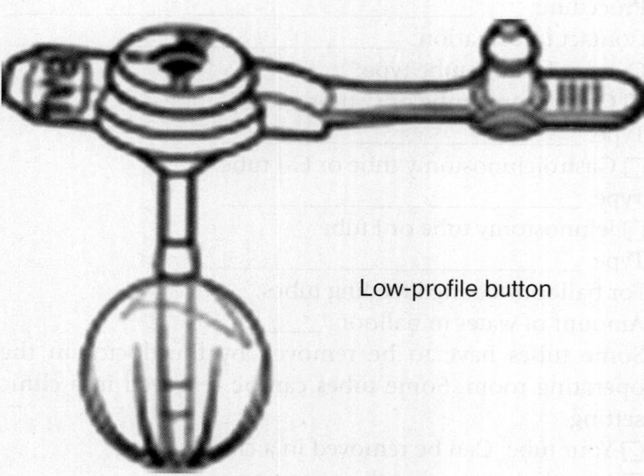

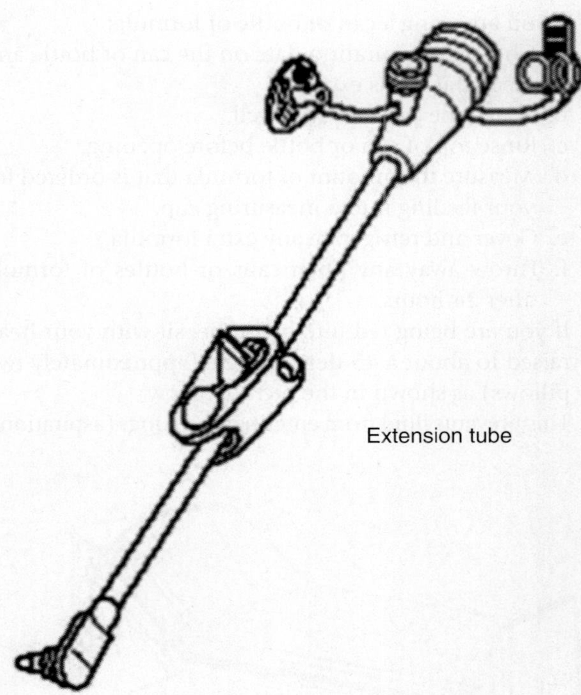

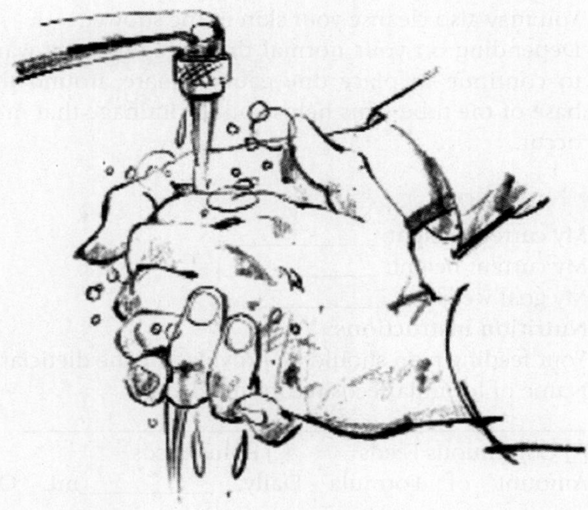

How does the feeding tube stay in?

The type of tube determines how the tube is secured. There may be a balloon on the end of the tube in your stomach that will keep it from coming out. Sometimes, the feeding tube is stitched to your skin. Your provider will explain how and when those sutures will be removed.

How do I protect the tube?

- Keep the tube inside your waist band or attached to your clothes.
- Do not pull on the tube.
- Be gentle with it.
- Do not let anyone else pull out the tube.

When should I return to the doctor?

Depending on the type of tube put in, you may need to come to the doctor's clinic. If so, the appointment will be made before you leave the hospital. It is often one week after your surgery if you have stitches that need to be removed. You may feel discomfort when the stitches are removed. Removing stitches is quick and your skin will feel better without them.

Next Appointment: ____________________

What are signs that the area around the tube may be infected?

- increasing redness of the skin
- thick yellow or green drainage around the tube that has an odor different from normal yellow-green mucus drainage
- increasing tenderness or soreness
- fever

Call your health care provider's office if you have these signs of infection.

Always wash your hands very well with soap and warm water before you touch the tube. Keep the supplies that you use to care for your tube clean. Wash your hands after you finish caring for your tube or feeding yourself.

How do I take care of my skin around the tube?

For the first few weeks you may notice a small amount of bloody or pale yellow drainage around the tube site. The fluid may be stomach juices. This is normal and should not alarm you.

- Clean around the base of the tube two times every day. Use a Q tip or regular wash cloth with soap and water to wash around the site. Cleaning around the feeding tube site will help remove any dried crust and fluid. It will also keep your skin clean while healing.
- If needed after each cleaning, put one small gauze square around the base of the tube. Cut a T-shape in the middle of the gauze. This helps the gauze fit around the base of the tube.

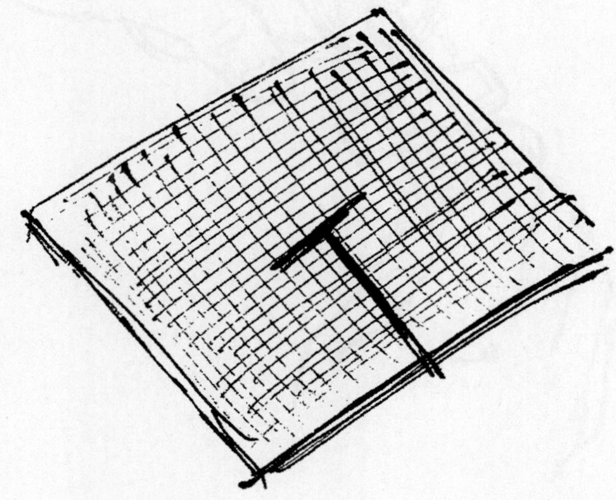

- You may also cleanse your skin in the shower.
- Depending on your normal drainage you may want to continue to place one gauze square around the base of the tube. This helps collect drainage that may occur.

My Nutrition

My current weight: ____________
My current height: ____________
My goal weight: ____________
Nutrition instructions:
Your feeding plan should be provided by the dietician.
Name of formula/feeds recommended:
____

☐ Continuous Feeds ☐ Bolus Feeds
Amount of Formula Daily: __________mL OR ______________ cans
Amount of Water flushes: ______________________mL
Amount of Additional Water: ___________________mL
Special Instructions: ______________________________
____
____

How do I do a bolus feeding through the tube?

1. Take the formula from the refrigerator. Allow it to come to room temperature. This is less likely to cause stomach upset.
2. Always wash your hands well before you touch the tube or can.
3. Pour 30 mL (1 ounce) of lukewarm water into a clean measuring cup.

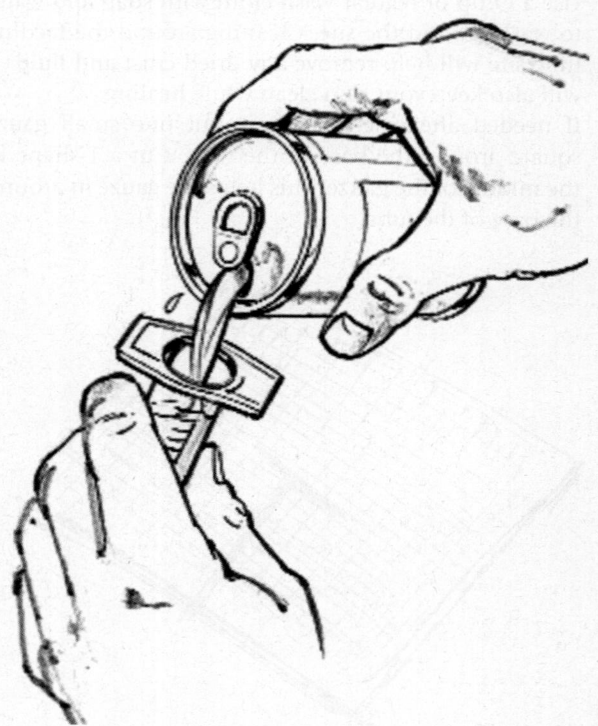

4. If you are using a can or bottle of formula:
   a. Check the expiration date on the can or bottle and discard if it has expired.
   b. Shake the can or bottle well.
   c. Rinse top of can or bottle before opening.
   d. Measure the amount of formula that is ordered for your feeding into a measuring cup.
   e. Cover and refrigerate any extra formula.
   f. Throw away any open cans or bottles of formula after 24 hours.
5. If you are being fed into a G-tube, sit with your head raised to about a 45-degree angle (approximately two pillows) as shown in the picture below.
6. This prevents fluid from entering your lungs (aspiration).

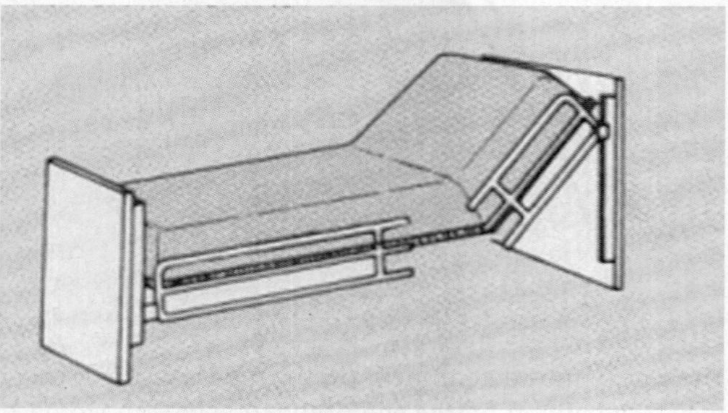

7. Clamp feeding tube. This prevents air from entering your stomach. Air causes too much fullness. It also prevents the fluid in your stomach from leaving your stomach.
8. Remove the plunger from the syringe. You do not need the plunger to feed yourself.
9. Put the tip of the syringe into tube.
10. Fill the syringe with the water. Unclamp the tube and allow the water to flow in by gravity. The flow goes more slowly if you lower the syringe. It goes more quickly if you raise the syringe.
11. Pour the formula into syringe when most of the water has gone in the stomach. This prevents air from entering your stomach.
12. After taking the right amount of formula, flush tubing with another 30 mL (1 ounce) of water. This helps prevent the feeding tube from clogging.
13. Remove the syringe and replace the plug in the end of the tube.
14. Wash your syringe and measuring cups with dish soap and warm water. Leave them on a clean towel to dry.
15. Keep your head up for 60 minutes after feeding is completed.

Note:

- Do not put hot or cold liquids through the feeding tube. Hot liquids may hurt the stomach lining. Cold liquids tend to upset the stomach.
- Do not add medicine to the formula unless you have discussed this with your health care provider.

How do I get water?

Water is important in taking care of yourself and your tube. You may put water through the feeding tube. The nutritionist will tell you how much water you need each day. Besides the water you use to flush the tube, this extra water prevents you from being:

- Too dry (dehydrated) in your mouth and skin and bowels
- Too thirsty (dry mouth)
- Constipated or irregular with your bowel movement.

Flushing water through your tube before and after each feeding keeps it clean and open. Put 30 mL of lukewarm water through the tube **before and after** every use each day.

How do I take my medicines?

Some medicines can be put through your feeding tube. *Check with your doctor* and pharmacist before putting any medicines through your tube. Your pharmacist can also talk to you about what types of medicines can be crushed or come in liquid form. Use liquid medicines when possible; crush pills well and mix with lukewarm water.

How do I check for residuals?

Your doctor may ask you to "check residuals." This is to measure how much fluid is still in your stomach from the last feeding. You check for residuals before giving yourself a feeding. Checking residuals assures that the formula is being emptied by the stomach.

If you have recently taken any food by mouth, wait approximately 60 minutes before checking residuals.

1. Unclamp and open your feeding tube.
2. Attach the syringe with the plunger.

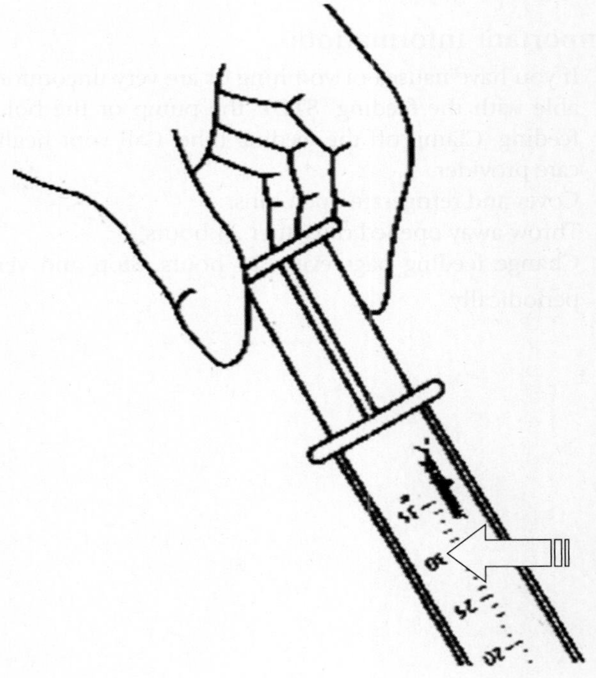

3. Slowly pull back on the plunger until it is harder to pull. The stomach contents will enter the syringe. If the stomach is empty, there may be no formula that comes back.
4. If the stomach is not empty, you may draw up some stomach juices. You may also draw up some formula from an earlier feeding. This is normal.
5. Check the numbers on the side of the syringe to determine the amount of residual. (If you withdraw more than the 60 mL of residual, you may need to empty this into a measuring cup until all of the residual is obtained and measured).
6. **Inject the residuals back into the stomach**. It is very important to return the gastric residuals back into the stomach. The gastric juices contain chemicals (enzymes and electrolytes) that your body needs to digest the feedings.
7. If the stomach residual is greater than 150 mL, wait 30 to 60 minutes, and check again before administering more formula. If you continually draw up high residuals (more than 150 mL), call your health care provider.

REMEMBER- When the tube is not in use:

Curl it up and tuck it into your clothing or clip it to your clothing

What are some problems I might have with tube feedings?

Clogged Tubes

- To prevent a clogged tube, always flush with at least 30 mL (1 ounce) of warm water after a feeding.
- Do not put whole pills or capsules into the tube. Crush all medicines until they are powder and dissolve in water. Ask your home care nurse or your health care provider for hints.
- If the tube gets clogged, try to loosen it by putting 30 mL of warm water in the tube. Then pull back and forth on the plunger.
- For tough clogs, call the doctor's office for advice.

Aspiration

Aspiration happens when food or fluids enter the lungs. Signs of aspiration include: coughing, gagging, change in skin color, increased temperature, rapid pulse, and noisy breathing. If this occurs: STOP the feeding and notify the doctor's office. To prevent aspiration:

- Sit or lie upright at a 30- to 45-degree angle (two pillows) during the feedings.
- Remain in this position for one hour after feedings.
- Administer feedings slowly.

Feeling sick

Nausea or bloating happens when formula:

- is given too fast
- is too concentrated
- is too cold

To prevent feeling sick:

- Feed slowly over 20 minutes.
- Relieve gas or bloating by allowing air out through the tube. Lie flat. Carefully open the cap and let the gas out. Massaging the belly will help get the air to the tube so that it can come out. Stomach contents may come out too.
- If nausea, bloating, or vomiting happens often with feedings, contact the doctor.

Leaking Tube

The most common complication of a feeding tube is leakage of stomach or intestinal contents around the tube. This is usually caused by a failure to secure the tube to prevent movement. A small amount of clear or pale yellow drainage around the tube can be normal.

You may have larger amounts of leakage if:

- The surrounding skin and tissues are not healing well
- The tube is in the wrong position
- The intestines are blocked
- The tube is not secured

Always make sure your tube is secured so it will not move side to side or in and out. Some tubes that do not have an external disc can be secured with a commercial tube stabilization device available from a medical supply company.

If your tube is leaking, you will need to protect your skin. Apply a layer of "diaper cream" containing zinc oxide before placing the gauze dressing. Wipe the drainage off the top of the cream and change the dressing whenever it is wet.

Hyperplasia

Hyperplasia is an overgrowth of red, raw tissue where the tube exits the skin. It can cause pain or bleeding. This tissue needs to be treated and can be treated with silver nitrate or a steroid cream. Ask your home health nurse or health care provider to help you with this.

Diarrhea

If you have loose stools for more than 3 days after beginning the tube feedings, contact your doctor.

- Diarrhea is common when starting new formula.
- It may also be a side effect of some medicines.

Constipation

Constipation happens when:

- physical activity is limited
- you take in too little water
- you take certain medications

Ask for advice from your home health nurse or health care provider. You may need to take a laxative or stool softener. More fiber in your feeding may also be needed.

How can I do a feeding using a pump?

Some people cannot tolerate bolus feedings that go in relatively fast. They will need a pump which will provide the feeding over several hours or continuously. This will allow a slower controlled rate. Below are the instructions for pump feeding. You will be trained to use your particular pump by the home health nurse or medical supply company. The instructions vary by manufacturer of the pumps.

- Gather your supplies and equipment.
- Wash your hands.
- Check the expiration date of the formula.
- Clean the top of the can.
- Vent or open your G-tube to allow air to come out (typically 1 to 2 minutes).
- Clamp the feeding bag.
- Pour formula into the feeding bag.
- Prime the feeding set—unclamp and allow the feeding to flow all the way to the end of the set. Then clamp.
- Place tubing into pump. Set pump rate.
- Attach the tubing to your tube.
- Unclamp the feeding set. Start the machine.
- When feeding is finished, flush tubing with water. Then disconnect.
- Some people require venting after feeding to help reduce excess air in belly.

Important Information:

- If you have nausea or vomiting or are very uncomfortable with the feeding, **STOP** the pump or the bolus feeding. Clamp off the feeding tube. Call your health care provider.
- Cover and refrigerate open cans.
- Throw away opened cans after 24 hours.
- Change feeding bags every 24 hours. Stop and vent periodically.

Notes

Feeding Tube Feeding Routine

Time	Flush (mL) Before	Formula (cans)	Mechanical Pump Rate (mL per hour)	Flush (mL) After

Feeding Tube Medicine Routine

Time	Flush (mL) Before	Medicine (Crushed)	Medicine (Liquid)	Flush (mL) After

GLOSSARY

Abdominal perineal resection (APR) a surgical procedure that includes the resection of the sigmoid colon, rectum, and anus; closure of perineum; and creation of end colostomy.

Anorectal malformation (ARM) a spectrum of congenital defects potentially occurring in the bowel and urinary and reproductive systems.

Anti–tumor necrosis factor (anti-TNF) antibodies a drug that suppresses response to tumor necrosis factor (TNF), which is part of the inflammatory response.

Body image a subjective picture of one's own physical appearance, usually based upon self-observation and by gauging the reactions of others.

Carcinoid tumors a type of neuroendocrine tumor originating from the crypts of Lieberkuhn.

Chromoendoscopy use of dye instilled into the GI tract via endoscopy to identify tissue type or pathology.

Colonic inertia a motility disorder, in which muscles or nerves in the colon fail to operate normally, preventing fecal matter from progressing normally through the colon.

Colostomy a surgically created opening into any section of the colon.

Convex skin barrier the interface between the skin and pouch of the pouching system that has curvature varying between a minimal amount of curvature (light convexity) to a maximum amount of curve (deep convexity).

Crohn's disease an inflammatory bowel disease in which the inflammation may occur anywhere within the GI tract, from the mouth to the anus, and may be continuous or patchy. The most commonly affected area is the terminal ileum, and many of those patients have cecal and/or right colonic involvement.

Diverticular disease pockets that develop in the colon wall, usually in the sigmoid or left colon, but may involve the entire colon. Diverticulosis describes the presence of these pockets. Diverticulitis describes inflammation or complications of these pockets.

Diverting fecal stoma a diversion that allows the fecal stream to be diverted from the diseased or injured portion of bowel.

Elastic skin barrier strip a piece of hydrocolloid with elastic used to secure the outer seal of the pouching system.

End stoma a stoma that is created by dividing the intestine, bringing the proximal end of the intestine through the abdominal wall, and maturing the stoma once outside of the abdominal wall to attach to the skin.

Extraintestinal manifestations inflammatory-type involvement of areas outside of the gastrointestinal tract found in some patients with ulcerative colitis or Crohn's disease.

Familial adenomatous polyposis (FAP) a condition caused by mutations in the oncogene *APC* and inherited in an autosomal dominant pattern with a 100% risk of developing colon cancer by age 40 years. Individuals with FAP develop hundreds to thousands of adenomatous polyps in the colon and in the duodenum and stomach.

Finney stricturoplasty a type of stricturoplasty (see below) that is performed for longer strictures up to 15 cm.

Fistula an abnormal connection between two epithelium-lined surfaces (i.e., two hollow organs or hollow organ and skin).

Folliculitis hair follicle inflammation, develops when there is inflammation due to injury or infection of skin; the mechanism of injury may be multidirectional shaving or pulling of hair when the adhesive skin barrier is removed.

Gardner's syndrome an inherited polyposis syndrome that, in addition to colonic polyposis, is associated with osteomas, epidermoid cysts, soft tissue tumors, fibromas, and/or desmoid tumors. Skin manifestations of Gardner's syndrome include epidermoid cysts, trichilemmal hybrid, or pilomatricomas developing on the face, scalp, or limbs of patients.

Hamartomas noncancerous (benign) masses of normal tissue that build up in the intestines or other places. These masses are called polyps if they develop inside a body structure, such as the intestines.

Hartmann's pouch consists of the anus and rectum that remain in place with the top of the rectum sewn closed as a defunctionalized segment.

Heineke-Mikulicz stricturoplasty a type of stricturoplasty (see below) that is performed for short strictures up to 10 cm.

Hereditary mixed polyposis syndrome a hereditary condition that is associated with an increased risk of developing polyps in the digestive tract.

Hirschsprung's disease (HD) the absence of intraneural ganglion cells and hypertrophic nerves of the bowel, which have created a functional partial or full obstruction. With the lack of ganglion cells, peristalsis does not occur and the stool cannot be pushed through the intestines properly and leads to a blockage.

HNPCC (Lynch syndrome) a type of colorectal cancer inherited by mutations in one of several mismatch repair genes (*MLH1*, *MSH2*, *MSH6*, and *PMS2*) leading to microsatellite instability. It is estimated that HNPCC accounts for 5% of colorectal cancers with a lifetime risk of developing CRC at a rate of 70% to 90%.

Ileal conduit a type of urinary diversion whereby ureters are implanted into a section of dissected ileum that is sutured closed on one end, while the other end is brought through the abdominal wall to create a stoma.

Ileal pouch anal anastomosis (IPAA) the removal of the entire colon and rectum while preserving the anal sphincter and the creation of an ileal pouch to serve as an internal pelvic reservoir of intestinal contents.

Ileocecectomy the removal of the terminal ileum and the cecum.

Ileostomy an opening into the last portion of the small intestine, the ileum.

Indiana pouch a continent catheterizable urinary diversion that is created from 10 to 12 cm of ileum (catheterizable channel), the ileocecal valve (continence mechanisms), and the right colon (reservoir).

Intussusception the process, more common in children, in which the intestine telescopes back on itself. The resulting blockage can result in bowel necrosis if left untreated.

Jejunostomy a surgically created opening into the jejunum.

Juvenile polyposis syndrome (JPS) a hereditary condition characterized by the presence of hamartomatous polyps in the digestive tract. The term "juvenile polyposis" refers to the type of polyp (juvenile polyp), not the age at which people are diagnosed. Most juvenile polyps are noncancerous, but there is an increased risk of cancer of the digestive tract (such as stomach, small intestine, colon, and rectum cancers) in families with JPS.

Kock pouch a high-volume, low-pressure intra-abdominal reservoir constructed from the terminal ileum that allows patients to maintain continence of stool and flatus without the need for an external stoma appliance. The internal pouch is emptied by intermittent self-catheterization when increasing volume of intestinal contents cause the pouch to expand, giving the sensation of fullness to indicate it should be emptied.

Learner readiness the degree to which a person is "ready to learn" and willingness to participate in behavior change.

Liquid skin barrier an acrylate copolymer or a cyanoacrylate clear film that can be placed on the peristomal skin to provide skin protection from stoma effluent, adhesive stripping or in some cases to seal the skin barrier.

Loop stoma a stoma that is created in the small or large intestine by mobilizing the side of the intestine up through the abdominal wall, making a transverse incision on the intestine, and maturing the mucosa. A supporting rod is placed under the stoma to prevent stoma retraction. The stoma will have two lumens, proximal and distal.

Loop-end stoma the intestine is transected from the lower bowel. After closing this end with a stapler, a loop of intestine approximately 10 cm proximal to this stapled end is brought to the abdominal surface through the premarked stoma site. Externally, there is no difference in how a loop or loop-end stoma looks. With loop-end construction, the distal lumen leads to a blind pouch. The blind segment is usually not very long and will produce mucus as the bowel is viable. Loop-end construction is used in bowel stomas when the person has a thick abdominal wall, shortened mesentery, or a combination, and there is concern about adequate blood supply to the distal end of the stoma.

Maturation the eversion of the bowel segment to expose the mucosa.

Michelassi side-to-side isoperistaltic stricturoplasty a type of stricturoplasty (see below) used for extensive and/or strictures occurring sequentially over long intestinal segments.

Mucocutaneous junction intersection between the bowel mucosa and the skin.

Mucocutaneous separation the detachment of stomal tissue from the surrounding peristomal skin of the stoma and mucocutaneous junction.

Mucosal transplantation seeding of viable intestinal mucosa along the suture line onto the peristomal skin.

Mucous fistula the end of a section of defunctionalized bowel is brought through the abdominal wall when a stoma is created.

Neobladder (also called an orthotopic urinary diversion) the creation of a low-pressure, high-volume reservoir that is anastomosed to the urethra. Patients rely on their urinary sphincter for continence and void by relaxing their sphincter and pelvic floor in combination with increasing intra-abdominal pressure by performing Valsalva or Credé maneuver.

Neurogenic bladder bladder dysfunction caused by neurologic impairment of the central and peripheral nervous system, which innervates the bladder.

One-piece pouching system a solid skin barrier and the pouch as one unit; the pouch is heat sealed onto the skin barrier.

Orthotopic urinary diversion (also called a neobladder) the creation of a low-pressure, high-volume reservoir that is anastomosed to the urethra. Patients rely on their urinary sphincter for continence and void by relaxing their sphincter and pelvic floor in combination with increasing intra-abdominal pressure by performing Valsalva or Credé maneuver.

Parastomal (peristomal) hernia a defect in abdominal fascia that allows the intestine to bulge into the parastomal area.

Percutaneous endoscopic gastrostomy (PEG) a tube placed into the stomach through the skin, aided by endoscopy.

Percutaneous nephrostomy tubes tubes that are inserted through the skin and into the renal pelvis of the kidney to facilitate drainage of urine after a partial or complete obstruction has occurred.

Peristomal allergic contact dermatitis an inflammatory skin response resulting from hypersensitivity to chemical elements.

Peristomal fungal/candidiasis infection a fungal rash that can occur beneath the skin barrier and/or beneath tape-bordered products and pouches.

Peristomal moisture–associated skin damage an inflammation and erosion of the skin adjacent to the stoma, associated with exposure to effluent such as urine or stool.

Peristomal psoriasis a chronic inflammatory and autoimmune disorder with many clinical variants. Peristomal and periwound skin is particularly vulnerable for patients with psoriasis because of the Koebner phenomenon, in which a flare of the disorder occurs in an area of localized skin trauma.

Peristomal varices enlarged blood vessels caused by portal hypertension. The varices may be visible as dilated veins in the submucosal area (referred to as caput medusa), bluish discoloration of the skin in the stoma area. These may also present as spontaneous bleeding from the mucocutaneous junction without any visible skin changes.

Peutz-Jeghers syndrome a condition characterized by the development of noncancerous growths called hamartomatous polyps in the gastrointestinal tract (particularly the stomach and intestines) and a greatly increased risk of developing certain types of cancer.

Permission, Limited Information, Specific Suggestions, Intensive Therapy (PLISSIT) four levels of response to issues with sexual health that encourages the nurse to intervene at the level he or she is most comfortable to provide counseling.

Pouching system products used to collect the stoma effluent, which provide a secure predictable seal and protect the peristomal skin.

Prebiotics plant fibers that promote healthy bowel flora growth.

Probiotics probiotic bacteria that arrive to the bowel in an active state. They interact with epithelial and immune cells boosting systemic immune activity and epithelial function.

Proctocolectomy with permanent end ileostomy the entire colon, rectum, and anus are removed, and an end ileostomy is created.

Prune belly syndrome (PBS) a severe congenital malformation with absence of abdominal musculature that present with wrinkly appearance of the abdominal skin and urinary tract anomalies.

Pseudoverrucous lesion an exuberant growth of benign papules that occur around a stoma when urine or stool irritates the skin, a type of chronic irritant contact dermatitis.

Pyoderma gangrenosum a neutrophilic dermatosis characterized by recurrent, painful ulcerations that present as pustules that enlarge and open into partial- or full-thickness wounds, sometimes with dark-colored, irregular borders and purulent exudate. These painful undermined ulcerations progress rapidly.

Radiation enteritis inflammation of the intestines that occurs after radiation therapy. Progressive loss of cells, villous atrophy, and cystic crypt dilation occur in the ensuing days and weeks. Occurs mostly in people receiving radiation to the abdomen and pelvic areas.

Retraction the disappearance of stoma tissue protrusion in line with or below skin level.

Skin barrier paste an adhesive hydrocolloid mixture available in a tube, used to enhance the seal of the pouching system by caulking the edge of the skin barrier closest to the stoma to help to prevent undermining of the seal. Also used to fill in uneven areas around and near the stoma to facilitate the seal of the solid skin barrier.

Skin barrier powder a hydrocolloid that is used to absorb moisture that can be utilized on denuded peristomal skin.

Skin barrier ring an adhesive hydrocolloid washer used around a stoma to enhance the seal by providing additional solid skin barrier and/or to level out the area around the stoma.

Skin barrier strip paste a band of adhesive hydrocolloid used to fit around a stoma to enhance the seal or to fill in uneven peristomal area.

Solid skin barrier the interface between the skin and the pouch of the pouching system that provides the seal (adhesion) and protects the peristomal skin.

Stamm gastrostomy a surgically placed tube into the stomach that involves circumferential purse-string sutures to stabilize the tube within the lumen of the stomach and affix the stomach to the anterior abdominal wall.

Stomal necrosis death of the stoma tissue resulting from impaired blood flow.

Stomal prolapse the telescoping of the intestine through the stoma.

Stomal stenosis the impairment of effluent drainage due to narrowing or contracting of the stoma tissue at the skin or fascial level.

Stomal trauma an injury to the stomal mucosa often related to pressure or physical force.

Stricture a narrowing of the bowel lumen caused by prolonged inflammation that can lead to scarring.

Stricturoplasty the creation of a longitudinal incision through the narrowed area of the intestine while closing the incision transversely, which widens the intestinal lumen used for the treatment of fibrotic strictures in Crohn's disease.

Synbiotics synergistic combinations of both probiotics and prebiotics.

TNM classification a cancer staging system that describes the following: tumor invasion, spread to lymph nodes, and distant metastatic spread.

Total pelvic exenteration a surgical procedure that includes the resection of pelvic structures including uterus, vagina, bladder, urethra, and rectum. This is indicated for rectal tumors with invasion to adjacent pelvic structures or gynecologic or urinary malignancies with involvement of the rectum.

Two-piece pouching system a solid skin barrier with a mechanism that accepts the pouch.

Ulcerative colitis an inflammation of the large bowel limited to the superficial mucosal lining of the bowel that follows a characteristic pattern: the rectum is always involved, and it extends proximally to include part of the colon or the entire colon.

Ureterostomy an opening in which the ureters, may be each brought to the skin in two separate stomas or one ureter anastomosed to the other and a single ureter brought out as a stoma.

Urostomy an opening into the urinary system that can be constructed from the small or large intestine. The term urostomy describes that there is an opening that drains urine and the type of stoma will be an ileal or colon conduit, or an ureterostomy. An ileal or colon conduit uses the ileum or colon to make a passage for the urine to exit the body.

Vesicostomy an opening is created above the symphysis pubis, the bladder opened, and the bladder mucosa approximated to the skin, generally seen in the pediatric population.

Volvulus a twisting of a portion of the gastrointestinal tract that can cause a blockage, impair blood flow, and damage part of the intestine.

Witzel gastrostomy technique surgical placement of a tube that involves creating a serosal tunnel as well as an abdominal wall tunnel through which the tube passes.

Index

Note: Page numbers followed by "f" refer to figures; page numbers followed by "t" refer to tables.